Hepatitis: An Issue of Clinics in Liver Disease

Hepatitis: An Issue of Clinics in Liver Disease

Edited by **Amelia Foster**

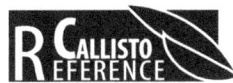

RCALLISTO REFERENCE

New York

Published by Callisto Reference,
106 Park Avenue, Suite 200,
New York, NY 10016, USA
www.callistoreference.com

Hepatitis: An Issue of Clinics in Liver Disease
Edited by Amelia Foster

International Standard Book Number: 978-1-63239-741-6 (Hardback)

Contents

Preface   IX

Chapter 1   **HD-03/ES: A Herbal Medicine Inhibits Hepatitis B Surface Antigen Secretion in Transfected Human Hepatocarcinoma PLC/PRF/5 Cells**   1
Sandeep R. Varma, R. Sundaram, S. Gopumadhavan, Satyakumar Vidyashankar and Pralhad S. Patki

Chapter 2   **Transplacental Transfer of Hepatitis B Neutralizing Antibody during Pregnancy in an Animal Model: Implications for Newborn and Maternal Health**   7
Li Ma, Malgorzata G. Norton, Iftekhar Mahmood, Zhong Zhao, Lilin Zhong, Pei Zhang and Evi B. Struble

Chapter 3   **Hepatitis B Vaccination and Screening Awareness in Primary Care Practitioners**   14
Adnan Said and Janice H. Jou

Chapter 4   **Tryptophan-Kynurenine Metabolism and Insulin Resistance in Hepatitis C Patients**   21
G. F. Oxenkrug, W. A. Turski, W. Zgrajka, J. V. Weinstock and P. Summergrad

Chapter 5   **Evaluation of the Significance of Pretreatment Liver Biopsy and Baseline Mental Health Disorder Diagnosis on Hepatitis C Treatment Completion Rates at a Veterans Affairs Medical Center**   25
Joseph Kluck, Rose M. O'Flynn, David E. Kaplan and Kyong-Mi Chang

Chapter 6   **Postinfantile Giant Cell Hepatitis: An Etiological and Prognostic Perspective**   31
Chhagan Bihari, Archana Rastogi and Shiv Kumar Sarin

Chapter 7   **Interleukin-16 Gene Polymorphisms are Considerable Host Genetic Factors for Patients' Susceptibility to Chronic Hepatitis B Infection**   38
Sara Romani, Seyed Masoud Hosseini, Seyed Reza Mohebbi, Shabnam Kazemian, Shaghayegh Derakhshani, Mahsa Khanyaghma, Pedram Azimzadeh, Afsaneh Sharifian and Mohammad Reza Zali

Chapter 8   **Interferon-α-Induced Changes to Natural Killer Cells are Associated with the Treatment Outcomes in Patients with HCV Infections**   43
Shinji Shimoda, Kosuke Sumida, Sho Iwasaka, Satomi Hisamoto, Hironori Tanimoto, Hideyuki Nomura, Kazufumi Dohmen, Kazuhiro Takahashi, Akira Kawano, Eiichi Ogawa, Norihiro Furusyo, Koichi Akashi and Jun Hayashi

Chapter 9   **Elevation in Serum Concentration of Bone-Specific Alkaline Phosphatase without Elevation in Serum Creatinine Concentration Secondary to Adefovir Dipivoxil Therapy in Chronic Hepatitis B Virus Infection**   50
Hiroshi Abe, Nobuyoshi Seki, Tomonori Sugita, Yuta Aida, Haruya Ishiguro, Tamihiro Miyazaki, Munenori Itagaki, Satoshi Sutoh and Yoshio Aizawa

Chapter 10   **High Dose of Lamivudine and Resistance in Patients with Chronic Hepatitis B**   59
Hamid Ullah Wani, Saad Al Kaabi, Manik Sharma, Rajvir Singh, Anil John,
Moutaz Derbala and Muneera J. Al-Mohannadi

Chapter 11   **Serum Inter-Alpha-Trypsin Inhibitor Heavy Chain 4 (ITIH4) in Children with
Chronic Hepatitis C: Relation to Liver Fibrosis and Viremia**   64
Mostafa M. Sira, Behairy E. Behairy, Azza M. Abd-Elaziz, Sameh A. Abd Elnaby
and Ehab E. Eltahan

Chapter 12   **Measuring the Response of Extrahepatic Symptoms and Quality of Life to
Antiviral Treatment in Patients with Hepatitis C**   71
David Isaacs, Nader Abdelaziz, Majella Keller, Jeremy Tibble and Inam Haq

Chapter 13   **Spectrum of Histomorphologic Findings in Liver in Patients with SLE: A Review**   78
Shrruti Grover, Archana Rastogi, Jyotsna Singh, Apurba Rajbongshi and
Chhagan Bihari

Chapter 14   **Hepatitis Viruses in Heamodialysis Patients: An Added Insult to Injury?**   85
Kranthi Kosaraju, Sameer Singh Faujdar, Aashima Singh and Ravindra Prabhu

Chapter 15   **MHC Class I Presented T Cell Epitopes as Potential Antigens for Therapeutic
Vaccine against HBV Chronic Infection**   89
Joseph D. Comber, Aykan Karabudak, Vivekananda Shetty, James S. Testa,
Xiaofang Huang and Ramila Philip

Chapter 16   **Hepatitis B Awareness among Medical Students and their Vaccination Status at
Syrian Private University**   100
Nazir Ibrahim and Amr Idris

Chapter 17   **Occult Hepatitis B: Clinical Viewpoint and Management**   107
Mehdi Zobeiri

Chapter 18   **Involvement of Differential Relationship between HCV Replication and Hepatic
PRR Signaling Gene Expression in Responsiveness to IFN-Based Therapy**   114
Nobukazu Yuki, Shinji Matsumoto, Michio Kato and Toshikazu Yamaguchi

Chapter 19   **Parvovirus B19 Associated Hepatitis**   120
Chhagan Bihari, Archana Rastogi, Priyanka Saxena, Devraj Rangegowda,
Ashok Chowdhury, Nalini Gupta and Shiv Kumar Sarin

Chapter 20   **Transforming Growth Factor-β1 Gene Polymorphism (T29C) in Egyptian Patients
with Hepatitis B Virus Infection: A Preliminary Study**   129
Roba M. Talaat, Mahmoud F. Dondeti, Soha Z. El-Shenawy and
Omaima A. Khamiss

Chapter 21   **Prevalence of *Hepatitis E Virus* among Adults in South-West of Iran**   135
Fatemeh Farshadpour, Reza Taherkhani and Manoochehr Makvandi

Chapter 22   **Prediction of Sustained Virological Response to Telaprevir-Based Triple Therapy
using Viral Response within 2 Weeks**   140
Hideyuki Tamai, Ryo Shimizu, Naoki Shingaki, Yoshiyuki Mori, Shuya Maeshima,
Junya Nuta, Yoshimasa Maeda, Kosaku Moribata, Yosuke Muraki, Hisanobu Deguchi,
Izumi Inoue, Takao Maekita, Mikitaka Iguchi, Jun Kato and Masao Ichinose

Chapter 23   **Portraying Persons who Inject Drugs Recently Infected with Hepatitis C Accessing Antiviral Treatment: A Cluster Analysis**   148
Jean-Marie Bamvita, Elise Roy, Geng Zang, Didier Jutras-Aswad, Andreea Adelina Artenie, Annie Levesque and Julie Bruneau

Chapter 24   **Predictors of Health-Related Quality of Life in Outpatients with Cirrhosis: Results from a Prospective Cohort**   155
Maja Thiele, Gro Askgaard, Hans B. Timm, Ole Hamberg and Lise L. Gluud

Chapter 25   **Seroepidemiology of Hepatitis B and C Viruses in the General Population of Burkina Faso**   161
Issoufou Tao, Tegwindé R. Compaoré, Birama Diarra, Florencia Djigma, Theodora M. Zohoncon, Maléki Assih, Djeneba Ouermi, Virginio Pietra, Simplice D. Karou and Jacques Simpore

Chapter 26   **Circulating Cytokines and Histological Liver Damage in Chronic Hepatitis B Infection**   166
Kittiyod Poovorawan, Pisit Tangkijvanich, Chintana Chirathaworn, Naruemon Wisedopas, Sombat Treeprasertsuk, Piyawat Komolmit and Yong Poovorawan

Chapter 27   **Knowledge of Hepatitis B Virus Infection, Immunization with Hepatitis B Vaccine, Risk Perception, and Challenges to Control Hepatitis among Hospital Workers in a Nigerian Tertiary Hospital**   173
Olusegun Adekanle, Dennis A. Ndububa, Samuel Anu Olowookere, Oluwasegun Ijarotimi and Kayode Thaddeus Ijadunola

Chapter 28   **A Novel Structurally Stable Multiepitope Protein for Detection of HCV**   179
Alexsandro S. Galdino, José C. Santos, Marilen Q. Souza, Yanna K. M. Nóbrega, Mary-Ann E. Xavier, Maria S. S. Felipe, Sonia M. Freitas and Fernando A. G. Torres

Chapter 29   **Atherosclerosis as Extrahepatic Manifestation of Chronic Infection with Hepatitis C Virus**   188
Theodoros Voulgaris and Vassilios A. Sevastianos

Chapter 30   **Seroprevalence and Predictors of Hepatitis B Virus Infection among Pregnant Women Attending Routine Antenatal Care in Arba Minch Hospital, South Ethiopia**   196
Tsegaye Yohanes, Zerihun Zerdo and Nega Chufamo

Chapter 31   **Prevalence of Hepatitis C Virus Genotypes in District Bannu, Khyber Pakhtunkhwa, Pakistan**   203
Shamim Saleha, Anwar Kamal, Farman Ullah, Nasar Khan, Asif Mahmood and Sanaullah Khan

Chapter 32   **Prevalence and Seroincidence of Hepatitis B and Hepatitis C Infection in High Risk People who Inject Drugs in China and Thailand**   208
J. Brooks Jackson, Liu Wei, Fu Liping, Apinun Aramrattana, David D. Celentano, Louise Walshe, Yi Xing, Paul Richardson, Ma Jun, Geetha Beauchamp, Deborah Donnell, Yuhua Ruan, Liying Ma, David Metzger and Yiming Shao

Chapter 33   **Histological and Clinical Characteristics of Patients with Chronic Hepatitis C**
               and Persistently Normal Alanine Aminotransferase Levels   213
               Bakht Roshan and Grace Guzman

               Permissions

               List of Contributors

Preface

This book aims to highlight the current researches and provides a platform to further the scope of innovations in this area. This book is a product of the combined efforts of many researchers and scientists from different parts of the world. The objective of this book is to provide the readers with the latest information in the field.

Hepatitis is the inflammatory condition of liver usually caused by viral, parasitic and bacterial infection but there may be other causes related to it. There can be different types of hepatitis depending upon the cause such as acute, fulminant and chronic hepatitis. Liver failure, fatigue, appetite loss, joint pain and yellowing of eyes are some of the common symptoms observed when a person suffers this disease. This book covers in detail all the aspects of this disease such as symptoms, causes, diagnosis, treatment, prevention, etc. It includes contributions of experts which will unfold innovative prospects and mechanisms related to hepatitis. This book provides comprehensive insights into this field. It will help new researchers by foregrounding their knowledge in this area.

I would like to express my sincere thanks to the authors for their dedicated efforts in the completion of this book. I acknowledge the efforts of the publisher for providing constant support. Lastly, I would like to thank my family for their support in all academic endeavors.

Editor

HD-03/ES: A Herbal Medicine Inhibits Hepatitis B Surface Antigen Secretion in Transfected Human Hepatocarcinoma PLC/PRF/5 Cells

Sandeep R. Varma, R. Sundaram, S. Gopumadhavan, Satyakumar Vidyashankar, and Pralhad S. Patki

Research and Development, The Himalaya Drug Company, Bangalore 562 123, India

Correspondence should be addressed to Sandeep R. Varma; dr.sandeepvarma@himalayahealthcare.com

Academic Editor: Yoichi Hiasa

HD-03/ES is a herbal formulation used for the treatment of hepatitis B. However, the molecular mechanism involved in the antihepatitis B (HBV) activity of this drug has not been studied using *in vitro* models. The effect of HD-03/ES on hepatitis B surface antigen (HBsAg) secretion and its gene expression was studied in transfected human hepatocarcinoma PLC/PRF/5 cells. The anti-HBV activity was tested based on the inhibition of HBsAg secretion into the culture media, as detected by HBsAg-specific antibody-mediated enzyme assay (ELISA) at concentrations ranging from 125 to 1000 μg/mL. The effect of HD-03/ES on HBsAg gene expression was analyzed using semiquantitative multiplex RT-PCR by employing specific primers. The results showed that HD-03/ES suppressed HBsAg production with an IC_{50} of 380 μg/mL in PLC/PRF/5 cells for a period of 24 h. HD-03/ES downregulated HBsAg gene expression in PLC/PRF/5 cells. In conclusion, HD-03/ES exhibits strong anti-HBV properties by inhibiting the secretion of hepatitis B surface antigen in PLC/PRF/5 cells, and this action is targeted at the transcription level. Thus, HD-03/ES could be beneficial in the treatment of acute and chronic hepatitis B infections.

1. Introduction

Hepatitis B virus (HBV) infection is a major health problem throughout the world, affecting more than 350 million people who are carriers of this virus that can cause chronic hepatitis, liver cirrhosis, and hepatocellular carcinoma [1]. A variety of serological markers appear following the infection with HBV, and first among these is HBsAg (hepatitis B surface antigen), which is observed two to three weeks before the clinical and biological symptoms appear. Prevalence of HBsAg in India varies from 1 to 13 percent with an average of 4.7 percent [2–4]. The molecular diagnosis which detects the HBsAg in the serum samples plays a significant role in the early diagnosis during hepatitis B (HB) infection.

PLC/PRF/5 is a continuous human hepatocarcinoma cell line whose genome contains integrated HBV DNA and secretes two of the hepatitis B virus envelope proteins [5]. The cells could secrete HBsAg continuously into the culture medium [6, 7]. These cells are suitable to study the effects of drugs on HBsAg expression and secretion [6]. Since the cells do not produce infectious virion particles, it is safe to handle the cell line with biosafety level 2 containment [8].

Several antivirals are currently available for the treatment of HBV, which include IFN-α, lamivudine, entecavir, telbivudine, and tenofovir. However, interferon therapy has limited efficacy, is slow-acting, and frequently causes adverse effects [9]. Interferon therapy is effective only for about 30 to 40 percent of the patients with chronic HBV infection. Undesirable side effects of interferon treatment are found such as fever, malaise, fatigue, depression, hair loss, neutropenia, and thrombocytopenia [10]. Lamivudine also produces response in a modest proportion of patients and causes a few side effects [11]. Moreover, antiviral drugs and interferon are expensive.

Herbal compounds from plant origin are leading for new drug discovery for infectious and noninfectious diseases. Several hundred plant species have been reported to possess antiviral properties and some have been utilized to treat patients [12]. HD-03/ES is a novel herbal formulation used for the treatment of HBV infections and is marketed as Liv.52 HB. HD-03/ES is a capsule formulation consisting of 125 mg each of hydroalcoholic extracts of the roots of herbs, *Cyperus rotundus* and *Cyperus scariosus*. The anti-HBV activity of HD-03/ES has been reported by several workers [13–15]. However, the molecular mechanism behind the anti-HBV activity of HD-03/ES has not been studied well *in vitro*. The present study investigated the effect of HD-03/ES on the inhibition of HBsAg secretion and its gene expression in PLC/PRF/5 cells.

2. Materials and Methods

2.1. Materials. PLC/PRF/5 cells were obtained from National Center for Cell Science (NCCS), Pune. Dulbecco's modified Eagle's medium (DMEM), fetal bovine serum (FBS), 3-(4,5-dimethylthiazol-2-yl)-2,5-diphenyl tetrazolium bromide (MTT), TRI reagent, and custom-prepared oligonucleotides, were obtained from Sigma Chemical Co. (St Louis, MO, USA). HBsAg Ultra ELISA kit was purchased from Bio-Rad, France. Penicillin and streptomycin were from Hi-media, Mumbai, India. Moloney murine leukemia virus (MMLV) reverse transcriptase, dNTP, and Taq DNA polymerase were from MBI Fermentas (Glen Burnie, MD, USA).

2.2. Extraction of HD-03/ES. HD-03/ES granules were obtained from the Formulation and Development Department, The Himalaya Drug Company, India. About 100 g of HD-03/ES granules was packed in a Soxhlet extraction apparatus. The material was extracted using methanol for 8 hours at 80°C. The extract was concentrated using a rotary evaporator. The dry residue was subjected to *in vitro* studies.

2.3. Cell Culture and Cytotoxicity Assay. PLC/PRF/5 cells were cultured in DMEM high glucose medium supplemented with 10% FBS, 100 IU penicillin, and 100 μg streptomycin per mL at 37°C and 5% CO_2. PLC/PRF/5 cells at density of 2×10^5 mL were seeded in 96-well plates and incubated overnight at 37°C and 5% CO_2. HD-03/ES was dissolved in 0.5% DMSO in DMEM high glucose medium and used for the experiments. The cells were treated with different concentrations of HD-03/ES in culture media and incubated for 24 h at 37°C and 5% CO_2 to determine cytotoxicity of the extract. Cell control and vehicle control were also maintained. Cell viability was tested by MTT assay after exposing the cells to 1 mg/mL MTT for 3 h at 37°C. The blue formazan product was solubilised in DMSO and optical density measured at 540 nm [16]. Nontoxic concentrations of HD-03/ES were used for further experiments.

2.4. HBsAg Detection. PLC/PRF/5 cells at the concentration of 5×10^4 mL were seeded in a 24-well plate and incubated overnight at 37°C. The cells were treated with four nontoxic concentrations of HD-03/ES and incubated for 24 h at 37°C and 5% CO_2. At the end of the incubation period, the supernatant was collected by centrifugation at 1000 rpm for 10 min at 4°C. The supernatant was collected in a fresh 1.5 mL microfuge tube and stored at −20°C for ELISA. The cell pellet was stored at −80°C for RNA isolation.

The diagnostic kit for HBsAg (ELISA) from BioRad, France, was used for the detection of HBsAg in the culture medium. The assay was carried out according to the manufacturer's protocol. The absorbance was measured at 450 nm for determining the HBsAg present in the samples. The percentage inhibition of HBV by HD-03/ES was calculated over the cell control.

2.5. RNA Isolation and RT-PCR. Total RNA was isolated from control cells and HD-03/ES-treated cells using TRI reagent and the RNA was stored at −80°C. RNA was subjected to DNase I treatment (10 μg DNase I for 5 min at 65°C and cooled in ice for 1 min). RNA was quantified using spectrophotometer and the quantity of RNA was determined. One microgram of RNA was reverse-transcribed using Oligo-dT Primer at 42°C as described by us earlier [17]. The cDNA was stored at −20°C for further PCR reactions. A semiquantitative multiplex PCR was designed to compare the RT-PCR products of S gene and pre-S gene with GAPDH gene products to determine the relative levels of expression of HBsAg. PCR was carried out to amplify the HBsAg (S and pre-S genes) using specific primers in the second-strand synthesis. The GAPDH primers were also added to the same tube for each PCR reaction. Since the annealing temperatures of HBsAg gene and GAPDH were similar (60°C), the annealing temperature of the reaction was fixed at 60°C. The primer sequence for S gene was 5′-CCCAATACCACATCATCC-3′ (sense) and 5′-GGATTGGGGACCCTGCGC-3′ (antisense). The primer sequences used for pre-S were 5′-GGGTCACCATATTCTTGG-3′ (sense) and 5′-GTCCTAGGAATCCTGATG-3′ (antisense). For GAPDH gene, the primer sequence used was 5′-ACCACAGTCCATGCCATCAC-3′ (sense) and 5′-TCCACCACCCTGTTGCTGTA-3′ (antisense). The PCR reaction was subjected to 36 seconds of denaturation at 95°C, followed by 25 cycles of denaturation at 95°C for 36 sec, annealing at 60°C for 30 sec and extension at 72°C for 90 sec. A final extension at 72°C for 10 min completed the PCR programme. The PCR products were analyzed on 2% agarose gel stained with ethidium bromide and photographed under exposure to UV light. A standard molecular weight marker was resolved along with the samples to differentiate the cDNA amplicons in the agarose gel. Densitometric analysis (Image J software, Rasband, USA) was carried out to find the differences in the expression of the selected genes.

3. Statistical Analysis

Data were analyzed to determine mean ± SD. Statistical analysis of the data was done by Student's unpaired *t*-test using GraphPad Prism software, (San Diego, USA). *P* value of less than 0.05 was considered significant.

4. Results

Prior to the investigation of the anti-HBV effects, any putative cytotoxic effects of the HD-03/ES extract on PLC/PRF/5 cells were studied by MTT assay. The result of the cytotoxicity measurement of HD-03/ES extract on PLC/PRF/5 cells is shown in Figure 1. The percentage toxicity of HD-03/ES at 2000, 1000, 500, 250, and 125 μg/mL was found to be 8.75, 1.25, 0.75, 0.25, and 0.00, respectively, in PLC/PRF/5 cells. The amount of HBsAg secreted into the cell culture medium was determined by ELISA. Four nontoxic concentrations (1000, 500, 250, and 125 μg/mL) were used for HBsAg detection in PLC/PRF/5 cells. The optical density (OD) was read at 450 nm using an ELISA plate reader and the percentage of HBsAg secretion by the drug-treated cells was calculated over cell control. Each experiment was repeated three times and the results showed that HD-03/ES at concentrations of 1000, 500, and 250 μg/mL inhibited HBsAg secretion by 86.38, 71.17, and 17.1%, respectively, as compared to the control (Figure 2). At 125 μg/mL, HD-03/ES did not inhibit HBsAg in PLC/PRF/5 cells. However, at higher concentrations, HD-03/ES suppressed HBsAg production in PLC/PRF/5 cells with an IC$_{50}$ of 380 μg/mL.

In order to check whether the inhibitory effect of HBsAg by HD-03/ES is targeted at the transcription level, semi-quantitative multiplex RT-PCR was carried out using the RNA isolated from HD-03/ES-treated/untreated cells. Both S-gene- and pre-S-gene-specific primers were employed to amplify the gene encoding HBsAg in PLC/PRF/5 cells. The amplification yielded specific cDNAs corresponding to S gene (625 bp) and pre-S gene (553 bp) (Figures 3 and 4). Densitometric analysis compared the gene expression levels of the amplicons in comparison with GAPDH, the internal control. The results showed that HD-03/ES at 1000 and 500 μg/mL suppressed the expression levels of HBsAg as compared to the cell control. The HBsAg expression levels in the cells treated with HD-03/ES extract were less than the control (Figures 3 and 4). The internal control, GAPDH, was uniformly amplified in all the samples.

5. Discussion

Chronic HBV infection remains a major public health problem worldwide as well as a therapeutic challenge. Various treatments for chronic HBV infections have had only limited success [18]. The long-term effects of the recent advanced techniques employed to eliminate the virus, including therapy with nucleoside analogs and other virus-replication inhibitors [19], are yet to be determined. Since HBV reverse transcriptase lacks proof-reading function, the virus shows rapid mutagenesis thus creating a large number of variants, some of which show resistance to antiviral drugs. This phenomenon is responsible for the low efficacy of the current drugs and the high rates of drug resistance [20, 21]. Therefore, there is an urgent need to develop new anti-HBV drugs.

HD-03/ES is a herbal medicine used for curing hepatitis B and contains the extracts of *Cyperus rotundus* and *Cyperus scariosus* roots. Several clinical trials and *in vitro* studies have been carried out which confirmed the anti-HBV activity of HD-03/ES [13–15, 22]. A previous study reported that HD-03/ES inhibited alanine aminotransferase and HBV DNA [14]. A recent study on HD-03/ES showed that the drug at

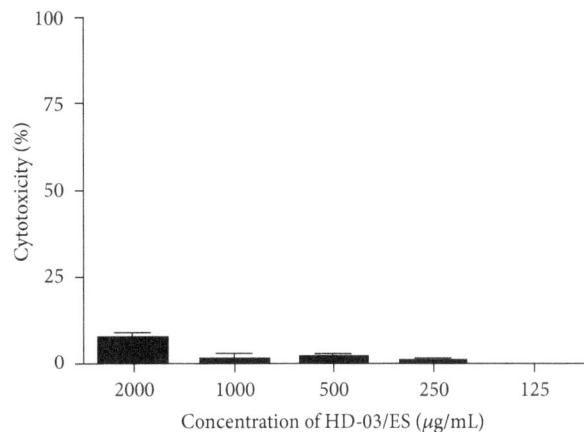

FIGURE 1: Cytotoxicity of HD-03/ES on PLC/PRF/5 cells. PLC/PRF/5 cells were incubated for 24 hr with different concentrations of HD-03/ES and the cell viability was then determined using an MTT assay. Data are expressed as percentage of control (n = 3).

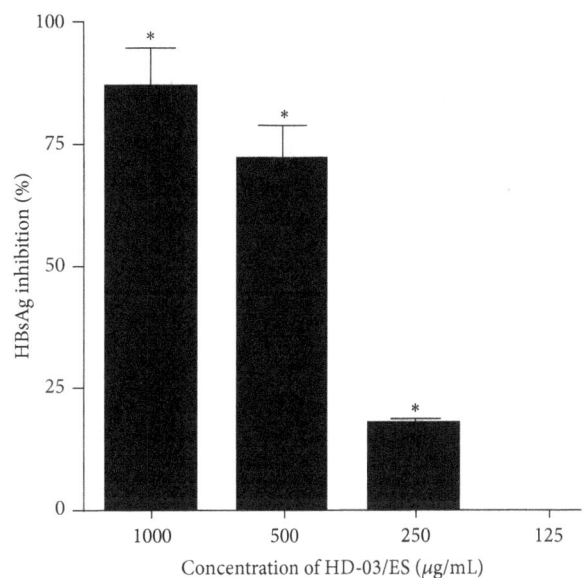

FIGURE 2: Effect of HD-03/ES on HBsAg secretion in PLC/PRF/5 cells by ELISA. PLC/PRF/5 cells were treated with four nontoxic concentrations of HD-03/ES for 24 hrs and the supernatant was assayed for ELISA using HBsAg Ultra ELISA kit. The percentage inhibition of HBsAg was calculated over control. Data is representative of three experiments. $^{*}P < 0.05$.

5 and 2.5 mg/mL inhibited 1.5 pg/mL of the HBV virus, and the drug prevents HBV infection by possibly interfering with the viral entry [13]. However, the molecular mechanism behind the anti-HBV activity of HD-03/ES has not been studied well. Though previous studies have shown that HD-03/ES suppresses HBsAg, [13, 14] the effect of HD-03/ES on the HBsAg gene expression has not been studied *in vitro*. The present study investigated the cellular and molecular effects of HD-03/ES on the HBsAg using PLC/PRF/5 cells.

Stable cell lines with integrated HBV genomes, namely, PLC/PRF/5 cells, are commonly used for assessing the action

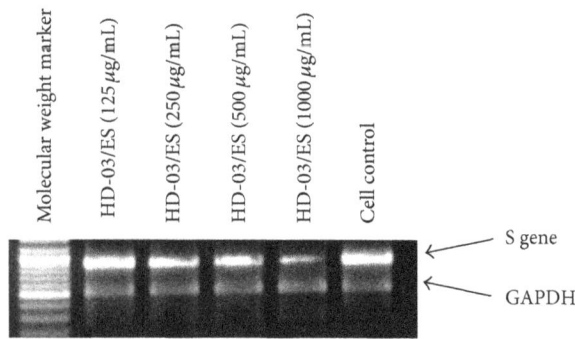

(a)

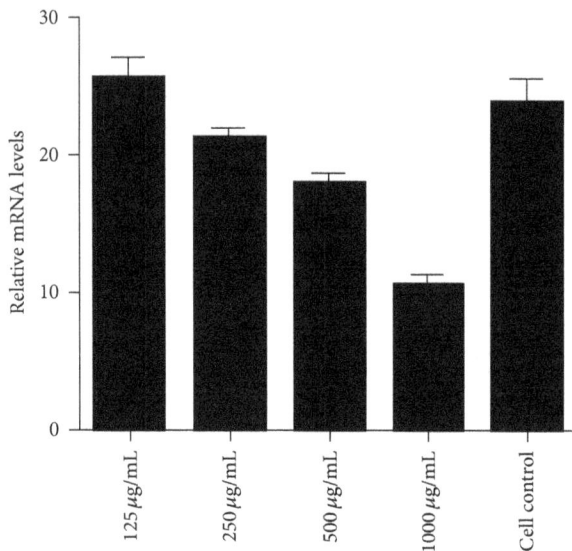

(b)

FIGURE 3: The effect of HD-03/ES on HBsAg gene expression. PLC/PRF/5 cells were treated with or without HD-03/ES at three nontoxic concentrations. RNA was isolated from drug-treated and -untreated cells and multiplex RT-PCR was performed using specific primers as described in the text. (a) RT-PCR product of S-gene and GAPDH resolved in 2% agarose gel. (b) Densitometric analysis of the gene transcripts and the values depict arbitrary units. Data is representative of two experiments.

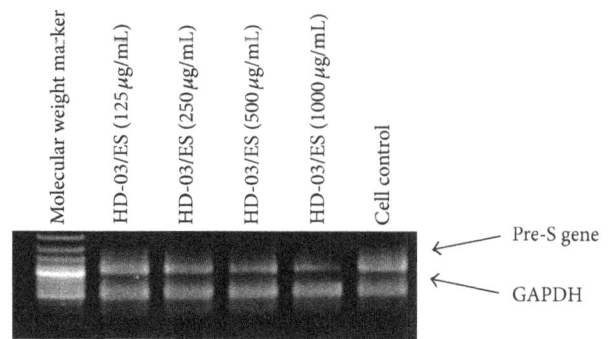

(a)

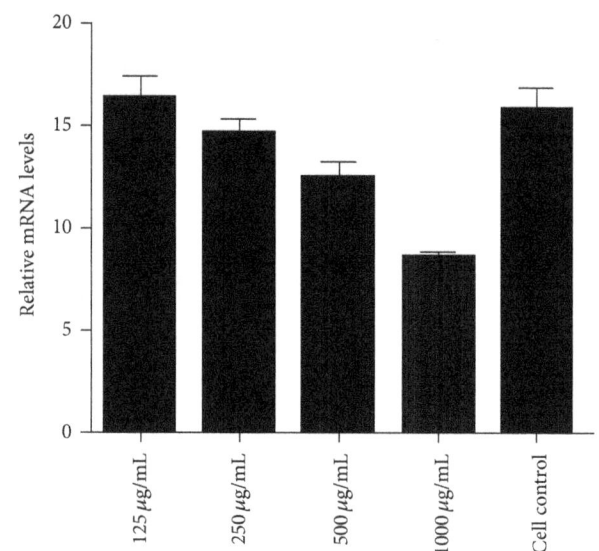

(b)

FIGURE 4: The effect of HD-03/ES on HBsAg gene expression. PLC/PRF/5 cells were treated with or without HD-03/ES at three nontoxic concentrations. RNA was isolated from drug-treated and -untreated cells and RT-PCR was performed using specific primers as described in the text ((a) RT-PCR product of pre-S gene and GAPDH resolved in 2% agarose gel; (b) densitometric analysis of the gene transcripts and the values depict arbitrary units). Data is representative of two experiments.

of drugs on HBsAg secretion [23, 24]. The property of PLC/PRF/5 cells to secrete HBsAg in the supernatant was used in the present study to evaluate the anti-HBV properties of HD-03/ES. HD-03/ES extract did not produce cytotoxic effect on PLC/PRF/5 cells within a reasonable dose range. It was seen that HD-03/ES at 1000 and 500 μg/mL concentrations inhibited the secretion of HBsAg by 86.38 and 71.17%, respectively, for a period of 24 hours. However the lower concentrations were not successful in inhibiting the HBsAg in PLC/PRF/5 cells. The lack of cytotoxicity on PLC/PRF/5 cells, at the concentrations tested, indicates that the decrease in HBsAg is not due to an adverse effect of the drug on cell viability. In order to further confirm that the inhibition is HBsAg specific, the secretion of albumin in cell culture supernatants was checked (data not shown). The results showed that the albumin content in the cell supernatants of

drug-treated/untreated cells was similar (data not shown). This study showed that the secretion of other cellular proteins like albumin was not altered by HD-03/ES at the doses tested. This result suggested that the antiviral effect of HD-03/ES might be more specific to the HBV.

PLC/PRF/5 cells contain six hepatitis B viral genomes integrated into the high molecular weight host DNA. The cells secrete only sAg and do not produce hepatitis B core antigen or free viral particles [25]. Both pre-S1 and pre-S2 proteins are expressed on the surface of HBsAg particles and are the essential components of complete virions and HBsAg filaments [26]. The expression of these envelope proteins originates from the HBV DNA coding for the respective genes, which is integrated into the cellular genome [23]. The pre-S2 mRNA encodes albumin receptors, which bind to pHSA and mediate viral attachment to the hepatocytes [27].

Pre-S1 and pre-S2 proteins are detectable in the serum of patients with acute and chronic hepatitis B virus infection when there are high levels of viral replication, and the clearance of these antigens from serum usually correlates with the prognosis of hepatitis B virus infection.

In order to assess whether the antiviral effect is due to the suppression of HBsAg gene, semiquantitative multiplex RT-PCR was carried out to amplify the regions coding the HBsAg gene in PLC/PRF/5 cells. The results showed that in drug-treated/control cells, HD-03/ES dose dependently suppressed the HBsAg gene expression. Densitometric analysis of the transcripts of S gene and Pre-S gene showed that HD-03/ES at higher concentrations, namely, 1000 and 500 μg/mL, has downregulated the HBsAg gene expression in PLC/PRF/5 cells. Thus, it could be concluded that HD-03/ES inhibits HBV by inhibiting HBsAg at the transcription level.

This study suggests that in liver cells which have integrated HBV DNA, both S and pre-S antigen secretion could be inhibited by HD-03/ES. Since truncated pre-S antigen has been shown to be a transactivation protein possibly involved in the oncogenic process, the effect of HD-03/ES on pre-S gene is of therapeutic relevance. The impact of HD-03/ES on HBV inhibition by proteins, such as core and polymerase associated with full replication, deserves further study.

6. Conclusion

In conclusion, we have studied the *in vitro* anti-HBV effect of HD-03/ES in transfected human hepatocarcinoma cells. HD-03/ES suppressed HBsAg production with an IC_{50} of 380 μg/mL in PLC/PRF/5 cells for a period of 24 h. HD-03/ES also downregulated HBsAg gene expression in PLC/PRF/5 cells. Previous reports have clearly indicated the anti-HBV activity of HD-03/ES. The main thrust of the present study is that, besides other methods of interference, HD-03/ES is capable of suppressing HBsAg, and the action is targeted at the transcription level.

Disclosure

The authors alone are responsible for the content and writing of the paper.

Conflict of Interests

The authors report no conflict of interests.

Acknowledgment

The authors are thankful to Dr. Shyam Ramakrishnan, Chief Scientific Officer, R&D, The Himalaya Drug Company, Bangalore, India, for his constant support and encouragement during this study.

References

[1] B. J. McMahon, "The natural history of chronic hepatitis B virus infection," *Seminars in Liver Disease*, vol. 24, no. 1, pp. 17–21, 2004.

[2] S. P. Thyagarajan, S. Jayaram, and B. Mohanavalli, "Prevalence of HBV in general population of India," in *Hepatitis in India: Problems and Prevention*, S. K. Sarin and A. K. Singhal, Eds., pp. 5–16, CBS, New Delhi, India, 1996.

[3] R. C. Jain, S. D. Bhat, and S. Sangle, "Prevalence of hepatitis surface antigen among rural population of Loni area in Ahmednagar district of Western Maharashtra," *The Journal of the Association of Physicians of India*, vol. 40, no. 6, pp. 390–391, 1992.

[4] B. N. Tandon, M. Irshad, M. Raju, G. P. Mathur, and M. N. Rao, "Prevalence of HBsAg and anti-HBs in children and strategy suggested for immunisation in India," *Indian Journal of Medical Research*, vol. 93, pp. 337–339, 1991.

[5] J. Alexander, E. Bey, J. M. Whitecutt, and J. H. Gear, "Adaptation of cells derived from human malignant tumors to growth *in vitro*," *South African Journal of Medical Sciences*, vol. 41, no. 2, pp. 89–98, 1976.

[6] R. Cattaneo, H. Will, N. Hernandez, and H. Schaller, "Signals regulating hepatitis B surface antigen transcription," *Nature*, vol. 305, no. 5932, pp. 336–338, 1983.

[7] J. H. Ou and W. J. Rutter, "Hybrid hepatitis B virus-host transcripts in a human hepatoma cell," *Proceedings of the National Academy of Sciences of the United States of America*, vol. 82, no. 1, pp. 83–87, 1985.

[8] W. Y. Lam, K. T. Leung, P. T. W. Law et al., "Antiviral effect of Phyllanthus nanus ethanolic extract against hepatitis B virus (HBV) by expression microarray analysis," *Journal of Cellular Biochemistry*, vol. 97, no. 4, pp. 795–812, 2006.

[9] T. Shaw and S. Locarini, "Entecavir for treatment of chronic hepatitis B," *Expert Review of Anti Infective Therapy*, vol. 2, no. 2, pp. 853–871, 2004.

[10] T. Vachirayonstein, S. Sirotamarat, K. Balachandra, and E. Saifah, "Cytotoxicity and inhibitory activity on hepatitis B surface antigen secretion from PLC/PRF/5 cells of medicinal plant extracts," *The Journal of Pharmaceutical Sciences*, vol. 30, no. 1-2, pp. 1–7, 2006.

[11] D. Lavanchy, "Hepatitis B virus epidemiology, disease burden, treatment, arid current and emerging prevention and control measures," *Journal of Viral Hepatitis*, vol. 11, no. 2, pp. 97–107, 2004.

[12] S. A. A. Jassim and M. A. Naji, "Novel antiviral agents: a medicinal plant perspective," *Journal of Applied Microbiology*, vol. 95, no. 3, pp. 412–427, 2003.

[13] M. Jeevan, N. Nasreen, S. Dinesh, M. V. Durgadevi, and E. Manickan, "Anti-HBV activity of HD-03/ES, a herbal medicine by interference of HBsAg binding to its receptor," *Journal of Pharmacy Research*, vol. 5, no. 8, pp. 4348–4352, 2012.

[14] P. Kar, M. Asim, M. P. Sarma, and P. S. Patki, "HD-03/ES: a promising herbal drug for HBV antiviral therapy," *Antiviral Research*, vol. 84, no. 3, pp. 249–253, 2009.

[15] J. S. Rajkumar, M. G. Sekar, and S. K. Mitra, "Safety and efficacy of oral HD-03/ES given for six months in patients with chronic hepatitis B virus infection," *World Journal of Gastroenterology*, vol. 13, no. 30, pp. 4103–4107, 2007.

[16] F. Denizot and R. Lang, "Rapid colorimetric assay for cell growth and survival—modifications to the tetrazolium dye procedure giving improved sensitivity and reliability," *Journal of Immunological Methods*, vol. 89, no. 2, pp. 271–277, 1986.

[17] R. S. Varma, G. Ashok, S. Vidyashankar, P. Patki, and K. S. Nandakumar, "Ethanol extract of Justicia gendarussa inhibits lipopolysaccharide stimulated nitric oxide and matrix metalloproteinase-9 expression in murine macrophage," *Pharmaceutical Biology*, vol. 49, no. 6, pp. 648–652, 2011.

[18] T. A. Shamliyan, R. MacDonald, A. Shaukat et al., "Antiviral therapy for adults with chronic hepatitis B: a systematic review for a National Institutes of Health Consensus Development Conference," *Annals of Internal Medicine*, vol. 150, no. 2, pp. 111–124, 2009.

[19] V. P. Papadopoulos, D. N. Chrysagis, A. N. Protopapas, I. G. Goulis, G. T. Dimitriadis, and K. P. Mimidis, "Peginterferon alfa-2b as monotherapy or in combination with lamivudine in patients with hbeag-negative chronic hepatitis B: a randomised study," *Medical Science Monitor*, vol. 15, no. 2, pp. CR56–CR61, 2009.

[20] S. Mauss and H. Wedemeyer, "Treatment of chronic hepatitis B and the implications of viral resistance to therapy," *Expert Review of Anti-Infective Therapy*, vol. 6, no. 2, pp. 191–199, 2008.

[21] S. Locarnini and N. Warner, "Major causes of antiviral drug resistance and implications for treatment of hepatitis B virus monoinfection and coinfection with HIV," *Antiviral Therapy*, vol. 12, no. 3, pp. H15–H23, 2007.

[22] A. K. Bhattacharya and S. P. Patki, "A preliminary study on the safety and efficacy of HD-03/ES therapy in patients with chronic hepatitis B: a prospective clinical study," *Journal of Herbal Medicine and Toxicology*, vol. 3, no. 2, pp. 137–141, 2009.

[23] P. Berthillon, J. M. Crance, F. Leveque et al., "Inhibition of the expression of hepatitis A and B viruses (HAV and HBV) proteins by interferon in a human hepatocarcinoma cell line (PLC/PRF/5)," *Journal of Hepatology*, vol. 25, no. 1, pp. 15–19, 1996.

[24] S. F. Yeh, M. Gupta, D. N. K. Sarma, and S. K. Mitra, "Down-regulation of hepatitis B surface antigen expression in human hepatocellular carcinoma cell lines by HD-03, a polyherbal formulation," *Phytotherapy Research*, vol. 17, no. 1, pp. 89–91, 2003.

[25] J. C. Edman, P. Gray, and P. Valenzuela, "Integration of hepatitis B virus sequences and their expression in a human hepatoma cell," *Nature*, vol. 286, no. 5772, pp. 535–538, 1980.

[26] E. R. Boulan and D. D. Sabatini, "Asymmetric budding of viruses in epithelial monolayers: a model system for study of epithelial polarity," *Proceedings of the National Academy of Sciences of the United States of America*, vol. 75, no. 10, pp. 5071–5075, 1978.

[27] H. Ohnuma, K. Takahashi, and S. Kishimoto, "Large hepatitis B surface antigen polypeptides of Dane particles with the receptor for polymerized human serum albumin," *Gastroenterology*, vol. 90, no. 3, pp. 695–701, 1986.

Transplacental Transfer of Hepatitis B Neutralizing Antibody during Pregnancy in an Animal Model: Implications for Newborn and Maternal Health

Li Ma,[1] Malgorzata G. Norton,[1] Iftekhar Mahmood,[2] Zhong Zhao,[1] Lilin Zhong,[1] Pei Zhang,[1] and Evi B. Struble[1]

[1] *Laboratory of Plasma Derivatives, Division of Hematology, Office of Blood Research and Review, Center for Biologics Evaluation and Research, FDA 1401 Rockville Pike, Rockville, MD 20852, USA*
[2] *Division of Hematology, Office of Blood Research and Review, Center for Biologics Evaluation and Research, FDA 1401 Rockville Pike, Rockville, MD 20852, USA*

Correspondence should be addressed to Evi B. Struble; evi.struble@fda.hhs.gov

Academic Editor: Yoichi Hiasa

Despite the success of postexposure prophylaxis (PEP) of the newborn in preventing mother-to-child transmission of hepatitis B virus), in non-US clinical trials, administering hepatitis B immune globulin (HBIG) to mothers at the end of pregnancy (in addition to passive-active PEP of the newborn) only partially improved outcomes. That is, a significant percentage of newborns became infected during their first year of life. We used a relevant animal model for human IgG transplacental transfer to study dose, time and subclass dependence of HBV neutralizing antibody (nAb) maternal, and fetal levels at the end of pregnancy. Pregnant guinea pigs received 50 or 100 IU/kg HBIGIV 2–5 days before delivery. Human total IgG, IgG subclasses, and nAb in mothers and their litters were measured.*In vitro* analyses of guinea pig Fc neonatal receptor binding to HBIGIV, as well as to all human IgG subclasses, were also performed. Our study showed that nAb transferred transplacentally from the pregnant guinea pigs to their litters; no transfer occurred during parturition. The amount of the transferred nAb was dose and time dependent. Thus, selection of an efficacious dose in the clinic is important: microdosing may be underdosing, particularly in cases of high viraemia.

1. Introduction

Chronic hepatitis B is a serious viral disease, associated with a high risk for developing liver cirrhosis and hepatocellular carcinoma [1–3]. Worldwide, two billion people have been infected with the virus and about 600,000 people die every year due to the consequences of hepatitis B [4]. HBV is endemic in China and other parts of Asia where 8–10% of the adult population is chronically infected, often since birth. Because 90% of infants infected at birth develop chronic HBV infection and 25% of those die prematurely from cirrhosis or liver cancer [5, 6], failure to prevent infection following perinatal exposure to HBV carries a heavy burden to the individual, family, and society at large.

Passive-active postexposure prophylaxis (PEP) with HBIG and hepatitis B vaccine is 85–95% effective in preventing vertical transmission of HBV compared to 70–95% prevention rate for the vaccine alone [6, 7]. Despite PEP, 3–13% of infants born to infected mothers acquire HBV [8]. The risk is particularly high for children born to mothers with a high viral load [9, 10]. Although pregnancy, especially the peripartum period, has been associated with an increase in hepatitis B viral load [11], maternal use of antiviral drugs, such as nucleoside analogs, as an adjunct to PEP of the newborn has not shown conclusive benefit over PEP alone [12]. Similarly, using HBIG at the end of pregnancy has not yielded significant reductions in HBV neonatal infection rates of vaccinated babies by the time they reach one year of age [10]. Intrigued by these reports, we set out to characterize HBV neutralizing antibody levels and pharmacokinetic characteristics in the mother and her newborn, respectively, after HBIG administration in an animal model of pregnancy.

TABLE 1: Summary of the *in vivo* study.

	Number of animals	Mean weight (range), g	Dose, IU/kg		Exposure, days	Mean litter size (range)	Mean litter weight (range), g
Pregnant	12	1206 (920–1360)	50 ($n = 6$)	100 ($n = 6$)	2–5	3 (1–5)	107 (82–150)
Nonpregnant	6	862 (764–924)	50 ($n = 3$)	100 ($n = 3$)	5	N/A	N/A

Our data shows that neutralizing antibody in HBIG can pass the placenta in a dose and time dependent manner. This finding has implications when considering an efficacious dose in the clinic.

2. Materials and Methods

2.1. Animal Study. All animal procedures were performed in accordance with protocols approved by the CBER Animal Care and Use Committee. Hartley Albino (Crl:HA) guinea pigs were purchased from commercial sources. The animals were housed in pairs or individually, and food and water were provided *ad libitum*. Female guinea pigs were mated in accordance with a published protocol [13] to produce timed pregnancies and HBIGIV was administered as previously described [14]. The *in vivo* study is summarized in Table 1. Briefly, twelve pregnant guinea pigs at an average age of 185 days, weighing on average 1206 g received HBIGIV on GD 65–69 at 50 IU/kg ($n = 6$) or 100 IU/kg ($n = 6$). An additional six nonpregnant controls, at a mean age 177 days, weighing on average 862 g received the same doses ($n = 3$/dose group). Blood samples were collected by percutaneous femoral vein puncture at 10, 30 and 60 minutes and then every day until farrowing or termination. All pregnant guinea pigs gave birth 2–5 days after test article administration, except one in the high dose group which delivered within four hours after receiving HBIGIV and was excluded from analysis. There were a total of 34 live and 3 stillborn piglets born, at an average weight of 107 g/piglet. Terminal blood samples were collected via cardiac puncture under anesthesia.

2.2. Serum Processing and ELISA. Blood samples were stored overnight at 4°C to coagulate and then spun in a benchtop centrifuge at 1500 ×g for 5 minutes. Serum was collected, transferred into fresh tubes, and then frozen at −80°C for storage. Total IgG and neutralizing antibody levels were determined by using Human IgG ELISA Kit (Bethyl Laboratories, Montgomery, TX) and ETI-AB-AUK PLUS (DiaSorin, Saluggia, Italy), respectively. IgG subclasses were measured by using human IgG subclass kits (Invitrogen). Each sample was run in duplicate and a standard curve was included in each plate.

2.3. Pharmacokinetic Analysis. Pharmacokinetic parameters from plasma concentration-time data in pregnant and nonpregnant guinea pigs were estimated by noncompartmental analysis. Half-life was calculated by regression analysis on the terminal phase of concentration-time data. Clearance (CL) was estimated as follows:

$$CL = \frac{Dose}{AUC}, \tag{1}$$

where AUC is the area under the curve calculated by the trapezoidal rule.

2.4. Guinea Pig FcRn and IgG Purification. A soluble version of human FcRn was constructed and purified as described [14]. Briefly, stably transfected Huh7 cells were grown in T-75 culture flasks (Fisher Scientific, Pittsburgh, PA) in GlutaMAX DMEM supplemented with 10% FBS until they reached confluence, at which point the medium was replaced with BD Cell MAB Serum Free Medium (Fisher) containing zeocin. The cultures were kept at 37°C in a CO_2 incubator for two weeks, then the growth medium was collected and its pH adjusted to 6.0 with 1 M HCl. The solution was loaded by gravity flow onto a column of 1 mL IgG Sepharose 6 Fast Flow resin (GE Healthcare Life Sciences, USA) equilibrated with binding buffer containing 50 mM Na phosphate pH 6, 150 mM NaCl, and 0.005% Tween 20. After being washed with 3 mL binding buffer, the column was eluted with elution buffer containing 50 mM Tris Cl pH 8.5 and 150 mM NaCl. The eluate was analyzed by western blot and then concentrated via ultrafiltration with a 30 KDa cutoff device (Millipore).

IgG subclasses purified from myeloma were obtained commercially (Sigma, 1 mg/mL) and then dialyzed overnight into binding buffer in a dialysis cassette (3 mL capacity, 10,000 KDa cutoff, Pierce). The concentration was determined by measuring absorption at 280 nm with a spectrophotometer (Molecular Systems), using a molar absorption coefficient 2×10^5 M^{-1} cm^{-1}. The samples were serially diluted threefold to obtain concentrations of 4000–48 nM which were then used in SPR measurements.

2.5. Surface Plasmon Resonance (SPR). Binding assays were performed at 25°C using the Biacore 3000 instrument (GE Healthcare, Piscataway, NJ, USA). Guinea pig soluble FcRn (GPFcRN) diluted in 10 mM sodium acetate, pH 4.0 was immobilized on a CM5 chip using an amine coupling kit (GE Healthcare, Piscataway, NJ, USA) to a density of 1000 resonance units (RU). A reference surface was also created by performing the amine coupling protocol with buffer only. IgG subclasses were dialyzed into the binding buffer and serially diluted threefold to obtain concentrations of 4000–48 nM. The diluted IgG subclasses were injected in duplicate across the reference and GPFcRn surface at 50 μL/min for 2 min.

After dissociating for 3 min with the binding buffer, the chip surface was regenerated using elution buffer.

The binding responses were double referenced by subtracting the signals from the reference cell and buffer-only injections from the analyte injections. Estimated K_D values were derived by fitting the binding and dissociation signals with a 1 : 1 (Langmuir) model using the BIA evaluation 4.1.1 software.

2.6. Anti-Human Immune Response. ELISA was used to measure guinea pig anti-human antibody formation. For this, strips precoated with anti-human IgG (Bethyl Laboratories, Montgomery, TX) were incubated with a 1 : 1000 dilution of HBIGIV in super block blocking buffer (thermoscientific) at room temperature for 1 h. The plate was washed four times with phosphate-buffered saline (PBS; pH 7.4) with 0.05% Tween 20 to remove unbound human IgG. Guinea pig serum samples were added to the plate, followed by incubation at 37°C for 1 h. The plate was then washed four times before adding goat anti-guinea pig antibodies (heavy chain and light chain, 1 : 100 dilution) conjugated to horse radish peroxidase (Abcam Inc.) and then incubated at 37°C for 1 h. After four washes, the reaction was developed with 1-step TMB-ELISA substrate solution (KPL) and stopped by adding 100 μL of 4 N sulfuric acid. The absorbance of each well was measured at 450 nm with a SpectraMax M2e microplate reader (Molecular Devices, Sunnyvale, CA).

2.7. Data Analysis. Absorbance values from ELISA were transformed into human antibody concentration or anti-HBs international units by fitting them to an equation derived from a five-parameter fit of the standard curve (SoftMax Pro). The values from all the siblings in each litter were averaged to obtain one single value. The fetal/maternal ratio for each litter was calculated by dividing the litter average by the concentration from its dam. This ratio for each litter over time was fitted using GraphPad Prism version 5.04 for Windows, GraphPad Software (San Diego, CA).

PK parameters from the pregnant and nonpregnant control guinea pigs were analyzed using unpaired, one tailed t-test and the P values reported; P values <0.05 were considered significant.

Differences in the mean nAb levels for the pregnant guinea pigs, nonpregnant controls, and piglets were analyzed using one way ANOVA with Bonferroni posttest for the high and low dose groups, respectively, using GraphPad Prism 5.04. P values <0.05 were considered significant.

3. Results

3.1. Human Antibody Transplacental Transfer. There was antibody transfer from the pregnant guinea pigs to all the fetuses in both dose groups. One notable exception was the one pregnant which delivered within four hours after HBIGIV administration. None of the piglets in her litter had measurable human antibody in their serum, indicating that no appreciable transfer of IgG occurs during delivery. Both total human IgG and neutralizing IgG were detected

TABLE 2: Serum neutralizing antibody levels (mIU/mL).

Dose	Nonpregnant controls (range)	Mothers (range)	Litter (range)
50 IU/kg	82 (67–96)****	101 (67–129)**	47 (11–110)*
100 IU/kg	209 (183–231)****	169 (114–201)**	90 (50–141)*

**** $P < 0.0001$; ** $P < 0.01$; * $P < 0.05$; P values were derived from *posthoc* comparisons between 50 and 100 IU/kg groups in each of the cohorts, respectively.

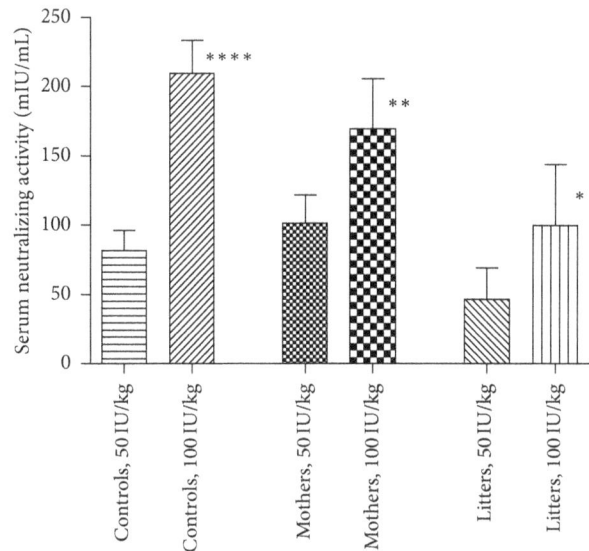

FIGURE 1: Neutralizing antibody in guinea pigs and their litters, averages group comparison.

in all the remaining guinea pigs and all the piglets in their litters at all the time points starting on day 2 (48 hours) after administration. The transfer of neutralizing antibody was dose dependent: the higher the administered dose is, the higher the average neutralizing antibody activity in the litter is (Table 2 and Figure 1). Regardless of the dose, the level of neutralizing antibody in all litters was higher than 10 mIU/mL, the accepted serological level for protection.

3.2. Human Antibody Transplacental Transfer Kinetics. As our preliminary data indicated [14], fetal concentration of neutralizing antibody increased with time. For each dose group, the litters born on day two had lower serum neutralizing activities than those born on subsequent days (Figure 2). The litter born five days after maternal HBIGIV administration had neutralizing antibody levels higher than their mothers'. The fetal : maternal ratio of the neutralizing antibody activity did not seem to depend on the dose and increased linearly with time in both dose groups (Figure 3). Based on a linear fit ($R^2 = 0.7$), the fetal : maternal ratio increased at a rate of ~0.2/day. A similar value was observed when the ratios of total IgG concentrations were fitted (data not shown). The data also fits well using an exponential growth curve ($r^2 = 0.8$), perhaps indicating that FcRn expression levels may be increasing with gestation age.

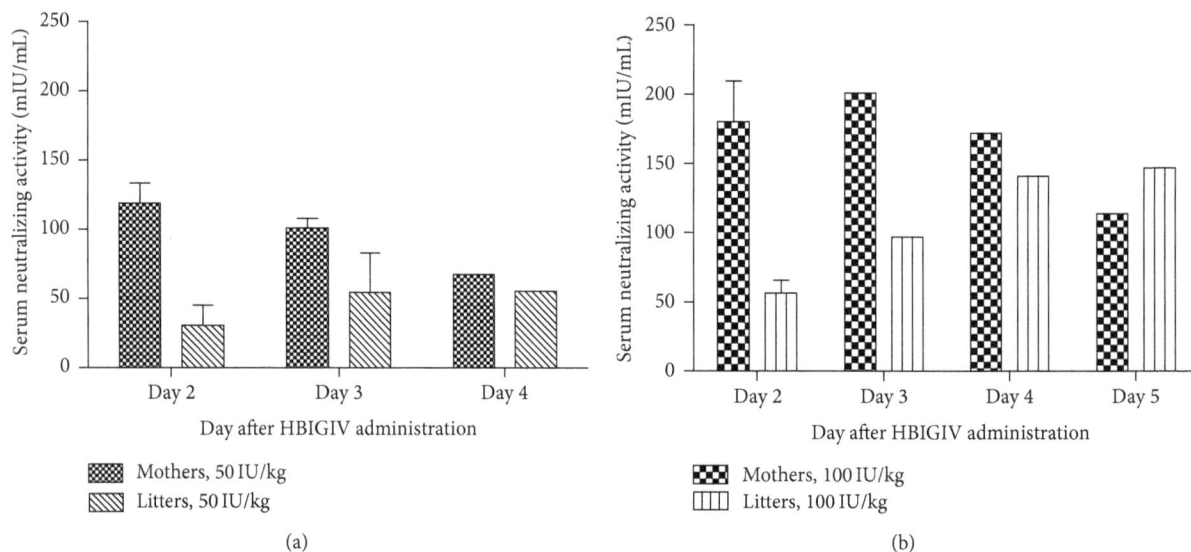

FIGURE 2: Neutralizing antibody in guinea pigs and their litters at 50 (a) and 100 IU/kg (b) dose.

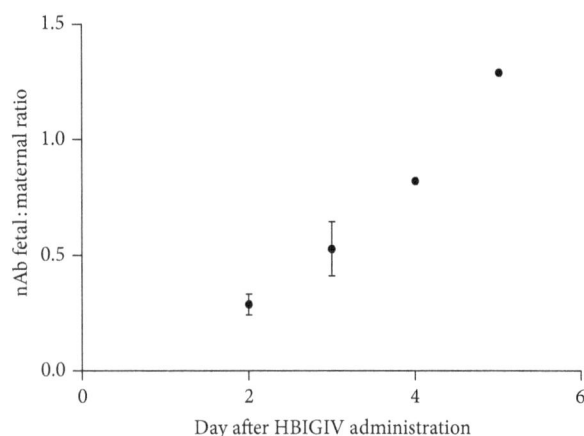

FIGURE 3: Kinetics of the neutralizing antibody fetal : maternal ratio.

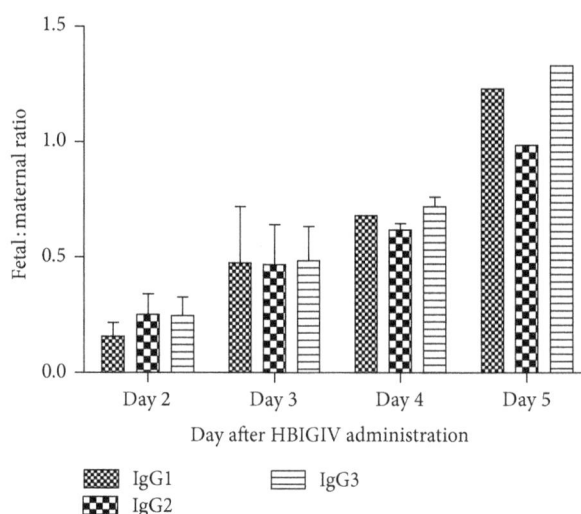

FIGURE 4: Kinetics of the fetal : maternal ratio for IgG subclasses.

3.3. IgG Subclass Transfer. IgG subclasses one through three were detected in all guinea pigs and litters. The amount of IgG4 in all animals, including nonpregnant controls, was below the detection limit because of the low concentration of IgG4 in the HBIGIV preparation used.

The fetal : maternal ratio for the other three subclasses paralleled that of the total and neutralizing antibody and was comparable for all subclasses (Figure 4).

3.4. Anti-Human Antibody Formation. As expected, there was no guinea pig anti-human antibody formation up to day 5 following HBIGIV administration. Anti-human IgG antibodies were measureable on one nonpregnant control on days 14 and 21 after administration, demonstrating the ability of our test system to detect these antibodies (data not shown).

3.5. Pharmacokinetics of Human IgG in the Guinea Pig Model. Human IgG had different PK characteristics in pregnant

guinea pigs compared to nonpregnant controls. On average, pregnant guinea pigs (Table 3) exhibited lower AUC, higher clearance ($P = 0.06$), and shorter half-life ($P = 0.03$) than the nonpregnant controls.

3.6. SPR of Guinea Pig FcRn Binding to Human IgG. All human IgG subclasses bound to the receptor (Figures 5(a)–5(d)) with dissociation constants (K_D) ranging from 3.4–6.8 μM.

4. Discussion

For more than two decades, WHO and CDC have recommended universal hepatitis B vaccination for all newborns during the first year(s) of life. This strategy is yielding results: in USA, it has been credited with an estimated 81% decline

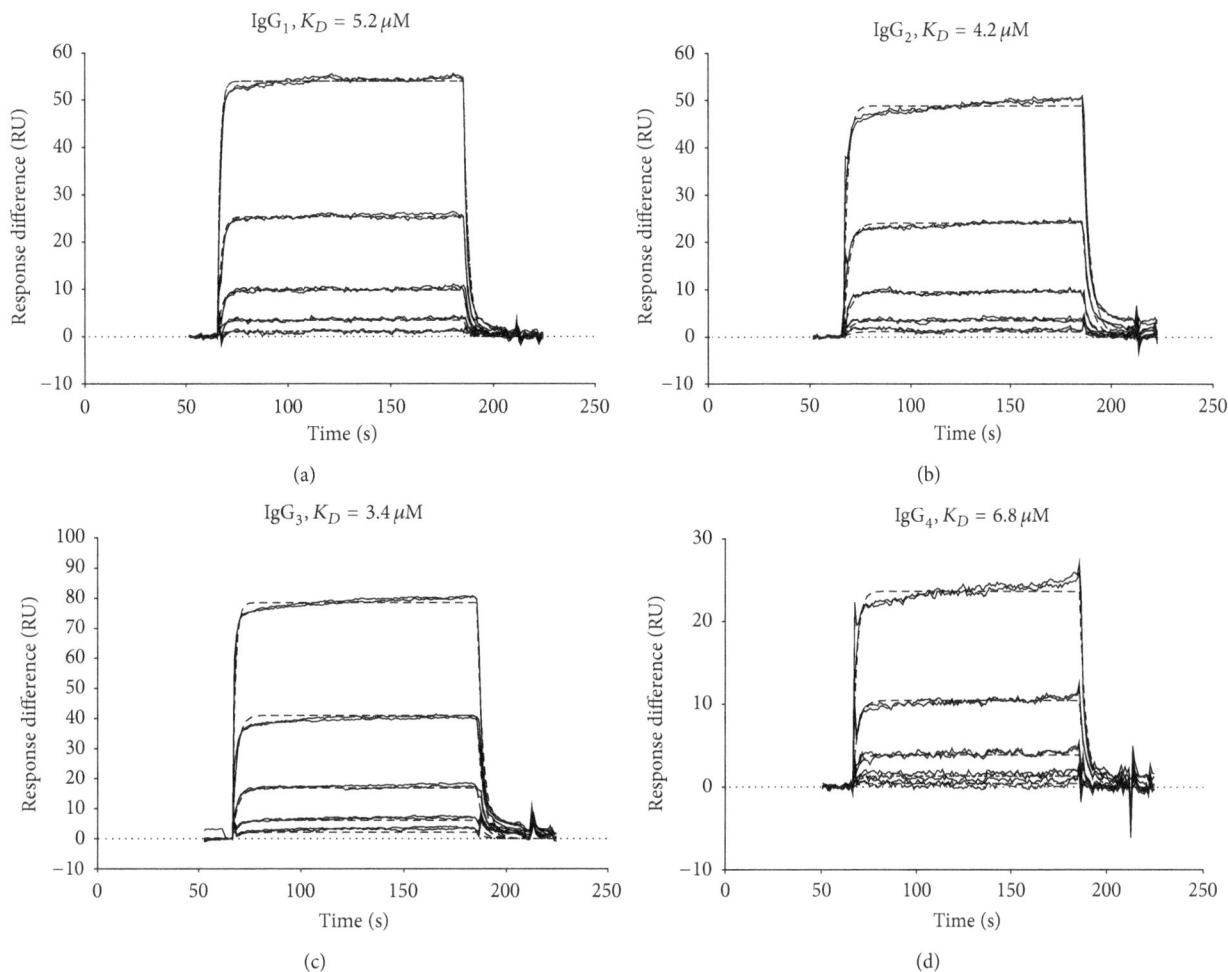

FIGURE 5: Binding of human IgG subclasses 1 through 4 to guinea pig FcRn receptor; panels (a) through (d), respectively. Dissociation constants (K_D) range from 3.4 to 6.8 mM.

TABLE 3: Average pharmacokinetic parameters for human IgG (50 IU/kg dose) in the pregnant guinea pigs and the nonpregnant controls.

	AUC[b] (μg*hr/mL)	CL[c] (mL/hr per kg)	Half-life (hours)
Pregnant, mean (STDEV)[a]	1819 (501)	1.396 (0.381)	59 (25)[*]
Nonpregnant, mean (STDEV)	2770 (846)	0.916 (0.245)	95 (4)[*]

[*]$P < 0.05$.

[a]One pregnant guinea pig was excluded from analysis due to abnormally high AUC (4-5 times higher than the other sows).

[b]Area under the curve.

[c]Clearance.

in new HBV infections since 1991 when it was first implemented [15]. With the ever-increasing number of countries, including the endemic areas [4, 16, 17], incorporating HBV vaccination in their national infant immunization programs, the overall burden of the disease is expected to decrease in the coming years. However, one subset of the vaccines has not shared the benefits of this global success story. Despite PEP,

a small but significant percentage of infants born to infected mothers still acquire HBV at birth [8]. The reasons for the prevention failure are not clear, but several factors play a role. For example, children of mothers who are HBeAg positive or with higher HBV DNA have significantly higher risk of becoming infected, showing that uncontrolled maternal infection is an important contributor [9]. Preterm infants weighing <2,000 g at birth do not respond well to the first dose of HBV vaccine given <24 hours after birth, indicating that immune immaturity may also be a contributing factor [18]. The two may also be linked, given that the risk of preterm labor is increased in women with exacerbation of chronic hepatitis B during pregnancy [12, 19].

If some or a combination of the enumerated factors are the cause for PEP failure, passive immune prophylaxis of the mothers with Hepatitis B Immune Globulin (i.e., HBIG and HBIGIV) would be beneficial. However, although HBIG has been used in pregnant women outside USA to help prevent vertical transmission of HBV, these studies have not shown clear efficacy.

Given the lack of data, we set out to gain a better understanding of the possible efficacious dose and kinetics of administered polyclonal antibody preparations during pregnancy. We administered two HBIGIV doses at the end of gestation in pregnant guinea pigs, both much higher than doses used in non-US clinical trials [10]. The low dose groups received 50 IU/kg HBIG, consistent with the label indication for prophylaxis following perinatal exposure [6]; the other dose was twice as high. Both doses resulted in neutralizing antibody concentrations in the newborns larger than 10 mIU/mL. Litters from the higher dose group had significantly more neutralizing antibodies than the lower dose group.

Newborn guinea pigs at birth had nAb levels that increased with the number of days from antibody administration to their mothers. Thus, for each dose group, litters born on day 2 had lower anti-HBs serum concentrations than those born on subsequent days (Figure 2). Consequently, each guinea pig litter essentially functioned as "a sink" for the human antibody product administered to their mother. This would imply altered pharmacokinetic parameters for HBIGIV during pregnancy in the guinea pig.

PK analysis of human IgG showed increased clearance and decreased AUC in pregnant compared to nonpregnant guinea pigs. The half-life was also decreased. Although statistically not significant, the difference in AUC between pregnant and nonpregnant guinea pigs indicates a physiological significance given the transplacental transfer of maternally administered antibodies to newborn guinea pigs.

The time-dependent accumulation of human IgG in the guinea pig fetal circulation at the end of pregnancy (Figures 2 and 3) is highly evocative of the increasing fetal : maternal IgG ratios derived from cord blood/maternal blood paired clinical samples [20–22].

A recent meta-analysis of Chinese clinical studies demonstrated that administering multiple small doses of HBIG, typically 200 IU on weeks 28, 32 and 36 of pregnancy, decreases the rate of infection for newborns [10]. A single 200 IU HBIG dose, depending on the specific lot, corresponds to a dose volume of 0.64 mL or less, and, for a 75 kg pregnant woman would be at least 7 times lower than 0.06 mL/kg, the recommended dose for post exposure prophylaxis. Thus, we refer to this dose as a "microdose". Interestingly, among infants for whom anti-HBs data was collected, a larger percentage had neutralizing antibodies after microdosing their mothers with HBIG *versus* controls, also demonstrating (as did our guinea pig studies) that nAbs in HBIG cross the placenta to reach pharmacologically active levels in the fetus.

Although this recent meta-analysis [10] adds strong support to the benefit of passive immunization strategies to help prevention of HBV vertical transmission before birth, the odds ratios are consistent with treatment failure for many infants. Our studies in the guinea pig prompt us to posit that maternal microdosing may not afford an adequate and sustained increase in maternal anti-Hbs levels. Given the dose-dependent nAb transplacental transfer we observed in our animal model, these lower maternal nAb would result in lower fetal concentrations. Furthermore, antibody pharmacokinetics in pregnant chronically infected women may be different from what we saw in our animal model in the absence of infection. For example, in women with

high viraemia or those experiencing pregnancy related HBV exacerbations, increased antibody clearance via antibody "sequestration" through opsonization, as seen in other antibody antiviral treatments [23, 24], could be occurring, thus further decreasing maternal (and fetal) neutralizing antibody levels. Our data leads us to believe that microdosing with HBIG during pregnancy may not be sufficient and, with or without exacerbations, higher or more frequent dosing at the end of gestation could improve outcomes for the newborns.

As with all antibody therapies during pregnancy, the risk for antibody facilitated, FcRn mediated transplacental viral transmission is a possibility. A recent clinical trial in HIV infected mothers receiving one dose of HIV hyperimmune globulin preparation during gestation weeks 36–38 considered but discounted its likelihood for HIV [25]. In the case of HBV, the odds ratios at birth favor HBIG usage during pregnancy [10], thus too excluding the possibility for antibody-mediated increased transmission.

It should be stressed that our study has inherent limitations. By using the pregnant guinea pig, a good model for transplacental transfer of human antibody, our study in guinea pigs does not account for HBV infection. It also is limited by a small sample size: twelve pregnant and six nonpregnant control guinea pigs, with one guinea pig and her litter excluded from analysis due to delivering within four hours of HBIGIV injection. Although transplacental transfer of nAb was evident in all the litters born two or more days after HBIGIV administration, in a statistically significant dose dependent manner, it is currently unknown if the same observation could be made in infected pregnant women. Despite being informative, animal studies such as this are not a replacement for clinical studies. The safety and efficacy of antibody preparations, including HBIG when used to prevent vertical transmission of HBV during pregnancy, will ultimately be determined in well-designed, adequately powered, randomized, controlled clinical studies.

Abbreviations

HBV:	Hepatitis B virus
HBIG:	Hepatitis B immune globulin
Anti-HBs:	Antihepatitis B surface antigen
HBeAg:	Hepatitis B e-antigen
PEP:	Postexposure prophylaxis
HBIGIV:	Hepatitis B immune globulin intravenous (human)
nAb:	Neutralizing antibody
SPR:	Surface plasmon resonance
RU:	Relative units
CL:	Clearance
AUC:	Area under the curve
MTCT:	Mother-to-child transmission.

Conflict of Interests

The authors have no conflict of interests regarding the publication of this paper.

Acknowledgments

The authors thank Dr. John Finlayson for discussions and editorial help. The study was partially funded by a grant from the FDA Office of Women's Health to EBS and PZ.

References

[1] C. M. Weinbaum, I. Williams, E. E. Mast et al., "Recommendations for identification and public health management of persons with chronic hepatitis B virus infection," *MMWR Recommendations and Reports*, vol. 57, article RR08, pp. 1–20, 2008.

[2] M. F. Sorrell, E. A. Belongia, J. Costa et al., "National Institutes of Health Consensus Development Conference Statement: management of hepatitis B," *Annals of Internal Medicine*, vol. 150, no. 2, pp. 104–110, 2009.

[3] C. W. Shepard, E. P. Simard, L. Finelli, A. E. Fiore, and B. P. Bell, "Hepatitis B virus infection: epidemiology and vaccination," *Epidemiologic Reviews*, vol. 28, no. 1, pp. 112–125, 2006.

[4] WHO, "Hepatitis B vaccines," *The Weekly Epidemiological Record*, vol. 84, no. 40, pp. 405–419, 2009.

[5] C. E. Stevens, R. P. Beasley, J. Tsui, and W. C. Lee, "Vertical transmission of hepatitis B antigen in Taiwan," *The New England Journal of Medicine*, vol. 292, no. 15, pp. 771–774, 1975.

[6] E. E. Mast, H. S. Margolis, A. E. Fiore et al., "A comprehensive immunization strategy to eliminate transmission of hepatitis B virus infection in the United States: recommendations of the Advisory Committee on Immunization Practices (ACIP) part 1: immunization of infants, children, and adolescents," *MMWR Recommendations and Reports*, vol. 54, article RR16, pp. 1–31, 2005.

[7] E. E. Mast, C. M. Weinbaum, A. E. Fiore et al., "A comprehensive immunization strategy to eliminate transmission of hepatitis B virus infection in the United States: recommendations of the Advisory Committee on Immunization Practices (ACIP) part II: immunization of adults," *MMWR Recommendations and Reports*, vol. 55, article RR16, pp. 1–25, 2006.

[8] G. Borgia, M. A. Carleo, G. B. Gaeta, and I. Gentile, "Hepatitis B in pregnancy," *World Journal of Gastroenterology*, vol. 18, no. 34, pp. 4677–4683, 2012.

[9] H. M. H. Ip, V. C. W. Wong, P. N. Lelie, M. C. Kuhns, and H. W. Reesink, "Prevention of hepatitis B virus carrier state in infants according to maternal serum levels of HBV DNA," *The Lancet*, vol. 1, no. 8635, pp. 406–410, 1989.

[10] Z. Shi, X. Li, L. Ma, and Y. Yang, "Hepatitis B immunoglobulin injection in pregnancy to interrupt hepatitis B virus mother-to-child transmission—a meta-analysis," *International Journal of Infectious Diseases*, vol. 14, no. 7, pp. e622–e634, 2010.

[11] A. Söderström, G. Norkrans, and M. Lindh, "Hepatitis B virus DNA during pregnancy and post partum: aspects on vertical transmission," *Scandinavian Journal of Infectious Diseases*, vol. 35, no. 11-12, pp. 814–819, 2003.

[12] N. Leung, "Chronic hepatitis B in Asian women of childbearing age," *Hepatology International*, vol. 3, no. 1, pp. 24–31, 2009.

[13] H. Elvidge, "Production of dated pregnant guinea pigs without post-partum matings," *Journal of the Institute of Animal Technicians*, vol. 23, no. 3, pp. 111–117, 1972.

[14] E. B. Struble, L. Ma, L. Zhong, A. Lesher, J. Beren, and P. Zhang, "Human antibodies can cross guinea pig placenta and bind its neonatal Fc receptor: implications for studying immune prophylaxis and therapy during pregnancy," *Clinical and Developmental Immunology*, vol. 2012, Article ID 538701, 9 pages, 2012.

[15] J. W. Ward, "Time for renewed commitment to viral hepatitis prevention," *American Journal of Public Health*, vol. 98, no. 5, pp. 779–781, 2008.

[16] D. FitzSimons, G. Hendrickx, A. Vorsters, and D. P. Van, "Hepatitis B vaccination: a completed schedule enough to control HBV lifelong? Milan, Italy, 17-18 November 2011," *Vaccine*, vol. 31, no. 4, pp. 584–590, 2013.

[17] A. Zidan, H. Scheuerlein, S. Schule, U. Settmacher, and F. Rauchfuss, "Epidemiological pattern of hepatitis B and hepatitis C as etiological agents for hepatocellular carcinoma in Iran and worldwide," *Hepatitis Monthly*, vol. 12, no. 10, Article ID e6894, 2012.

[18] N. Linder, T. H. Vishne, E. Levin et al., "Hepatitis B vaccination: long-term follow-up of the immune response of preterm infants and comparison of two vaccination protocols," *Infection*, vol. 30, no. 3, pp. 136–139, 2002.

[19] J. P. Hieber, D. Dalton, J. Shorey, and B. Combes, "Hepatitis and pregnancy," *Journal of Pediatrics*, vol. 91, no. 4, pp. 545–549, 1977.

[20] R. W. Pitcher-Wilmott, P. Hindocha, and C. B. S. Wood, "The placental transfer of IgG subclasses in human pregnancy," *Clinical and Experimental Immunology*, vol. 41, no. 2, pp. 303–308, 1980.

[21] A. Malek, R. Sager, and H. Schneider, "Maternal-fetal transport of immunoglobulin G and its subclasses during the third trimester of human pregnancy," *American Journal of Reproductive Immunology*, vol. 32, no. 1, pp. 8–14, 1994.

[22] N. E. Simister, "Placental transport of immunoglobulin G," *Vaccine*, vol. 21, no. 24, pp. 3365–3369, 2003.

[23] W. A. Marasco and J. Sui, "The growth and potential of human antiviral monoclonal antibody therapeutics," *Nature Biotechnology*, vol. 25, no. 12, pp. 1421–1434, 2007.

[24] J. Schupbach, H. Gunthard, M. S. C. Fung et al., "Pharmacokinetics of an HIV-1 gp120-specific chimeric antibody in patients with HIV-1 disease," *Biotherapy*, vol. 6, no. 3, pp. 205–215, 1993.

[25] C. Onyango-Makumbi, S. B. Omer, M. Mubiru et al., "Safety and efficacy of HIV hyperimmune globulin for prevention of mother-to-child HIV transmission in HIV-1-infected pregnant women and their infants in Kampala, Uganda (HIVIGLOB/NVP STUDY)," *Journal of Acquired Immune Deficiency Syndromes*, vol. 58, no. 4, pp. 399–407, 2011.

Hepatitis B Vaccination and Screening Awareness in Primary Care Practitioners

Adnan Said[1] and Janice H. Jou[2]

[1] Division of Gastroenterology and Hepatology, University of Wisconsin School of Medicine and
   Public Health and William S. Middleton VAMC, Madison, WI 53705, USA
[2] Division of Gastroenterology and Hepatology, Oregon Health Sciences University and Portland VAMC, Portland, OR 97239, USA

Correspondence should be addressed to Adnan Said; axs@medicine.wisc.edu

Academic Editor: Annagiulia Gramenzi

Introduction. The goals of *Healthy People US* 2020 have called for increased screening and vaccination of high-risk groups for Hepatitis B (HBV). *Methods.* We performed a survey of 400 randomly chosen primary care practitioners (PCPs) in Wisconsin to assess their knowledge, attitudes, and practices regarding screening and vaccination for HBV. *Results.* Screening rates of patients at risk of sexual transmission were low, with 61% of respondents stating that they screen patients who had more than 1 sex partner in 6 months and 86% screening patients with a history of sex with prostitutes. Screening rate for persons with a history of intravenous drug use was 94%. Children of immigrants were screened by 65%, persons on hemodialysis by 73%, and prison inmates by 69%. Screening increased with provider experience with HBV. Deficiencies in vaccination rates mirrored screening practices. Major barriers to screening were cost, someone else's responsibility, time constraints, or lack of knowledge. *Conclusions.* Without improved education and practices of PCPs about HBV screening and vaccination, the goals of healthy people 2020 regarding HBV will not be met. Barriers to screening and vaccination need to be addressed. Cost-effectiveness of alternative strategies such as universal vaccination under the age of 50 should be explored.

1. Introduction

Worldwide over 400 million people are carriers of hepatitis B; in the United States an estimated 1.25 million people are chronically infected and an estimated 51,000 new cases occurred in 2005 [1, 2]. Although the incidence of HBV has declined since the 1980s in all age groups, the decline has been slower in adults, particularly in males from ages 25–44 [2].

1.1. Vaccination Guidelines. Immunization Guidelines from the Centers for Disease Control (CDC) published in 1991 and updated in 1995 and 1999 call for universal vaccination of all persons younger than 18 years of age and adults older than 18 who are at risk for hepatitis B infection [3]. In December 2006, the Advisory Committee on Immunization Practices from the CDC released the first comprehensive statement on hepatitis B immunization since universal vaccination was advocated in 1991 [4]. These updated guidelines apart from reemphasizing the recommendations from previous iterations emphasized the importance of administering hepatitis B vaccination in primary care clinics as part of routine clinical care and to remove barriers for this care.

Although guidelines abound, 10% of practitioners are completely unaware of the existence of 78% of the guidelines [5] and current vaccination rates for adults and children at risk are less than optimal. A national survey of adults at risk for HBV found that only 30-31% had received the first dose of the HBV vaccine although 80% reported visiting a clinician during the past year [6]. There are missed opportunities for HBV vaccination in patients at risk as many of these subjects had multiple visits in one year. Data on vaccination rates for patients with specific risk factors tell a similar story.

1.2. Sexual Risk Factors. Among noninjection drug users, predictors of HBV seroconversion include females who engage in unprotected receptive anal sex, men who have sex with men (MSM), persons having a sex partner known for less than 6 months, and males and females who receive money or drugs for sex [7]. Vaccination rates in groups at risk of sexual transmission of HBV however remain low although recommendations for vaccination have been longstanding. In young men who have sex with men (MSM) the vaccination rates were only 9% with a prevalence of infection of 11% over the last two decades. Of this group, 96% had consistent contact with the health care system [8]. In recent years, the vaccination rates have improved somewhat although they are still far below acceptable levels. In a survey of MSM from 1999 to 2000, the vaccination rate for HBV was only 38.9% [9].

1.3. Immigration from Endemic Areas. The incidence of HBV is high in immigrants to the US from endemic areas of the world. Approximately 40,000 immigrants infected with chronic HBV are granted permanent residence in the United States annually [10]. A demographic group at particular risk is thus children of immigrants born in the United States, particularly those born before universal vaccination of neonates was instituted in 1991. Furthermore access to perinatal and neonatal healthcare is limited and these groups may not seek healthcare at these times reducing the opportunity for screening and vaccination and leading to increased rates of perinatal and horizontal transmission of HBV.

In a study of Korean-Americans from 1988 to 1990, males had a carrier rate of 8% for HBV while females had a rate of 4.4%. The rate of HBV carrier status in children of immigrants born in the United States was almost 3%. Furthermore, all mothers who had HBsAg and HBeAg had offspring who were HBsAg positive, underscoring the risk of perinatal transmission in immigrant populations [11]. In the Hmong population in Wisconsin who migrated from Laos, the overall prevalence of chronic HBV in Hmong children born in the United States between 1984 and 1989 was 14% [12]. Eleven percent of the HBsAg positive children were born to mothers who were HBsAg negative. Vaccination rates in this population vary widely from 12% to 86% [13, 14]. Household contacts of HBsAg carriers should be considered for screening and subsequent vaccination if they are susceptible [3, 4].

1.4. Incarceration. The risk in prison inmates is thought to be related to the high risk behaviors associated with this demographic including injection drug use and having multiple sex partners. In a correctional facility in Georgia, the prevalence of HBV infection was 2 percent, with an incidence in the facility in one year of almost 3 percent in inmates identified as high risk. The annual incidence of HBV in this facility (3579 per 100,000) was 120 times the national incidence. Additionally, clustering of unique HBV nucleotide sequencing in groups of newly infected inmates suggested that there was transmission between individuals at the correctional institution [15]. Investigation of two community outbreaks in Tennessee found that 60% of those infected had a history of incarceration. There was a prevalence of 4% for chronic HBV and 3% for acute HBV in this cohort.

1.5. Hemodialysis Patients. In dialysis patients the incidence and prevalence of HBV is high due to multiple parenteral exposures during dialysis and the immunosuppressed state associated with end stage renal disease [4, 16, 17]. Since 1982, HBV vaccination has been recommended for hemodialysis patients [18]. Although there have been significant improvements in the vaccination rates since that time, HBV vaccination rates in hemodialysis patients actually decreased in 14 of the 18 End Stage Renal Disease Network states, districts, and territories between 2001 and 2002. Furthermore, only 36.8–66.5% of hemodialysis patients in 2002 were vaccinated [19]. Dialysis centers are settings in which practitioners see high risk patients, and therefore further efforts should be undertaken to achieve 100% compliance with vaccination and to encourage periodic screening for HBV.

1.6. Role of Primary Care Practitioners. Primary care practitioners have a critical role in identifying and screening patients at high risk for acquisition for hepatitis B and subsequent vaccination of these patients [4]. However, our review of the medical literature suggests that little is known about primary care practitioners' awareness of guidelines for hepatitis B screening and vaccination, identifying the risk factors for transmission of hepatitis B, or experience of barriers to adherence to the guidelines [3, 20–22]. Our study sought to assess the knowledge, attitudes, and practices of primary care practitioners in Wisconsin regarding screening and vaccination guidelines for HBV and to identify barriers to these practices.

2. Methods

2.1. Study Sample. A master list of primary care physicians in Internal Medicine, Family Medicine, Pediatrics, and Obstetrics was obtained from the Wisconsin Department of Regulation and Licensing and used to select a random sample of 400 physicians from all over Wisconsin. A total of 166 practitioners responded to the survey. Forty-seven did not have a valid address or forwarding address, yielding a final response rate of 47%.

2.2. Survey Instrument. A 20-question survey (available upon request) was developed to assess clinician knowledge, attitudes, and practices in regard to hepatitis B vaccination and screening. Practitioners were asked about whether they offer HBV vaccinations, the number of patients seen with HBV, the number of patients vaccinated for HBV, screening practices, and barriers to screening. In addition, the practitioners were asked about their knowledge of the hepatitis B guidelines and attitudes toward HBV as a public health problem. Demographic data collected were practice type, patient population, years in practice, and country of residency training. The survey was tested for construct and content validity by expert review and by pretesting in a local group of PCPs.

2.3. Procedures. The study protocol was approved by the institutional review board of the University of Wisconsin School of Medicine and Public Health.

2.4. Data Collection. The first mailing was sent out without an incentive in November 2005. Included in the mailings were a self addressed stamped envelope, a survey with a code to permit tracking and follow-up, and a separate reply postcard. The post asked practitioners about their interest in participating in a future focus group to discuss barriers to hepatitis B vaccination and a CME program addressing hepatitis B vaccination and screening. A second mailing was sent in February 2007 to increase the response rate and included a five-dollar cash incentive.

2.5. Data Analysis. Question responses were initially reported as frequencies and percentages. For cross tabulations of discrete data chi-square statistics were used and a 2-sided P value of <0.05 was considered statistically significant. Binary logistic regression was used to examine independent predictors of discrete outcomes.

3. Results

3.1. Respondent Characteristics. Of the 166 respondents, 95 (57%) were in private practice, 25 (15%) were in Hospital-affiliated private practice, 13 (8%) were in a University Hospital Clinic, 25 (15%) responded "Other" (e.g., Community Health Clinic), and 8 (5%) did not answer the question. Thirty-one percent had been in practice for 0–10 years, 33% for 11–20 years, 25% for 21–30 years, and 11% for greater than 30 years. Forty percent of practitioners saw adults only, 40% saw both adults and children, and 20% saw children only.

More than half (53%) reported that they had not seen any patients with HBV infection in the past year, 40% had seen between 1 to 5 patients, 4% had seen 6–10 patients, and 3% had seen more than 10 patients with HBV. Residency training was completed in the United States for 97% of the respondents and internationally for three percent.

3.2. Current Practices for Screening for HBV Status. Overall, 59% felt that their current HBV screening practices were adequate. Practitioners were asked what proportion of their patients at risk for HBV were screened for infection in the past year: 19% responded that they screened all patients, 36% screened some but less than half, 31% screened more than half, and 14% did not screen any of their patients for HBV.

The proportion of practitioners who screen various groups of patients is depicted in Figures 1 and 2. Ninety percent of practitioners stated they screen pregnant women. Sixty-one percent said that they screen persons with a history of more than one sex partner in six months and 80% screen men who have sex with men. The number of practitioners reporting that they screen persons with a history of sex with prostitutes was higher at 86% and for screening sex workers it was 87%.

Only 37% of PCPs stated that they screen everybody under the age of 18 and 65% screen US-born children of immigrants. Intravenous drug users are screened by 94% of the respondents. Prison inmates are screened by 69% and hemodialysis patients by 73%. Household members of HBV patients are screened by 78%.

Other groups not recommended in screening guidelines (distractor groups in the survey) such as day care workers are screened by 42% of providers, people drinking well water by 9%, and people eating sushi by 12%.

Screening of patients at risk for HBV increased with provider's experience with hepatitis B such that those who saw greater than 5 patients per year were more likely to screen at risk groups including sex workers, persons who have sex with prostitutes, sex partners of HBV carriers, prison inmates, and hemodialysis patients than were their counterparts in the study who saw less than 5 patients with HBV each year ($P < 0.0001$).

3.3. Vaccination Practices. Ninety-one percent of respondents were in a practice that offered HBV vaccination while 9% of the respondents were not. In the past year, 16% of practitioners had not vaccinated any patients for HBV, 14% had vaccinated 1–5 patients, 10% had vaccinated 6–10, and 60% had vaccinated more than 10 patients. When the practitioners were asked if they routinely asked their patients at risk for HBV if they had been vaccinated for HBV, 66% stated that they did, and 33% reported that they did not.

3.4. Knowledge of the HBV Guidelines and Etiology. Of the groups identified by the CDC guidelines as populations who should receive vaccinations for HBV, several groups were correctly identified by a majority of respondents (Figures 3 and 4): persons with more than one sex partner in six months (72%), men who have sex with men (82%), intravenous drug users (92%), prison inmates (52%), and hemodialysis patients (72%). Persons who have sex with prostitutes would be vaccinated by 82% of providers and sex workers by 85%. Sexual partners of HBV positive patients would be vaccinated by 94%. Neonates born to mothers with HBV would be vaccinated by 92% of providers. A smaller number identified children 18 years old and younger (73%) as an appropriate group for HBV vaccination. Children of immigrants born in the United States would be vaccinated by only 50% of respondents.

Persons working in the health care field would be vaccinated by 92% of providers.

Other groups that are not recommended for vaccination such as persons exposed to ill-prepared food would be vaccinated by 22% of respondents, day care workers by 54%, and pregnant women by 42%.

The responses to the question asking for the most common cause of chronic viral hepatitis in the United States (HCV followed by HBV) were as follows: 4% hepatitis A (HAV), 39% HBV, 56% hepatitis C (HCV), and 1% hepatitis E (HEV). Another question was asked regarding the most common cause of chronic hepatitis worldwide and 16% replied that it was HAV, 70% HBV (correct answer), 13% HCV, and 1% HEV.

Identification of serum tests for HBV screening are shown in Figure 5 with the majority of practitioners selecting HBsAg followed by HBcAb as the screening tests of choice.

Practitioners screening selected patient groups (%)

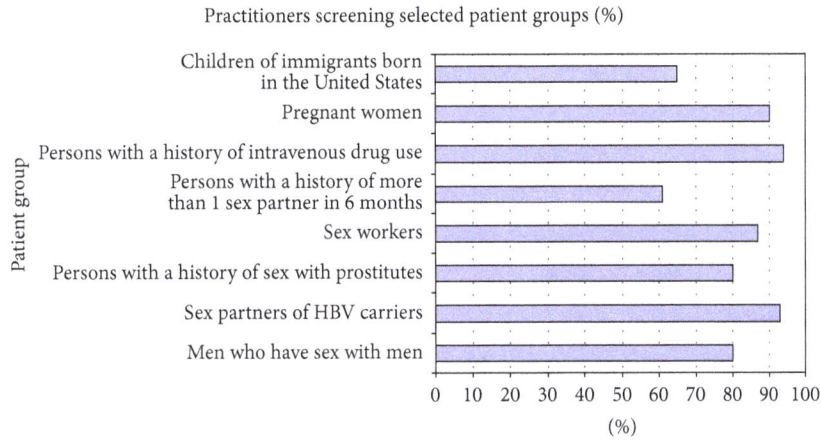

FIGURE 1: Percent of practitioners who would screen for HBV in selected groups.

Practitioners screening selected patient groups (%)

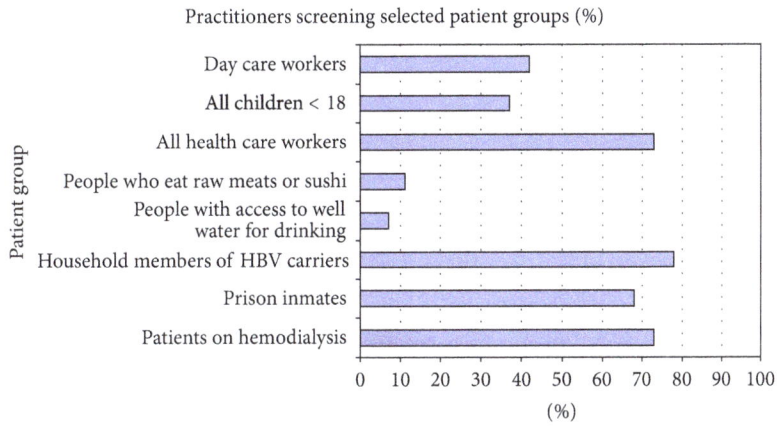

FIGURE 2: Percent of practitioners who would screen for HBV in selected groups.

Practitioners vaccinating for HBV in selected patient groups (%)

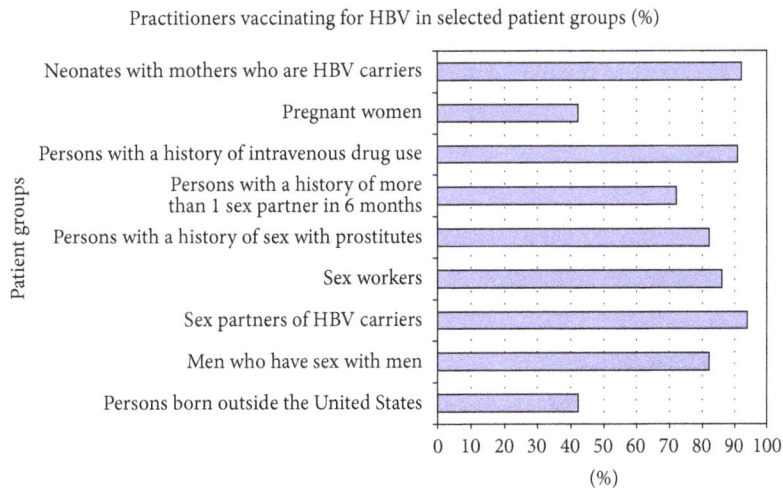

FIGURE 3: Percent of practitioners who would vaccinate for HBV in selected groups.

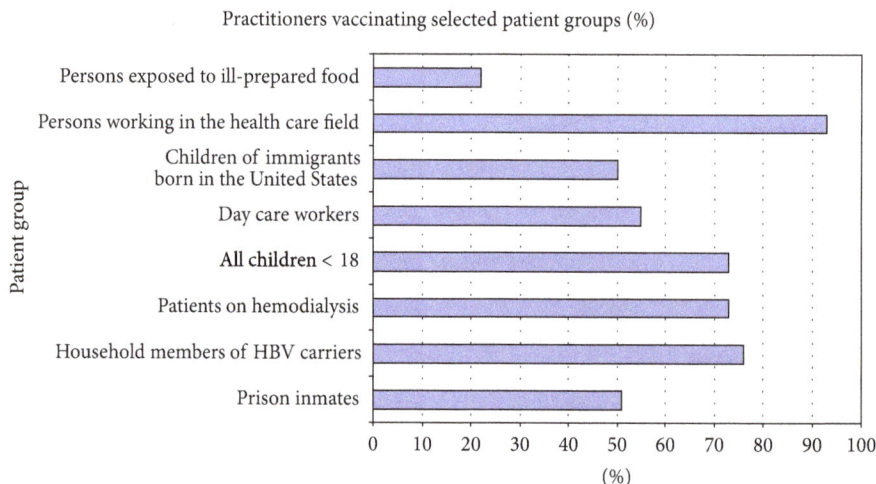

FIGURE 4: Percent of practitioners who would vaccinate for HBV in selected groups.

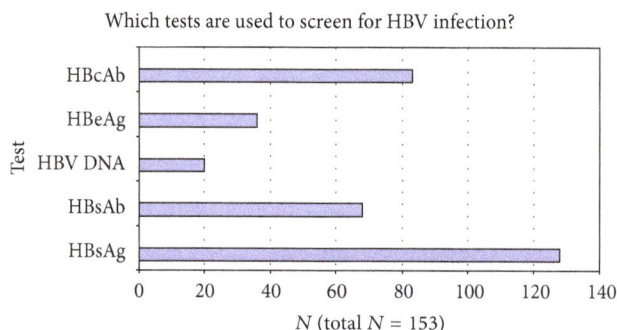

FIGURE 5: Which tests are used to screen for HBV infection?

3.5. Barriers to Screening. Regarding barriers to screening patients for HBV status, 11% percent responded that the cost of screening for HBV was too great, 7% felt that someone else was responsible for screening, and 3% felt that screening for HBV was not relevant to a patient's health care maintenance. Other barriers identified by respondents were lack of knowledge about HBV risk factors, vaccination and screening (9%), time constraints (5%), and forgetting or not making a point to ask (3%). Three percent felt that since they were pediatricians all of their patients must have been immunized and therefore it was unnecessary to screen their patients for HBV.

3.6. Attitudes toward HBV as a Public Health Issue. Practitioners were also asked how important HBV is as a public health problem in general with 48% responding that it was very important, 49% responding that it was somewhat important, and 3% felt that it was not important. In contrast, when asked whether or not they felt that HBV is an important public health problem in their own practice, only 18% believed it was very important, 44% somewhat important, and 38% not important.

4. Discussion

Despite being a vaccine preventable disease HBV remains prevalent worldwide. *Healthy People 2020* called for increased vaccination rates for susceptible individuals [23]. Clearly, without adequate identification of patients who are at risk, HBV is unlikely to be eradicated [24]. Identification of all groups at risk for HBV is difficult as there are many modes of transmission including sexual, percutaneous, and mucosal exposures [10]. This requires an investment of time inquiring about these exposures and a process that would offer appropriate screening tests and vaccinations to eligible patients. Such a plan would rely heavily on the participation of primary care physicians who have the best opportunity for screening a broad cohort of patients.

Current screening practices emphasize the importance of risk factor identification particularly high risk sexual practices, intravenous drug use, and other risk groups such as prison inmates and hemodialysis patients. However, the cohort represented in this survey of PCPs was unable to consistently identify relevant risk factors. Intravenous drug use was identified as a risk factor by a majority of the respondents. The practitioners in our survey less consistently identified sexual risk factors for transmission of HBV; they were less attuned to HBV risks associated with being a child born in the United States to immigrants, a prison inmate, and a patient on hemodialysis.

Clearly these at risk populations need to be highlighted in educational screening and vaccination programs as well.

Even if risk factors are known, routine screening may not occur due to a variety of barriers. Many practitioners indicated that they were uncomfortable with inquiring about these risk factors from their patients, cost, time constraints, and lack of awareness and knowledge about groups at risk for HBV infection. In the medical literature, other barriers to adherence to practice guidelines are lack of self-efficacy, lack of outcome expectancy, inertia of previous practice, external barriers, and patient-related barriers. Many of those who responded to this survey did not feel that there were any areas of improvement in their practices in regard to hepatitis B vaccination and screening.

Funding is another barrier as many patients at risk for HBV are uninsured or underinsured.

4.1. Future Directions. There are options for interventions to increase HBV vaccination and screening rates. One would be educational programs for practitioners to increase knowledge of high risk groups for HBV to consider for screening and vaccination. Programs to implement the CDC guidelines can be established in medical institutions and primary care clinics. Additionally, correctional facilities are in great need of funding to vaccinate their inmates and dialysis centers need to vaccinate 100% of their susceptible patients. Follow-up surveys are being planned in the future to determine if over time HBV screening and vaccination rates have changed.

Since guidelines are difficult to keep up with and implement, an alternative strategy at a national level would be a reconsidering of the guidelines to vaccinate all persons under age of 50 to cast a wider net. The cost-effectiveness of this approach versus the current strategy (vaccinating everyone under 18 and adults at high risk) needs to be worked out.

The *Healthy People 2020* disease reduction goals have been established for achieving the prevention of HBV transmission in the United States. Disease reduction goals for infants and children include reducing the estimated number of chronic HBV infections in infants and young children to 400 cases and the number of new hepatitis B cases reported among persons 2–18 years of age to zero cases. Healthy People 2020 vaccination goals for infants and children include setting a target coverage level for infants of age of 0–3 days receiving the initial birth dose of hepatitis B vaccine to 85% and for children of age of 19–35 months completing the three-dose hepatitis B vaccination series to 90%.

Disease reduction goals for adults include reducing the rate of acute hepatitis B to 1.5 cases per 100,000 in persons of age of 19 years and older. Among adults in high-risk groups, disease reduction goals include reducing the number of cases of acute hepatitis B to 215 cases in injection-drug users and to 45 new infections among men who have sex with men [23]. Without educational intervention to increase awareness, and changing attitudes and practice, these goals will not be met.

Conflict of Interests

The authors declare that they have no conflict of interests regarding the publication of this paper.

References

[1] B. J. McMahon, "Epidemiology and natural history of hepatitis B," *Seminars in Liver Disease*, vol. 25, supplement 1, pp. 3–8, 2005.

[2] A. Wasley, J. T. Miller, and L. Finelli, "Surveillance for acute viral hepatitis-United States, 2005," *MMWR: Morbidity and Mortality Weekly Report*, vol. 56, no. 3, pp. 1–24, 2007.

[3] Centers for Disease Control and Prevention (CDC)., "Update: recommendations to prevent hepatitis B virus transmission-United States," *MMWR: Morbidity and Mortality Weekly Report*, vol. 48, no. 2, pp. 33–34, 1999.

[4] E. E. Mast, C. M. Weinbaum, A. E. Fiore et al., "A comprehensive immunization strategy to eliminate transmission of hepatitis B virus infection in the United States: recommendations of the Advisory Committee on Immunization Practices (ACIP) Part II: immunization of adults," *MMWR: Morbidity and Mortality Weekly Report*, vol. 55, no. 16, pp. 1–33, 2006.

[5] M. D. Cabana, C. S. Rand, N. R. Powe et al., "Why don't physicians follow clinical practice guidelines?: a framework for improvement," *Journal of the American Medical Association*, vol. 282, no. 15, pp. 1458–1465, 1999.

[6] N. Jain, H. Yusuf, P. M. Wortley, G. L. Euler, S. Walton, and S. Stokley, "Factors associated with receiving hepatitis B vaccination among high-risk adults in the United States: an analysis of the National Health Interview Survey, 2000," *Family Medicine*, vol. 36, no. 7, pp. 480–486, 2004.

[7] A. Neaigus, V. A. Gyarmathy, M. Zhao, M. Miller, S. R. Friedman, and D. C. Des Jarlais, "Sexual and other noninjection risks for HBV and HCV seroconversions among noninjecting heroin users," *Journal of Infectious Diseases*, vol. 195, no. 7, pp. 1052–1061, 2007.

[8] D. A. MacKellar, L. A. Valleroy, G. M. Secura et al., "Two decades after vaccine license: hepatitis B immunization and infection among young men who have sex with men," *The American Journal of Public Health*, vol. 91, no. 6, pp. 965–971, 2001.

[9] "Hepatitis A and Hepatitis B vaccination rates improve: majority of gay and bi men still not protected," *Gay and Lesbian Medical Association (GMLA) News Release*, 2000.

[10] G. A. Poland, "Evaluating existing recommendations for hepatitis A and B vaccination," *The American Journal of Medicine*, vol. 118, supplement 10, pp. 16S–20S, 2005.

[11] H.-W. L. Hann, R. S. Hann, and W. C. Maddrey, "Hepatitis B virus infection in 6,130 unvaccinated Korean-Americans surveyed between 1988 and 1990," *The American Journal of Gastroenterology*, vol. 102, no. 4, pp. 767–772, 2007.

[12] M. B. Hurie, E. E. Mast, and J. P. Davis, "Horizontal transmission of hepatitis B virus infection to United States-born children of Hmong refugees," *Pediatrics*, vol. 89, no. 2, pp. 269–273, 1992.

[13] L. M. Butler, P. K. Mills, R. C. Yang, and M. S. Chen Jr., "Hepatitis B knowledge and vaccination levels in California Hmong youth: implications for liver cancer prevention strategies," *Asian Pacific Journal of Cancer Prevention*, vol. 6, no. 3, pp. 401–403, 2005.

[14] R. E. Vryheid, "A survey of vaccinations of immigrants and refugees in San Diego County, California," *Asian American and Pacific Islander journal of health*, vol. 9, no. 2, pp. 221–230, 2001.

[15] A. J. Khan, E. P. Simard, W. A. Bower et al., "Ongoing transmission of hepatitis B virus infection among inmates at a state correctional facility," *The American Journal of Public Health*, vol. 95, no. 10, pp. 1793–1799, 2005.

[16] Y.-L. Cao, S.-X. Wang, and Z.-M. Zhu, "Hepatitis B viral infection in maintenance hemodialysis patients: a three year follow-up," *World Journal of Gastroenterology*, vol. 13, no. 45, pp. 6037–6040, 2007.

[17] F. Fabrizi, S. Bunnapradist, and P. Martin, "HBV infection in patients with end-stage renal disease," *Seminars in Liver Disease*, vol. 24, supplement 1, pp. 63–70, 2004.

[18] "Recommendations for preventing transmission of infections among chronic hemodialysis patients," *MMWR: Morbidity and Mortality Weekly Report*, vol. 50, no. 5, pp. 1–43, 2001.

[19] L. Finelli, J. T. Miller, J. I. Tokars, M. J. Alter, and M. J. Arduino, "National surveillance of dialysis-associated diseases in the United States, 2002," *Seminars in Dialysis*, vol. 18, no. 1, pp. 52–61, 2005.

[20] S. S. Bull, C. Rietmeijer, J. D. Fortenberry et al., "Practice patterns for the elicitation of sexual history, education, and counseling among providers of STD services: results from the gonorrhea community action project (GCAP)," *Sexually Transmitted Diseases*, vol. 26, no. 10, pp. 584–589, 1999.

[21] N. Masters, A. Livingstone, and V. Cencora, "Hepatitis B: prevention in primary care," *British Medical Journal*, vol. 298, no. 6678, p. 908, 1989.

[22] B. Maheux, N. Haley, M. Rivard, and A. Gervais, "STD risk assessment and risk-reduction counseling by recently trained family physicians," *Academic Medicine*, vol. 70, no. 8, pp. 726–728, 1995.

[23] http://www.healthypeople.gov/2020/topicsobjectives2020/default.aspx.

[24] S. T. Goldstein, M. J. Alter, I. T. Williams et al., "Incidence and risk factors for acute hepatitis B in the United States, 1982–1998: Implications for vaccination programs," *Journal of Infectious Diseases*, vol. 185, no. 6, pp. 713–719, 2002.

Tryptophan-Kynurenine Metabolism and Insulin Resistance in Hepatitis C Patients

G. F. Oxenkrug,[1] W. A. Turski,[2] W. Zgrajka,[3] J. V. Weinstock,[4] and P. Summergrad[1]

[1] Psychiatry and Inflammation Program, Department of Psychiatry, Tufts Medical Center, Tufts University, Boston, MA 02111, USA
[2] Department of Experimental and Clinical Pharmacology, Medical University, 20-090 Lublin, Poland
[3] Department of Toxicology, Institute of Rural Health, 20-090 Lublin, Poland
[4] Division of Gastroenterology/Hepatology, Tufts Medical Center, Tufts University, Boston, MA 02111, USA

Correspondence should be addressed to G. F. Oxenkrug; goxenkrug@tuftsmedicalcenter.org

Academic Editor: Alessandro Antonelli

Chronic hepatitis C virus (HCV) infection is associated with 50% incidence of insulin resistance (IR) that is fourfold higher than that in non-HCV population. IR impairs the outcome of antiviral treatment. The molecular mechanisms of IR in HCV are not entirely clear. Experimental and clinical data suggested that hepatitis C virus per se is diabetogenic. However, presence of HCV alone does not affect IR. It was proposed that IR is mediated by proinflammatory cytokines, mainly by TNF-alpha. TNF-alpha potentiates interferon-gamma-induced transcriptional activation of indoleamine 2,3-dioxygenase, the rate-limiting enzyme of tryptophan- (TRP-) kynurenine (KYN) metabolism. Upregulation of TRP-KYN metabolism was reported in HCV patients. KYN and some of its derivatives affect insulin signaling pathways. We hypothesized that upregulation of TRP-KYN metabolism might contribute to the development of IR in HCV. To check this suggestion, we evaluated serum concentrations of TRP and KYN and HOMA-IR and HOMA-beta in 60 chronic HCV patients considered for the treatment with IFN-alpha. KYN and TRP concentrations correlated with HOMA-IR and HOMA-beta scores. Our data suggest the involvement of KYN and its metabolites in the development of IR in HCV patients. TRP-KYN metabolism might be a new target for prevention and treatment of IR in HCV patients.

1. Introduction

Hepatitis C patients have fourfold higher incidence of insulin resistance (IR) than non-HCV population, that is, healthy controls or chronic hepatitis B patients [1]. IR is the major feature of the metabolic syndrome (diabetes type 2, obesity, hypertension, and cardiovascular disorders). HCV-associated IR may lead to resistance to antiviral therapy, hepatocarcinogenesis, and extrahepatic complications [2, 3].

The molecular mechanisms whereby HCV infection leads to IR are not entirely clear. Experimental and clinical findings indicated that hepatitis C virus per se is diabetogenic [4, 5]. However, presence of HCV alone does not affect IR [6]. It was suggested that increased production of proinflammatory cytokines, especially TNF-alpha, contributes to the development of IR in HCV patients [7]. TNF-alpha potentiates interferon-gamma- (IFNG-) triggered transcriptional induction of indoleamine 2,3-dioxygenase (IDO), the rate-limiting enzyme of tryptophan- (TRP-) kynurenine (KYN)

metabolism [8]. Upregulated IDO expression in the dendritic cells [9] and in the liver [10] and increased serum KYN : TRP ratio (KTR) [10] were reported for HCV patients. Review of clinical and experimental data suggested that KYN and some of its derivatives affect biosynthesis, release, and activity of insulin [11]. We suggested that upregulated TRP-KYN metabolism might be one of the mechanisms of IR in HCV patients [12]. To check this suggestion, we evaluated serum TRP and KYN concentrations and IR and pancreatic beta-cell function in HCV patients.

2. Methods

Participants were recruited from HCV patients considered for starting a treatment with pegylated interferon-alpha and ribavirin. The study was approved by Tufts Medical Center IRB, and written consents were obtained for participation in the study. Blood samples were collected after 12 hrs of fasting.

TABLE 1: Kynurenines and insulin resistance in intent-to-treatment HCV patients.

$N = 60$	HOMA2-IR 1.3 (0.4–3.4)[*]	HOMA-beta 153 (57–395)[*]	KYN 1030 (480–3100)[**]	TRP 13550 (7000–27000)[**]	KTR 7.5 (3.2–14.2)[*]	KYNA 10 (4.3–36)
HOMA2-IR		$r = 0.81$ $P < 0.0001$	$r = 0.32$ $P = 0.01$	$r = 0.31$ $P = 0.01$	Not significant	Not significant
HOMA-beta	$r = 0.81$ $P < 0.0001$		$r = 0.3$ $P = 0.02$	$r = 0.35$ $P = 0.01$	Not significant	Not significant
KYN	$r = 0.32$ $P = 0.01$	$r = 0.30$ $P = 0.02$		$r = 0.42$ $P < 0.0003$	$r = 0.62$ $P < 0.0001$	$r = 0.47$ $P = 0.0001$
TRP	$r = 0.31$ $P = 0.01$	$r = 0.35$ $P = 0.01$	$r = 0.42$ $P < 0.0003$		$r = -0.30$ $P = 0.005$	Not significant
KTR	Not significant	Not significant	$r = 0.62$ $P < 0.0001$	$r = -0.30$ $P = 0.005$		Not significant
KYNA	Not significant	Not significant	$r = 0.47$ $P = 0.0001$	Not significant	Not significant	

[*] Median (50th percentile) (minimum-maximum).
[**] pmol/mL (50th percentile) (minimum-maximum).

2.1. Assessment of IDO Activity. IDO activation results in decrease of TRP and increase of KYN and, therefore, in elevation of KTR that is used as a marker of IDO activity in clinical studies [13]. However, there are some peculiarities related to the use of KTR as a marker of IDO activity in HCV patients. Increased KTR was reported in HCV patients but without data on serum TRP and KYN levels [10]. On the other hand, the decreased concentrations of both TRP and KYN in serum and macrophages and, consequently, decreased KTR were observed in HCV [14]. In the largest, so far, study, concentrations of KYN in 176 patients were significantly higher those than in healthy controls, whereas the levels of TRP were comparable in the two groups. Authors suggested that in HCV patients serum KYN level can be used as a marker of IDO activity [9].

Serum TRP, KYN, and kynurenic acid (KYNA) concentrations were evaluated by HPLC-UV-fluorimetric method [15].

2.2. Assessment of IR. IR was assessed by homeostatic model assessment index, version 2 (HOMA2-IR), and pancreatic beta-cell function by HOMA-beta index, based on fasting glucose and insulin levels, using the computer-based solution of the model provided by the Diabetes Trials Unit, Oxford Center for Diabetes, Endocrinology, and Metabolism (http://www.dtu.ox.ac.uk/index.php?maindoc=/homa/history.php) [16]. Serum glucose was measured using an enzymatic, kinetic reaction on the Olympus AU400e with Olympus Glucose Reagents (OSCR6121) (Olympus America Inc., Melville, NY, USA). Serum insulin is measured using the Immulite 1000 Insulin Kit (LKIN1) on the Immulite 1000 (Siemens Medical Solutions Diagnostics, Los Angeles, CA, USA).

2.3. Statistical Treatment. Quantitative data are presented using median (50th percentile) and minimum-maximum range. Nonparametric tests (Wilcoxon and Mann-Whitney U) were used to assess correlations for nonnormally distributed data.

3. Results

There were 42 male and 18 female American Caucasian HCV patients, 52.2 ± 7.45 years of age. Forty-eight patients had HCV genotype 1 or 4, and twelve patients had HCV genotype 2 or 3. None of the patients have been diagnosed with diabetes mellitus. 20 out of 60 patients had HOMA2-IR >2.

Serum KYN concentrations correlated with scores of HOMA2-IR and HOMA-beta (Table 1). TRP (KYN precursor) but not KYNA (immediate metabolite of KYN) [17, 18] correlated with HOMA2-IR and HOMA-beta. HOMA2-IR strongly correlated with HOMA-beta scores (Table 1). There was no correlation between serum KTR and both of the HOMA indexes. Serum KYNA concentrations correlated with KYN but not with TRP concentrations (Table 1).

4. Discussion

The major findings of the present study are the correlations between serum concentration of KYN and scores of HOMA2-IR and HOMA-beta in HCV patients. As far as we are aware, this is the first observation of such a correlation. Considering that serum KYN concentrations used an index of IDO activity in HCV patients [9], our data suggested a possible involvement of upregulated of TRP-KYN metabolism in the development of IR in HCV patients.

We did not find correlation between IR indexes and KTR, a marker of IDO activity in clinical studies [13]. As it was indicated earlier (see Section 2), in HCV patients, serum KYN concentrations might be considered as an index of IDO activity [9].

Present finding of correlation between serum KYN and TRP with both HOMA-2-IR and HOMA-beta is in line with the reported induction of IR by surplus dietary TRP in pigs [19] and with recent observation of increased serum KYN in diabetes retinopathy patients [20].

Association between elevated KYN and TRP concentrations and IR might be a result or a cause of IR. It was considered that TRP-KYN metabolism might contribute to mechanisms of diabetes [11]. Recent review of clinical and

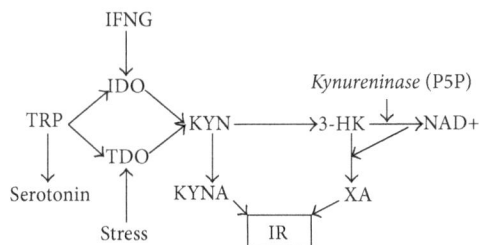

FIGURE 1: Kynurenic pathway of tryptophan metabolism and insulin resistance. Abbreviations: TRP: tryptophan; IFNG: interferon gamma; IDO: indoleamine 2,3-dioxygenase; TDO: TRP 2,3-dioxygenase; KYN: kynurenine; 3-HK: 3-hydroxyKYN; P5P: pyridoxal 5′-phosphate; NAD+: nicotinamide adenine dinucleotide; KYNA: kynurenic acid; XA: xanthurenic acid; IR: insulin resistance.

experimental data suggested the involvement of KYN pathway of TRP metabolism in the development of IR since KYN and some of its derivatives affect biosynthesis, release, and activity of insulin [12].

Diabetogenic effect of KYN and its derivatives, XA, 3-HK, and KYNA, (Figure 1) may be mediated by inhibition of pro-insulin synthesis in isolated rat pancreatic islets [21] and of insulin release from rat pancreas [22]. However, the effective concentrations (millimolar) of KYNA were much higher than its concentrations (micromolar) in pig's pancreatic juice [23]. The most plausible candidate for mediation of diabetogenic effect of upregulated TRY-KYN metabolism is XA. Increased urine excretion of XA was reported in type 2 diabetes patients in comparison with healthy subjects [24], while XA induced experimental diabetes in rats [25]. XA might contribute to the development of diabetes via formation of chelate complexes with insulin (XA-In) [26, 27] and induction of pathological apoptosis of pancreatic beta cells through caspase-3-dependent mechanism [28, 29]. Formation of XA from 3-HK depends on the vitamin B6 since its active metabolite, pyridoxal 5′-phosphate (P5P), is a cofactor of kynureninase, the enzyme, catalyzing 3-HK metabolism to NAD+ (Figure 1). P5P deficiency shifts 3-HK metabolism from formation of NAD+ to production of XA [30]. It is noteworthy that HCV infection is associated with significantly lowered P5P [31].

Evaluation of XA should be included in future studies of the role of TRP-KYN metabolism in mechanisms of HCV-associated IR.

Mechanisms of IR in HCV might be different from those in non-HCV patients. Thus, we observed in agreement with previous finding that a positive correlation between HOMA-IR and HOMA-beta was reported in HCV patients [32], in comparison with negative correlation between HOAM-2IR and HOMA-beta in non-HCV patients [16]. In the present study, a strong positive correlation between HOAM-2IR and HOMA-beta was observed as well (Table 1).

5. Conclusions

Our data of correlation between KYN and IR suggested the involvement of TRP-KYN metabolism in the development

of IR in HCV patients. Detection and treatment of HCV-associated IR are of importance considering that HCV-associated IR may lead to resistance to antiviral therapy, hepatocarcinogenesis, and extrahepatic manifestations, including an increased risk of cardiovascular disorders [33]. TRP-KYN metabolism might be a new target for prevention and treatment of IR in HCV patients.

Disclosure

P. Summergrad is a nonpromotional speaker for CME Outfitters, Inc., and consultant and nonpromotional speaker for PriMed, Inc.

Conflict of interests

All other authors declare no conflict of interests regarding this study.

Acknowledgments

The authors appreciate the excellent technical assistance of J. Curcuru. G. F. Oxenkrug is a recipient of NIMH099517 Grant.

References

[1] M. Romero-Gómez, "Insulin resistance and hepatitis C," *World Journal of Gastroenterology*, vol. 12, no. 44, pp. 7075–7080, 2006.

[2] R. Moucari, T. Asselah, D. Cazals-Hatem et al., "Insulin Resistance in chronic hepatitis C: association with genotypes 1 and 4, serum HCV RNA level, and liver fibrosis," *Gastroenterology*, vol. 134, no. 2, pp. 416–423, 2008.

[3] H. S. Conjeevaram, A. S. Wahed, N. Afdhal, C. D. Howell, J. E. Everhart, and J. H. Hoofnagle, "Changes in insulin sensitivity and body weight during and after peginterferon and ribavirin therapy for hepatitis C," *Gastroenterology*, vol. 140, no. 2, pp. 469–477, 2011.

[4] J. F. Huang, M. L. Yu, C. Y. Dai et al., "Glucose abnormalities in hepatitis C virus infection," *Kaohsiung Journal of Medical Sciences*, vol. 29, no. 2, pp. 61–68, 2013.

[5] A. Shlomai, M. Mouler, E. Rechtma et al., "The metabolic regulator PGC-1a links hepatitis C virus infection to hepatic insulin resistance," *Journal of Hepatology*, vol. 57, pp. 867–873, 2012.

[6] A. Lecube, C. Hernández, J. Genescà et al., "Proinflammatory cytokines, insulin resistance, and insulin secretion in chronic hepatitis C patients: a case-control study," *Diabetes Care*, vol. 29, no. 5, pp. 1096–1101, 2006.

[7] N. Tanaka, T. Nagaya, M. Komatsu et al., "Insulin resistance and hepatitis C virus: a case-control study of non-obese, non-alcoholic and non-steatotic hepatitis virus carriers with persistently normal serum aminotransferase," *Liver International*, vol. 28, no. 8, pp. 1104–1111, 2008.

[8] C. M. Robinson, P. T. Hale, and J. M. Carlin, "The role of IFN-γ and TNF-α-responsive regulatory elements in the synergistic induction of indoleamine dioxygenase," *Journal of Interferon and Cytokine Research*, vol. 25, no. 1, pp. 20–30, 2005.

[9] K. Higashitani, T. Kanto, S. Kuroda et al., "Association of enhanced activity of indoleamine 2, 3-dioxygenase in dendritic cells with the induction of regulatory T cells in chronic hepatitis C infection," *Journal of Gastroenterology*, vol. 48, no. 5, pp. 660–670, 2013.

[10] E. Larrea, J. I. Riezu-Boj, L. Gil-Guerrero et al., "Upregulation of indoleamine 2,3-dioxygenase in hepatitis C virus infection," *Journal of Virology*, vol. 81, no. 7, pp. 3662–3666, 2007.

[11] J. H. Connick and T. W. Stone, "The role of kynurenines in diabetes mellitus," *Medical Hypotheses*, vol. 18, no. 4, pp. 371–376, 1985.

[12] G. Oxenkrug, "Insulin resistance and dysregulation of tryptophan—kynurenine and kynurenine—nicotinamide adenine dinucleotide metabolic pathways," *Molecular Neurobiology*, 2013.

[13] K. Schroecksnadel, B. Frick, C. Winkler, and D. Fuchs, "Crucial role of interferon-γ and stimulated macrophages in cardiovascular disease," *Current Vascular Pharmacology*, vol. 4, no. 3, pp. 205–213, 2006.

[14] A. Cozzi, A. L. Zignego, R. Carpendo et al., "Low serum tryptophan levels, reduced macrophage IDO activity and high frequency of psychopathology in HCV patients," *Journal of Viral Hepatitis*, vol. 13, no. 6, pp. 402–408, 2006.

[15] W. A. Turski, M. Nakamura, W. P. Todd, B. K. Carpenter, W. O. Whetsell Jr., and R. Schwarcz, "Identification and quantification of kynurenic acid in human brain tissue," *Brain Research*, vol. 454, no. 1-2, pp. 164–169, 1988.

[16] T. M. Wallace, J. C. Levy, and D. R. Matthews, "Use and abuse of HOMA modeling," *Diabetes Care*, vol. 27, no. 6, pp. 1487–1495, 2004.

[17] R. . Schwarcz, J. P. Bruno, and P. J. Muchowski, "Kynurenines in the mammalian brain: when physiology meets pathology," *Nature Reviews Neuroscience*, vol. 13, no. 7, pp. 465–477, 2012.

[18] G. F. Oxenkrug, "Genetic and hormonal regulation of tryptophan—kynurenine metabolism implications for vascular cognitive impairment, major depressive disorder, and aging," *Annals of the New York Academy of Sciences*, vol. 1122, pp. 35–49, 2007.

[19] S. J. Koopmans, M. Ruis, R. Dekker, and M. Korte, "Surplus dietary tryptophan inhibits stress hormone kinetics and induces insulin resistance in pigs," *Physiology and Behavior*, vol. 98, no. 4, pp. 402–410, 2009.

[20] P. K. Munipally, S. G. Agraharm, V. K. Valavala, S. Gundae, and N. R. Turlapati, "Evaluation of indoleamine 2,3-dioxygenase expression and kynurenine pathway metabolites levels in serum samples of diabetic retinopathy patients," *Archives of Physiology and Biochemistry*, vol. 117, no. 5, pp. 254–258, 2011.

[21] Y. Noto and H. Okamoto, "Inhibition by kynurenine metabolites of proinsulin synthesis in isolated pancreatic islets," *Acta Diabetologica Latina*, vol. 15, no. 5-6, pp. 273–282, 1978.

[22] K. S. Rogers and S. J. Evangelista, "3-hydroxykynurenine, 3-hydroxyanthranilic acid, and o-aminophenol inhibit leucine-stimulated insulin release from rat pancreatic islets," *Proceedings of the Society for Experimental Biology and Medicine*, vol. 178, no. 2, pp. 275–278, 1985.

[23] D. Kuc, W. Zgrajka, J. Parada-Turska, T. Urbanik-Sypniewska, and W. A. Turski, "Micromolar concentration of kynurenic acid in rat small intestine," *Amino Acids*, vol. 35, no. 2, pp. 503–505, 2008.

[24] M. Hattori, Y. Kotake, and Y. Kotake, "Studies on the urinary excretion of xanthurenic acid in diabetics," *Acta Vitaminologica et Enzymologica*, vol. 6, no. 3, pp. 221–228, 1984.

[25] Y. Kotake, T. Ueda, and T. Mori, "Abnormal tryptophan metabolism and experimental diabetes by xanthurenic acid (XA)," *Acta Vitaminologica et Enzymologica*, vol. 29, no. 1-6, pp. 236–239, 1975.

[26] S. Ikeda and Y. Kotake, "Urinary excretion of xanthurenic acid and zinc in diabetes: (3) occurrence of xanthurenic acid-Zn2+ complex in urine of diabetic patients and of experimentally-diabetic rats," *Italian Journal of Biochemistry*, vol. 35, no. 4, pp. 232–241, 1986.

[27] G. Meyramov, V. Korchin, and N. Kocheryzkina, "Diabetogenic activity of xanturenic acid determined by its chelating properties," *Transplantation Proceedings*, vol. 30, no. 6, pp. 2682–2684, 1998.

[28] H. Z. Malina, C. Richter, M. Mehl, and O. M. Hess, "Pathological apoptosis by xanthurenic acid, a tryptophan metabolite: activation of cell caspases but not cytoskeleton breakdown," *BMC Physiology*, vol. 1, no. 1, pp. 7–11, 2001.

[29] Q. Wang, J. Chen, Y. Wang et al., "Hepatitis C virus induced a novel apoptosis like death of pancreatic beta cells through a caspase 3-dependent pathway," *PLoS ONE*, vol. 7, no. 6, Article ID e38522, 2012.

[30] D. A. Bender, E. N. M. Njagi, and P. S. Danielian, "Tryptophan metabolism in vitamin B6-deficient mice," *British Journal of Nutrition*, vol. 63, no. 1, pp. 27–36, 1990.

[31] C. C. Lin and M. C. Yin, "Vitamins B depletion, lower iron status and decreased antioxidative defense in patients with chronic hepatitis C treated by pegylated interferon alfa and ribavirin," *Clinical Nutrition*, vol. 28, no. 1, pp. 34–38, 2009.

[32] G. F. Helaly, N. G. Hussein, W. Refai, and M. Ibrahim, "Relation of serum insulin-like growth factor-1 (IGF-1) levels with hepatitis C virus infection and insulin resistance," *Translational Research*, vol. 158, no. 3, pp. 155–162, 2011.

[33] A. Trpkovic, E. Stokic, D. Radak, S. Mousa, D. P. Mikhailidis, and E. R. Isenovic, "Chronic hepatitis C, insulin resistance and vascular disease," *Current Pharmaceutical Design*, vol. 16, no. 34, pp. 3823–3829, 2010.

5

Evaluation of the Significance of Pretreatment Liver Biopsy and Baseline Mental Health Disorder Diagnosis on Hepatitis C Treatment Completion Rates at a Veterans Affairs Medical Center

Joseph Kluck,[1,2] Rose M. O'Flynn,[1] David E. Kaplan,[3,4] and Kyong-Mi Chang[3,4]

[1] Department of Pharmacy, Philadelphia Veterans Affairs Medical Center, 3900 Woodland Avenue, Philadelphia, PA 19104, USA
[2] Department of Pharmacy, Hospital of the University of Pennsylvania, 3400 Spruce Street, Philadelphia, PA 19104, USA
[3] Gastroenterology Section, Philadelphia Veterans Affairs Medical Center, 3900 Woodland Avenue, Philadelphia, PA 19104, USA
[4] Division of Gastroenterology, University of Pennsylvania Perelman School of Medicine, 421 Curie Boulevard, 9th Floor, Philadelphia, PA 19104, USA

Correspondence should be addressed to Joseph Kluck; joseph.kluck@uphs.upenn.edu

Academic Editor: Tatehiro Kagawa

Objectives. This study was performed to define the overall treatment response rates and treatment completion rates among the population of Hepatitis C infected patients at an urban VA Medical Center. Additionally, we examined whether pretreatment liver biopsy is a positive predictor for treatment completion and if the presence of mental health disorders is a negative predictor for treatment completion. *Methods.* Retrospective chart review was performed on the 375 patients that were treated for HCV and met the study inclusion parameters between January 1, 2003 and April 1, 2008 at our institution. Clinical data was obtained from the computerized patient record system and was analyzed for respective parameters. *Results.* Sustained virological response was achieved in 116 (31%) patients. 169 (45%) patients completed a full treatment course. Also, 44% of patients who received a pretreatment liver biopsy completed treatment versus 46% completion rates for patients who did not receive a pretreatment liver biopsy. Baseline ICD9 diagnosis of a mental health disorder was not associated with higher treatment discontinuation rates. *Conclusions.* In conclusion, pretreatment liver biopsy was not a positive predictor for treatment completion, and the presence of mental health disorders was not a negative predictor for treatment completion.

1. Background

Hepatitis C virus (HCV) is a highly persistent, hepatotropic RNA virus that causes chronic necroinflammatory liver disease [1]. HCV seroprevalence is 2.2% in the world, 1.6% in the USA and as high as 15-16% in select Veterans Affairs Medical Centers (VAMC) [2–6]. Comorbid factors common among the US veteran population, such as advanced age, obesity, HIV coinfection, immunosuppression, and alcohol intake, are associated with accelerated liver disease and progression to cirrhosis in chronically HCV-infected patients [7–9]. HCV-associated cirrhosis (occurring in 20–30% of HCV-infected individuals) results in increased morbidity and mortality due to end stage liver failure and hepatocellular carcinoma (HCC) that may warrant liver transplantation [10–12].

Thus, the goal of HCV therapy is to clear HCV RNA in an effort to prevent or delay liver-related death and/or complications [7, 9].

The desired objective outcome of HCV-directed therapy is a sustained virologic response (SVR), which is defined as an undetectable HCV viral load (VL) 24 weeks after therapy completion and denotes a cure of the infection [7]. Several variables are known to predict the likelihood of SVR with pegylated interferon and ribavirin treatment. Other than HCV genotype, which has the strongest impact on SVR rates, favorable treatment response is associated with pretreatment HCV VL below 600,000 IU/mL, female gender, age less than 40 years old, race/ethnicity other than black/African American, body weight less than 75 kg, absence of insulin resistance, elevated ALT levels, and absence of bridging fibrosis or cirrhosis [7]. In the VA system, the characteristics associated with a favorable treatment response are underrepresented, as a high proportion of patients are males, greater than 50 years of age, of African American background, cirrhotic, have high HCV viral loads, and weigh more than 75 kg [13]. In addition, many HCV-infected patients in the VA system display other comorbidities that limit HCV treatment tolerability and efficacy, such as HIV coinfection, poorly controlled diabetes, morbid obesity, and psychiatric disorders including depression, posttraumatic stress disorder, and schizophrenia, or recent substance abuse [13–15]. Since these comorbidities are not well represented in most large randomized clinical trials for HCV therapy [16–20], it is difficult to extrapolate the findings in the published literature to the veteran population [13].

At the time of our study protocol development and throughout the evaluation period, the accepted standard treatment of HCV involved combination pegylated interferon plus ribavirin for a total of 24 weeks for HCV genotypes 2 and 3, or 48 weeks for HCV genotypes 1 and 4 [7, 21–23]. SVR has been shown to occur more often in patients that complete a full course of treatment compared to patients that discontinue treatment early [13, 22, 24].

The main goals of this study were to define the overall treatment response and treatment completion rates among our population of HCV-infected veterans at the Philadelphia VA Medical Center. Additionally, we examined how completion rates were influenced by psychological factors. Two different concepts were proposed for evaluating this domain. The first concept aimed to determine whether or not patients that began therapy within one year of receiving a liver biopsy would be more likely to complete treatment. The second focused on evaluating if the diagnosis of a mental health disorder at baseline affected HCV therapy completion rates.

We hypothesized that patients may be more likely to complete therapy if they undergo staging of liver disease by means of biopsy. Does having a biopsy, which is an invasive procedure, psychologically motivate patients to complete therapy [25]? A patient's willingness to undergo a liver biopsy may indicate that the patient is mentally prepared to initiate and complete the extensive treatment for HCV. One might also predict that patients who do not receive liver biopsy might be less aware of their disease severity and may be less likely to see treatment to completion.

HCV-drug therapy has been widely associated with causing psychiatric side effects, often leading to early discontinuation of treatment [13]. To determine if the presence of mental health disorders is a negative predictor for treatment completion, we assessed whether the number of mental health disorders at baseline affected rates of HCV therapy completion. We also evaluated the rates of therapy discontinuation, specifically due to psychiatric adverse effects, amongst patients with and without a mental health disorder.

2. Patients and Methods

2.1. Study Population. HCV-infected veterans who were initiated on pegylated interferon alpha- (PEG-IFN-) based therapy at the Philadelphia VAMC between January 1, 2003

and April 1, 2008 were retrospectively identified by using the pharmacy database and examined for baseline demographic, clinical, and HCV treatment information using the Computerized Patient Record System (CPRS). Given the evolving nature of HCV therapy, we excluded patients whose HCV treatment prescriptions were filled within the study period but had initiated treatment before January 1, 2003. We also excluded patients whose prescriptions were filled within the desired timeline but were documented as either having received fewer than four weeks of antiviral therapy, or having never initiated therapy. This study protocol was reviewed and approved by the Institutional Review Board at the Philadelphia Veterans Affairs Medical Center (VAMC).

If a patient received multiple courses of HCV treatment, information on the most recent course of therapy was collected since retreatment would only occur if the patient failed therapy due to intolerance or lack of efficacy.

2.2. Clinical Data Collection from CPRS. Baseline patient information included age, race, gender, weight, HCV genotype, liver transplantation status, hepatic fibrosis (by liver biopsy or Fibrosure, when available), and significant comorbid illnesses recorded at baseline before HCV therapy. Race was obtained by chart documentation based on patient self-report. Mental health disorder diagnoses and diabetes diagnosis were determined by ICD9 codes, progress notes, and/or pharmacy medication records. HIV status was determined by laboratory screening when available. Baseline laboratory data was recorded as the most recent value documented within 12 months prior to the first dose of interferon and ribavirin. Concomitant alcohol or substance abuse was documented based on progress notes.

Initial treatment regimen and on-treatment alterations were retrieved from pharmacy records and/or in progress notes. Stop dates for treatment were defined as 4 weeks after the last prescription fill date for interferon or ribavirin, unless specifically stated otherwise in progress notes. The number of treatment courses was determined using pharmacy records, unless the number of treatment courses was specifically mentioned in progress notes since some patients may have previously been treated outside of the VA system. Completion rates were determined by the occurrence of treatment ending earlier than the specified treatment length, as determined by individual viral genotype and by provider comments in progress notes. Reasons for early termination of treatment were recorded if specifically stated in progress notes.

2.3. Definition of HCV Treatment Responses. HCV treatment responses were based on Roche Cobas Amplicor Taqman HCV RNA assay used in the clinical laboratory. The starting date of treatment was used as a marker to assess the monitoring of viral load for rapid virological response (RVR), early virological response (EVR), end-of-treatment response (ETR), and sustained virological response (SVR) per the definition of HCV diagnosis, management, and treatment guidelines [7]. Treatment failure was defined as less than a 2 log decrease in HCV RNA at week 12 or if HCV RNA was greater than 0 at week 24 [7].

Laboratory data, pharmacy records, and progress notes were used to retrieve data for adverse effects. Anemia, neutropenia, and thrombocytopenia occurring during the studied course of treatment were recorded. Pharmacy records were used to determine if growth factors such as erythropoietin or filgrastim were utilized to treat respective adverse effects.

3. Results

3.1. Patient Selection and Characteristics. Between January 1, 2003 and April 1, 2008 at the PVAMC, a total of 463 patients were identified as receiving prescriptions for pegylated-interferon and ribavirin. Eighty-eight of the 463 subjects were excluded for the following reasons: 24 (27.3%) initiated therapy before January 2003; 36 (40.9%) filled their first prescription but reported never initiating therapy; 16 (18.2%) stopped therapy within 4 weeks due to adverse effects; 12 (13.6%) filled the first prescription but had fewer than 4 weeks of followup documented. Thus, a total of 375 HCV-treated patients were included in the study.

3.2. Baseline Results. Among the 375 total subjects, 98% were male, 51% were of black racial background, and 80% had genotype 1 or 4 infections (Table 1). Median age among included subjects was 53 years (range 27–77). Median BMI was 29.2 kg/m^2 (95% CI 18.7–59.5) where 37% of patients were overweight, 40% of patients were obese, and 4% of patients were morbidly obese. Median pretreatment HCV viral titers were 1,350,000 IU/mL (range 344–25,400,000). Diabetes was common in the cohort, affecting 97 (26%) patients. HIV coinfection was present in 35 (9%) while 87 (23%) did not have a documented HIV assessment. A total of 252 (67%) patients received only one course of HCV treatment, as compared to 33% of patients who received two or more courses of therapy. Concomitant substance abuse was reported by 11 (3%) patients while 30 (8%) patients reported use of alcohol during treatment.

Mental health disorders were common, with 224 (59.7%) patients having at least one mental health disorder (Table 2). Subjects were found to commonly have multiple mental health disorders with depressive disorders, posttraumatic stress disorders, and anxiety disorders, most frequently represented.

3.3. Sustained Virological Response (SVR) Relative to HCV Genotype, Ethnicity, and Treatment Completion. SVR was achieved in 116/375 (31%) patients. The remaining patients were either well-documented nonresponders (187 (50%)) or lacked documentation of response (72 (19%)). As expected, SVR rate was lower for patients infected with genotypes 1 and 4 than genotypes 2 and 3 (23% versus 59%, $P < 0.0001$). However, SVR rates did not differ significantly by ethnicities in patients with HCV genotypes 1 and 4 (21.1% white versus 23.6% black, $P = 0.7580$) or HCV genotypes 2 and 3 (66.7% white versus 37.5% black, $P = 0.2317$). Overall, 169 (45%) patients completed a full treatment course, respective for specific HCV genotype. Median duration of therapy among genotypes 1 and 4 was 48.3 weeks for patients that achieved

Table 1: Baseline characteristics.

Variables	Cohort ($n = 375$)
Gender	
Male, n (%)	367 (98%)
Female, n (%)	8 (2%)
Race/ethnicity	
Black, n (%)	192 (52%)
White, n (%)	141 (38%)
Unknown, n (%)	22 (6%)
Other, n (%)	20 (5%)
Genotype	
1 and 4, n (%)	301 (80%)
2 and 3, n (%)	58 (15%)
Not documented, n (%)	12 (3%)
Mixed, n (%)	4 (1%)
Age (years), median (range)	53 (27–77)
BMI (kg/m^2)	29.2 (18.7–59.5)
Obese (BMI 30 to 39.9), n (%)	149 (40%)
Overweight (BMI 25 to 29.9), n (%)	137 (37%)
Morbidly obese (BMI $\geq$ 40), n (%)	15 (4%)
HCV VL RNA (IU/mL), median (range)	1,350,000 (344–25,400,000)
Diabetes diagnosis, n (%)	97 (26%)
HIV diagnosis	
No, n (%)	253 (68%)
Not assessed or not documented, n (%)	87 (23%)
Yes, n (%)	35 (9%)
Course of therapy	
1st, n (%)	252 (67%)
2nd, n (%)	92 (25%)
3rd or more, n (%)	31 (8%)
Concomitant substance abuse, n (%)	11 (3%)
Concomitant alcohol use, n (%)	30 (8%)
Alb (g/dL), median (range)	4.2 (2.7–5.3)
Hgb (g/dL), median (range)	14.6 (9.8–18.2)
INR, median (range)	1.0 (0.86–1.78)
PLT (THO/uL), median (range)	197.5 (42–439)
SCr (mg/dL), median (range)	1.0 (0.6–3.5)
Tbili (mg/dL), median (range)	0.8 (0.1–2.9)
WBC (THO/uL), median (range)	6.2 (2.2–14.9)

SVR and 30.1 weeks for patients that did not respond to therapy. Median duration of therapy among genotypes 2 and 3 was 24.7 weeks for patients that achieved SVR and 20.7 weeks for patients that did not achieve SVR.

3.4. Is Pretreatment Liver Biopsy a Positive Predictor of Treatment Completion? Eighty-five (23%) patients received a liver biopsy within one year of starting HCV treatment. Of these 85 patients, 37 (44%) completed the full course of therapy. Of the 290 included patients that did not receive a liver

TABLE 2: Frequency of specific mental health disorder.

Mental health disorder, ICD-9 diagnosis	Frequency, n	%
Depressive disorder	125	42
Posttraumatic stress disorder	90	30
Anxiety disorder (not specified)/panic disorder/social phobia/obsessive compulsive disorder	37	12
Schizophrenia/psychosis/thought disorder	24	8
Bipolar disorder	13	4
Mood disorder (not specified)	7	2
Cognitive disorder/organic brain disorder	4	1
Personality disorder	4	1

TABLE 3: Summary of completion rate by the number of mental health disorders.

Mental health disorder at baseline	n (%), patients completed HCV treatment course[**]
0	62/151 (41%)
1	70/152 (46%)
2 or more	37/72 (51%)

[**]Chi-square analysis shows that no statistical difference was found for completion rates across these strata ($P = 0.33$).

biopsy within one year of starting HCV treatment, 132 (46%) completed therapy (χ^2, $P = 0.81$). Therefore, there was no statistical difference found regarding treatment completion rates in patients who received a biopsy when compared to patients who did not receive a biopsy prior to initiation of treatment.

3.5. Does Having a Mental Health Disorder Affect Completion of Antiviral Therapy? Early discontinuation of HCV therapy was common with more than half of the patients (206/375 (55%)) stopping therapy prior to completion of the full course. The most common reasons for early discontinuation were (1) medication-related side effects (46%), (2) virological failure (32%), and (3) loss to followup (15%). To determine the impact of mental health disorders on completion rates, we assessed treatment completion rates across three groups: patients without a mental health disorder at baseline, patients with one mental health disorder at baseline, and patients with two or more mental health disorders at baseline (Table 3). No statistical difference was found for completion rates for these groups ($P = 0.33$).

Additionally, we assessed early termination of treatment rates involving psychiatric related adverse drug effects. Of the 94 patients that stopped treatment early due to any medication related side effects, 59 (63%) had at least one documented mental health disorder prior to the start of HCV treatment, whereas 35 (37%) had no history of a mental health diagnosis. Twenty-four (41%) of these 59 patients stopped treatment early specifically due to psychiatric related adverse drug effects, compared with 10 of these 35 (29%) who did not have a mental health disorder at the start of HCV treatment ($P = 0.27$). Thus, the baseline diagnosis of a mental health disorder was not associated with higher treatment discontinuation rates in our patients.

4. Discussion

Our results indicate that there is no difference in rates of completion when considering biopsy status within one year of starting HCV treatment. While biopsy status had no impact on treatment completion rates, it is likely that biopsy status correlated with treatment uptake as the biopsy rate of this

cohort (23%) was significantly greater than the rate of liver biopsy in the untreated chronic hepatitis C population at our center (3.8%). We did not collect provider level information in this analysis, but it is also highly likely that provider practice style might strongly influence patient persistence during therapy.

In theory, patients with mental health disorders, at baseline, would seem less likely to tolerate and complete a full course of HCV treatment, as they may be more sensitive to the psychiatric adverse effect profile of interferon-alpha. To assess the impact of a mental health disorder at baseline on HCV therapy completion rates, we assessed whether the number of mental health disorders at baseline affected rates of HCV therapy completion and rates of therapy discontinuation related to psychiatric adverse effects for patients with relative to those without mental health disorders. Pegylated interferon and ribavirin can cause symptoms of anxiety and depression at an incidence of 20–30% [26–28]. Some studies have shown that almost 50% of patients undergoing antiviral treatment can experience symptoms of anxiety, depression, or irritability [29]. Additional studies have shown that interferon induced depression significantly contributes to early discontinuation of treatment and subsequently lower incidence of SVR [30–32]. Interestingly, our study showed that the rates of HCV therapy discontinuation due to psychiatric-related adverse drug effects were similar between patients with a mental health disorder at baseline and with no mental health disorder at baseline.

Since complete information on patients lost to follow-up was not available, it is possible that psychiatric adverse effects contributed to these discontinuations. Therefore, we determined that it was necessary to evaluate overall completion rates for patients with mental health disorders at baseline. We also intended to determine if there was any difference in completion rates among patients with different numbers of mental health diagnoses at baseline. Liu et al. evaluated a random sample of patients treated in the HCV clinic and noted that patients with a diagnosis of depression at baseline had lower rates of completion than patients without preexisting depression [33]. Previous studies have also shown that patients with schizophrenia have similar completion rates as patients without schizophrenia [34]. Our study revealed that patients with one or more mental health disorders at baseline had similar rates of completion when compared to patients without any diagnosed mental health disorder.

Our study found that discontinuation of treatment due to psychiatric related adverse drug effects was similar among all patients, regardless of mental health disorder diagnosis at baseline. Additionally, patients with any number of mental health disorders at baseline have similar rates of completion as patients without a mental health disorder. With this being said, it is difficult to ignore the role that mental health plays with HCV treatment. Mental health disorders should not necessarily be seen as a barrier to HCV treatment. It may be more important for all patients, regardless of psychiatric history, to have close monitoring and individualization of their care, as supported by a recent study and treatment guidelines [7, 35].

Several quality improvement measures were identified for our HCV clinic, as a result of this evaluation. This study did indicate that it is necessary to standardize the monitoring and followup of HCV-treated patients at our institution, so that 100% of patients are consistently assessed for adverse drug effects, HIV-status, reason for early discontinuation of treatment, and viral load at appropriate time points.

There were several potential limitations of our study. Our study contained many variables over a large span in time. Specific changes in HCV therapy identified between the study dates included adherence to checking viral load, aggressiveness in management of adverse effects, practice styles, treatment guidelines, and the actual viral assay. In addition, data was not collected regarding patients' mental health stability or use of psychiatric medications at baseline. This potential for bias was known prior to preparation of the study, as this was a retrospective analysis. Some data was self-reported by patients, such as concomitant alcohol and substance abuse during the treatment course, and this information is potentially biased to underreporting. Another limitation was also attributed to the study design. Incomplete data was occasionally observed, due to lack of documentation and patients lost to follow-up.

In conclusion, in this retrospective analysis, liver biopsy within one year of starting HCV therapy was not associated with increased rates of therapy completion. Similar completion rates were found between patients without a mental health disorder at baseline, with one mental health disorder prior to treatment, and with two or more mental health disorders at baseline. Treatment discontinuation due to psychiatric-related adverse drug effects was found to be similar among patients, regardless of psychiatric history.

Abbreviations

BMI: Body mass index
CPRS: Computerized patient record system
ETR: End of treatment response
EVR: Early virologic response
HCC: Hepatocellular carcinoma
HCV: Hepatitis C virus
HIV: Human immunodeficiency virus
PEG-INF: Pegylated interferon
RVR: Rapid virologic response
SVR: Sustained virologic response
VA: Veterans affairs
VAMC: Veterans Affairs Medical Center
VL: Viral load.

Disclaimer

The content of this article does not reflect the views of the VA or of the US Government.

References

[1] R. Williams, "Global challenges in liver disease," *Hepatology*, vol. 44, no. 3, pp. 521–526, 2006.

[2] M. J. Alter, "Epidemiology of hepatitis C virus infection," *World Journal of Gastroenterology*, vol. 13, no. 17, pp. 2436–2441, 2007.

[3] G. L. Armstrong, A. Wasley, E. P. Simard, G. M. McQuillan, W. L. Kuhnert, and M. J. Alter, "The prevalence of hepatitis C virus infection in the United States, 1999 through 2002," *Annals of Internal Medicine*, vol. 144, no. 10, pp. 705–714, 2006.

[4] R. C. Cheung, "Epidemiology of hepatitis C virus infection in American Veterans," *American Journal of Gastroenterology*, vol. 95, no. 3, pp. 740–747, 2000.

[5] J. A. Dominitz, E. J. Boyko, T. D. Koepsell, P. J. Heagerty, C. Maynard, and J. L. Sporleder, "Elevated prevalence of hepatitis C infection in users of United States veterans medical centers," *Hepatology*, vol. 41, no. 1, pp. 88–96, 2005.

[6] K. L. Sloan, K. A. Straits-Tröster, J. A. Dominitz, and D. R. Kivlahan, "Hepatitis C Tested Prevalence and Comorbidities among Veterans in the US Northwest," *Journal of Clinical Gastroenterology*, vol. 38, no. 3, pp. 279–284, 2004.

[7] M. G. Ghany, D. B. Strader, D. L. Thomas, and L. B. Seeff, "Diagnosis, management, and treatment of hepatitis C: an update," *Hepatology*, vol. 49, no. 4, pp. 1335–1374, 2009.

[8] M. G. Ghany, D. R. Nelson, D. B. Strader, D. L. Thomas, and L. B. Seeff, "An update on treatment of genotype 1 chronic hepatitis C virus infection: 2011 practice guideline by the American Association for the Study of Liver Diseases," *Hepatology*, vol. 54, no. 4, pp. 1433–1444, 2011.

[9] G. M. Lauer and B. D. Walker, "Hepatitis C virus infection," *The New England Journal of Medicine*, vol. 345, no. 1, pp. 41–52, 2001.

[10] G. Fattovich, G. Giustina, F. Degos et al., "Morbidity and mortality in compensated cirrhosis type C: a retrospective follow-up study of 384 patients," *Gastroenterology*, vol. 112, no. 2, pp. 463–472, 1997.

[11] T. Poynard, P. Bedossa, and P. Opolon, "Natural history of liver fibrosis progression in patients with chronic hepatitis C," *The Lancet*, vol. 349, no. 9055, pp. 825–832, 1997.

[12] C. Global Burden of Hepatitis C Working Group, "Global burden of disease (GBD) for hepatitis C," *The Journal of Clinical Pharmacology*, vol. 44, no. 1, pp. 20–29, 2004.

[13] L. I. Backus, D. B. Boothroyd, B. R. Phillips, and L. A. Mole, "Predictors of response of U.S. veterans to treatment for the hepatitis C virus," *Hepatology*, vol. 46, no. 1, pp. 37–47, 2007.

[14] B. A. Piasecki, J. D. Lewis, K. R. Reddy et al., "Influence of alcohol use, race, and viral coinfections on spontaneous HCV clearance in a US veteran population," *Hepatology*, vol. 40, no. 4, pp. 892–899, 2004.

[15] H. S. Yee, S. L. Currie, J. M. Darling, and T. L. Wright, "Management and treatment of hepatitis C viral infection: recommendations from the Department of Veterans Affairs Hepatitis C Resource Center Program and the National Hepatitis C Program Office," *American Journal of Gastroenterology*, vol. 101, no. 10, pp. 2360–2378, 2006.

[16] G. L. Davis, R. Esteban-Mur, V. Rustgi et al., "Interferon alfa-2b alone or in combination with ribavirin for the treatment

of relapse of chronic hepatitis C," *The New England Journal of Medicine*, vol. 339, no. 21, pp. 1493–1499, 1998.

[17] E. J. Heathcote, M. L. Shiffman, W. G. E. Cooksley et al., "Peginterferon alfa-2a in patients with chronic hepatitis C and cirrhosis," *The New England Journal of Medicine*, vol. 343, no. 23, pp. 1673–1680, 2000.

[18] J. H. Hoofnagle and L. B. Seeff, "Peginterferon and ribavirin for chronic hepatitis C," *The New England Journal of Medicine*, vol. 355, no. 23, pp. 2444–2451, 2006.

[19] J. G. Mchutchison, S. C. Gordon, E. R. Schiff et al., "Interferon alfa-2b alone or in combination with ribavirin as initial treatment for chronic hepatitis C," *The New England Journal of Medicine*, vol. 339, no. 21, pp. 1485–1492, 1998.

[20] S. Zeuzem, S. V. Feinman, J. Rasenack et al., "Peginterferon alfa-2a in patients with chronic hepatitis C," *The New England Journal of Medicine*, vol. 343, no. 23, pp. 1666–1672, 2000.

[21] M. W. Fried, M. L. Shiffman, K. R. Reddy et al., "Peginterferon alfa-2a plus ribavirin for chronic hepatitis C virus infection," *The New England Journal of Medicine*, vol. 347, no. 13, pp. 975–982, 2002.

[22] S. J. Hadziyannis, H. Sette, T. R. Morgan et al., "Peginterferon-α2a and ribavirin combination therapy in chronic hepatitis C: a randomized study of treatment duration and ribavirin dose," *Annals of Internal Medicine*, vol. 140, no. 5, pp. 346–167, 2004.

[23] M. P. Manns, J. G. McHutchison, S. C. Gordon et al., "Peginterferon alfa-2b plus ribavirin compared with interferonalfa-2b plus ribavirin for initial treatment of chronic hepatitis C: a randomised trial," *The Lancet*, vol. 358, no. 9286, pp. 958–965, 2001.

[24] V. L. Re, V. K. Amorosa, A. R. Localio et al., "Adherence to hepatitis C virus therapy and early virologic outcomes," *Clinical Infectious Diseases*, vol. 48, no. 2, pp. 186–193, 2009.

[25] J. L. Dienstag, "The role of liver biopsy in chronic hepatitis C," *Hepatology*, vol. 36, no. 5, pp. S152–S160, 2002.

[26] "Pegasys package insert," September 2012, http://www.accessdata.fda.gov/drugsatfda_docs/label/2011/103964s5204lbl.pdf.

[27] "Peg-Intron package insert," September 2012, http://www.accessdata.fda.gov/drugsatfda_docs/label/2011/103949s5217s5222lbl.pdf.

[28] "Ribavirin package insert," September 2012, http://www.accessdata.fda.gov/drugsatfda_docs/label/2011/021511s023lbl.pdf.

[29] E. Dieperink, M. Willenbring, and S. B. Ho, "Neuropsychiatric symptoms associated with hepatitis C and interferon alpha: a review," *American Journal of Psychiatry*, vol. 157, no. 6, pp. 867–876, 2000.

[30] M. W. Fried, "Side effects of therapy of hepatitis C and their management," *Hepatology*, vol. 36, no. 5, pp. S237–S244, 2002.

[31] P. Hauser, "Neuropsychiatric side effects of HCV therapy and their treatment: focus on IFNα-induced depression," *Gastroenterology Clinics of North America*, vol. 33, no. 1, pp. S37–S50, 2004.

[32] C. L. Raison, S. D. Broadwell, A. S. Borisov et al., "Depressive symptoms and viral clearance in patients receiving interferon-α and ribavirin for hepatitis C," *Brain, Behavior, and Immunity*, vol. 19, no. 1, pp. 23–27, 2005.

[33] S. S. Liu, T. D. Schneekloth, J. A. Talwalkar et al., "Impact of depressive symptoms and their treatment on completing antiviral treatment in patients with chronic hepatitis C," *Journal of Clinical Gastroenterology*, vol. 44, no. 8, pp. e178–e185, 2010.

[34] M. Huckans, A. Mitchell, S. Ruimy, J. Loftis, and P. Hauser, "Antiviral therapy completion and response rates among hepatitis c patients with and without schizophrenia," *Schizophrenia Bulletin*, vol. 36, no. 1, pp. 165–172, 2010.

[35] B. T. Clark, G. Garcia-Tsao, and L. Fraenkel, "Patterns and predictors of treatment initiation and completion in patients with chronic hepatitis C virus infection," *Patient Preference and Adherence*, vol. 6, pp. 285–295, 2012.

6

Postinfantile Giant Cell Hepatitis: An Etiological and Prognostic Perspective

Chhagan Bihari,[1] **Archana Rastogi,**[1] **and Shiv Kumar Sarin**[2]

[1] *Department of Pathology, Institute of Liver and Biliary Sciences (ILBS), D-1 Vasant Kunj, New Delhi 110070, India*
[2] *Department of Hepatology, Institute of Liver and Biliary Sciences (ILBS), New Delhi 110070, India*

Correspondence should be addressed to Archana Rastogi; drarchanarastogi@gmail.com

Academic Editor: Tatehiro Kagawa

Giant cell hepatitis is common manifestation in pediatric liver diseases, but quite uncommon in adults, only about 100 cases reported in the English literature in the last two decades. Data for the present review were identified by a structured PubMed/MEDLINE search from 1963 to December 2012, using keywords postinfantile giant cell hepatitis (PIGCH), adult giant cell hepatitis, and syncytial giant cell hepatitis in adults and liver. We report a case of postinfantile giant cell hepatitis along with the review related to the etiology and respective outcome, as the literature in the last 20 years suggests. This condition is probably due to idiosyncratic or cytopathic response of individual to various hepatocytic stimuli. It is purely a histomorphological diagnosis and does not establish the etiology. Autoimmune liver diseases are most common etiology, in around 40% of cases, but various viruses, drugs, posttransplant condition, and other causes also have been reported. Prognosis depends upon the etiology. In this paper, we emphasized various causative factors of PIGCH and their respective outcome in patients affected by them. We also highlighted the possible pathogenesis and histopathological spectrum of this entity on the basis of description given in various studies and our limited experience of few cases.

1. Introduction

Giant cell hepatitis is a condition characterized by inflammation and large multinucleated hepatocytes in the hepatic parenchyma. Giant cell transformation of hepatocytes along with extramedullary hematopoiesis is a common response in the newborn liver diseases [1–4]. Postinfantile giant cell hepatitis is a rare disorder. It is an unusual regenerative or degenerative hepatocytes response to various noxious stimuli, characterized by the presence of multinucleated cells in liver with generally dismal clinical outcome [1–4]. We report a case of postinfantile hepatitis with review of the literature regarding various etiological agents and their respective prognostic outcome.

2. Methods

Postinfantile giant cell hepatitis (PIGCH) is defined as acute or chronic hepatitis in adults with extensive hepatocyte multinucleation. These cases can be heterogeneous in terms of their clinical, serological, and histological features [1, 3]. PIGCH is purely a histological diagnosis which is based on morphological criteria of conspicuous presence of giant cell hepatocytes; therefore, it is a descriptive term and does not speak about the etiology in any individual case [1]. Facts for the present paper were collected from the structured PUBMED/MEDLINE search from 1963 to 2012. The search was carried out by combining the keywords postinfantile giant cell hepatitis, adult giant cell hepatitis, and syncytial giant cell hepatitis in adults and liver. We have comprehensively categorized the prognostic outcome of various studies into poor, moderate, and good prognosis groups. In poor prognostic group, we have included the patients who had acute liver failure, acute decompensation on chronic liver disease, and death with due diagnosis of this entity. In moderate prognosis group we have put those patients who had rapid onset of cirrhosis following the diagnosis of PIGCH, and in good prognosis category, we have grouped

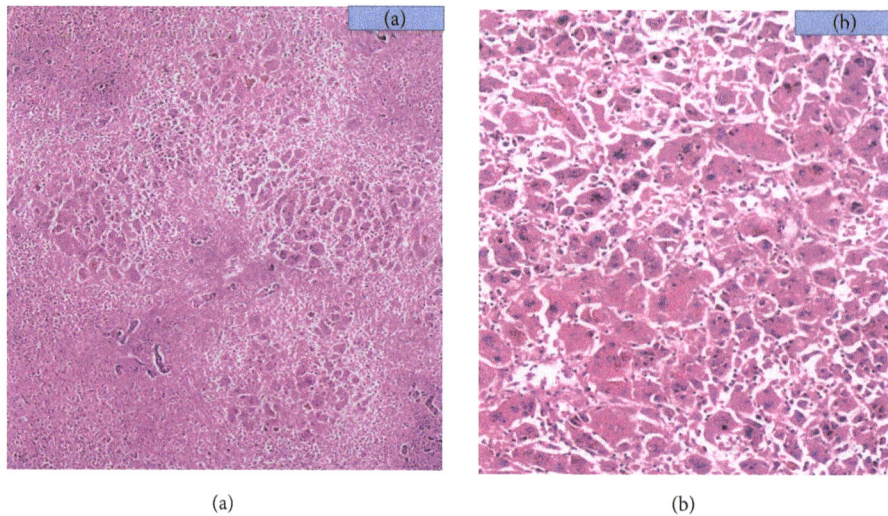

FIGURE 1: (a) H&E stained section (40x) of explant liver showing massive parenchymal loss and remaining hepatocytes with giant cell transformation. (b) H&E stained section (200x) showing giant cell transformation of hepatocytes.

those patients who had mild hepatitis. Here, we report a case of postinfantile giant cell hepatitis that had acute liver failure and undergone living donor related liver transplant.

3. Report

21-year-old male presented with complaints of fever, myalgia, and arthralgia of one-month duration. Fever was continuous high grade. Myalgia and arthralgia subsided within a week. He had progressive jaundice for 2-3 weeks. On examination, patient had deep icterus, fever, and enlarged liver of 3 cm below right costal margin, and it was tender on palpation. Contrast enhanced computed tomography (CECT) and magnetic resonance imaging (MRI) abdomen showed hepatomegaly, ascites, and bilateral pleural effusion. His serum was positive for anti-HAV IgM, and antinuclear antibody (ANA) titer was 1 : 80. Serum ceruloplasmin and 24-hour urinary copper were normal. His liver function test got worsened within 6 days of hospital course, and his total bilirubin raised from 4.5 to 19.17 mg/dL (normal value 0.2–1 mg/dL), aspartate aminotransferase (AST) raised from 830 to 1490 U/L (normal value 6–40 U/L), alanine aminotransferase (ALT) from 459 to 744 U/L (normal value 4–40 U/L), and international normalized ratio (INR) for prothrombin time raised from 1.5 to 6.2. His serum ammonia level reached 211 microgram/dl, and he developed hepatic encephalopathy. The clinical diagnosis was hepatitis A related acute liver failure. The patient was transplanted according to King's College criteria for acute liver failure, and explant liver on histopathological examination showed submassive necrosis with focal sparing of the portal areas. There was prominent giant cell transformation of viable hepatocytes (Figures 1(a) and 1(b)). Histopathological diagnosis was submassive hepatic necrosis with postinfantile giant cell hepatitis. Patient is on regular followup for 6 months and is doing well.

4. Discussion

PIGCH is very rare in adults (0.1%–0.25% of all hepatic diseases); approximately 100 cases have been reported so far [1–3, 28]. Age and gender do not show any significant preponderance in the series described by Johnson et al., Devaney et al., Phillips et al., Tordjmann et al., and by Micchelli et al. [1–3, 7, 29]. It has been reported from 5 to 80 years of age.

In our institute, total adult liver biopsies were done; only three had postinfantile giant cell hepatitis till date.

Various etiologies associated with postinfantile giant cell hepatitis are summarized in Table 1 and their respective prognosis in Table 2.

Medications which can cause PIGCH are methotrexate, 6-mercaptopurine, clometacine, amitriptyline, chlordiazepoxide, p-amino salicylic acid, vinyl chloride, chlorpromazine, herbal medicines, and amoxicillin + clavulanate and doxycycline. These drugs presumed to injure the hepatocytes and cause degenerating effect and formation of giant hepatocytes in certain individuals [1, 3, 5–9]. Most of the reported cases in the literature presented as mild hepatitis [1, 3, 5, 6] except in three; one died due to clometacine induced liver failure [7]; one was a known case of autoimmune hepatitis and was treated with amoxicillin + clavulanate for cellulitis of thigh and clinically deteriorated and required liver transplant [8]. Another case was treated with doxycycline for one week for bacterial bronchitis, and soon he developed acute liver failure and required liver transplant [9].

A variety of autoimmune disorders have been reported as potential cause of PIGCH. It has been reported in cases of autoimmune hepatitis (AIH), systemic lupus erythematosus, autoimmune hemolytic anemia rheumatoid arthritis, primary sclerosing cholangitis, polyarthritis, ulcerative colitis, polyarteritis nodosa, and primary biliary cirrhosis [1, 2, 5, 7, 10–23, 44].

TABLE 1: Various etiological agents of post infantile giant cell hepatitis.

Drugs and medication	Methotrexate, clometacin, 6-mercaptapurine, p-aminosalicylic acid, vinyl chloride, amitriptyline, chlordiazepoxide, and chlorpromazine and herbal medicine
Autoimmune diseases	Systemic lupus erythematosus, rheumatoid arthritis, polyarthritis, ulcerative colitis, autoimmune hemolytic anemia, primary sclerosing cholangitis, and autoimmune hepatitis (AIH), polyarteritis nodosa, and primary biliary cirrhosis
Viral causes	Hepatitis A, B, C, E Epstein-Barr virus (EBV), HIV, paramyxo-like virus. herpesvirus 6A infection, and human papillomavirus.
Miscellaneous	Hypereosinophilia, chronic lymphocytic leukaemia, lymphoma, sarcoidosis, Kugelberg-Welander syndrome, hypoparathyroidism, Sickle cell anaemia, and post transplant

In autoimmune diseases, autoimmune hepatitis (AIH) mainly type I with ANA (ANF) positivity is one of the major cause of PIGCH, accounting for 40% of all autoimmune related cases. The mechanism of giant cell formation in cases of autoimmune disorders is still unknown. Fusion of mononuclear hepatocytes or nuclear proliferation not followed by cell division represents the two prevailing pathogenetic hypotheses [31]. This may be due to autoimmune disease per se or due to both immune complexes, vascular pathology in autoimmune cases creating nutritional challenge to hepatocytes [19]. Clinical course varies from normalization of hepatic histology to progression to cirrhosis and liver failure. The prognosis is dictated by the underlying liver disease. Clinical course is usually severe with most of the patients progressing to rapid onset of cirrhosis [1, 2, 5, 7, 10–23, 31, 44].

Hepatitis A, B, C, E Epstein-Barr virus (EBV), HIV, Cytomegalovirus, and a potentially unidentified paramyxo-like virus have been found to be associated with entity. In a study, human herpes virus 6A infection in a liver transplant recipient was a cause of giant cell hepatitis [1–3, 7, 24–30, 32–34, 36, 37, 45, 46].

In HAV infection, PIGCH is a morphological reaction pattern due to the immunoreactivity of viral agents to the hepatocytes. Hepatitis A is an acute infectious disease caused by the hepatitis A virus (HAV), an RNA virus, usually spread by the fecal-oral route. In developing countries and in regions with poor hygiene standards, the incidence of infection with this virus is high. HAV infection produces a self-limited disease that does not result in chronic infection or chronic liver disease. Hepatitis A infection is diagnosed by Anti-HAV IgM antibody. Acute liver failure from Hepatitis A is rare < 0.5%. Hepatitis A infection is diagnosed by Anti-HAV IgM antibody [46]. Four cases of PIGCH were reported out of which one had coexistence of positive ANA.

All four had fatal course (acute liver failure) [1, 24–26]. The reported cases had Anti-HAV IgM positivity and ANA positivity had acute fulminant PIGCH, which required an orthotopic liver transplant. Three cases with HBV infection were reported; two had acute hepatitis, and another one had chronic hepatitis, and all three had favorable outcomes [2, 7].

In association to HCV infection, a largest study of 22 biopsies of 18 cases with PIGCH was done by Micchelli et al. Out of these 18 cases, 12 had coinfection with HIV. In addition, there were 2 cases of PIGCH; in HIV/HCV coinfection were also reported. In one patient, there was a progressive clinical worsening after three-month course of prednisone, leading to liver failure and death. His postmortem liver biopsy showed more abundant giant hepatocytes accompanied with the development of a histological pattern of severe fibrosing cholestatic hepatitis. The second patient received a prolonged course of pegylated interferon-alpha-2b and ribavirin with clearance of syncytial giant hepatocytes despite HCV-RNA persistence [30]. Histologically, giant cells were located in zone 3 hepatocytes, were persisted over time, and did not appear to be a marker of aggressive hepatitis [28, 29].

In three cases EBV was suggested a possible etiology of giant cell hepatitis resulting in fulminant hepatic failure [31–33].

Paramyxo viral infection including parainfluenza 1, 2, and 3, measles virus, respiratory syncytial virus and distemper virus has been increasingly linked to Postinfantile giant cell hepatitis. Evidence of paramyxo-like viral particles was first reported by Phillips et al. in a series of 10 patients. Five patients' required liver transplantation and the other five died. Other two cases of PIGCH out of which in one patient with CLL presented as an acute hepatitis which lead to cirrhosis in 18 months and other case lead to fulminant course. In these cases also, high-resolution electron micrographs revealed the existence of nucleocapsid-like particles forming aggregates in the cytoplasm of syncytial hepatocytes resembling paramyxo-like viral particles [26, 34, 35].

In one patient etiology of PIGCH was suggested as human herpes virus-6A (HHV-6A), who underwent liver transplant for Caroli's disease. He originally had latent infection of human herpes virus-6B (HHV-6B). He developed PICGH at the 13th day of liver transplant. He received organ from a donor with latent infection of human herpes virus-6A. Extensive serologic, molecular and immunohistochemical investigations were done to search for an infectious cause of giant-cell hepatitis. At the onset of the disease, the detection of HHV-6A specific early protein p41/38 in giant cells and later on follow-up samples of plasma, and affected liver tissue suggested that HHV-6A may be a cause of PIGCH. This patient improved clinically, serologically, and histomorphologically after 4 months of treatment [27]. A case of Wilson's disease reported by Welte et al. presented with acute liver failure with presence of syncytial hepatocytes in the liver biopsy. On investigation, this patient was found to be serologically positive for cytomegalovirus [37].

TABLE 2: Cases of post infantile Giant hepatitis with their prognostic outcome.

Etiology	Number of cases	Prognostic outcome	References
Drugs			
Methotrexate	2	Good (mild hepatitis)	[1, 5]
Chlorpromazine	1	Good (mild hepatitis)	[1]
ISABGOL	1	Good (mild hepatitis)	[6]
Clometacine	1	Poor (acute liver failure)	[7]
Amoxicillin and Clavulanate	1	Poor (chronic hepatitis with acute decompensation)	[8]
Doxycycline	1	Poor (acute liver failure) Treated for a week for bacterial bronchitis	[9]
Autoimmune			
AIH	5	1 (died) 4 Good (clinically improved)	[1]
	2	1 Moderate (rapid onset of cirrhosis died) 1 Moderate (rapid onset of cirrhosis)	[5]
	10	Moderate 25% (acute hepatitis), 42% moderate (chronic active hepatitis), 33% moderate to poor cirrhosis, >1-month duration	[2]
	13	4 Poor (liver failure) 5 Moderate (rapid cirrhosis) 4 Good (responded to immunosuppressants)	[7]
AIH	1	Moderate (rapid onset of cirrhosis)	[10]
	1	Good (responded to immunossupresion)	[11]
SLE	2	Moderate	[2, 12]
Autoimmune hemolytic anemia	3	Poor	[13–15]
PSC + AIH	2	Moderate (rapid onset of cirrhosis) Good (mild hepatitis)	[16, 17]
AIH + polyarthritis	1	Moderate (early cirrhosis)	[18]
AIH + polyarteritis	1	Moderate (early cirrhosis)	[19]
AIH + UC	1	Moderate (early cirrhosis)	[20]
PBC	2	1 Poor, (liver failure) 1 moderate (early cirrhosis)	[21, 22]
AIH II	1	Poor (died)	[23]
Viral			
HAV	4	Poor (fatal liver failure)	[1, 24–26]
HEV	1	Good (mild hepatitis)	[27]
HBV	3	Good (1 acute hepatitis, 2 chronic hepatitis)	[2, 7]
HCV	22	Good (chronic hepatitis)	[5, 28–30]
EBV	3	Poor (fatal liver failure)	[31–33]
Paramyxoviruses	13	Poor (7 fatal liver failure, 6 died)	[3, 26, 34, 35]
HIV + HCV	2	Good (chronic hepatitis)	[30]
HIV	2	Good (chronic hepatitis)	[36]
HHV-6A	1	Good (chronic hepatitis)	[27]
CMV	1	Poor (acute liver failure with underlying Wilson's diseases)	[37]
Hypereosinophilia	3	2 Poor (liver failure) 1 Good	[24, 32, 38]
CLL	3	2 Poor (liver failure) 1 Good (responded to immunosuppression)	[39]
Posttransplant	10	Poor (recurrent disease, mostly required retransplant)	[40–43]

Associations with three eosinophilia cases were reported. Two of them had fatal disease course [24, 38], and one had better outcome [32].

Concomitant malignancies have occasionally been described in patients with PIGCH [2]. Two patients with CLL have been reported. A common etiology suggested in both cases was paramyxovirus particles found in giant cells on electron microscopy [34, 39].

Cases with liver transplantation, early recurrence of giant cell hepatitis after liver transplantation favors the hypothesis of a transmissible agent as the etiology of the disease. In a study of seven patients who developed giant cell hepatitis (GCH) after liver transplantation, five of these patients also had GCH as their original liver disease and experienced a particularly aggressive course because of recurrent giant cell hepatitis, beginning 1–21 months after transplantation. Two died and another two required hepatic retransplantation because of recurrent GCH (one of them had GCH recurrence in a second liver allograft). A remaining patient with recurrent GCH is alive for 6 years after transplantation. Followup of the two patients who developed de novo GCH 8 and 24 months after hepatic transplantation showed active micronodular cirrhosis. All of these cases were serologically negative for hepatitis viruses. None had a history of drug exposure. Two patients had an associated autoimmune syndrome, which could have been the cause of GCH. Human papilloma virus (HPV) type 6 was detected in liver tissues with GCH from one of three cases before and three of four cases after transplantation. Recurrent disease in five of seven patients suggested that this entity may be related to a transmissible agent or that a particular recipient may injure liver in a way that elicits a giant cell reaction [40]. Routine follow-up liver biopsy is necessary in these cases in order to gain more information about the precise incidence and aggressively of disease recurrence in the allograft [38, 40–42].

Postinfantile giant cell hepatitis clinical spectrum varies from acute hepatitis to mild chronic liver in the form of icteric disease, [7, 29] to rapid progression of cirrhosis, and to subacute hepatic failure to fatal hepatic failure [1–40, 44–47]. Adult giant-cell hepatitis has been shown to be progressive and often fatal disease process, with a survival rate of only approximately 50% without orthotopic liver transplantation [3, 5, 7, 26, 29, 38–42]. The high mortality rate is often due to severe liver failure, or sepsis in the setting of aggressive use of immunosuppressant [3, 5, 7, 26, 29, 38–42].

Raised bilirubin, slightly raised to markedly raised transaminases autoantibody markers are positive in around 50% cases mostly ANA/ANF [1, 5, 7, 10–23, 44]. In other cases, viral markers are positive where etiology viral [1–3, 5, 7, 24–30, 32–37, 39, 45, 46].

Gross examination liver biopsy may be of uniformly dark green to grayish brown in color [3]. Liver is usually shrunken, but in some acute cases it can be enlarged [3]. Microscopically, diagnostic giant cells are the common pathological finding. Other biopsy findings are periportal lymphocytic infiltrate (T lymphocytes), massive necrosis, bridging necrosis, "activated" perisinusoidal cells, bilirubinostasis, and Mallory hyaline bodies, often associated with neutrophilic infiltrate and severe fibrosis [1–3, 7, 29].

In most cases, the giant cell change found more than two-thirds of the parenchyma. Giant cell transformation is most pronounced in zone 3. The giant cells often contain 4 to 20 centrally allocated nuclei [1] (Figures 1(a) and 1(b)). In cases of HAV, Paramyxo virus, EBV, few autoimmune related cases, and hypereosinophilia related and post transplant HPV-6 related cases show giant cell predominance in periportal periseptal areas with muliti-acinar necrosis and increased inflammation [1, 3, 23–26, 32–35, 38–42]. Cases showed some degree of periportal fibrosis to severe fibrosis [1, 2, 5, 7, 29]. Progression to rapid onset of cirrhosis was evident in the biopsy specimens in cases particularly with autoimmune diseases [24–27, 30, 32–37, 39, 45, 46], and submassive to massive necrosis of liver parenchyma were seen in cases with HAV, paramyxo virus infection, those with positive EBV serology, hypereosinophilia, and post transplant recurrence of PIGCH [1, 3, 24–26, 32–35, 38–41].

The mechanisms by which the characteristic multinucleated hepatocytes syncytia formed are unknown. Two processes have been proposed: increased hepatocytes nuclear proliferation that is not followed by cell division or the membrane fusion of neighboring hepatocytes [2, 13, 15, 44, 48]. In adults, giant cell change of hepatocytes represents an unusual and idiosyncratic regenerative response to a wide variety of hepatic stimuli [4, 48, 49].

There is no established treatment for paramyxo virus induced PIGCH. There are a few sporadic case reports in the literature where ribavirin treatment was successful but failed in another cases [41]. This drug, which has been shown to be quite effective against paramyxo virus, needs further clinical evaluation for this particular viral cause related to PIGCH [39, 48–51].

In PIGCH in HCV-HIV coinfection and isolated HCV positive cases, specific treatment with pegylated interferon and ribavirin can lead to histological resolution and biochemical improvement, even in the absence of HCV-RNA clearance [11]. A considerable number of patients exhibit autoimmune features and they respond to prednisone therapy alone or in combination with immunosuppressant such as Azathioprine as recommended by AASLD 2002 (American Association for the Study of Liver Diseases) [5, 12–22, 44, 52]. In posttransplant cases of PIGCH cyclophosphamide therapy claimed to be life saving and effective by few [51].

5. Conclusion

Autoimmune causes account for approximately 40% of PIGCH, which commonly presents as chronic liver disease while 25% of cases can have an acute presentation and few of them have rapid onset of cirrhosis [2, 4, 12–22, 28, 44]. Autoimmune diseases with presentation of giant cell hepatitis have moderate sort of prognosis [12–22, 44]. Those with paramyxo virus, EBV, HAV, and post transplant HPV induced PIGCH have subfulminant to fulminant course and required orthotopic liver transplant [1, 3, 24–26, 33–35, 38–42]. In HCV, HBV, HEV, HCV-HIV induced PIGCH have relatively better outcome [5, 7, 28, 29]. Overall PIGCH presents clinically as severe form of hepatitis [53].

Conflict of Interests

The authors declare no conflict of interests.

Authors' Contributions

All authors contributed in conceiving and developing the paper.

References

[1] S. J. Johnson, J. Mathew, R. N. M. MacSween, M. K. Bennett, and A. D. Burt, "Post-infantile giant cell hepatitis: histological and immunohistochemical study," *Journal of Clinical Pathology*, vol. 47, no. 11, pp. 1022–1027, 1994.

[2] K. Devaney, Z. D. Goodman, and K. G. Ishak, "Postinfantile giant-cell transformation in hepatitis," *Hepatology*, vol. 16, no. 2, pp. 327–333, 1992.

[3] M. J. Phillips, L. M. Blendis, S. Poucell et al., "Sporadic hepatitis with distinctive pathological features, a severe clinical course, and paramyxoviral features," *The New England Journal of Medicine*, vol. 324, no. 7, pp. 455–460, 1991.

[4] J. Y. N. Lau, G. Koukoulis, G. Mieli-Vergani, B. C. Portmann, and R. Williams, "Syncytial giant-cell hepatitis—a specific disease entity?" *Journal of Hepatology*, vol. 15, no. 1-2, pp. 216–219, 1992.

[5] L. Gabor, K. Pal, and S. Zsuzsa, "Giant cell hepatitis in adults," *Pathology and Oncology Research*, vol. 3, no. 3, pp. 215–218, 1997.

[6] M. Fraquelli, A. Colli, M. Cocciolo, and D. Conte, "Adult syncytial giant cell chronic hepatitis due to herbal remedy," *Journal of Hepatology*, vol. 33, no. 3, pp. 505–508, 2000.

[7] T. Tordjmann, S. Grimbert, C. Genestie et al., "Adult multi-nuclear cell hepatitis. A study in 17 patients," *Gastroenterologie Clinique et Biologique*, vol. 22, no. 3, pp. 305–310, 1998.

[8] V. Singh, M. Rudraraju, E. J. Carey et al., "An unusual occurrence of giant cell hepatitis," *Liver Transplantation*, vol. 15, no. 12, pp. 1888–1890, 2009.

[9] J. Hartl, R. Buettner, F. Rockmann et al., "Giant cell hepatitis: an unusual cause of fulminant liver failure," *Zeitschrift fur Gastroenterologie*, vol. 48, no. 11, pp. 1293–1296, 2010.

[10] H. Hayashi, R. Narita, M. Hiura et al., "A case of adult autoimmune hepatitis with histological features of giant cell hepatitis," *Internal Medicine*, vol. 50, no. 4, pp. 315–319, 2011.

[11] K. Tajiri, Y. Shimizu, Y. Tokimitsu et al., "An elderly man with syncytial giant cell hepatitis successfully treated by immuno-suppressants," *Internal Medicine*, vol. 51, no. 16, pp. 2141–2144, 2012.

[12] K. Dohmen, S. Ohtsuka, H. Nakamura et al., "Post-infantile giant cell hepatitis in an elderly female patient with systemic lupus erythematosus," *Journal of Gastroenterology*, vol. 29, no. 3, pp. 362–368, 1994.

[13] M. Gorelik, R. Debski, and H. Frangoul, "Autoimmune hemolytic anemia with giant cell hepatitis: case report and review of the literature," *Journal of Pediatric Hematology/Oncology*, vol. 26, no. 12, pp. 837–839, 2004.

[14] P. Vajro, F. Migliaro, C. Ruggeri et al., "Life saving cyclophos-phamide treatment in a girl with giant cell hepatitis and autoimmune haemolytic anaemia: case report and up-to-date on therapeutical options," *Digestive and Liver Disease*, vol. 38, no. 11, pp. 846–850, 2006.

[15] A. R. Perez-Atayde, S. M. Sirlin, and M. Jonas, "Coombs-positive autoimmune hemolytic anemia and postinfantile giant cell hepatitis in children," *Pediatric Pathology*, vol. 14, no. 1, pp. 69–77, 1994.

[16] U. Protzer, H. P. Dienes, L. Bianchi et al., "Post-infantile giant cell hepatitis in patients with primary sclerosing cholangitis and autoimmune hepatitis," *Liver*, vol. 16, no. 4, pp. 274–282, 1996.

[17] M. P. Stoffel, H. M. Steffen, V. Dries, H. P. Dienes, and C. A. Baldamus, "Acute exacerbation overlapping autoimmune liver disease with development of giant cell hepatitis after 14 years' disease duration," *Journal of Internal Medicine*, vol. 244, no. 4, pp. 355–356, 1998.

[18] J. Estradas, V. Pascual-Ramos, B. Martínez et al., "Autoimmune hepatitis with giant-cell transformation," *Annals of Hepatology*, vol. 8, no. 1, pp. 68–70, 2009.

[19] J. Koskinas, M. Deutsch, C. Papaioannou, G. Kafiri, and S. Hadziyannis, "Post-infantile giant cell hepatitis associated with autoimmune hepatitis and polyarteritis nodosa," *Scandinavian Journal of Gastroenterology*, vol. 37, no. 1, pp. 120–123, 2002.

[20] J. Labowitz, S. Finklestein, and M. Rabinovitz, "Postinfantile giant cell hepatitis complicating ulcerative colitis: a case report and review of the literature," *The American Journal of Gastroenterology*, vol. 96, no. 4, pp. 1274–1277, 2001.

[21] N. Watanabe, S. Takashimizu, K. Shiraishi et al., "Primary biliary cirrhosis with multinucleated hepatocellular giant cells: implications for pathogenesis of primary biliary cirrhosis," *The European Journal of Gastroenterology and Hepatology*, vol. 18, no. 9, pp. 1023–1027, 2006.

[22] M. Rabinovitz and A. J. Demetris, "Postinfantile giant cell hepatitis associated with anti-M2 mitochondrial antibodies," *Gastroenterology*, vol. 107, no. 4, pp. 1162–1164, 1994.

[23] Z. Ben-Ari, E. Broida, Y. Monselise et al., "Syncytial giant-cell hepatitis due to autoimmune hepatitis type II (LKM$_1$+) presenting as subfulminant hepatitis," *The American Journal of Gastroenterology*, vol. 95, no. 3, pp. 799–801, 2000.

[24] P. Kinra and B. M. John, "Hepatitis—a induced non infantile giant cell hepatitis," *Medical Journal Armed Forces India*, vol. 63, no. 2, pp. 182–183, 2007.

[25] R. H. Krech, V. Geenen, H. Maschek, and B. Högemann, "Adult giant cell hepatitis with fatal course. Clinical pathology case report and reflections on the pathogenesis," *Pathologe*, vol. 19, no. 3, pp. 221–225, 1998.

[26] M. A. Khan, J. Ahn, N. Shah et al., "Fulminant hepatic failure in an adult patient with giant-cell hepatitis," *Gastroenterology and Hepatology*, vol. 5, no. 7, pp. 502–504, 2009.

[27] L. Potenza, M. Luppi, P. Barozzi et al., "HHV-6A in syncytial giant-cell hepatitis," *The New England Journal of Medicine*, vol. 359, no. 6, pp. 593–602, 2008.

[28] W. Kryczka, B. Walewska-Zielecka, and E. Dutkiewicz, "Acute seronegative hepatitis C manifesting itself as adult giant cell hepatitis: a case report and review of literature," *Medical Science Monitor*, vol. 9, supplement 6, pp. 29–31, 2003.

[29] S. T. L. Micchelli, D. Thomas, J. K. Boitnott, and M. Torbenson, "Hepatic giant cells in hepatitis C virus (HCV) mono-infection and HCV/HIV co-infection," *Journal of Clinical Pathology*, vol. 61, no. 9, pp. 1058–1061, 2008.

[30] A. Moreno, A. Moreno, M. J. Pérez-Elías et al., "Syncytial giant cell hepatitis in human immunodeficiency virus-infected patients with chronic hepatitis C: 2 cases and review of the literature," *Human Pathology*, vol. 37, no. 10, pp. 1344–1349, 2006.

[31] H. Thaler, "Post-infantile giant cell hepatitis," *Liver*, vol. 2, no. 4, pp. 393–403, 1982.

[32] N. Kerkar, D. Gold, S. N. Thung, and B. L. Shneider, "Jaundice accompanied by giant cell hepatitis and eosinophilia in childhood," *Seminars in Liver Disease*, vol. 24, no. 1, pp. 107–111, 2004.

[33] M. Lazzarino, E. Orlandi, F. Baldanti et al., "The immunosuppression and potential for EBV reactivation of fludarabine combined with cyclophosphamide and dexamethasone in patients with lymphoproliferative disorders," *The British Journal of Haematology*, vol. 107, no. 4, pp. 877–882, 1999.

[34] C. J. Fimmel, L. Guo, R. W. Compans et al., "A case of syncytial giant cell hepatitis with features of a paramyxoviral infection," *The American Journal of Gastroenterology*, vol. 93, no. 10, pp. 1931–1937, 1998.

[35] C. J. Fimmel and S. Robertazzi.., "Fulminant hepatic failure in an adult patient with giant-cell hepatitis," *Gastroenterology and Hepatology*, vol. 5, no. 7, pp. 504–506, 2009.

[36] L. Falasca, F. D. Nonno, F. Palmieri et al., "Two cases of giant cell hepatitis in HIV-infected patients," *International Journal of STD & AIDS*, vol. 23, no. 7, pp. 3–4, 2012.

[37] S. Welte, M. Gagesch, A. Weber et al., "Fulminant liver failure in Wilson's disease with histologic features of postinfantile giant cell hepatitis, cytomegalovirus as the trigger for both?" *The European Journal of Gastroenterology and Hepatology*, vol. 24, no. 3, pp. 328–331, 2012.

[38] A. Kumar and G. Y. Minuk, "Postinfantile giant cell hepatitis in association with hypereosinophilia," *Gastroenterology*, vol. 101, no. 5, pp. 1417–1419, 1991.

[39] E. Gupta, M. Yacoub, M. Higgins, and A. M. Al-Katib, "Syncytial giant cell hepatitis associated with chronic lymphocytic leukemia: a case report," *BMC Blood Disorders*, vol. 19, article 8, no. 12, 2012.

[40] J. P. Lerut, N. Claeys, O. Ciccarelli et al., "Recurrent postinfantile syncytial giant cell hepatitis after orthotopic liver transplantation," *Transplant International*, vol. 11, no. 4, pp. 320–322, 1998.

[41] O. Pappo, E. Yunis, J. A. Jordan et al., "Recurrent and de novo giant cell hepatitis after orthotopic liver transplantation," *The American Journal of Surgical Pathology*, vol. 18, no. 8, pp. 804–813, 1994.

[42] F. Durand, C. Degott, A. Sauvanet et al., "Subfulminant syncytial giant cell hepatitis: recurrence after liver transplantation treated with ribavirin," *Journal of Hepatology*, vol. 26, no. 3, pp. 722–726, 1997.

[43] S. Nair, B. Baisden, J. Boitnott, A. Klein, and P. J. Thuluvath, "Recurrent, progressive giant cell hepatitis in two consecutive liver allografts in a middle-aged woman," *Journal of Clinical Gastroenterology*, vol. 32, no. 5, pp. 454–456, 2001.

[44] J. C. Thijs, A. Bosma, S. C. Henzen-Logmans, and S. G. M. Meuwissen, "Postinfantile giant cell hepatitis in a patient with multiple autoimmune features," *The American Journal of Gastroenterology*, vol. 80, no. 4, pp. 294–297, 1985.

[45] O. Harmanci, I. K. Önal, O. Ersoy, B. Gürel, C. Sökmensüer, and Y. Bayraktar, "Post infantile giant cell hepatitis due to hepatitis E virus along with the presence of autoantibodies," *Digestive Diseases and Sciences*, vol. 52, no. 12, pp. 3521–3523, 2007.

[46] A. Wasley, A. Fiore, and B. P. Bell, "Hepatitis A in the era of vaccination," *Epidemiologic Reviews*, vol. 28, no. 1, pp. 101–111, 2006.

[47] G. Koukoulis, G. Mieli-Vergani, and B. Portmann, "Infantile liver giant cells: immunohistological study of their proliferative state and possible mechanisms of formation," *Pediatric and Developmental Pathology*, vol. 2, no. 4, pp. 353–359, 1999.

[48] K. Aterman, "Neonatal hepatitis and its relation to viral hepatitis of mother. A review of the problem," *The American Journal of Diseases of Children*, vol. 105, pp. 395–416, 1963.

[49] E. Roberts, E. L. Ford-Jones, and M. J. Phillips, "Ribavirin for syncytial giant cell hepatitis," *The Lancet*, vol. 341, no. 8845, pp. 640–641, 1993.

[50] H. P. . Dienes, U. Protzer, G. Gerken et al., "Pathogenesis and clinical relevance of post infantile giant cell hepatitis (PIGCH)," *Hepatology*, vol. 18, article 175A, 1993.

[51] Y. Horsmans, C. Galant, M. L. Nicholas, M. Lamy, and A. P. Geubel, "Failure of ribavarin or immunosupressive therapy to alter the course of post-inflantile giant-cell hepatitis," *Journal of Hepatology*, vol. 22, article 382, no. 3, 1995.

[52] A. J. Czaja and D. K. Freese, "Diagnosis and treatment of autoimmune hepatitis," *Hepatology*, vol. 36, no. 2, pp. 479–497, 2002.

[53] L. Bianchi and L. M. Terracciano, "Giant cell hepatitis in adult," *Praxis*, vol. 83, no. 44, pp. 1237–1241, 1994.

7

Interleukin-16 Gene Polymorphisms Are Considerable Host Genetic Factors for Patients' Susceptibility to Chronic Hepatitis B Infection

Sara Romani,[1,2] **Seyed Masoud Hosseini,**[2] **Seyed Reza Mohebbi,**[1] **Shabnam Kazemian,**[3] **Shaghayegh Derakhshani,**[1] **Mahsa Khanyaghma,**[1] **Pedram Azimzadeh,**[1,3] **Afsaneh Sharifian,**[1] **and Mohammad Reza Zali**[1]

[1] *Gastroenterology and Liver Diseases Research Center, Shahid Beheshti University of Medical Sciences, Tehran, Iran*
[2] *Department of Microbiology, Faculty of Biological Sciences, Shahid Beheshti University, Tehran, Iran*
[3] *Basic and Molecular Epidemiology of Gastroenterology Disorders Research Center, Shahid Beheshti University of Medical Sciences, Tehran, Iran*

Correspondence should be addressed to Pedram Azimzadeh; azimzadeh.pedram@gmail.com

Academic Editor: Piero Luigi Almasio

Host genetic background is known as an important factor in patients' susceptibility to infectious diseases such as viral hepatitis. The aim of this study was to determine the effect of genetic polymorphisms of interleukin-16 (IL-16) cytokine on susceptibility of hepatitis B virus (HBV) infected patients to develop chronic HBV infection. Genotyping was conducted using PCR followed by enzymatic digestion and RFLP (restriction fragment length polymorphism) analysis. We genotyped three single nucleotide polymorphisms (SNPs) in the *Il-16* gene (rs11556218 T>G, rs4778889 T>C, and rs4072111 C>T) to test for relationship between variation at these loci and patients' susceptibility to chronic HBV infection. Allele frequency of *Il-16* gene rs4072111 and rs11556218 was significantly different between chronic HBV patients and healthy blood donors. Genotype frequency of rs4778889 polymorphism of *Il-16* gene was significantly different when chronic HBV patients and HBV clearance subjects were compared. Our results showed that *Il-16* gene polymorphisms are considerable host genetic factors when we chase biomarkers for prognosis of HBV infected patients.

1. Background and Objectives

More than 350 million individuals around the world are infected with hepatitis B virus. The diagnosis of chronic infection is made by a combination of serology, viral, and biochemical markers [1]. Prevalence of anti-HBc and HBsAg in the United States at 2006 is estimated to be 4.7% and 0.27%, respectively [2].

Iran is located on intermediate endemic region for hepatitis B infection and prevalence of HBsAg positivity among general adult population in about 3 to 10 percent in different regions [3]. World Health Organization (WHO) and Center for Disease Control and Prevention (CDC) reported that prevalence of chronic hepatitis B infection in Iran ranges between 2 and 7 percent [4].

Occult HBV infection is reported among 7 to 13 percent of anti-HBc positive and/or anti-HBs positive subjects, but this type of viral hepatitis is seen in 0 to 17 percent of healthy blood donors. When we investigate the susceptibility factors for HBV clearance this phenomenon could have confounder effect. So HBV-DNA PCR test must be performed for all study subjects to obviate this issue [5].

Interleukin-16 (*Il-16*) is a multifunctional cytokine with the role of immune response synchronization and direction [6]. The mature secreted form of this protein acts as a ligand for CD4$^+$ cells and this ligand-receptor binding leads to activation of a key intracellular pathway that regulates T cell proliferation [7]. The major *Il-16* related functional proteins are STAT6, interleukin-4 (*Il-4*), and tumor necrosis factor-α (TNF-α) [8].

TABLE 1: PCR and RFLP information for the SNPs of interleukin-16 gene.

Polymorphism	Primer	PCR (bp)	Restriction enzyme (incubation temp °C)	Restricted fragments' size (bp)
rs4072111 C/T	F: 5′-CACTGTGATCCCGGTCCAGTC-3′ R: 5′-TTCAGGTACAAACCCAGCCAG C-3′	164	BsmAI (55)	C: 164 T: 140 + 24
rs11556218 T/G	F: 5′-GCTCAGGTTCACAGAGTGTTTCCATA-3′ R: 5′-TGTGACAATCACAGCTTGCCTG-3′	171	Nde I (37)	T: 171 G: 147 + 24
rs4778889 T/C	F: 5′-CTCCACACTCAAAGCCTTTTGTTCCTAT$\underline{G}^{a}$ A-3′ R: 5′-CCATGTCAAAACGGTAGCCTCAAGC-3′	280	AhdI (37)	T: 280 C: 246 + 34

[a]The underlined base in the forward primer is different from that of the original sequence and serves as the introduction of a recognition site for the restriction enzyme AhdI.

Some current efforts to prevent the populations from the infectious diseases such as viral hepatitis have focused on finding powerful genetic susceptibility biomarkers [9]. In recent years few polymorphism markers have been found in association with viral hepatitis. SNPs located in *HLA-DPA1* and *HLA-DPB1* genes were identified as protective factors for chronic hepatitis B infection [10] and SNPs of *IL28B* gene were significantly related to spontaneous clearance of hepatitis C infection [11].

HBV clearance is in connection with powerful CD4^{+} T cells and *Il-16* plays a critical role in T cell regulation [12]. Due to this, phenomenon variations occurring in *Il-16* gene sequence could affect its function and cause deregulation in immune response against viral hepatitis [13].

Present study was designed to investigate the relationship between three SNPs of *Il-16* gene and patients' susceptibility to chronic hepatitis B infection and to determine the effect of *Il-16* gene polymorphisms on development of chronic HBV infection.

2. Methods

2.1. Study Population. Seven hundred and forty-four individuals were enrolled in the genotyping procedure including 245 chronic HBV patients, 105 HBV clearance subjects, and 394 healthy controls. Inclusion criteria for chronic hepatitis B patients group were HBsAg positive test for at least 6 months and HBV infection was confirmed by detection of serum HBV DNA using PCR method. The patients with these characteristics were excluded from study: HCV or HIV coinfection and history of autoimmune diseases. HBV clearance group consisted of individuals with anti-HBc positive and HBs-antigen negative tests. All healthy control subjects were anti-HBc, HBs-antigen, and HBV-DNA PCR negative and have not met these criteria, any history of hepatitis or liver dysfunction, autoimmune diseases, and HCV or HIV.

2.2. Single Nucleotide Polymorphisms. According to literature review and basic information about the *Il-16* cytokine, we selected three SNPs in the *Il-16* gene sequence including rs11556218 T>G, rs4778889 T>C, and rs4072111 C>T. The minor allele frequency (MAF) of all three selected SNPs was greater than 0.05 according to previous studies.

2.3. Genomic DNA Purification and Genotyping. Blood samples were collected from all study subjects in EDTA coated tubes. Genomic DNA was extracted from whole blood using standard phenol chloroform method as previously described by Sambrook [14]. Genotype determination for three selected SNPs was performed by PCR-RFLP method as previously described by Gao et al. [15] Primer sequences and RFLP material are presented in Table 1. In brief pure PCR products were obtained using specific primer pairs (Bioneer, South Korea) for each SNP; and enzymatic digestion for each one was performed using specific restriction endonucleases (Fermentas, Latvia). Digested DNA was analyzed on 3% low electroendosmosis agarose gel (Agarose LE, Roche, Germany).

2.4. Direct Sequencing. To confirm the results of RFLP analysis we performed direct sequencing using chain termination method and 3130*xl* genetic analyzer instrument (Applied Biosystems, USA) for 5% of our samples as duplicate genotyping.

2.5. Statistical Analysis. Statistical analyses were carried out using IBM SPSS software version 20 (IBM SPSS Statistics 20; SPSS, Chicago, IL). *P* values less than 0.05 were considered as significant. To compare three included groups (HBV cases, HBV clearance, and healthy controls) for their genotype and allele status we performed Chi square test and to consider the simultaneous effect of genotype and allele along with gender and age (as probable confounder variables) we conducted a logistic regression test. To compare the mean age between three studied groups we used one-way ANNOVA.

3. Results

Among 245 chronic HBV patients 157 (64.1%) individuals were male and 88 (35.9%) were female and from 394 healthy controls 205 (52%) were male and 189 (48%) were female; so our third group (HBV clearance) consisted of 64 male and 41 female, total 105 subjects. Mean age in chronic HBV group was 49.15 ± 15.50 years, in healthy control group was 45.26 ± 16.42 years, and in HBV clearance group was 42.2 ± 14.96 years; there was a significant difference between three groups according to age and gender status (*P* value < 0.05). In order

TABLE 2: Allele and genotype frequency of three SNPs among chronic HBV patients versus healthy control subjects.

SNP	Variable	Healthy control ($n = 394$) n (%)	HBV patient ($n = 245$) n (%)	Adjusted* OR (95% CI), P_{value}
	Genotypes			
	CC	316 (80.2)	181 (73.9)	1.00 (reference)
	CT	74 (18.8)	58 (23.7)	1.391 (0.937–2.066), 0.102
rs4072111	TT	4 (1.0)	6 (2.4)	2.929 (0.787–10.894), 0.109
	Alleles			
	C	706 (89.6)	420 (85.7)	1.00 (reference)
	T	82 (10.4)	70 (14.3)	**1.471 (1.039–2.081), 0.029**
	Genotypes			
	TT	124 (31.5)	43 (17.6)	1.00 (reference)
	TG	215 (54.6)	147 (60)	**2.028 (1.344–3.061), 0.001**
rs11556218	GG	55 (14)	55 (22.4)	**2.894 (1.722–4.864), 0.000**
	Alleles			
	T	463 (58.8)	233 (47.6)	1.00 (reference)
	G	325 (41.2)	257 (52.4)	**1.574 (1.250–1.982), 0.000**
	Genotypes			
	TT	264 (67)	156 (63.7)	1.00 (reference)
	TC	111 (28.2)	84 (34.3)	1.303 (0.916–1.853), 0.140
rs4778889	CC	19 (4.8)	5 (2)	0.439 (0.159–1.216), 0.113
	Alleles			
	T	639 (81.1)	396 (80.8)	1.00 (reference)
	C	149 (18.9)	94 (19.2)	1.027 (0.767–1.375), 0.860

*Adjusted for confounder variables: age and gender.

to control the probable confounding effects of age and gender we performed data adjustment using logistic regression.

All subjects were genotyped for three SNPs of *Il-16* gene sequence. When comparing chronic HBV patients with healthy blood donors, we found a significant association between T allele of rs4072111 polymorphism and higher risk of chronic disease development (*P* value: 0.029, OR: 1.471, and 95% CI: 1.039–2.081). Frequency of TG and GG genotypes and G allele distribution in rs11556218 polymorphism were also significantly different between two study groups, but our results showed no statistically significant difference between allele and genotype frequency of rs4778889 polymorphism between chronic HBV patients and healthy control group. These data are summarized in Table 2. Despite these findings, we found a statistically significant relationship between the rs4778889 CC genotype (rare genotype) and three times higher risk for chronic HBV infection, when we compare chronic HBV and HBV clearance groups (*P* value: 0.035, OR: 3.723, and 95% CI: 1.100–12.602). Summary of genotyping data of chronic HBV and HBV clearance groups is shown in Table 3.

4. Discussion

The mechanisms involved in the patients' susceptibility to chronic hepatitis B infection are not well understood. Clearance or pathogenesis of HBV infection is expected to be multifactorial affected by environment, viral factors, and host genetic variations. The products of many human genes and their downstream effectors influence host defense against HBV infection and person to person differences in susceptibility to chronic hepatitis disease.

Precursor of human *Il-16* protein contains 631 amino acids and is constitutively synthesized in unstimulated T cells. This peptide goes through proteolytic processing that results in a 121-amino acid bioactive molecule [5]. Almost all 121 amino acids of this peptide are involved in PDZ domains and this phenomenon makes it a unique structure [16].

Il-16 is secreted by several types of cells and its association with recruitment of CD4$^+$ immune cells to location of inflammation. Involvement of *Il-16* in pathogenesis of viral hepatitis is in connection with its receptor (CD4) [17]. *Il-16* is produced by a variety of immune cells in addition to CD4$^+$ and CD8$^+$ T cells [18]. Biological activities of *Il-16* cytokine are chemotaxis of CD4$^+$ cells, upregulation of CD25 protein, and secretion of interleukin-1b (*Il-1b*), interleukin-4 (*Il-4*), and tumor necrosis factor-α (*TNF-α*). On the other hand, activation of STAT6 protein is a common function in CD4$^+$ cells, and STAT6 together with *Il-4* are involved in T cell mediated hepatitis. This pathway of events is consistent with the fact that immune responses related to T lymphocytes are important in viral hepatitis [19, 20].

There is limited data about the association of SNPs in the *Il-16* gene sequence and risk of chronic hepatitis B infection, whereas the role of cellular immunity in dealing with hepatitis HBV infection is clear and on the other hand CD4 (receptor of *Il-16*) is involved in this process [21, 22]. So it might be considered that *Il-16* plays a role in immune response against HBV infection.

TABLE 3: Allele and genotype frequency of three SNPs among chronic HBV patients versus HBV clearance subjects.

SNP	Variable	HBV clearance ($n = 105$) n (%)	HBV patient ($n = 245$) n (%)	Adjusted* OR (95% CI), P_{value}
	Genotypes			
	CC	86 (81.9)	181 (73.9)	1.00 (reference)
	CT	17 (16.2)	58 (23.7)	0.577 (0.307–1.082), 0.086
rs4072111	TT	2 (1.9)	6 (2.4)	0.814 (0.142–4.672), 0.817
	Alleles			
	C	189 (89.6)	420 (85.7)	1.00 (reference)
	T	21 (10.4)	70 (14.3)	0.651 (0.378–1.121), 0.122
	Genotypes			
	TT	16 (15.2)	43 (17.6)	1.00 (reference)
	TG	63 (60)	147 (60)	1.118 (0.567–2.203), 0.748
rs11556218	GG	26 (24.8)	55 (22.4)	1.298 (0.594–2.836), 0.513
	Alleles			
	T	95 (45.2)	233 (47.6)	1.00 (reference)
	G	115 (54.8)	257 (52.4)	1.109 (0.788–1.561), 0.509
	Genotypes			
	TT	68 (64.8)	156 (63.7)	1.00 (reference)
	TC	29 (27.6)	84 (34.3)	0.785 (0.459–1.342), 0.376
rs4778889	CC	8 (7.6)	5 (2)	**3.723 (1.100–12.602), 0.035**
	Alleles			
	T	165 (78.6)	396 (80.8)	1.00 (reference)
	C	45 (21.4)	94 (19.2)	1.144 (0.751–1.744), 0.531

*Adjusted for confounder variables: age and gender.

According to the results of our study, rs11556218 T>G, rs4778889 T>C, and rs4072111 C>T polymorphisms of *Il-16* gene are associated with patients' susceptibility to chronic hepatitis B infection. As we showed in the results section rs4072111 and rs11556218 polymorphisms are in relationship with higher susceptibility of general population for development of chronic HBV and rs4778889 polymorphism which is associated with higher risk of chronic HBV among HBV infected individuals.

A recent published study on Chinese patients suffering from hepatitis C virus (HCV) disease revealed that there is an association between STAT6 SNPs and patients' susceptibility to sustained viral response. These outcomes suggest that STAT6 SNPs are prospective genetic biomarkers for HCV prognosis [23].

Li et al. reported that the genetic variations (SNPs) of *Il-16* are significantly related to chronic HBV related hepatocellular carcinoma (HCC). These results also showed that rs11556218 TG and GG genotypes of the *Il-16* gene contributed in patients' susceptibility to chronic hepatitis B when using healthy subjects as controls [24].

In our previous study we have shown that there is a significant relationship between the micro-RNA binding site polymorphism of the *Il-16* gene and risk of colorectal cancer (CRC) [25]. Our previous study also suggested that rs11556218 T>G and rs4778889 T>C polymorphisms have influence on the altered risk of CRC [26].

In conclusion, HBV infected patients with anti-HBc Ab positive test who have had CC genotype rs4778889 are more susceptible to establish a chronic disease. We can also conclude that rs4072111 and rs11556218 polymorphisms are suitable susceptibility biomarkers for development of chronic HBV infection. Our results are in concordance with previous studies and we suggest that *Il-16* is related to hepatitis B infection and *Il-16* gene polymorphisms are considerable host genetic factors for patients' susceptibility to chronic hepatitis B infection.

Conflict of Interests

The authors declare that they have no potential conflict of interests.

Acknowledgments

This project was supported by the Gastroenterology and Liver Diseases Research Center, Shahid Beheshti University of Medical Sciences, Tehran, Iran. The authors would like to thank the lab staff Seyedeh Mina Seyedi, Hanieh Mirtalebi, and Farahnaz Jabbarian for their kind assistance.

References

[1] B. Custer, S. D. Sullivan, T. K. Hazlet et al., "Global epidemiology of hepatitis B virus," *Journal of Clinical Gastroenterology*, vol. 38, no. 10, supplement 3, pp. S158–S168, 2004.

[2] A. Wasley, D. Kruszon-Moran, W. Kuhnert et al., "The prevalence of hepatitis B virus infection in the united states in the era of vaccination," *The Journal of Infectious Diseases*, vol. 202, no. 2, pp. 192–201, 2010.

[3] S. Amini, M. F. Mahmoodi, S. Andalibi, and A. Solati, "Seroepidemiology of hepatitis B, Delta and human immunodeficiency virus infections in Hamadan province, Iran: a population based study," *The Journal of Tropical Medicine and Hygiene*, vol. 96, no. 5, pp. 277–287, 1993.

[4] J. Poorolajal and R. Majdzadeh, "Prevalence of chronic hepatitis B infection in Iran: a review article," *Journal of Research in Medical Sciences*, vol. 14, no. 4, pp. 249–258, 2009.

[5] W. W. Cruikshank, D. M. Center, N. Nisar et al., "Molecular and functional analysis of a lymphocyte chemoattractant factor: association of biologic function with CD4 expression," *Proceedings of the National Academy of Sciences of the United States of America*, vol. 91, no. 11, pp. 5109–5113, 1994.

[6] J. Richmond, M. Tuzova, W. Cruikshank, and D. Center, "Regulation of cellular processes by interleukin-16 in homeostasis and cancer," *Journal of Cellular Physiology*, vol. 229, no. 2, pp. 139–147, 2014.

[7] W. W. Cruikshank, D. M. Center, N. Nisar et al., "Molecular and functional analysis of a lymphocyte chemoattractant factor: association of biologic function with CD4 expression," *Proceedings of the National Academy of Sciences of the United States of America*, vol. 91, no. 11, pp. 5109–5113, 1994.

[8] C. Liu, J. Mills, K. Dixon et al., "IL-16 signaling specifically induces STAT6 activation through CD4," *Cytokine*, vol. 38, no. 3, pp. 145–150, 2007.

[9] S. J. Chapman and A. V. S. Hill, "Human genetic susceptibility to infectious disease," *Nature Reviews Genetics*, vol. 13, no. 3, pp. 175–188, 2012.

[10] Y. Kamatani, S. Wattanapokayakit, H. Ochi et al., "A genome-wide association study identifies variants in the HLA-DP locus associated with chronic hepatitis B in Asians," *Nature Genetics*, vol. 41, no. 5, pp. 591–595, 2009.

[11] A. Rauch, Z. Kutalik, P. Descombes et al., "Genetic variation in IL28B is associated with chronic hepatitis C and treatment failure: a genome-wide association study," *Gastroenterology*, vol. 138, no. 4, pp. 1338–1345, 2010.

[12] S. Urbani, C. Boni, B. Amadei et al., "Acute phase HBV-specific T cell responses associated with HBV persistence after HBV/HCV coinfection," *Hepatology*, vol. 41, no. 4, pp. 826–831, 2005.

[13] K. C. Wilson, D. M. Center, and W. W. Cruikshank, "The effect of interleukin-16 and its precursor on T lymphocyte activation and growth," *Growth Factors*, vol. 22, no. 2, pp. 97–104, 2004.

[14] J. Sambrook, *Molecular Cloning: A Laboratory Manual*, edited by J. Sambrook, D. W. Russell, Cold Spring Harbor Laboratory, Cold Spring Harbor, NY, USA, 2001.

[15] L.-B. Gao, L. Rao, Y.-Y. Wang et al., "The association of interleukin-16 polymorphisms with IL-16 serum levels and risk of colorectal and gastric cancer," *Carcinogenesis*, vol. 30, no. 2, pp. 295–299, 2009.

[16] N. Bannert, K. Vollhardt, B. Asomuddinov et al., "PDZ Domain-mediated interaction of interleukin-16 precursor proteins with myosin phosphatase targeting subunits," *Journal of Biological Chemistry*, vol. 278, no. 43, pp. 42190–42199, 2003.

[17] E. A. Lynch, C. A. W. Heijens, N. F. Horst, D. M. Center, and W. W. Cruikshank, "Cutting edge: IL-16/CD4 preferentially induces Th1 cell migration: requirement of CCR5," *The Journal of Immunology*, vol. 171, no. 10, pp. 4965–4968, 2003.

[18] K. Bowers, C. Pitcher, and M. Marsh, "CD4: a co-receptor in the immune response and HIV infection," *The International Journal of Biochemistry and Cell Biology*, vol. 29, no. 6, pp. 871–875, 1997.

[19] B. Jaruga, F. Hong, R. Sun, S. Radaeva, and B. Gao, "Crucial role of IL-4/STAT6 in T cell-mediated hepatitis: up-regulating eotaxins and IL-5 and recruiting leukocytes," *The Journal of Immunology*, vol. 171, no. 6, pp. 3233–3244, 2003.

[20] A. Durán, A. Rodriguez, P. Martin et al., "Crosstalk between PKCζ and the IL4/Stat6 pathway during T-cell-mediated hepatitis," *EMBO Journal*, vol. 23, no. 23, pp. 4595–4605, 2004.

[21] T. Manigold and V. Racanelli, "T-cell regulation by CD4 regulatory T cells during hepatitis B and C virus infections: facts and controversies," *The Lancet Infectious Diseases*, vol. 7, no. 12, pp. 804–813, 2007.

[22] H. M. Diepolder, M.-C. Jung, E. Keller et al., "A vigorous virus-specific CD4$^+$ T cell response may contribute to the association of HLA-DR13 with viral clearance in hepatitis B," *Clinical & Experimental Immunology*, vol. 113, no. 2, pp. 244–251, 1998.

[23] Y. P. Lim, Y. A. Hsu, K. H. Tsai et al., "The impact of polymorphisms in STAT6 on treatment outcome in HCV infected Taiwanese Chinese," *BMC Immunology*, vol. 14, no. 1, article 21, 2013.

[24] S. Li, Y. Deng, Z.-P. Chen et al., "Genetic polymorphism of interleukin-16 influences susceptibility to HBV-related hepatocellular carcinoma in a Chinese population," *Infection, Genetics and Evolution*, vol. 11, no. 8, pp. 2083–2088, 2011.

[25] P. Azimzadeh, S. Romani, S. R. Mohebbi et al., "Association of polymorphisms in microRNA-binding sites and colorectal cancer in an Iranian population," *Cancer Genetics*, vol. 205, no. 10, pp. 501–507, 2012.

[26] P. Azimzadeh, S. Romani, S. R. Mohebbi et al., "Interleukin-16 (IL-16) gene polymorphisms in Iranian patients with colorectal cancer," *Journal of Gastrointestinal and Liver Diseases*, vol. 20, no. 4, pp. 371–376, 2011.

Interferon-α-Induced Changes to Natural Killer Cells Are Associated with the Treatment Outcomes in Patients with HCV Infections

Shinji Shimoda,[1] Kosuke Sumida,[1] Sho Iwasaka,[1] Satomi Hisamoto,[1] Hironori Tanimoto,[2] Hideyuki Nomura,[2] Kazufumi Dohmen,[3] Kazuhiro Takahashi,[4] Akira Kawano,[5] Eiichi Ogawa,[6] Norihiro Furusyo,[6] Koichi Akashi,[1] and Jun Hayashi[6]

[1] Department of Medicine and Biosystemic Science, Graduate School of Medical Science, Kyushu University, Fukuoka 812-8252, Japan
[2] The Center for Liver Disease, Shin-Kokura Hospital, Kitakyushu 803-8505, Japan
[3] Department of Internal Medicine, Chihaya Hospital, Fukuoka 813-8501, Japan
[4] Department of Medicine, Hamanomachi Hospital, Fukuoka 810-8539, Japan
[5] Department of Medicine, Kitakyushu Municipal Medical Center, Kitakyushu 802-0077, Japan
[6] Department of General Internal Medicine, Kyushu University Hospital, Fukuoka 812-8582, Japan

Correspondence should be addressed to Shinji Shimoda; sshimoda@intmed1.med.kyushu-u.ac.jp

Academic Editor: Tatehiro Kagawa

Aim. We analyzed the pretreatment natural killer (NK) cell functions with the aim of predicting the sustained virological response (SVR) or the interleukin (IL) 28B polymorphism that is strongly associated with the treatment response. *Methods*. The peripheral NK cells from chronic hepatitis patients with HCV genotype 1 and high virus titers were activated using a Toll-like receptor (TLR) 4 ligand and IFN-α. The cell surface markers were evaluated using a flow cytometric analysis, and IFN-γ production was evaluated using an enzyme-linked immunosorbent assay (ELISA). The genotyping of the polymorphisms in the *IL28B* gene region (rs8099917) on chromosome 19 was performed on the DNA collected from each patient. *Results*. The production of IFN-γ was significantly higher in the SVR patients compared with the no-response (NR) patients, whereas the cell surface markers were similar between the SVR and the NR patients. There were no significant differences found in the *IL28B* genotype distribution associated with the production of IFN-γ. *Conclusion*. Differences in the NK cell functions were observed between the SVR patients and the NR patients, suggesting that NK cells play a potential role in the treatment response independent of the *IL28B* genotype.

1. Introduction

The hepatitis C virus (HCV) is the major cause of chronic liver disease, with an estimated global prevalence of 2.5%, that is, 170 million people infected worldwide [1], and is a leading cause of cirrhosis, hepatocellular carcinoma, and liver transplantation [2]. Antiviral treatment, which is based on the combination of pegylated interferon- (IFN-) α and the nucleoside analog ribavirin (RBV), is associated with a sustained virologic response (SVR), that is, serum HCV RNA negatively for 6 months after the cessation of the antiviral therapy.

The HCV genotype, viral load, age, and fibrosis stage are well known as pretreatment variables [3–6]; moreover, single nucleotide polymorphisms (SNPs) located in the region of the interleukin (IL) 28B gene have been strongly associated with an SVR [7, 8]. Although the *IL28B* genotype can be useful when making treatment decisions, this variable alone is not a perfect predictor of the treatment outcome.

The natural killer (NK) cells involved in innate immunity play central roles of defense against viral infections through a direct cytotoxic effect in the destruction of the virus-infected target cells and the production of inflammatory cytokines [9].

Furthermore, in contrast to T cells, NK cells do not require priming for the recognition of the target cells. There has been growing evidence that NK cells have an important role in mediating the IFN-induced viral clearance of chronic HCV infections when the cell surface markers or the cytotoxicity of NK cells is evaluated [10]. Furthermore, we previously demonstrated that activated NK cells have cytotoxity against autologous biliary epithelial cells in the presence of IFN-α [11].

We hypothesize that because NK cells rapidly produce IFN-γ using several cytokines including IFN-α, pretreated changes of NK cells in the presence of an *ex vivo* IFN-α stimulation would become an indicator for the virological response; likewise, insulin resistance is another pretreatment predictor as we previously reported [12]. Furthermore, since the *IL28B* gene has been strongly associated with an acute HCV clearance [13], the relationship between the *IL28B* genotype and the NK cell functions that play a central role in the early phase viral clearance was investigated.

2. Materials and Methods

2.1. Study Subjects. A total of 20 patients with a chronic HCV genotype 1 infection and high viral load (>5.0 log IU/mL) were studied. All of the patients were treatment-naïve prior to their enrollment. The study samples were collected prior to the start of a standard pegylated IFN-α and RBV therapy. The patients who had undetectable HCV RNA for at least 6 months after treatment were classified as sustained viral responders (SVR, $n = 8$); those who had undetectable HCV RNA in the end of the treatment, however, detectable after the treatment, were classified as partial responders (PR, $n = 8$), and those who had persistently detectable HCV RNA during the therapy were classified as null responders (NR, $n = 4$).

All of the subjects gave their written informed consent and the experimental protocols were conducted under the Guidelines of the Research Ethics Committee of Kyushu University.

2.2. IL28B Polymorphism Analysis. The single nucleotide polymorphism (SNP) testing of the *IL28B* gene (rs8099917) was completed for all of the patients using a real-time PCR method on the genomic DNA extracted from the whole blood samples. The heterozygotes (TGs) or the homozygotes (GGs) of the minor allele (G) were described as having the *IL28B* minor allele, whereas the homozygotes for the major allele (TT) were described as having the *IL28B* major allele [7].

2.3. Isolation of Peripheral Blood Mononuclear Cells and NK Cells. The peripheral blood mononuclear cells (PBMCs) were separated from the heparinized fresh blood using a Ficoll-Isopaque gradient centrifugation technique. The NK cells were negatively isolated from the PBMC using magnetic beads (NK isolation kit; Miltenyi Biotec, Auburn, CA, USA). A viability of >95% using a trypan blue dye exclusion technique and a purity of >90% using flow cytometry for CD56 positives were considered to be acceptable [11].

2.4. IFN-γ Production from NK Cells. In an effort to identify the nature of the cytokines that were involved in promoting the NK cell effector function, the supernatants from the NK cells that have been cultured for 2 days with or without pegylated IFN-α (3 μg/mL, Schering-Plough, Kenilworth, NJ, USA) and lipopolysaccharide (LPS) (10 μg/mL, Invitrogen, San Diego, CA, USA) were analyzed for the production of IFN-γ. Pegylated IFN-α instead of IFN-α was used as pegylated IFN-α working *in vivo* during the standard pegylated IFN-α and RBV therapy. The assays were performed using a sandwich ELISA (R&D Systems, Minneapolis, MN, USA) with a combination of unlabeled and biotin-coupled or enzyme-coupled monoclonal antibodies to each cytokine. Both of the activated and the resting NK cells were evaluated for cell surface markers.

2.5. Flow Cytometric Analysis of the Cell Surface Antigens. In order to evaluate the cell surface antigen expression in the PBMC and NK cells (1×10^6), the cells were stained at 4°C in the dark for 30 min, washed twice in 2 mL of a phosphate-buffered saline containing 1% bovine serum albumin and 0.01% sodium azide, and were fixed in 500 μL of 1% paraformaldehyde. The cells were stained for CD3, CD16, and CD56 (BD Biosciences, San Diego, CA, USA). A two-color flow cytometry was performed using an FACSnCalibur Flow Cytometer (BD Biosciences).

2.6. Statistical Analysis. All of the experiments were performed in triplicate and the data points shown are the mean values of the results of these triplicates. The comparisons between the points for certain data sets were expressed as the mean ± standard deviation (SD), and the significance of differences was determined by Student's t-test. All of the analyses were 2-tailed and the P values <0.05 were considered to be significant. The statistical analyses were performed using the Intercooled Stata 8.0 software program (StataCorp, College Station, TX, USA).

3. Results

3.1. Subjects. The characteristics of patients who were undergoing the standard pegylated IFN-α and RBV combined therapy are summarized in Table 1. Patients who experienced a relapse following the administration of the standard therapy (partial responders) were excluded from this study. As expected, the *IL28B* TT genotype was dominant in the SVR patients (75%) and not dominant in the PR patients (50%) or the NR patients (50%).

3.2. Phenotypes and IFN-γ Production in NK Cells before and after IFN-α Stimulation. In order to evaluate the role of NK cells, we enriched the NK cells from the PBMC using magnetic beads. The CD3 positive fraction was completely eliminated during the isolation of the NK cells (Figure 1). The NK cells were incubated with or without LPS and IFN-α for 2 days, as the NK cells could not produce detectable amounts of IFN-γ solely with IFN-α. CD56 bright NK cells increased after stimulation (Figures 2(a) and 2(b)).

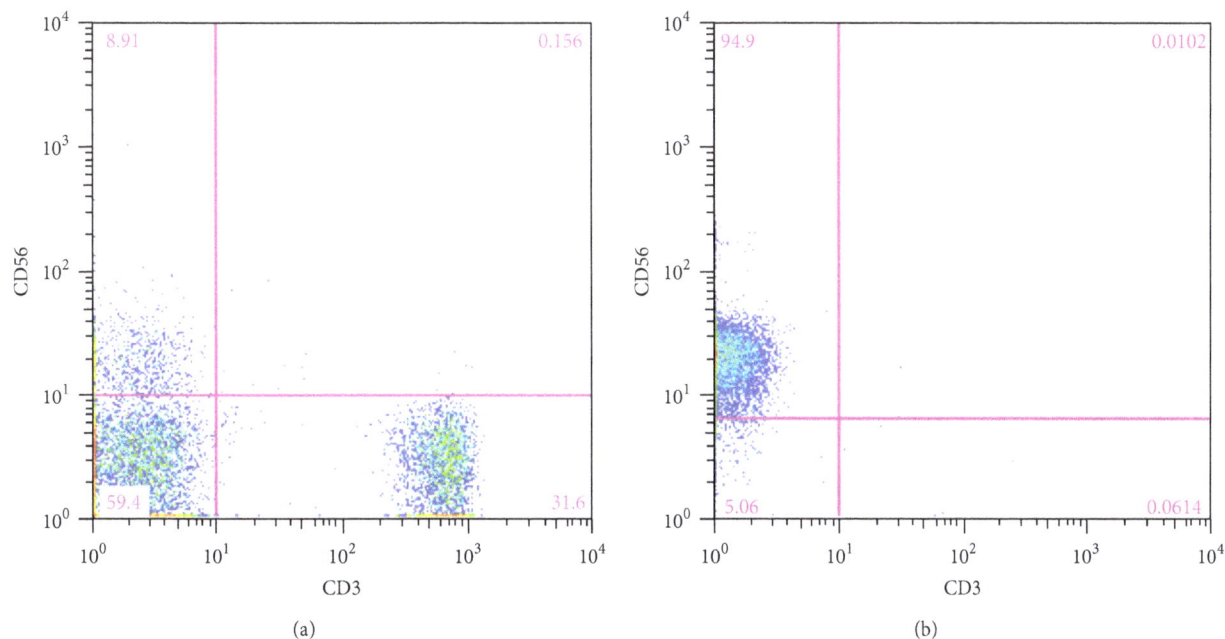

(a)   (b)

FIGURE 1: The isolation of the NK cells. The cell surface markers were determined in the PBMC using flow cytometry. (a) The PBMC constituted of CD3+CD56− cells (31.6%), CD3−CD56− cells (59.4%), CD3−CD56+ cells (8.91%), and CD3+CD56+ cells (0.2%). (b) Following the NK cell isolation, the number of CD3 positive cells had clearly decreased.

TABLE 1: Clinical features classified by the SVR status of chronic hepatitis C patients with genotype 1.

Sex	Age (yr)	ALT (IU/L)	g-GTP (IU/L)	Plt (10⁹/L)	IL-28B (rs8099917)	Response
M	59	63	33	20	TT	SVR
M	50	31	31	20.2	TT	SVR
M	69	35	27	17.3	TT	SVR
M	31	61	25	18.5	TT	SVR
F	69	125	157	16.3	TT	SVR
M	55	66	132	18.4	TT	SVR
M	67	119	61	20.2	TG	SVR
F	52	178	101	16.1	TG	SVR
F	37	45	65	18.7	TT	NR
F	43	65	128	13.4	TT	NR
M	29	79	147	20.2	TG	NR
F	68	76	76	7.9	TG	NR
M	43	112	62	18.2	TT	PR
M	51	84	59	17.7	TT	PR
F	38	31	30	20.1	TT	PR
F	63	72	33	15.9	TT	PR
M	62	44	48	12.2	TG	PR
M	66	38	52	11.8	TG	PR
M	54	50	32	18.8	TG	PR
F	60	77	43	13.8	GG	PR

The NK cells were classified as CD56+CD16−, CD56−CD16+, and CD56+CD16+ phenotypes (Figure 2(c)) and these phenotypes changed after stimulation (Figure 2(d)).

The frequency of the CD56+CD16+ NK cells was similar in SVR patients (before stimulation: 81.1 ± 4.2%, after stimulation: 61.7 ± 8.0%), PR patients (before stimulation: 69.4 ± 7.9%, after stimulation: 71.8 ± 7.4%), and NR patients (before stimulation: 81.6 ± 5.7%, after stimulation: 62.7 ± 14.2%) (Figure 3(a)). The same tendency was observed for CD56+CD16− in SVR patients (before stimulation: 7.3 ± 3.0%, after stimulation: 19.4 ± 6.1%), PR patients (before stimulation: 7.8±2.5%, after stimulation: 16.5±3.6%), and NR patients (before stimulation: 10.3 ± 4.3%, after stimulation: 28.8 ± 13.7%) (Figure 3(b)) and for CD56−CD16+ in SVR patients (before stimulation: 9.5 ± 2.6%, after stimulation: 4.5 ± 2.7%), PR patients (before stimulation: 6.3 ± 2.0%, after stimulation: 7.1 ± 1.8%), and NR patients (before stimulation: 6.1 ± 4.4%, after stimulation: 5.6 ± 3.2%) (Figure 3(c)). In the CD56+CD16− fraction, the frequency was increased after stimulation regardless of the treatment response. Conversely, the IFN-γ production from the stimulated NK cells was higher in the SVR patients (894 ± 215 pg/mL) compared with the NR patients (668 ± 119 pg/mL; $P < 0.05$) and similar to the PR patients (804 ± 225 pg/mL) (Figure 3(d)). Prior to the IFN-α stimulation, the NK cells from the SVR, PR, and NR patients did not produce any detectable IFN-γ levels (data not shown).

3.3. Phenotypes and IFN-γ Production in NK Cells according to the IL28B Genotype.

We also classified the above results according to IL28B genotype. The frequency of CD56+CD16+ NK cells was similar in patients with IL28B TT (before stimulation: 77.1 ± 8.4%, after stimulation: 71.5 ± 6.2%) and patients with IL28B TG (before stimulation: 71.4 ± 12.4%, after stimulation: 61.9 ± 11.8%) (Figure 4(a)). The same

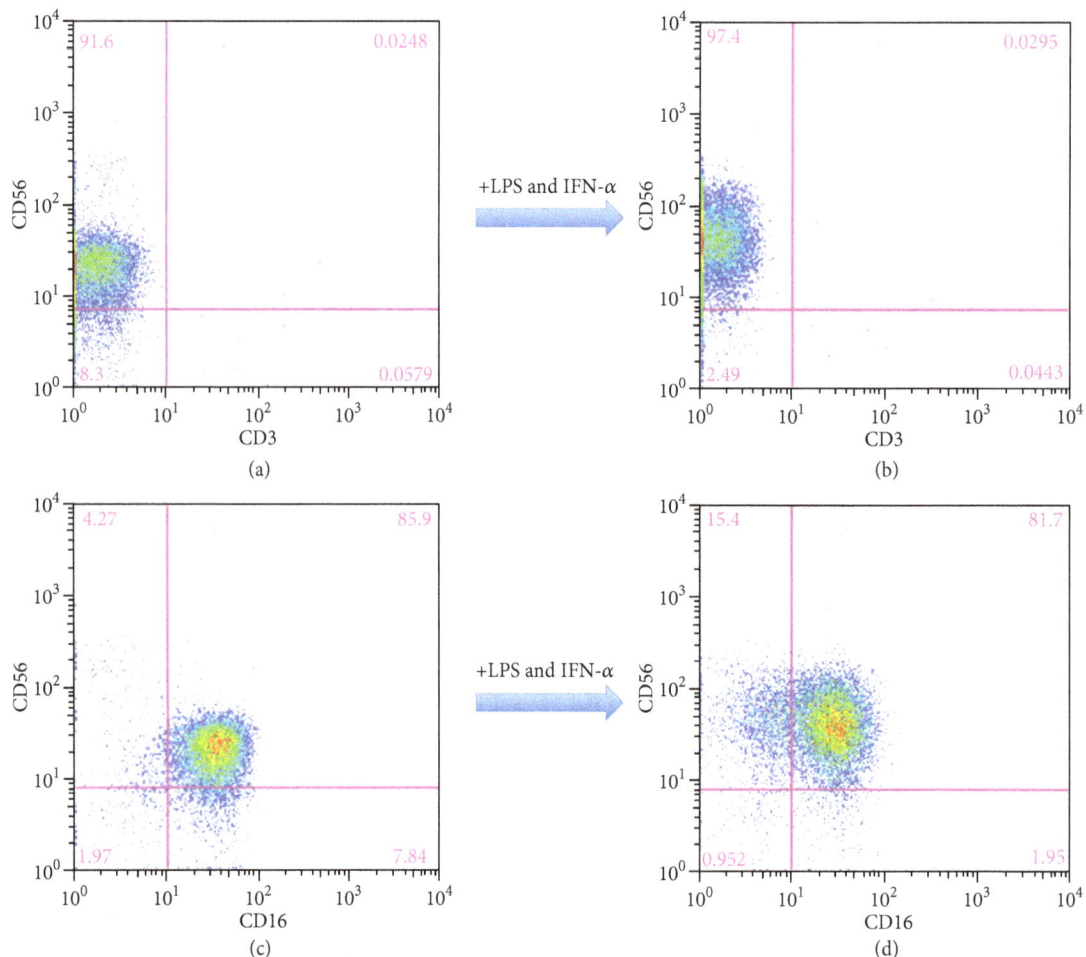

FIGURE 2: The surface markers of the NK cells before and after stimulation. The isolated NK cells were rested or stimulated with LPS and IFN-α for 2 days. Between (a) and (b), the CD3 and CD56 markers on the NK cells were not changed after stimulation. At (c), the resting NK cells were characterized as CD56+CD16− cells (4.3%), CD56+CD16+ cells (85.9%), and CD56−CD16+ cells (7.8%). At (d), the stimulated NK cells were characterized as CD56+CD16− cells (15.4%), CD56+CD16+ cells (81.7%), and CD56−CD16+ cells (2.0%).

tendency was observed for CD56+CD16− in patients with *IL28B* TT (before stimulation: 8.2 ± 2.8%, after stimulation: 15.1 ± 7.3%) and patients with *IL28B* TG (before stimulation: 12.7 ± 5.6%, after stimulation: 22.9 ± 12.0%) (Figure 4(b)). The same tendency was observed for CD56−CD16+ in patients with *IL28B* TT (before stimulation: 8.2 ± 3.1%, after stimulation: 4.9 ± 2.6%) and patients with *IL28B* TG (before stimulation: 6.9 ± 2.7%, after stimulation: 6.7 ± 2.6%) (Figure 3(c)). Regardless of the SVR, PR, or NR classification, the IFN-γ production from activated NK cells was similar in patients with *IL28B* TT (833 ± 225 pg/mL) and patients with *IL28B* TG (783 ± 204 pg/mL) (Figure 4(d)).

4. Discussion

Because the NK cell cytotoxicity and the presence of cell surface markers correlate with the virological response, NK cells can serve as biomarkers of a patient's IFN-α responsiveness [14, 15]. In addition, the IFN-α-induced modulation of the signal transducer and activator of transcription (STAT) 1 and STAT 4 phosphorylation underlies the polarization of the NK cells

in an HCV infection [16–18]. During the IFN-α treatment, the polarized NK cells are recruited from the peripheral blood into the liver [19]. Therefore, it may be inappropriate to evaluate the peripheral NK cells for the general functions of the NK cells that are undergoing treatment. To this end, we collected the peripheral NK cells prior to treatment and evaluated the NK cell functions with IFN-α *ex vivo* with the aim of predicting the virological responses. Although the interactions between the killer cell Ig-like receptors (KIRs) expressed on NK cells and the HLA expressed on target cells are well known to play a key role in NK cell activation, it is difficult to obtain HCV-infected autologous target cells for the evaluation of the cytotoxicity of the NK cells. Therefore, we instead evaluated the IFN-γ production relating to the NK cell functions.

It has been previously reported that a polarized NK cell phenotype can be induced by a chronic exposure to HCV-induced IFN-α, contributing to liver injury through tumor necrosis factor-related apoptosis inducing ligand (TRAIL) expression and cytotoxicity [20]. Therefore, we hypothesized that we could predict an outcome of SVR or NR according

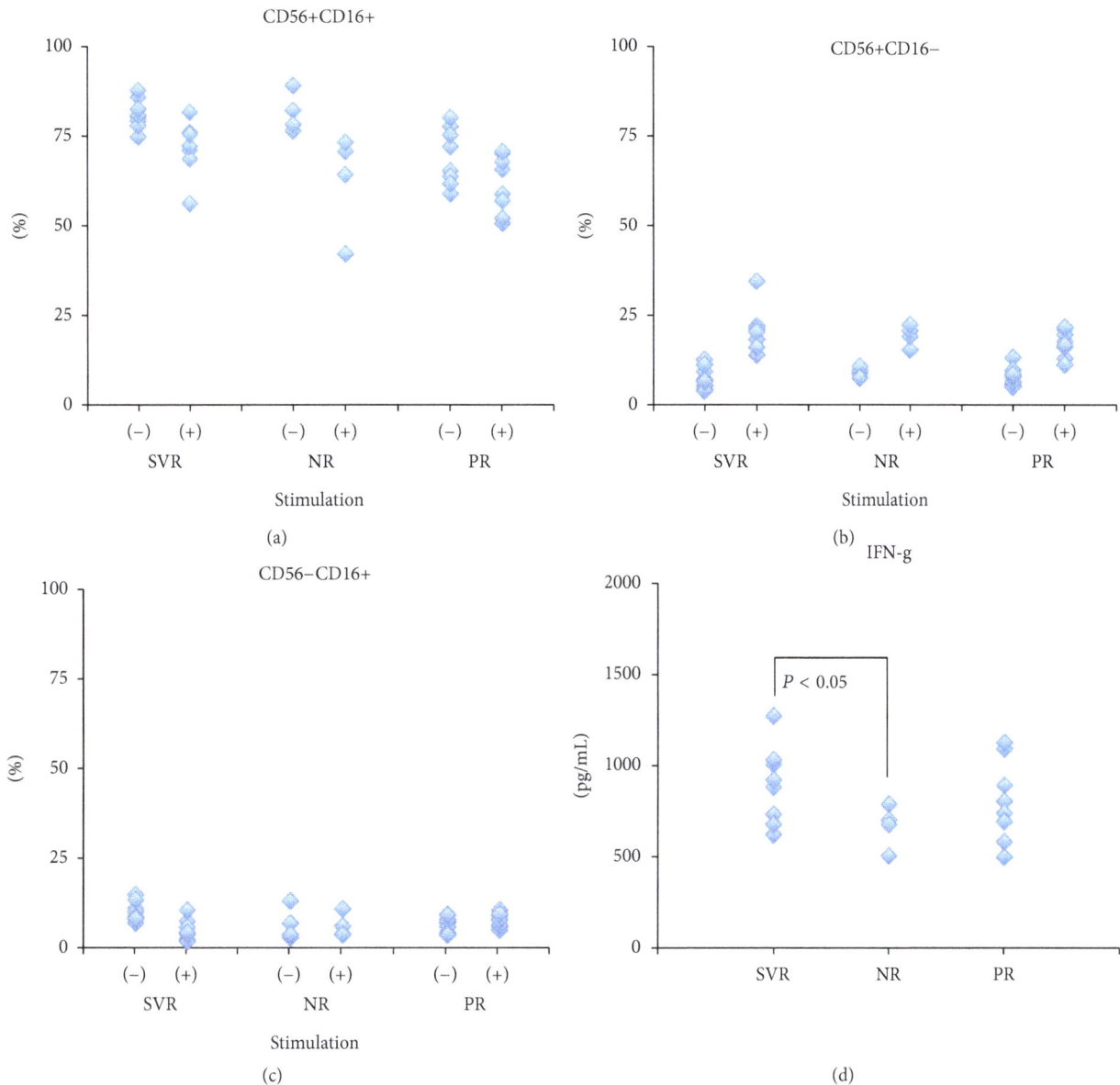

FIGURE 3: The characterization of the before and after stimulation NK cells, as classified by the SVR and NR grouping. Between (a) and (c), there were no statistically significant differences between the SVR and NR groups associated with the cell surface markers on the NK cells. However, the NK cells from the SVR group did produce higher amounts of IFN-γ than those from the NR group ($P < 0.05$) (d).

to the INF-γ production from NK cells with or without LPS and IFN-α exposure. Previous reports have compared the effects of the IL-12 and IL-15 induction of NK cells, and, to this end, we prepared nonstimulated NK cells and IFN-α stimulated NK cells with LPS. We evaluated NK cell function in 20 patients (8 SVR, 8 PR, and 4 NR patients). The study size was small to evaluate NK cell function fully; however, we found that we could not predict an outcome of SVR according to the changes in cell surface markers, and, furthermore, the NK cell phenotype and function did not differ among the subgroups with different *IL28B* genotypes as had been previously reported [21]. These findings are consistent with the fact that NK cells do not respond to IFN-α via different signal transductions of type III IFN (including

IL28B) [22, 23]. Additionally, there were no differences of this IFN-γ production between the patients with early virologic response (EVR) and no-EVR or rapid virologic response RVR and no-RVR (data not shown). This suggests that IFN-γ production from peripheral NK cells does not correlate sharply with the declining dose of HCV-RNA for the initial 2 or 4 weeks of pegylated IFN-α and RBV treatment.

As the NK cells kill the target cells through the directed release of perforin, granzyme-containing granules, and TRAIL which is associated with the control of an HCV infection [24], the combined effects of KIR, TRAIL, and *IL28B* in the context of IFN treatment are possible [25]. However, the evaluation of these effects would require additional studies with a larger number of patients. In addition, while

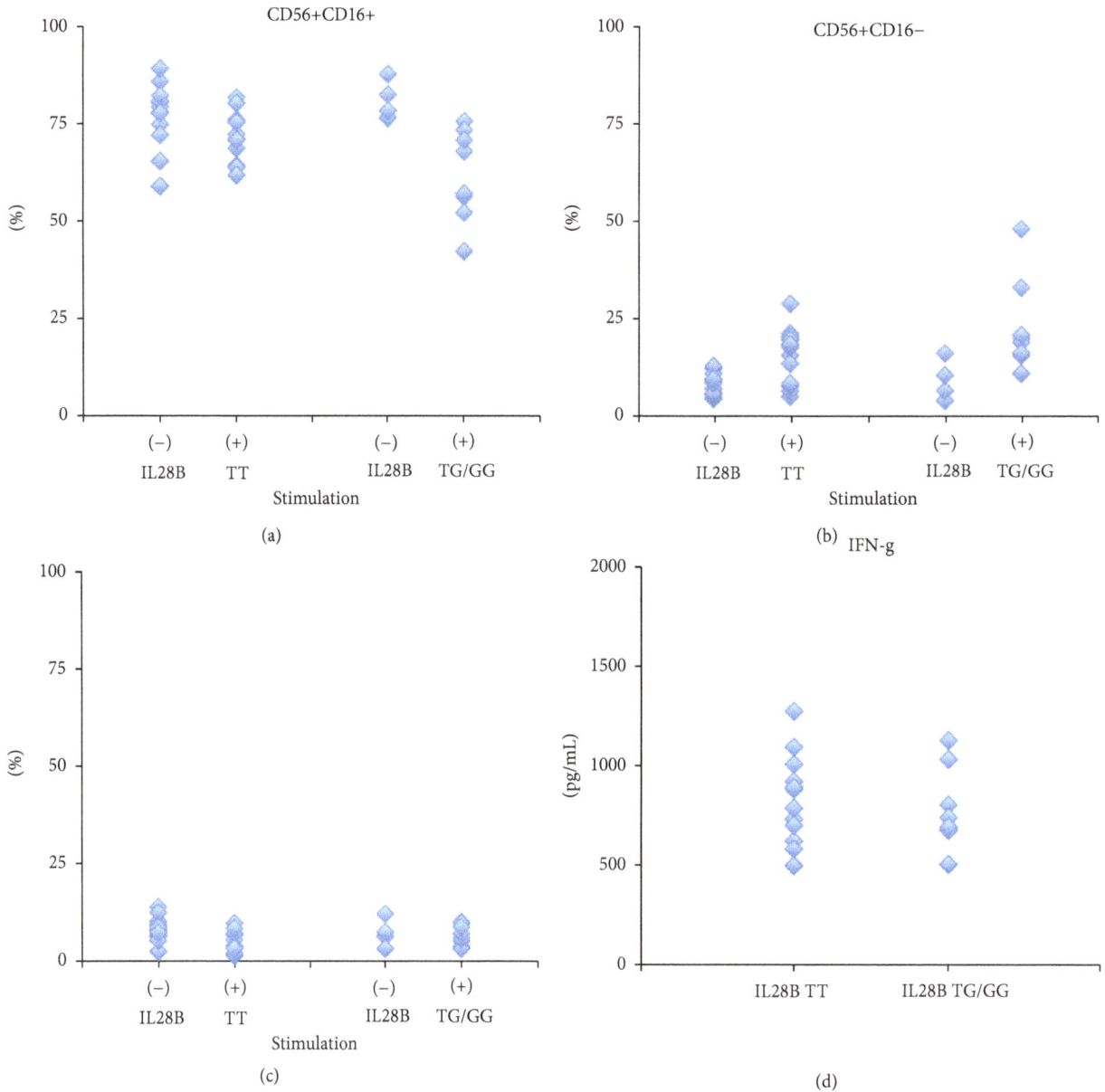

FIGURE 4: The characterization of the before and after stimulation NK cells, as classified by the *IL28B* TT and *IL28B* TG grouping. Between (a) and (c), there were no statistically significant differences noted between the *IL28B* TT and *IL28B* TG groups for the cell surface markers on the NK cells. Additionally, the NK cells from the *IL28B* TT group do not produce high amounts of IFN-γ when compared to the members of the *IL28B* TG group (d).

the different inhibitory/activating receptors on the NK cells are well known to be associated with antiviral activity [26–29], further evaluations of the related cell surface markers must be performed.

In conclusion, these results demonstrate that the *ex vivo* NK cell response may serve as a biomarker for IFN-α treatment responsiveness independent of the *IL28B* genotype.

References

[1] C. W. Shepard, L. Finelli, and M. J. Alter, "Global epidemiology of hepatitis C virus infection," *Lancet Infectious Diseases*, vol. 5, no. 9, pp. 558–567, 2005.

[2] G. L. Davis, J. E. Albright, S. F. Cook, and D. M. Rosenberg, "Projecting future complications of chronic hepatitis C in the United States," *Liver Transplantation*, vol. 9, no. 4, pp. 331–338, 2003.

[3] E. Ogawa, N. Furusyo, K. Toyoda, H. Takeoka, S. Maeda, and J. Hayashi, "The longitudinal quantitative assessment by transient elastography of chronic hepatitis C patients treated with pegylated interferon alpha-2b and ribavirin," *Antiviral Research*, vol. 83, no. 2, pp. 127–134, 2009.

[4] M. Kainuma, N. Furusyo, E. Kajiwara et al., "Pegylated interferon α-2b plus ribavirin for older patients with chronic hepatitis C," *World Journal of Gastroenterology*, vol. 16, no. 35, pp. 4400–4409, 2010.

[5] M. Kainuma, N. Furusyo, K. Azuma et al., "Pegylated interferon α-2b plus ribavirin for Japanese chronic hepatitis C patients with normal alanine aminotransferase," *Hepatology Research*, vol. 42, no. 1, pp. 33–41, 2012.

[6] N. Furusyo, M. Katoh, Y. Tanabe et al., "Interferon alpha plus ribavirin combination treatment of Japanese chronic hepatitis C patients with HCV genotype 2: a project of the Kyushu University Liver Disease Study Group," *World Journal of Gastroenterology*, vol. 12, no. 5, pp. 784–790, 2006.

[7] Y. Tanaka, N. Nishida, M. Sugiyama et al., "Genome-wide association of IL28B with response to pegylated interferon-α and ribavirin therapy for chronic hepatitis C," *Nature Genetics*, vol. 41, no. 10, pp. 1105–1109, 2009.

[8] D. Ge, J. Fellay, A. J. Thompson et al., "Genetic variation in IL28B predicts hepatitis C treatment-induced viral clearance," *Nature*, vol. 461, no. 7262, pp. 399–401, 2009.

[9] M. B. Lodoen and L. L. Lanier, "Viral modulation of NK cell immunity," *Nature Reviews Microbiology*, vol. 3, no. 1, pp. 59–69, 2005.

[10] A. Ahmad and F. Alvarez, "Role of NK and NKT cells in the immunopathogenesis of HCV-induced hepatitis," *Journal of Leukocyte Biology*, vol. 76, no. 4, pp. 743–759, 2004.

[11] S. Shimoda, K. Harada, H. Niiro et al., "Interaction between Toll-like receptors and natural killer cells in the destruction of bile ducts in primary biliary cirrhosis," *Hepatology*, vol. 53, no. 4, pp. 1270–1281, 2011.

[12] E. Ogawa, N. Furusyo, M. Murata et al., "Insulin resistance undermines the advantages of IL28B polymorphism in the pegylated interferon alpha-2b and ribavirin treatment of chronic hepatitis C patients with genotype 1," *Journal of Hepatology*, vol. 57, no. 3, pp. 534–540, 2012.

[13] D. L. Thomas, C. L. Thio, M. P. Martin et al., "Genetic variation in IL28B and spontaneous clearance of hepatitis C virus," *Nature*, vol. 461, no. 7265, pp. 798–801, 2009.

[14] K. Cheent and S. I. Khakoo, "Natural killer cells and hepatitis C: action and reaction," *Gut*, vol. 60, no. 2, pp. 268–278, 2011.

[15] S. Jost and M. Altfeld, "Control of human viral infections by natural killer cells," *Annual Review of Immunology*, vol. 31, pp. 163–194, 2013.

[16] T. Miyagi, T. Takehara, K. Nishio et al., "Altered interferon-α-signaling in natural killer cells from patients with chronic hepatitis C virus infection," *Journal of Hepatology*, vol. 53, no. 3, pp. 424–430, 2010.

[17] B. Edlich, G. Ahlenstiel, A. Z. Azpiroz et al., "Early changes in interferon signaling define natural killer cell response and refractoriness to interferon-based therapy of hepatitis C patients," *Hepatology*, vol. 55, no. 1, pp. 39–48, 2012.

[18] D. D. Anthony, S. J. Conry, K. Medvik et al., "Baseline levels of soluble CD14 and CD16+56– natural killer cells are negatively associated with response to interferon/ribavirin therapy during HCV-HIV-1 coinfection," *Journal of Infectious Diseases*, vol. 206, no. 6, pp. 969–973, 2012.

[19] G. Ahlenstiel, B. Edlich, L. J. Hogdal et al., "Early changes in natural killer cell function indicate virologic response to interferon therapy for hepatitis C," *Gastroenterology*, vol. 141, no. 4, pp. 1231–e2, 2011.

[20] G. Ahlenstiel, R. H. Titerence, C. Koh et al., "Natural killer cells are polarized toward cytotoxicity in chronic hepatitis C in an interferon-alfa-dependent manner," *Gastroenterology*, vol. 138, no. 1, pp. 325–335, 2010.

[21] B. Oliviero, D. Mele, E. Degasperi et al., "Natural killer cell dynamic profile is associated with treatment outcome in patients with chronic HCV infection," *Journal of Hepatology*, vol. 59, no. 1, pp. 38–44, 2013.

[22] S. I. Khakoo, C. L. Thio, M. P. Martin et al., "HLA and NK cell inhibitory receptor genes in resolving hepatitis C virus infection," *Science*, vol. 305, no. 5685, pp. 872–874, 2004.

[23] T. Marcello, A. Grakoui, G. Barba-Spaeth et al., "Interferons alpha and lambda inhibit hepatitis C virus replication with distinct signal transduction and gene regulation kinetics," *Gastroenterology*, vol. 131, no. 6, pp. 1887–1898, 2006.

[24] K. A. Stegmann, N. K. Björkström, H. Veber et al., "Interferon-alpha-induced TRAIL on natural killer cells is associated with control of hepatitis C virus infection," *Gastroenterology*, vol. 138, no. 5, pp. 1885–e10, 2010.

[25] M. M. Dring, M. H. Morrison, B. P. McSharry et al., "Innate immune genes synergize to predict increased risk of chronic disease in hepatitis C virus infection," *Proceedings of the National Academy of Sciences of the United States of America*, vol. 108, no. 14, pp. 5736–5741, 2011.

[26] L. Golden-Mason, A. E. Stone, K. M. Bambha, L. Cheng, and H. R. Rosen, "Race- and gender-related variation in natural killer p46 expression associated with differential anti-hepatitis C virus immunity," *Hepatology*, vol. 56, no. 4, pp. 1214–1222, 2012.

[27] B. Krämer, C. Körner, M. Kebschull et al., "Natural killer p46High expression defines a natural killer cell subset that is potentially involved in control of hepatitis C virus replication and modulation of liver fibrosis," *Hepatology*, vol. 56, no. 4, pp. 1201–1213, 2012.

[28] L. Golden-Mason, K. M. Bambha, L. Cheng et al., "Natural killer inhibitory receptor expression associated with treatment failure and interleukin-28B genotype in patients with chronic hepatitis C," *Hepatology*, vol. 54, no. 5, pp. 1559–1569, 2011.

[29] F. Bozzano, A. Picciotto, P. Costa et al., "Activating NK cell receptor expression/function (NKp30, NKp46, DNAM-1) during chronic viraemic HCV infection is associated with the outcome of combined treatment," *European Journal of Immunology*, vol. 41, no. 10, pp. 2905–2914, 2011.

Elevation in Serum Concentration of Bone-Specific Alkaline Phosphatase without Elevation in Serum Creatinine Concentration Secondary to Adefovir Dipivoxil Therapy in Chronic Hepatitis B Virus Infection

Hiroshi Abe, Nobuyoshi Seki, Tomonori Sugita, Yuta Aida, Haruya Ishiguro, Tamihiro Miyazaki, Munenori Itagaki, Satoshi Sutoh, and Yoshio Aizawa

Division of Gastroenterology and Hepatology, Department of Internal Medicine, Jikei University School of Medicine Katsushika Medical Center, Katsushika-ku, Tokyo 125-8506, Japan

Correspondence should be addressed to Hiroshi Abe; hiroshiabe43222@yahoo.co.jp

Academic Editor: Piero Luigi Almasio

Of 168 patients with chronic hepatitis B virus (HBV) infection-related liver disease, 20 patients who had received 100 mg of lamivudine plus 10 mg/day of adefovir dipivoxil (ADV) (ADV group) and 124 patients who had received 0.5 mg/day of entecavir or 100 mg/day of lamivudine (non-ADV group) for >1 year were enrolled. For comparative analyses, 19 well-matched pairs were obtained from the groups by propensity scores. At the time of enrollment, serum creatinine and phosphate concentrations were similar between the ADV and non-ADV groups; however, urinary phosphate ($P = 0.0424$) and serum bone-specific alkaline phosphatase (BAP) ($P = 0.0228$) concentrations were significantly higher in the ADV group than in the non-ADV group. Serum BAP was significantly higher at the time of enrollment than before ADV administration in the ADV group ($P = 0.0001$), although there was no significant change in serum BAP concentration in the non-ADV group. There was a significant positive correlation between the period of ADV therapy and ΔBAP ($R^2 = 0.2959$, $P = 0.0160$). Serum BAP concentration increased before increase in serum creatinine concentration and was useful for early detection of adverse events and for developing adequate measures for continuing ADV for chronic HBV infection-related liver disease.

1. Introduction

Chronic hepatitis B virus (HBV) infection causing chronic hepatitis, cirrhosis, and hepatocellular carcinoma affects more than 350 million people worldwide [1, 2]. Antiviral therapies that contain interferon and nucleos(t)ide analogues are used in patients who are infected with HBV and are at a higher risk of developing cirrhosis and hepatocellular carcinoma [1, 3, 4]. The purpose of the treatment is to suppress HBV replication and to prevent mortality associated with disease progression to end-stage liver disease and major complications [4, 5]. Currently, 5 oral nucleos(t)ide analogues are approved for the treatment of liver disease related to chronic HBV infection in Europe and USA, although only 3 nucleos(t)ide analogues, namely, lamivudine (LAM), entecavir (ETV), and adefovir dipivoxil (ADV), are approved for

use in Japan. LAM, the first approved nucleoside analogue for chronic HBV infection-related liver disease, suppresses HBV replication and improves hepatic inflammation in most patients [6]. However, more than 60% of patients with chronic HBV infection who receive long-term LAM therapy become resistant to the agent within 4 years of starting the therapy [7]. For patients with LAM resistance, virological breakthrough due to development of ADV-resistant mutations occurred in 21% of 14 patients within 18 months after changing to ADV monotherapy [8]; ETV-resistant mutations were found in 8% of 151 patients 2 years after changing to ETV monotherapy (1 mg once per day) [9]. Therefore, LAM monotherapy has not been used for patients with chronic HBV infection since ETV was approved. In patients with LAM resistance, tenofovir (TDF, not yet approved for use in Japan) or ADV therapy is advised [10].

The appearance of virological and biochemical breakthroughs during combination therapy with ADV and LAM is very rare in patients with LAM resistance; therefore, combination therapy is recommended in such cases [11, 12]. At present, combination therapy with ADV and LAM must be continued for a long period of time, even though long-term use of ADV is associated with a slight risk of renal toxicity [13, 14]. Although ADV has a favorable risk/benefit profile with little or no evidence of renal toxicity after 48 weeks of low-dose treatment (10 mg per day) [15, 16], some studies have reported development of severe osteomalacia caused by renal tubular dysfunction (Fanconi syndrome) after long-term use of ADV [17, 18]. Therefore, establishment of a protocol is required for early identification of osteomalacia caused by renal tubular dysfunction during the administration of ADV. Serum bone-specific alkaline phosphatase (BAP) is the most commonly used bone disease marker in hemodialyzed patients [19]. Serum BAP levels increase gradually in osteomalacia secondary to the administration of ADV, without increase in serum creatinine concentration [17, 18]. Therefore, serum BAP concentration may be a potentially useful marker for early detection of osteomalacia caused by renal impairment secondary to the administration of ADV.

To determine the significance of these indicators for the management of patients receiving long-term ADV plus LAM therapy, we evaluated bone metabolism markers, including serum and urinary phosphate concentrations and serum BAP, in chronic hepatitis B (CHB) patients receiving nucleos(t)ide analogues.

2. Materials and Methods

2.1. Patients. This study complies with the standards of the 1975 Declaration of Helsinki and current ethical guidelines; written informed consent was obtained from each patient.

Between August 2003 and January 2012, 168 consecutive patients positive for hepatitis B surface antigen (HBsAg), who presented to the Division of Gastroenterology and Hepatology of our institution, received nucleos(t)ide analogue therapy. Among them, 144 consecutive patients who received ADV or the other nucleoside analogues (LAM or ETV) for more than 1 year were enrolled. Most patients had HBV genotype B or C, as seen in a previous Japanese study [12]. Of these, 20 patients had received a combination of 100 mg of LAM plus 10 mg of ADV per day (ADV group), and 124 patients had received either 100 mg of LAM per day or 0.5 mg of ETV (non-ADV group). Patients in the ADV group received additional ADV because of increase in serum HBV DNA levels ($\geq 1 \log_{10}$ copies/mL) during LAM monotherapy. The non-ADV group included 34 patients who started LAM therapy (100 mg per day) but had been subsequently switched to ETV therapy (0.5 mg per day) to avoid the appearance of LAM-refractory HBV. This group also included 90 patients who had received 0.5 mg of ETV per day as a first-line therapy. Exclusion criteria were as follows: presence of antibodies to hepatitis C virus or HIV; a current alcohol consumption of >20 g/day; and presence of hepatocellular carcinoma, other liver diseases, progressive decompensated liver cirrhosis, or renal dysfunction at the time of starting nucleos(t)ide analogue therapy (serum creatinine: male, >1.3 mg/dL; female, >1.1 mg/dL). Patients who had hypertension [20] and/or diabetes mellitus [21] were also excluded from this study owing to the risk of renal impairment. In addition, patients who were receiving vitamin D were excluded from this study because this therapy may affect bone turnover. All blood samples were obtained from patients after fasting.

To reduce the confounding effects of covariates, we used propensity scores [22, 23] to match the ADV group to the non-ADV group during nucleos(t)ide analogue therapy based on the stage of liver disease at the time of enrollment and renal function at the time of receiving the nucleos(t)ide analogue. Variables that may have influenced the treatment outcomes, including age, sex, the duration of nucleos(t)ide analogue therapy, platelet count, serum alanine aminotransferase (ALT), serum albumin at the time of enrollment (nucleos(t)ide analogue therapy for >1 year), and serum creatinine level at the time of receiving nucleos(t)ide analogues, were used to generate a propensity score ranging from 0 to 1 by logistic regression. The nearest available match on the estimated propensity score was used to select participants in the ADV group and find participants in the non-ADV group with the closest propensity scores. Nineteen well-matched pairs of patients in the ADV and non-ADV groups were obtained.

2.2. Analysis of Serological and DNA Markers for HBV. HBsAg in patients' sera was tested by enzyme immunoassay using commercially available kits (Dainabott, Tokyo, Japan). The serum HBV DNA concentration was monitored using a polymerase chain reaction assay (COBAS Amplicor HBV monitor test, Roche Diagnostics K. K., Tokyo, Japan; lower limit of detection, 2.6 log copies/mL) before November 2007 and by another polymerase chain reaction assay (COBAS AmpliPrep-COBAS Taqman HBV Test, Roche Diagnostics K. K.; lower limit of detection, 2.1 log copies/mL) after December 2007. YMDD mutations were detected using a line probe assay (INNO-LiPA HBV DR assay, Innogenetics NV).

2.3. Examination of Bone Turnover Markers. Serum BAP was measured at the time of enrollment and before nucleos(t)ide analogue administration using a commercially available polyacrylamide-gel (PAG) disk electrophoresis kit designed for use in humans (AlkPhor System, Jokoh Co. Ltd, Tokyo, Japan) using serum stored at −30°C.

Serum levels of intact parathyroid hormone (PTH) were measured using an electrochemiluminescence immunoassay (Roche Diagnostics K. K.), and urinary cross-linked N-telopeptide of type I collagen (NTX) was measured using an ELISA (Osteomark, Inverness Medical Innovations Inc., Waltham, MA, USA) at the time of enrollment.

ΔBAP, a sensitive marker reflecting the changes in bone metabolism, was calculated as follows: serum BAP concentration at the time of enrollment minus serum BAP concentration before administration of nucleos(t)ide analogues. ΔBAP was then compared with the length of nucleos(t)ide analogue therapy.

TABLE 1: Baseline clinical characteristics of 144 patients received nucleos(t)de analogues with chronic HBV-infected liver disease at the time of enrollment.

	Median (range)		P value
	ADV group ($n = 20$)	Non-ADV group ($n = 124$)	
At the time of enrollment			
Age (yr)	52 (29–78)	55 (28–83)	0.8368
Sex (male/female)	15/5	82/42	0.5974
HBV genotype (A/B/C/F/n.d)	2/2/12/1/3	3/26/65/0/30	0.8671
HBV DNA ($\log_{10}$ copies/mL)	2.1 > (negative–3.0)	2.1 > (negative–6.2)	0.1896
Platelet count ($\times 10^3/m^3$)	16.5 (10.2–31.0)	16.8 (3.4–31.5)	0.1987
ALT (IU/L)	26 (10–60)	20 (8–124)	0.1117
Alb (g/dL)	4.4 (4–5.3)	4.4 (1.8–5.2)	0.9154
Cirrhosis (presence/absence)	5/15	30/94	0.8392
At the time of starting ADV or ETV			
Serum creatinine (mg/dL)	0.8 (0.6–1.2)	0.76 (0.52–1.30)	0.3853
Follow-up duration (month)	103 (37–141)	40 (12–152)	$8.1E - 09$
Duration of nucleos(t)ide analogue therapy (month)	103 (37–141)	34 (12–117)	$9.8E - 10$
Duration of adefovir administration (month)	73 (12–107)		
Propensity score	0.197 (0.068–0.553)	0.108 ($3.49E - 05$–0.514)	0.0018

ADV: adefovir dipivoxil; non-ADV: lamivudine or entecavir.

2.4. Other Markers in Serum and Urine. Levels of phosphate and creatinine were examined at the time of enrollment and before nucleos(t)ide analogue administration using serum stored at −30°C. Levels of urinary phosphate were examined at the time of enrollment.

2.5. Statistical Analysis. Data are presented as median values (range). The Mann-Whitney U test and Wilcoxon rank-sum test were used to analyze continuous variables. Fisher's exact test was used for analysis of categorical data. All tests of significance were two tailed, and a P value of <0.05 was considered significant. All statistical analyses were performed using STATISTICA for Windows version 6 (StatSoft, Oklahoma, USA).

3. Results

3.1. Characteristics of 19 Well-Matched Pairs in the ADV and Non-ADV Groups. The baseline characteristics of the 144 patients enrolled in the study are summarized in Table 1. There were no significant differences with respect to age, sex, duration of nucleos(t)ide analogue therapy, platelet count, serum ALT, serum albumin, total bilirubin at the time of enrollment, and serum creatinine level at the time of nucleos(t)ide analogue administration between the ADV and non-ADV groups (Table 2).

3.2. Markers in Serum and Urine at the Time of Enrollment. There was no difference in serum creatinine concentration between the ADV and non-ADV groups at the time of enrollment. Serum phosphate concentration tended to be lower in the ADV group, although the difference was not statistically significant. In contrast, urinary phosphate concentration was

significantly higher in the ADV group than in the non-ADV group ($P = 0.0424$). There was no significant difference between the ADV and non-ADV groups in the concentration of serum alkaline phosphatase (ALP) isoenzyme 2, which is liver specific; however, serum BAP concentration was significantly higher in the ADV group than in the non-ADV group ($P = 0.0228$) (Figure 1).

There were no significant differences in serum intact PTH, 25-hydroxyvitamin D, and urinary NTX concentrations between the ADV and non-ADV groups (Figure 2).

3.3. Changes in Serum Creatinine, Phosphate, and ALP Isoenzymes before and after Administration of Nucleos(t)ide Analogues. There were no significant changes in serum creatinine or serum phosphate concentration with the administration of ADV or the other nucleoside analogues (LAM or ETV) (Figure 3). Serum ALP2 concentrations were significantly lower at the time of enrollment than before drug administration in both ADV group ($P = 0.0126$) and non-ADV group ($P = 0.0025$). Serum BAP was significantly higher at the time of enrollment than before nucleos(t)ide analogue administration in the ADV group ($P = 0.0001$). There was no significant change in serum BAP concentration in the non-ADV group (Figure 4).

3.4. Correlation between the Duration of Nucleos(t)ide Analogues Therapy and the Change in Serum ALP Isoenzyme Component. Although there was no correlation between the length of nucleoside analogue therapy and ΔBAP in the non-ADV group, there was a significant positive correlation between the period of ADV therapy and ΔBAP in the ADV group ($R^2 = 0.2959$; $P = 0.0160$, R: correlation coefficient) (Figure 5).

TABLE 2: Clinical characteristics of 19 well-matched pairs of ADV group and non-ADV group at the time of enrollment obtained by propensity score.

	Median (range)		P value
	ADV group ($n = 19$)	Non-ADV group ($n = 19$)	
At the time of enrollment			
Age (yr)	42 (29–68)	45 (34–68)	0.8940
Sex (male/female)	14/5	14/5	0.7126
HBV genotype (A/B/C/F/n.d)	1/3/11/1/3	1/4/10/0/4	0.7945
HBV DNA ($\log_{10}$ copies/mL)	2.1 > (negative–2.6)	2.1 > (negative–3.2)	0.2868
Platelet count ($\times 10^3/m^3$)	16.2 (10.2–31.0)	16.0 (9.8–28.3)	0.1675
ALT (IU/L)	26 (15–49)	25 (9–60)	0.8742
Alb (g/dL)	4.4 (4–5.3)	4.4 (3.9–5.3)	0.8714
Cirrhosis (presence/absence)	5/14	5/14	0.7126
Child Pugh score of cirrhosis cases	All 5 cases: 5	All 5 cases: 5	
At the time of starting ADV or ETV			
Serum creatinine (mg/dL)	0.8 (0.6–1.2)	0.78 (0.57–1.2)	0.7692
Follow-up duration (month)	96 (29–134)	90 (55–102)	0.1323
Duration of nucleos(t)ide analogue therapy (month)	96 (29–134)	90 (55–102)	0.1323
Duration of Adefovir administration (month)	73 (12–107)		
Propensity score	0.197 (0.068–0.553)	0.205 (0.067–0.514)	0.8267

ADV: adefovir dipivoxil; non-ADV: lamivudine or entecavir.

4. Discussion

In the present study, we found that serum BAP concentration was significantly elevated after the administration of ADV for more than 1 year. This finding was not observed after the administration of the other nucleoside analogues. Because serum BAP concentration reflects bone metabolism and is increased in osteomalacia, this finding suggests a tendency for subclinical osteomalacia in patients using ADV. However, we did not observe significant differences between the ADV and non-ADV treatment groups with respect to intact serum PTH concentration, 25-hydroxyvitamin D, and urinary NTX concentration, which are important markers of hyperparathyroidism, osteomalacia, and osteoporosis, respectively. This result may have been obtained because these bone turnover markers were examined in patients who did not develop symptomatic renal impairment or osteomalacia related to ADV treatment in this study.

A study evaluating long-term ADV therapy reported that 5% of the patients who received therapy up to 5 years had a slight elevation in serum creatinine concentration [24]. Although renal impairment is one of the most important side effects of ADV, we did not find a significant elevation in serum creatinine concentration among patients in that treatment group. However, we did observe that serum phosphate concentration tended to be lower and urinary phosphate concentration was significantly higher at the time of enrollment (≥1 year after starting ADV therapy) than before starting nucleos(t)ide analogue therapy. Therefore, it was difficult to detect potential renal dysfunction on the basis of elevation in serum creatinine concentration alone. According to a recent report, the maximal reabsorption of phosphate in the renal tubules and serum phosphate concentration were low in several patients receiving ADV;

however, after changing therapy to ETV, serum phosphate concentration improved [25]. In the present study, urinary phosphate concentration was significantly higher in the ADV group than in the non-ADV group, although there was no significant difference in serum phosphate concentration. These findings may be attributed to the increase in urinary phosphate that occurs before a decrease in serum phosphate. Therefore, monitoring for an increase in urinary phosphate may be critical for earlier detection of osteomalacia caused by renal tubular impairment.

Given that BAP is a bone turnover marker, we examined change in serum BAP concentration to determine the potential risks of osteomalacia caused by renal tubular impairment. Serum BAP concentration increased significantly after administration of ADV for >1 year. However, this finding was not observed after administration of the other nucleoside analogues. Therefore, osteomalacia caused by renal tubular impairment may be a unique side effect of ADV, especially after long-term use of ADV.

ADV plus LAM combination therapy is very useful in patients with LAM-resistant chronic HBV infection, and it is recommended as the first-line therapy for LAM-resistant disease in Japan [26]. However, because the criteria for discontinuation of nucleos(t)ide analogue therapy are not clear, long-term ADV plus LAM combination therapy is required in these patients to avoid risk of relapse. Long-term ADV plus LAM combination therapy carries a potential risk of renal impairment and development of Fanconi syndrome [17]. However, in the present study, patients did not present with symptoms of Fanconi syndrome; this finding may indicate that ADV plus LAM combination therapy is fairly safe for almost all patients if appropriate monitoring is provided for adverse effects of ADV.

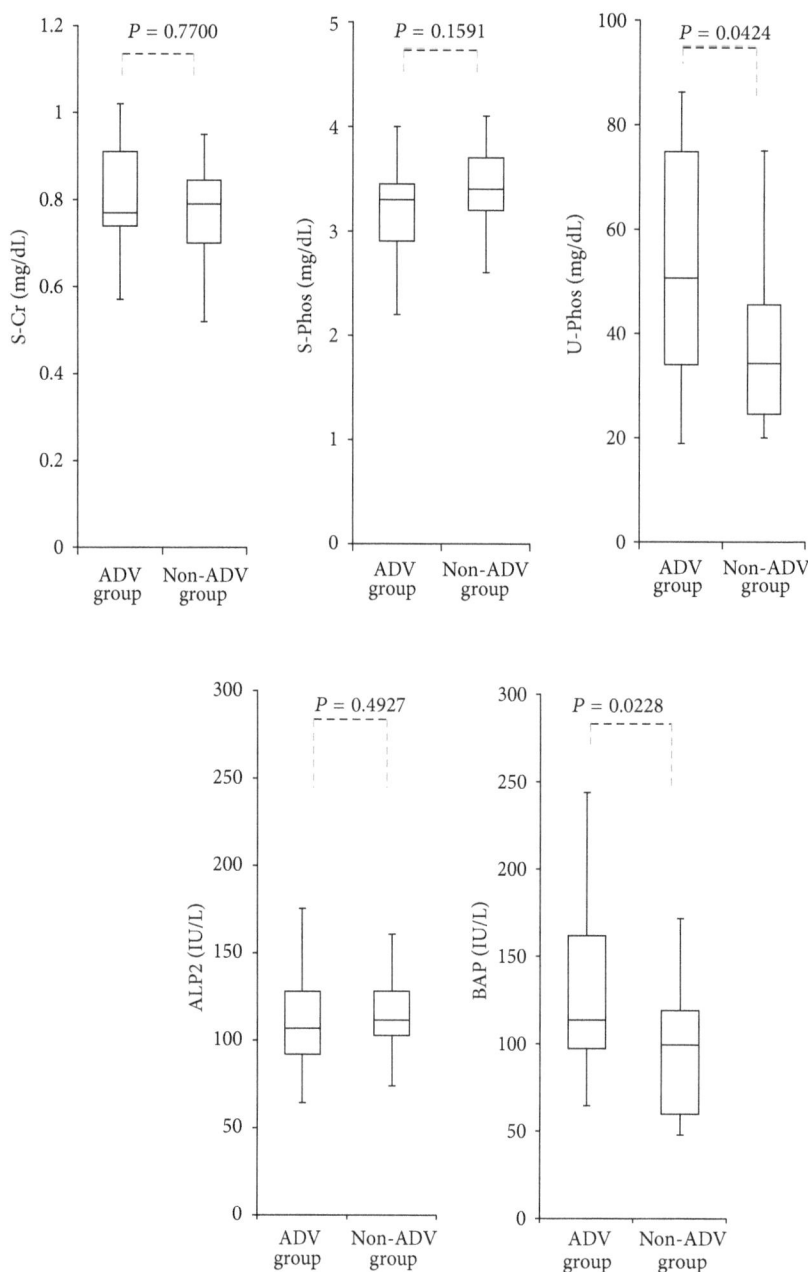

FIGURE 1: Serum creatinine, serum phosphate, urinary phosphate, serum ALP2, and BAP concentration at the time of at least 1 year or more after starting nucleos(t)ide analogue therapy in ADV group and non-ADV group (S-Cr; serum creatinine, S-Phos; serum phosphate, U-Phos; urinary phosphate, ALP; alkaline phosphatase, BAP; bone specific alkaline phosphatase).

Our results suggest that compared to serum creatinine and/or phosphate concentration, increases in concentrations of urinary phosphate and serum BAP are more useful indicators for early identification of renal tubular impairment. Further, serum BAP concentration increased before serum phosphate decreased; this finding may indicate that serum phosphate was being released from the bones, even though it was being lost through the kidneys. In addition, ΔBAP, a sensitive maker for detecting bone metabolism abnormalities, increased with the duration of ADV plus LAM therapy.

Therefore, the risk of osteomalacia may increase with long-term use of ADV.

A previous report suggested that dose reduction of ADV to 10 mg every other day leads to improvement of renal function without compromising treatment efficacy [27]. In our experience, serum creatinine concentration increased from 0.9 mg/dL to 1.3 mg/dL after the addition of ADV (10 mg/day) to LAM monotherapy (100 mg/day) in 1 patient; subsequently, after 3 months of reducing the dose of ADV to 10 mg every other day, serum creatinine concentration

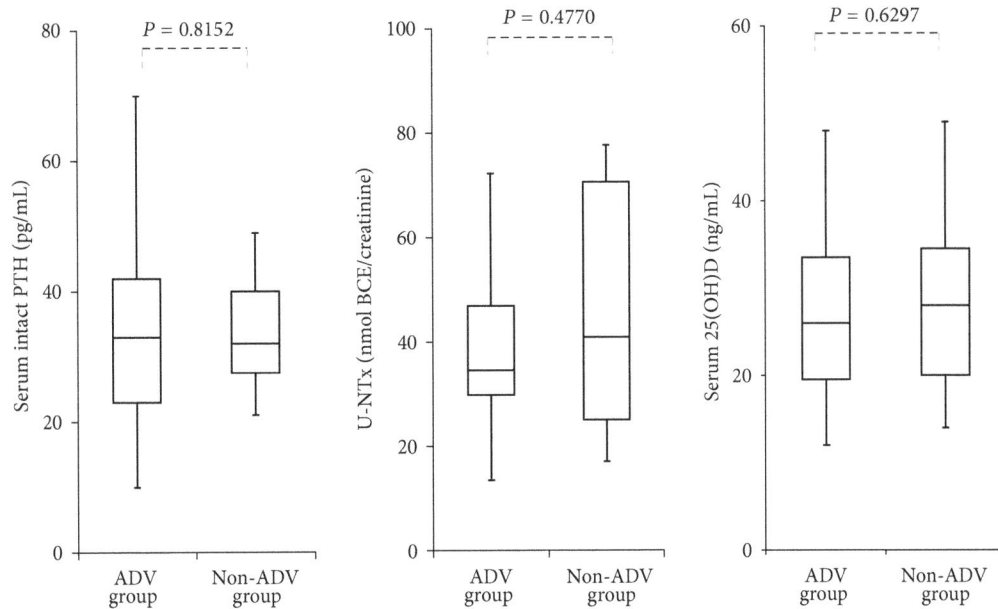

FIGURE 2: Serum intact PTH, U-NTx, and 25(OH)D concentrations at the time of at least 1 year or more after starting nucleos(t)ide analogue therapy in ADV group and non-ADV group (U-NTx: urinary N-telopeptide of type I collagen; intact PTH: intact parathyroid hormone; 25(OH)D:25-hydroxyvitamin D).

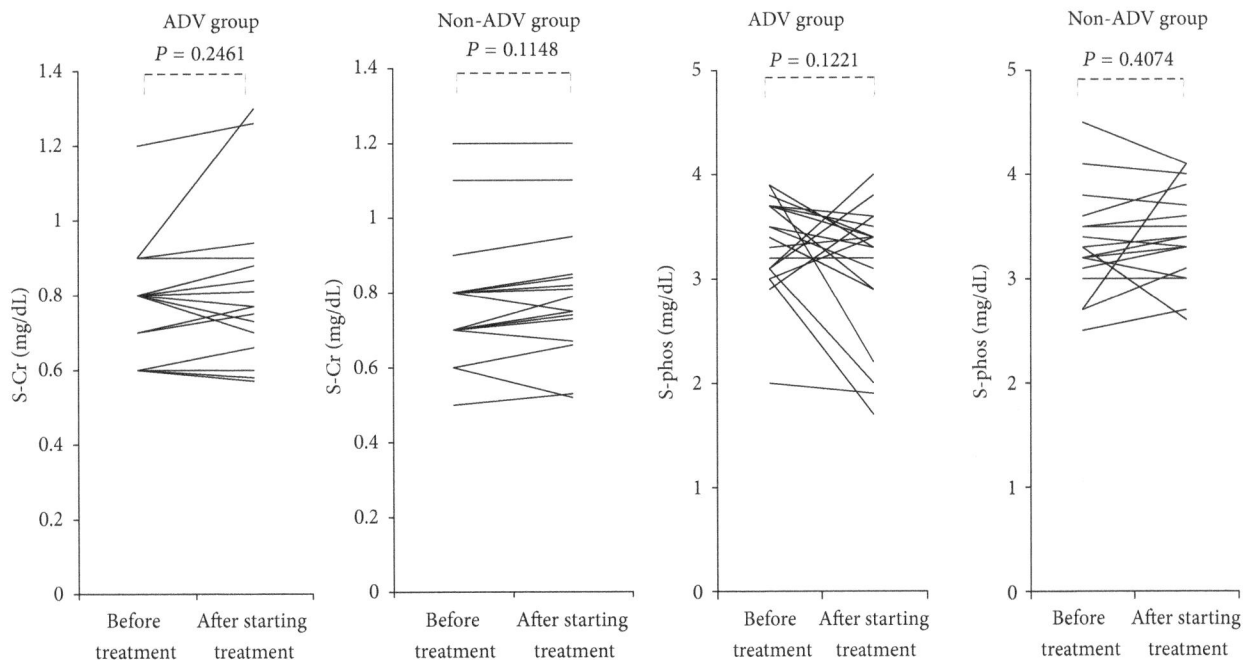

FIGURE 3: Transition of serum creatinine and phosphate concentrations from before treatment to at the time of at least 1 year or more after starting nucleos(t)ide analogue therapy in ADV group and non-ADV group (S-Cr; serum creatinine, S-Phos; serum phosphate, after starting treatment; at the time of at least one year or more after starting nucleos(t)ide analogue therapy).

improved to 1.0 mg/dL. However, because there is no obvious standard procedure for dose reduction, further studies are required to establish when and how to reduce ADV dose for patients whose serum ALP and/or urinary phosphate concentrations increase after long-term administration of ADV.

Furthermore, 2 adult patients with acquired immunodeficiency syndrome presented with severe bone pain associated with TDF [28], which is also used for the treatment of chronic HBV infection-related liver disease in Japan and is associated with an increase in serum ALP [29]. Although the relatively high rate of ETV resistance is a concern [30],

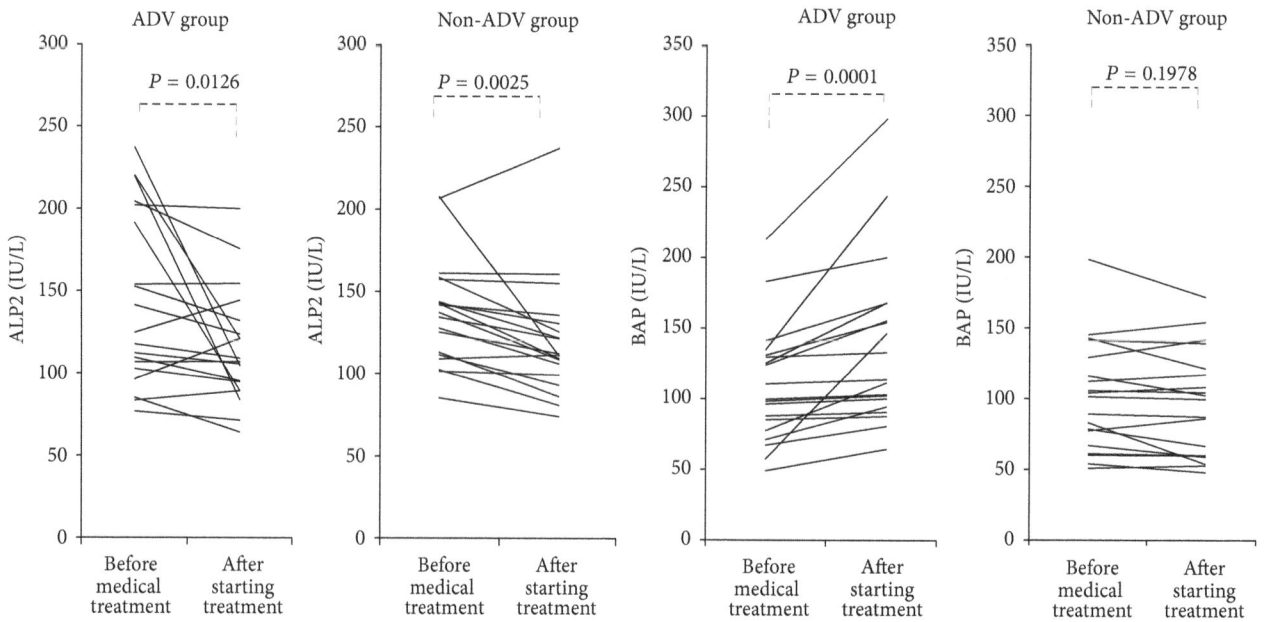

FIGURE 4: Transition of serum ALP2 and BAP concentrations from before medical treatment to at the time of at least 1 year or more after starting nucleos(t)ide analogue therapy in ADV group and non-ADV group.

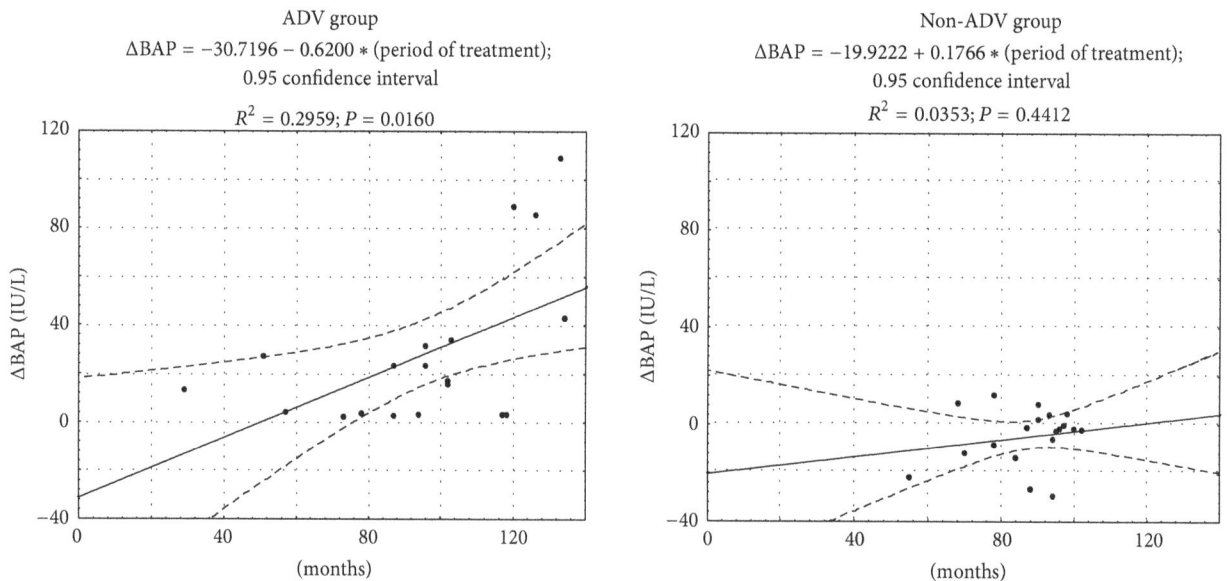

FIGURE 5: Relation between period of nucleos(t)ide analogue therapy and ΔBAP. ΔBAP; (serum BAP concentration at the time of at least 1 year or more after starting nucleos(t)ide analogue therapy)-(serum BAP concentration before treatment).

therapy with 1.0 mg of ETV per day may be considered when ADV and TDF are contraindicated in patients with LAM resistance because of treatment-induced renal impairment and osteomalacia.

Nucleos(t)ide analogue therapies are very useful for the treatment of chronic HBV infection-related liver disease, have few adverse effects with subjective symptoms, and are often used in long-term treatment. However, patients receiving these therapies should be supervised and monitored carefully for the early detection of adverse effects. Periodic measurement of serum BAP may be helpful in the early detection of osteomalacia in the absence of elevation of serum creatinine concentration.

5. Conclusions

In conclusion, examination of serum BAP concentration is useful for predicting osteomalacia caused by renal impairment in the absence of subjective symptoms and is essential for the establishment of adequate measures for determining the continuation of nucleos(t)ide analogue therapy for chronic HBV infection-related liver disease.

Conflict of Interests

The authors declare that there are no conflicts of interest to declare.

References

[1] D. Ganem and A. M. Prince, "Hepatitis B virus infection—natural history and clinical consequences," *The New England Journal of Medicine*, vol. 350, no. 11, pp. 1118–1129, 2004.

[2] A. S. F. Lok and B. J. McMahon, "Chronic hepatitis B: update of recommendations," *Hepatology*, vol. 39, no. 3, pp. 857–861, 2004.

[3] J. L. Dienstag, "Drug therapy: hepatitis B virus infection," *The New England Journal of Medicine*, vol. 359, no. 14, pp. 1486–1500, 2008.

[4] E. B. Keeffe, D. T. Dieterich, S.-H. B. Han et al., "A treatment algorithm for the management of chronic hepatitis B virus infection in the united states: 2008 update," *Clinical Gastroenterology and Hepatology*, vol. 6, no. 12, pp. 1315–1341, 2008.

[5] C.-Y. Dai, W.-L. Chuang, M.-Y. Hsieh et al., "Adefovir dipivoxil treatment of lamivudine-resistant chronic hepatitis B," *Antiviral Research*, vol. 75, no. 2, pp. 146–151, 2007.

[6] C.-L. Lai, R.-N. Chien, N. W. Y. Leung et al., "A one-year trial of lamivudine for chronic hepatitis B," *The New England Journal of Medicine*, vol. 339, no. 2, pp. 61–68, 1998.

[7] C.-H. Chen, C.-M. Lee, S.-N. Lu et al., "Comparison of clinical outcome between patients continuing and discontinuing lamivudine therapy after biochemical breakthrough of YMDD mutants," *Journal of Hepatology*, vol. 41, no. 3, pp. 454–461, 2004.

[8] I. Rapti, E. Dimou, P. Mitsoula, and S. J. Hadziyannis, "Adding-on versus switching-to adefovir therapy in lamivudine-resistant HBeAg-negative chronic hepatitis B," *Hepatology*, vol. 45, no. 2, pp. 307–313, 2007.

[9] D. J. Tenney, R. E. Rose, C. J. Baldick et al., "Two-year assessment of entecavir resistance in lamivudine-refractory hepatitis B virus patients reveals different clinical outcomes depending on the resistance substitutions present," *Antimicrobial Agents and Chemotherapy*, vol. 51, no. 3, pp. 902–911, 2007.

[10] European Association for the Study of the Liver, "EASL clinical practice guidelines: management of chronic hepatitis B," *Journal of Hepatology*, vol. 50, no. 2, pp. 227–242, 2009.

[11] P. Lampertico, M. Viganò, E. Manenti, M. Iavarone, E. Sablon, and M. Colombo, "Low resistance to adefovir combined with lamivudine: a 3-year study of 145 lamivudine-resistant hepatitis B patients," *Gastroenterology*, vol. 133, no. 5, pp. 1445–1451, 2007.

[12] H. Yatsuji, F. Suzuki, H. Sezaki et al., "Low risk of adefovir resistance in lamivudine-resistant chronic hepatitis B patients treated with adefovir plus lamivudine combination therapy: two-year follow-up," *Journal of Hepatology*, vol. 48, no. 6, pp. 923–931, 2008.

[13] S. K. Fung and A. S. F. Lok, "Drug insight: nucleoside and nucleotide analog inhibitors for hepatitis B," *Nature Clinical Practice Gastroenterology and Hepatology*, vol. 1, no. 2, pp. 90–97, 2004.

[14] N. B. Ha, N. B. Ha, R. T. Garcia et al., "Renal dysfunction in chronic hepatitis B patients treated with adefovir dipivoxil," *Hepatology*, vol. 50, no. 3, pp. 727–734, 2009.

[15] S. J. Hadziyannis, N. C. Tassopoulos, E. J. Heathcote et al., "Adefovir dipivoxil for the treatment of hepatitis B e antigen-negative chronic hepatitis B," *The New England Journal of Medicine*, vol. 348, no. 9, pp. 800–807, 2003.

[16] S. J. Hadziyannis, N. C. Tassopoulos, E. Jenny Heathcote et al., "Long-term therapy with adefovir dipivoxil for HBeAg-negative chronic hepatitis B," *The New England Journal of Medicine*, vol. 352, no. 26, pp. 2673–2681, 2005.

[17] A. Tamori, M. Enomoto, S. Kobayashi et al., "Add-on combination therapy with adefovir dipivoxil induces renal impairment in patients with lamivudine-refractory hepatitis B virus," *Journal of Viral Hepatitis*, vol. 17, no. 2, pp. 123–129, 2010.

[18] C. M. Girgis, T. Wong, M. C. Ngu et al., "Hypophosphataemic osteomalacia in patients on adefovir dipivoxil," *Journal of Clinical Gastroenterology*, vol. 45, no. 5, pp. 468–473, 2011.

[19] P. Ureña, M. Hruby, A. Ferreira, K. S. Ang, and M.-C. De Vernejoul, "Plasma total versus bone alkaline phosphatase as markers of bone turnover in hemodialysis patients," *Journal of the American Society of Nephrology*, vol. 7, no. 3, pp. 506–512, 1996.

[20] J. A. Whitworth, "2003 World Health Organization (WHO)/International Society of Hypertension (ISH) statement on management of hypertension," *Journal of Hypertension*, vol. 21, no. 11, pp. 1983–1992, 2003.

[21] T. Kuzuya, S. Nakagawa, J. Satoh et al., "Report of the committee on the classification and diagnostic criteria of diabetes mellitus," *Diabetes Research and Clinical Practice*, vol. 55, no. 1, pp. 65–85, 2002.

[22] R. B. D'Agostino Jr., "Propensity score methods for bias reduction in the comparison of a treatment to a non-randomized control group," *Statistics in Medicine*, vol. 17, pp. 2265–2281, 1998.

[23] M. M. Joffe and P. R. Rosenbaum, "Invited commentary: propensity scores," *American Journal of Epidemiology*, vol. 150, no. 4, pp. 327–333, 1999.

[24] S. J. Hadziyannis, N. C. Tassopoulos, E. J. Heathcote et al., "Long-term therapy with adefovir dipivoxil for HBeAg-negative chronic hepatitis B for up to 5 years," *Gastroenterology*, vol. 131, no. 6, pp. 1743–1751, 2006.

[25] N. Gara, X. Zhao, M. T. Collins et al., "Renal tubular dysfunction during long-term adefovir or tenofovir therapy in chronic hepatitis B," *Alimentary Pharmacology and Therapeutics*, vol. 35, no. 11, pp. 1317–1325, 2012.

[26] H. Yatsuji, F. Suzuki, H. Sezaki et al., "Low risk of adefovir resistance in lamivudine-resistant chronic hepatitis B patients treated with adefovir plus lamivudine combination therapy: two-year follow-up," *Journal of Hepatology*, vol. 48, no. 6, pp. 923–931, 2008.

[27] J. L. Hartono, M. O. Aung, Y. Y. Dan et al., "Resolution of adefovir-related nephrotoxicity by adefovir dose-reduction in patients with chronic hepatitis B," *Alimentary Pharmacology & Therapeutics*, vol. 37, pp. 710–719, 2013.

[28] M. A. Jhaveri, H. W. Mawad, A. C. Thornton, N. W. Mullen, and R. N. Greenberg, "Tenofovir-associated severe bone pain: i cannot walk!," *Journal of the International Association of Physicians in AIDS Care*, vol. 9, no. 5, pp. 328–334, 2010.

[29] C. A. Fux, A. Rauch, M. Simcock et al., "Tenofovir use is associated with an increase in serum alkaline phosphatase in the Swiss HIV Cohort Study," *Antiviral Therapy*, vol. 13, no. 8, pp. 1077–1082, 2008.

[30] Y. Suzuki, F. Suzuki, Y. Kawamura et al., "Efficacy of entecavir treatment for lamivudine-resistant hepatitis B over 3 years: histological improvement or entecavir resistance?" *Journal of Gastroenterology and Hepatology*, vol. 24, no. 3, pp. 429–435, 2009.

High Dose of Lamivudine and Resistance in Patients with Chronic Hepatitis B

Hamid Ullah Wani, Saad Al Kaabi, Manik Sharma, Rajvir Singh, Anil John, Moutaz Derbala, and Muneera J. Al-Mohannadi

Department of Medicine, Division of Gastroenterology, Hamad Medical Corporation (HMC), 2 South 2, P.O. Box 3050, Doha, Qatar

Correspondence should be addressed to Hamid Ullah Wani; doch95@yahoo.com

Academic Editor: Piero Luigi Almasio

Background. Lamivudine is the most affordable drug used for chronic hepatitis B and has a high safety profile. With the daily dose of 100 mg there is progressive appearance of resistance to lamivudine therapy. In our study we used 150 mg of lamivudine daily as a standard dose which warrants further exploration for the efficacy of the drug. *Aims of the Study.* To assess the efficacy of lamivudine 150 mg daily on resistance in patients with chronic hepatitis B. *Methods.* This retrospective study consists of 53 patients with chronic hepatitis B treated with 150 mg of lamivudine daily. The biochemical and virological response to the treatment were recorded at a 1-year and 2-, 3-, 4-, and 5-year period and time of emergence of resistance to the treatment was noted. *Results.* The mean age of the patients was 54 years with 80% being males. The resistance to lamivudine 150 mg daily at 1 year and 2, 3, and 5 years was 12.5%, 22.5%, 37.5%, and 60%, respectively, which is much less compared to the standard dose of 100 mg of lamivudine. *Conclusions.* Lamivudine is safe and a higher dose of 150 mg daily delays the resistance in patients with chronic hepatitis B.

1. Introduction

Chronic hepatitis B remains the most common serious health problem in the world, especially in the Asia Pacific region. Worldwide, there are 350 million people with chronic carrier of HBV. Treatment of HBV is relatively safe and easy compared to hepatitis C treatment, but the drug resistance is the main problem. The lamivudine and telbivudine are prone to develop resistance rapidly. Since the introduction of lamivudine, treatment of chronic hepatitis B has been characterized by a rapid increase in the number of available antiviral drugs, all belonging to the class of HBV polymerase inhibitors. Due to better tolerance and more convenient administration compared to interferon, HBV polymerase inhibitors today account for the vast majority of prescribed therapies for chronic hepatitis B in Western countries [1, 2]. However, long-term suppression of HBV is needed, particularly in HBeAg-negative patients harboring the precore mutant.

Lamivudine (LAM) was the first approved HBV polymerase inhibitor. It is characterized by good clinical tolerability, moderate antiviral efficacy, and rather quick development of resistance. Approximately 20% of patients treated with LAM develop resistance to LAM by 1 year and 70% to 80% by 5 years after the start of treatment [3].

Preliminary data indicate that the development of multiple lamivudine associated mutations may even reduce the efficacy of tenofovir therapy [4]. However, we have a good number of patients who are on lamivudine therapy with excellent viral response who need a continuous followup to observe the development of LAM resistance.

The clinical endpoints of chronic hepatitis B treatment are still not well defined [5, 6]. In HBeAg-positive patients, HBeAg seroconversion has been shown to be associated with a reduction in liver-associated morbidity and increased survival [7]. Thus, HBeAg seroconversion is considered a clinical endpoint in this group of patient population and discontinuation of HBV polymerase inhibitors is recommended 6–12 months after HBeAg seroconversion in patients who have not developed liver cirrhosis [8–10]. Treatment endpoints in HBeAg-negative hepatitis B in most cases are restricted to sustained normalization of ALT levels and suppression of HBV DNA, as HBsAg seroconversion is rare with current treatment options [3, 7]. Consequently, treatment duration and endpoints are more difficult to define in these patients. Most guidelines therefore recommend indefinite treatment of patients with HBeAg-negative chronic hepatitis B.

2. Materials and Methods

This retrospective study included 53 patients with chronic hepatitis B who were on lamivudine treatment since June 2005 at the Department of Gastroenterology, Hamad Medical Corporation. Before the start of lamivudine treatment all patients were HBsAg positive, had detectable levels of HBV DNA level >5 to 10 log copies/mL, and had elevated liver enzymes about 3 to 5 times the upper limit of normal. All patients received lamivudine in a single daily dose of 150 mg.

The patients with the following conditions were excluded from the study:

(1) coinfection with hepatitis C, hepatitis D, and human immunodeficiency virus,

(2) association with other forms of liver diseases, such as alcoholic liver disease, drug-induced hepatitis, or autoimmune hepatitis,

(3) previous treatment of HBV with interferon and nucleos(t)ide analogs other than LAM.

The patients who did not have a regular followup on the medical records and the patients who had no clinical and laboratory assessments at regular intervals were excluded.

All of these patients had a followup after every 3 to 6 months with routine biochemical liver function tests and serum HBV DNA levels. Serum HBV DNA levels were quantified at baseline and at each follow-up visit using the COBAS Ampli Prep or COBAS Taqman HBV test (Roche Molecular System) [11, 12].

The (i) biochemical response (normalization of serum alanine aminotransferase (ALT) level), (ii) complete virological response (undetectable serum HBV DNA by real-time polymerase chain reaction, <100 copies/mL), and (iii) virological breakthrough were recorded in all patients. Out of 50 patients, 40 patients had a regular five-year followup available in the medical records.

Virological breakthrough was defined as an increase in serum HBV DNA of more than 1 log copies/mL from the nadir of the initial response. A flare-up of hepatitis was defined as an increase in ALT level to more than 3 times the upper limit of normal.

In this study we do not have molecular studies available for lamivudine resistance. The time of "virological breakthrough" and "flare-up" of hepatitis was taken as resistance to lamivudine.

The study protocol was reviewed and approved by the Institutional Review Board of Hamad Medical Corporation.

3. Statistical Methods

Descriptive statistics in the form of mean, standard deviations, and range are calculated for interval variables, whereas counts and percentages are performed for categorical

TABLE 1: Demographic and clinical characteristics of the patients.

	Number	Range
Age	40	27–79 years Mean 54 years ± SD 8.94
Gender	40	Male 32 (80%) Female 8 (20%)
HBSAg	40	40 positive (100%)
HBSAb	40	32 positive (80%) 8 negative (20%)
HBeAg	40	25 positive (62.5%) 15 negative (37.5%)
HBeAb	40	15 positive (37.5%) 25 negative (62.5%)

TABLE 2: Biochemical and virological characteristics of the patient prior to treatment.

Disease duration	Years 5 (1–10) years
ALT IU/L	120 (80–150) IU/L
Duration of treatment	60 months
HBV DNA IU/mL	$2.0 \times 10^{3-10}$ IU/mL
Previous interferon therapy	0

variables. Kaplan Meier curve has been performed to see probability of not having resistance to lamivudine at different points of months. SPSS 20.0 Statistical Package is used for the analysis.

4. Results

The study population consists of 53 patients with chronic hepatitis B who were on lamivudine since June 2005. Out of 53 patients, 40 patients fulfilled the inclusion criteria. The mean age was 54 years with 80% being males. Fourteen patients (35%) were from the state of Qatar and 26 patients (65%) were expatriates. Twenty-five patients (62.5%) were HBeAg + and 15 patients (37.5%) were HBeAg − (Table 1). Before starting lamivudine treatment, all patients were having elevated liver enzyme ranging from 3 to 5 times the upper limit of normal and HBVDNA levels >2,000 IU/mL. Mean duration of lamivudine treatment was 60 months. None of the patients received interferon therapy or any other antiviral drug during this period. Seven patients had liver biopsy which was showing fibrosis stages 1 to 2 and inflammation grades 2 to 3 on Metavir Score system (Table 2).

All patients (Table 3) had biochemical normalization within 3 to 6 months of initiation of lamivudine therapy. Overall (87%) patients were having a virological and biochemical response at 12 months of lamivudine treatment and 2 patients were having early viral breakthrough at 6 months after a partial HBV-DNA suppression. The response to lamivudine treatment was 77.4% at 24 months, 62.5% at 36 months, 50% at 48 months, and 40% at 60 months (Table 3).

There is progressive evolution of lamivudine resistance reaching up to 50% at 48 months and 60% at 60 months (Figure 1). Three patients achieved HBeAg seroconversion to

TABLE 3: Treatment (biochemical and virological response).

	12 months	24 months	36 months	48 months	60 Months
HBV DNA IU/mL Below detection level	35/40 (87.5%)	31/40 (77.4%)	25/40 (62.5%)	20/40 (50%)	16/40 (40%)
Biochemical activity (high ALT)	2/40	normal	normal	normal	normal
HBsAg seroconversion	0%	0%	0%	0%	0%
HBeAg seroconversion	0%	0%	1	2	3
Viral breakthrough	5/40 (12.5%)	9/40 (22.5%)	15/40 (37.5%)	20/40 (50%)	24/40 (60%)

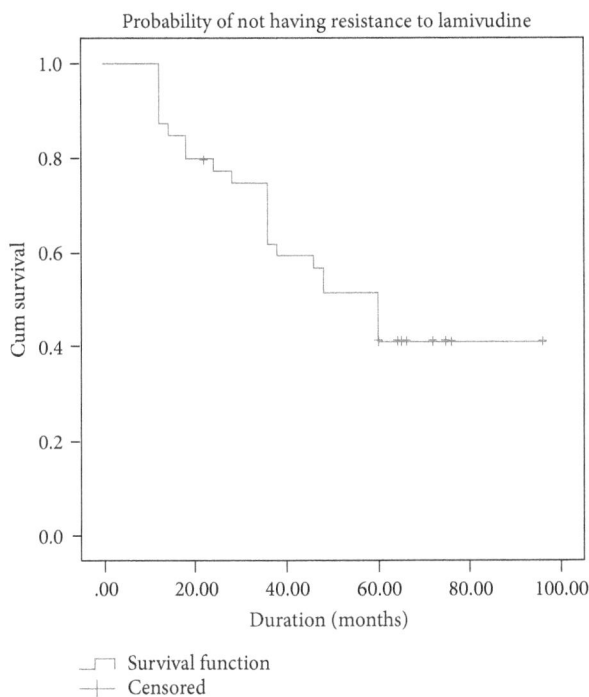

FIGURE 1: Kaplan-Meier curve showing probability of not having resistance to lamivudine.

anti-HBeAg, none had HBsAg seroconversion to antiHBs antibody positivity during these 5 years of treatment. Two patients died with multifocal hepatocellular carcinoma even after HBV-DNA suppression.

5. Discussion

Lamivudine was the first approved polymerase inhibitor for chronic hepatitis B. It is characterized by excellent tolerability with minimal or no side effects [2, 13]. There is rapid development of antiviral resistance to the standard dose of 100 mg of lamivudine in patients with chronic hepatitis B. Twenty (20%) patients developed resistance within one year of treatment which can progress to 70 to 80% at 4 to 5 years [6, 14]. The resistance rates have been higher in HBeAg

positive patients [15, 16]. HBsAg loss and seroconversion to anti-HBsAg antibody may occur spontaneously in 1–3% of cases per year, usually after several years with persistently undetectable HBV DNA [3, 14].

In our study with the lamivudine dose of 150 mg daily the resistance at 1 year was only 12.5% compared to 20 to 24% with standard lamivudine dose. The resistance was also delayed at 2 and 3 years with the 150 mg lamivudine treatment and was 22.5% and 37.5% which is much less compared to the standard dose of 100 mg of lamivudine. The main result of our study is that patients who received high dose of lamivudine have lower rate of resistance (60%) over a mean duration of 60 months.

Torre et al. showed more profound suppression of viral replication with a lamivudine dose of 300 mg once daily [17]. Ha et al. showed that an initial high dose of 300 mg of lamivudine over a period of 2 weeks followed by 100 mg daily, compared to standard dose, has a lower rate of resistance (60% versus 76%) [18].

Adefovir, entecavir, and tenofovir are commonly used antivirals in patients with lamivudine resistance, although the development of the resistance is delayed and is less extent compared to lamivudine and telbivudine [19–21]. The lamivudine, even with dose of 150 mg, is safe in patients with end stage renal disease. Lamivudine mutations have been shown to confer cross-resistance to telbivudine, emtricitabine, and entecavir [22, 23].

The treatment endpoints of chronic hepatitis B are also not well defined. HBe antigen and hepatitis B surface antigen (HBsAg) seroconversion are markers of disease control and immunity. In our study, 7.5% achieved HBeAg seroconversion but none had HBsAg seroconversion during these 5 years of lamivudine treatment.

Lamivudine is the most cost-effective treatment for the chronic HBV [24, 25]. Although the new agents, like entecavir and tenofovir, appear more effective, they are more expensive than lamivudine. Selecting between these agents completely depends upon the available health care budget and willingness to pay. For poor patients, like in our study, who cannot afford the costly drugs, it appears more cost-effective to start with lamivudine than adefovir and entecavir. In one meta-analysis of cost-effective strategy, 3/6 studies that evaluated the lamivudine against other drugs find it as a dominant strategy [26]. As recommended by current management guidelines, lamivudine once daily is used for an indefinite period in patients with cirrhosis [27–29].

The important limitation of our study is that being a retrospective study there is no other available group for the comparison; however, the objective of the study was to see the effect of high dose of lamivudine on the resistant pattern of chronic hepatitis B.

6. Conclusions

Our study showed that 150 mg of lamivudine delayed the appearance of resistance in chronic hepatitis B. Lamivudine is very cheap compared to new antiviral drugs, has high safety profile, and has good compliance as compared to other new drugs. With this current available evidence, we consider that lamivudine as an antiviral treatment for chronic hepatitis B is a cost-effective intervention for many health care systems, including ours.

Conflict of Interests

The authors declare that there is no conflict of interests regarding the publication of this paper.

References

[1] N. Leung, "Treatment of chronic hepatitis B: case selection and duration of therapy," *Journal of Gastroenterology and Hepatology*, vol. 17, no. 4, pp. 409–414, 2002.

[2] T.-T. Chang, C.-L. Lai, R.-N. Chien et al., "Four years of lamivudine treatment in Chinese patients with chronic hepatitis B," *Journal of Gastroenterology and Hepatology*, vol. 19, no. 11, pp. 1276–1282, 2004.

[3] C. Pramoolsinsup, "Management of viral hepatitis B," *Journal of Gastroenterology and Hepatology*, vol. 17, no. 1, pp. S125–S145, 2002.

[4] L. Martín-Carbonero and E. Poveda, "Hepatitis B virus and HIV infection," *Seminars in Liver Disease*, vol. 32, no. 2, pp. 114–119, 2012.

[5] C. Wang, R. Fan, J. Sun, and J. Hou, "Prevention and management of drug resistant hepatitis B virus infections," *Journal of Gastroenterology and Hepatology*, vol. 27, no. 9, pp. 1432–1440, 2012.

[6] S. Manolakopoulos, S. Bethanis, J. Elefsiniotis et al., "Lamivudine monotherapy in HBeAg-negative chronic hepatitis B: prediction of response-breakthrough and long-term clinical outcome," *Alimentary Pharmacology and Therapeutics*, vol. 23, no. 6, pp. 787–795, 2006.

[7] Y. Tanaka, A. E. T. Yeo, E. Orito et al., "Prognostic indicators of breakthrough hepatitis during lamivudine monotherapy for chronic hepatitis B virus infection," *Journal of Gastroenterology*, vol. 39, no. 8, pp. 769–775, 2004.

[8] M.-J. Sheu, H.-T. Kuo, C.-Y. Lin et al., "Lamivudine monotherapy for chronic hepatitis B infection with acute exacerbation revisited," *European Journal of Gastroenterology and Hepatology*, vol. 21, no. 4, pp. 447–451, 2009.

[9] A. Tsubota, Y. Arase, Y. Suzuki et al., "Lamivudine monotherapy for spontaneous severe acute exacerbation of chronic hepatitis B," *Journal of Gastroenterology and Hepatology*, vol. 20, no. 3, pp. 426–432, 2005.

[10] L. J. Sun, J. W. Yu, Y. H. Zhao, P. Kang, and S. C. Li, "Influential factors of prognosis in lamivudine treatment for patients with acute-on-chronic hepatitis B liver failure," *Journal of Gastroenterology and Hepatology*, vol. 25, no. 3, pp. 583–590, 2010.

[11] M. Buti, F. Sánchez, M. Cotrina et al., "Quantitative hepatitis B virus DNA testing for the early prediction of the maintenance of response during lamivudine therapy in patients with chronic hepatitis B," *Journal of Infectious Diseases*, vol. 183, no. 8, pp. 1277–1280, 2001.

[12] T. Ide, R. Kumashiro, Y. Koga et al., "A real-time quantitative polymerase chain reaction method for hepatitis B virus in patients with chronic hepatitis B treated with lamivudine," *The American Journal of Gastroenterology*, vol. 98, no. 9, pp. 2048–2051, 2003.

[13] J. H. Kim, S. K. Yu, Y. S. Seo et al., "Clinical outcomes of chronic hepatitis B patients with persistently detectable serum hepatitis B virus DNA during lamivudine therapy," *Journal of Gastroenterology and Hepatology*, vol. 22, no. 8, pp. 1220–1225, 2007.

[14] S. K. Fung, F. Wong, M. Hussain, and A. S. F. Lok, "Sustained response after a 2-year course of lamivudine treatment of hepatitis B e antigen-negative chronic hepatitis B," *Journal of Viral Hepatitis*, vol. 11, no. 5, pp. 432–438, 2004.

[15] A. Marrone, R. Zampino, P. Karayannis et al., "Clinical reactivation during lamivudine treatment correlates with mutations in the precore/core promoter and polymerase regions of hepatitis B virus in patients with anti-hepatitis B e-positive chronic hepatitis," *Alimentary Pharmacology and Therapeutics*, vol. 22, no. 8, pp. 707–714, 2005.

[16] P. Honkoop, H. G. M. Niesters, R. A. M. de Man, A. D. M. E. Osterhaus, and S. W. Schalm, "Lamivudine resistance in immunocompetent chronic hepatitis B: incidence and patterns," *Journal of Hepatology*, vol. 26, no. 6, pp. 1393–1395, 1997.

[17] F. Torre, E. G. Giannini, M. Basso, V. Fazio, V. Savarino, and A. Picciotto, "Initial high dose of lamivudine delays the appearance of viral resistance in chronic hepatitis B patients," *Journal of Gastrointestinal and Liver Diseases*, vol. 20, no. 1, pp. 47–50, 2011.

[18] M. Ha, G. Zhang, S. Diao et al., "Rescue therapy for lamivudine-resistant chronic hepatitis B: adefovir monotherapy, adefovir plus lamivudine or entecavir combination therapy," *Internal Medicine*, vol. 51, no. 12, pp. 1509–1515, 2012.

[19] H. L. Y. Chan, Y. C. Chen, E. J. Gane et al., "Randomized clinical trial: efficacy and safety of telbivudine and lamivudine in treatment-naïve patients with HBV-related decompensated cirrhosis," *Journal of Viral Hepatitis*, vol. 19, no. 10, pp. 732–743, 2012.

[20] H. Jiang, J. Wang, and W. Zhao, "Lamivudine versus telbivudine in the treatment of chronic hepatitis B: a systematic review and meta-analysis," *European Journal of Clinical Microbiology & Infectious Diseases*, vol. 32, no. 1, pp. 11–18, 2013.

[21] M. G. Peters, H. W. Hann, P. Martin et al., "Adefovir dipivoxil alone or in combination with lamivudine in patients with lamivudine-resistant chronic hepatitis B," *Gastroenterology*, vol. 126, no. 1, pp. 91–101, 2004.

[22] H. J. Kim, J. H. Park, D. I. Park et al., "Rescue therapy for lamivudine-resistant chronic hepatitis B: Comparison between entecavir 1.0 mg monotherapy, adefovir monotherapy and adefovir add-on lamivudine combination therapy," *Journal of Gastroenterology and Hepatology*, vol. 25, no. 8, pp. 1374–1380, 2010.

[23] M. Sherman, C. Yurdaydin, H. Simsek et al., "Entecavir therapy for lamivudine-refractory chronic hepatitis B: improved virologic, biochemical, and serology outcomes through 96 weeks," *Hepatology*, vol. 48, no. 1, pp. 99–108, 2008.

[24] F. Kanwal, I. M. Gralnek, P. Martin, G. S. Dulai, M. Farid, and B. M. R. Spiegel, "Treatment alternatives for chronic hepatitis B virus infection: a cost-effectiveness analysis," *Annals of Internal Medicine*, vol. 142, no. 10, pp. 821–831, 2005.

[25] L. Solari, G. Hijar, R. Zavala, and J. M. Ureta, "Economic evaluation of antiviral treatment for chronic hepatitis B: a systematic review," *Revista Peruana de Medicina Experimental y Salud Publica*, vol. 27, no. 1, pp. 68–79, 2010.

[26] X. Sun, W.-X. Qin, Y.-P. Li, and X.-H. Jiang, "Comparative cost-effectiveness of antiviral therapies in patients with chronic hepatitis B: a systematic review of economic evidence," *Journal of Gastroenterology and Hepatology*, vol. 22, no. 9, pp. 1369–1377, 2007.

[27] C. Y. Peng, R. N. Chien, and Y. F. Liaw, "Hepatitis B virus-related decompensated liver cirrhosis: benefits of antiviral therapy," *Journal of Hepatology*, vol. 57, no. 2, pp. 442–450, 2012.

[28] S. K. Fung and A. S. F. Lok, "Management of patients with hepatitis B virus-induced cirrhosis," *Journal of Hepatology*, vol. 42, no. 1, pp. S54–S64, 2005.

[29] E. B. Keeffe, D. T. Dieterich, S.-H. B. Han et al., "A treatment algorithm for the management of chronic hepatitis B virus infection in the United States," *Clinical Gastroenterology and Hepatology*, vol. 2, no. 2, pp. 87–106, 2004.

Serum Inter-Alpha-Trypsin Inhibitor Heavy Chain 4 (ITIH4) in Children with Chronic Hepatitis C: Relation to Liver Fibrosis and Viremia

Mostafa M. Sira,[1] Behairy E. Behairy,[1] Azza M. Abd-Elaziz,[2] Sameh A. Abd Elnaby,[3] and Ehab E. Eltahan[3]

[1] Department of Pediatric Hepatology, National Liver Institute, Menofiya University, Shebin El-koom, Menofiya 32511, Egypt
[2] Department of Microbiology and Immunology, National Liver Institute, Menofiya University, Shebin El-koom, Menofiya 32511, Egypt
[3] Department of Pediatrics, Faculty of Medicine, Menofiya University, Shebin El-koom, Menofiya 32511, Egypt

Correspondence should be addressed to Mostafa M. Sira; msira@liver-eg.org

Academic Editor: Piero Luigi Almasio

Liver fibrosis and viremia are determinant factors for the treatment policy and its outcome in chronic hepatitis C virus (HCV) infection. We aimed to investigate serum level of inter-alpha-trypsin inhibitor heavy chain 4 (ITIH4) and its relation to liver fibrosis and viremia in children with chronic HCV. ITIH4 was measured by ELISA in 33 treatment-naive children with proved chronic HCV and compared according to different clinical, laboratory and histopathological parameters. Liver histopathological changes were assessed using Ishak score and compared with aspartate transaminase-to-platelet ratio (APRI) and FIB-4 indices as simple noninvasive markers of fibrosis. ITIH4 was measured in a group of 30 age- and sex-matched healthy controls. ITIH4 was significantly higher in patients than in controls (54.2 ± 30.78 pg/mL versus 37.21 ± 5.39 pg/mL; $P = 0.021$). ITIH4, but not APRI or FIB-4, had a significant direct correlation with fibrosis stage ($P = 0.015$, 0.961, and 0.389, resp.), whereas, the negative correlation of ITIH4 with HCV viremia was of marginal significance ($P = 0.071$). In conclusion, ITIH4 significantly correlated with higher stages of fibrosis indicating a possible relation to liver fibrogenesis. The trend of higher ITIH4 with lower viremia points out a potential antiviral properties and further studies in this regard are worthwhile.

1. Introduction

Hepatitis C virus (HCV) infection is a serious health problem that may result in chronic hepatitis, cirrhosis, and hepatocellular carcinoma. It is estimated that over 200 million people are infected worldwide, while 80% develop a chronic form [1]. HCV prevalence varies geographically, with rates of 1.7% in the United States, 2.1% in Southeast Asia, and 5.3% in Africa [2]. In children younger than 11 years, worldwide seroprevalence of HCV is 0.2% and in those older than 11 years it is 0.4% [3].

Egypt reports the highest prevalence worldwide ranging from 8.7% in upper Egypt to 24.3% in lower Egypt with genotype 4 in more than 90% of those infected [4]. Studies of the magnitude of HCV infection in Egyptian children revealed a prevalence of 3% in upper Egypt and 9% in lower Egypt [5]. Liver disease seems to be milder in children than in adults; however, the natural history of HCV infection acquired in infancy and childhood remains poorly characterized and the long-term outcome of the disease is still a matter of debate [2].

Although liver biopsy represents the gold standard for evaluating presence, type, and stage of liver fibrosis and for characterizing necroinflammation, it remains an invasive procedure with inherent risks. Thus, it cannot be performed frequently to monitor therapeutic outcomes [6, 7]. Moreover, in children, biopsy is still perceived to carry a higher risk of complications, so it is less accepted than in adults. Therefore, developing noninvasive tests that can predict initial disease stage and progression over time represents a high priority and a growing medical need [8, 9].

A recent study, using proteomic analysis of serum from adult patients with chronic HCV infection, revealed that inter-alpha-trypsin heavy chain 4 (ITIH4) was a candidate to predict liver fibrosis [10]. ITIH4 was found to be higher in HCV patients with mild to moderate fibrosis compared to healthy controls, while in those with cirrhosis, the net production of ITIH4 was found to be downregulated [11].

ITIH4 is a plasma glycoprotein that is expressed mainly in the liver [12]. It is one of the inter-alpha-trypsin inhibitors (ITI) family which are found in human plasma in relatively high concentrations. As their original names suggest, the family molecules were studied extensively as protease inhibitors [13]. It was reported that influenza viral replication was inhibited by the protease inhibitor; trypsin inhibitor [14].

We aimed to investigate serum level of ITIH4 and its relation to liver fibrosis and viremia in children with chronic HCV infection.

2. Materials and Methods

2.1. Study Population. The study included 33 children with proved chronic HCV infection recruited from the outpatient and inpatient of Pediatric Hepatology department, National Liver Institute, Menofiya University. Diagnosis of chronic hepatitis C was based on the presence of serum anti-HCV antibody (Ab) and persistently positive HCV-RNA as detected by polymerase chain reaction (PCR) for more than 6 months [15, 16], negative hepatitis B viral markers, and absence of any associated liver disease, supported by the histopathological feature of HCV infection in liver biopsy. A second group of 30 healthy children with no signs or symptoms of liver disease or any other diseases, normal liver transaminases, and negative anti-HCV Ab served as controls. A signed informed consent was obtained from the legal guardians of all the patients and controls before enrollment in the study. The study was approved by the Research Ethics Committee of the National Liver Institute.

2.2. Laboratory Investigations. Laboratory investigations, including liver function tests, complete blood count (CBC), kidney function tests, serum autoantibodies (anti-nuclear antibodies, anti-smooth muscle antibodies, and liver-kidney microsomal antibodies) and prothrombin time were performed for all the patients. Serum viral markers were performed using enzyme-linked immunosorbent assay (ELISA) according to the manufacturer instructions, HCV Ab (Innogenetics, Ghent, Belgium), hepatitis B virus surface antigen, hepatitis B virus core immunoglobulin (Ig)M, and IgG Abs (all from Dia Sorin, Saluggia, Italy). Real-time PCR for HCV-RNA was performed using COBAS Ampliprep/COBAS TaqMan, Roche Molecular Systems, Inc., Branchburg, NJ, 08876 USA (detection limit was 15 IU/mL). According to the viral load, viremia was classified arbitrarily into low ($<2 \times 10^5$ IU/mL), moderate ($\geq 2 \times 10^5 - 2 \times 10^6$ IU/mL), and high viremia ($\geq 2 \times 10^6$ IU/mL) [17]. Serum ITIH4 levels

were assayed using ELISA kit (WKEA Med Supplies Corp, NY 10123, United States) according to the manufacturer instructions. Serum samples of the patients were collected, maximally, within 6 months of liver biopsy [18]. All the controls were tested for aspartate transaminase (AST), alanine transaminase (ALT), CBC, HCV Ab, and serum ITIH4.

2.3. Liver Biopsy and Histopathological Evaluation. Liver biopsy was performed using an ultrasonography-guided true cut needle for all the patients. The mean length of the biopsy core provided was 1.16 ± 0.18 cm, ranging from 1.0 cm to 1.6 cm with a median of 1.0 cm. Specimens were fixed in formalin, embedded in paraffin, and stained with hematoxylin and eosin, Masson's trichrome, reticulin, and Perl's stains. Hepatic necroinflammatory activity and liver fibrosis were evaluated according to Ishak staging and grading score. Necroinflammatory activity was classified into minimal (score 1–3), mild (score 4–8), moderate (score 9–12), and severe (score 13–18) [19]. Fibrosis was classified into mild (stage 1), moderate (stages 2-3), and severe fibrosis or cirrhosis (stages 4-6) [5]. Significant fibrosis was defined as Ishak score of 3 or more (presence of bridging fibrosis) [20]. AST-to-platelet ratio index (APRI) and FIB-4 index were calculated according to the formula APRI = AST/upper limit of normal $\times 100$/platelet count (10^9/L), FIB-4 = Age (years) $\times$ AST/platelet count (10^9/L) $\times$ (ALT)$^{1/2}$ [21] and compared in different stages of fibrosis.

2.4. Statistical Analysis. Descriptive results were expressed as mean $\pm$ standard deviation (SD) or number (percentage) of individuals with a condition. For quantitative data, statistical significance was tested by Mann-Whitney U nonparametric test. For qualitative data, significance between groups was tested by Chi-square test. Correlation was tested by Spearman's test. Results were considered significant if P value $\leq$ 0.05. Statistical analysis was performed using SPSS statistical package version 13 (SPSS Inc., Chicago, IL, USA).

3. Results

3.1. Study Population Characteristics. The study included 33 children with chronic HCV infection. They were 12 females and 21 males. Their mean age was 10.95 ± 4.53 ranging from 3.5 to 18 years. A second group of 30 age- and sex-matched ($P > 0.05$ for both) healthy children served as controls. They were 11 females and 19 males. Their mean age was 11.13 ± 4.04 ranging from 4 to 17 years. The major possible modes of infection were male circumcision (63.6%) followed by presence of a family member with HCV infection (60.6%), surgery (42.42%), blood transfusion (27.27%), and dental procedures (15.15%). Many children had more than one possible mode of infection. The majority of patients (87.9%) were asymptomatic while four (12.1%) children presented with abdominal enlargement. Clinically, four (12.1%) children had hepatomegaly, one child (3.0%) had splenomegaly, and none had jaundice or ascites. Fibrosis stage ranged from F1 to F3 and activity grade ranged from A1 to A8. The majority of patients (84.8%) had either F1 or F2 fibrosis and mild activity (66.7%), and 8 out of 33 (24.2%) had steatosis (Table 1).

3.2. Histopathological Findings in Patients with Normal versus Elevated Transaminases.

All the patients had mild to moderate fibrosis and minimal to mild activity in liver biopsy. Yet, nearly half of them had normal transaminases (46.2%, 45.0%, 45.5%, and 45.5% with mild fibrosis, moderate fibrosis, minimal activity, and mild activity, resp.) (Table 2).

3.3. ITIH4 according to Disease Severity and Correlation with Laboratory and Histopathological Parameters.

The mean value of serum ITIH4 was significantly higher in patients than in controls (54.2 ± 30.78 pg/mL versus 37.21 ± 5.39 pg/mL; $P = 0.021$). There was no statistical significant difference in the mean level of ITIH4 when comparing patients with different activity grades and patients with normal transaminases versus those with elevated transaminases ($P > 0.05$ for both; Table 3) but it was slightly higher in those with moderate fibrosis and in those with elevated transaminases. In addition, there was a significant direct correlation between ITIH4 and the stage of fibrosis ($P = 0.015$) while there was no significant correlation with the other studied laboratory parameters, yet, the negative correlation with HCV viremia was of marginal significance ($P = 0.071$) (Table 4). On the other hand, there was no correlation between APRI ($r = -0.009$ and $P = 0.961$) and FIB-4 ($r = 0.155$ and $P = 0.389$) with the stage of fibrosis.

3.4. ITIH4, but Not APRI or FIB-4 Is Significantly Higher in Patients with Significant Fibrosis (Ishak Score ≥ 3).

Serum ITIH4 was at its lowest (41.63 ± 13.15 pg/mL) in patients with F1, increasing in patients with F2 (53.03 ± 35.75 pg/mL) and reaching the highest level in F3 (90.42 ± 20.67 pg/mL). Though the levels in F1 and F2 had no significant difference from those in healthy controls, the levels in F3 were significantly higher than those in F1, F2, and the controls (Figure 1(a)). On the other hand, there was no statistically significant difference in the mean values of APRI ($P = 0.949$) and FIB-4 ($P = 0.253$) according to different stages of fibrosis, yet, FIB-4 tended to increase with higher stages of fibrosis (Figures 1(b) and 1(c), resp.).

3.5. ITIH4 according to Hepatitis C Viral Load.

Serum ITIH4, though not statistically significant ($P = 0.356$), was negatively associated with the level of viremia. It was higher (57.29 ± 34.13 pg/mL) in patient with low viremia trending to be successively lower in patients with moderate and low viremia (51.95 ± 27.41 pg/mL and 42.51 ± 18.03 pg/mL resp.). The levels in patients with low viremia were significantly higher compared to that in controls ($P = 0.016$) (Figure 2).

4. Discussion

The natural history of chronic hepatitis C in children differs from that in adults since HCV infection is relatively benign, induces mild changes in the liver with a low level of fibrosis and a low rate of progression, and is rarely associated with severe or decompensate liver disease [22]. Bortolotti et al. [23]

TABLE 1: Laboratory and histopathological characteristics of the studied patients.

Parameter	HCV patients ($n = 33$)
Liver function tests	
Total bilirubin (mg/dL)	0.98 ± 0.39
Direct bilirubin (mg/dL)	0.29 ± 0.25
Albumin (g/dL)	4.25 ± 0.72
Alanine transaminase (U/L)	69.45 ± 125.89
Aspartate transaminase (U/L)	52.79 ± 120.49
Gamma glutamyl transpeptidase (U/L)	46.38 ± 16.38
Alkaline phosphatase (U/L)	257.79 ± 94.92
Fibrosis stage	
F1	13 (39.4)
F2	15 (45.4)
F3	5 (15.2)
Activity grade	
Minimal (A1–A3)	11 (33.3)
Mild (A4–A8)	22 (66.7)
Steatosis	8 (24.2)

reported that hepatitis C in children is usually asymptomatic. Most of our patients (87.9%) were asymptomatic, while the other patients sought medical advice because of abdominal enlargement. Clinically, 4 (12.1%) had hepatomegaly and only one had splenomegaly but none had jaundice or ascites. A similar finding was reported by El-Raziky et al. [5] since soft enlargement of the liver was found in two (11%) children with HCV infection and none had splenomegaly or ascites.

In the current study, although all the patients had mild to moderate fibrosis and minimal to mild activity in liver biopsy, nearly half of them had normal transaminases. It has been reported that alanine transaminase levels were normal in half of the subjects, yet, histological abnormalities were detectable in three quarters of HCV-RNA positive cases [5]. This means that liver enzymes in chronic HCV infection do not necessarily reflect the histopathological abnormalities in the majority of cases and liver biopsy would be essential for evaluation of the disease state and extent of liver injury.

APRI and FIB-4 have been of interest to clinicians because they are simple to calculate and readily available from hospital or clinic laboratories during usual patient care [21]. In our study, APRI and FIB-4 showed no statistically significant difference ($P > 0.05$ for both) among fibrosis stages; however, FIB-4 tended to increase successively from F1 to F3. In hand with our results, Díaz et al. [24] reported that APRI significantly predicts cirrhosis but not fibrosis in pediatric patients. de Lédinghen et al. [25] found that APRI was of benefit in predicting cirrhosis in children with various chronic liver diseases. The majority of reports using APRI and FIB-4 showed a significant performance in discriminating F0–F2 from F3-F4 Metavir score [21], or discriminating F0–F3 from F4–F6 Ishak score [26]. Such advanced stages of fibrosis or cirrhosis were not detected in our study population.

TABLE 2: Histopathological findings in patients with normal versus elevated transaminases.

Histopathology	Normal transaminases $n = 15$	Elevated transaminases $n = 18$	P value
Fibrosis stage			
Mild fibrosis ($n = 13$)	6 (46.2)	7 (53.8)	0.948
Moderate fibrosis ($n = 20$)	9 (45.0)	11 (55.0)	
Activity grade			
Minimal activity ($n = 11$)	5 (45.5)	6 (54.5)	1.0
Mild activity ($n = 22$)	10 (40)	12 (54.5)	

TABLE 3: Serum ITIH4 according to disease activity.

Parameter	ITIH4 (pg/mL)	P value
Activity grade		
Minimal ($n = 11$)	47.17 ± 14.36	0.566
Mild ($n = 22$)	57.72 ± 36.15	
Transaminases level		
Normal ($n = 15$)	53.02 ± 25.27	0.856
Elevated ($n = 18$)	55.19 ± 35.43	

TABLE 4: Correlation of ITIH4 with laboratory and histopathological parameters in liver biopsy.

Parameter	ITIH4 (pg/mL)	
	r	P-value
Total bilirubin (mg/dL)	−0.233	0.193
Direct bilirubin (mg/dL)	−0.204	0.254
Albumin (g/dL)	−0.232	0.194
Alanine transaminase (U/L)	−0.03	0.867
Aspartate transaminase (U/L)	−0.141	0.434
Gamma glutamyl transpeptidase (U/L)	−0.316	0.684
Alkaline phosphatase (U/L)	−0.143	0.506
HCV-RNA (IU/mL)	−0.318	0.071
Fibrosis stage	0.422	0.015
Activity grade	0.082	0.650

APRI and FIB4 reflect alterations in hepatic functions rather than in extracellular matrix (ECM) metabolism. Since, several HCV reports have described normal transaminase levels in about 25%–30% of chronic HCV patients, there may be a potential advantage in assessing serum direct fibrosis markers that do not involve transaminases [27], of which ITIH4 can be considered as one. In our study, 45.5% (15/33) of patients had normal transaminases despite the presence of mild or moderate fibrosis. This may explain the unsatisfactory results of APRI and FIB-4 for detection of significant fibrosis in our study compared to that of ITIH4.

There have been many studies on the biological effects of the ITI molecules, proposing an involvement in various acute-phase processes such as inflammation and cancer [28]. Inhibition of tumor growth and spreading mediated by ITIH genes most likely relates to their stabilizing effects on the extracellular matrix, as well as their covalent linkage of hyaluronic acid [29]. The anti-inflammatory role for ITI has

been suggested by the discovery of stable complexes between these proteins and tumor necrosis factor-stimulated gene 6 [30].

The main target of the current study was to evaluate serum ITIH4 level in children with chronic HCV infection and its relation to liver fibrosis and the level of viremia. Our results showed that ITIH4 serum levels increased successively as fibrosis progresses from F1 to F3. This is in agreement with Yang et al. [10] who reported that ITIH4 was in its lowest value in Metavir F1 and increased as fibrosis progresses then decreased at F4 (cirrhosis). In addition, Gangadharan et al. [11] reported that ITIH4 appears to be candidate to discriminate Metavir F3 from F4 fibrosis.

In patients with no or minimal fibrosis at presentation, antiviral treatment could possibly be delayed due to the mild nature of the disease and the slow progression of liver fibrosis, while in those with significant fibrosis, antiviral treatment is a priority [31]. For that, identifying patients with significant fibrosis is of utmost importance. In the current study, ITIH4 was significantly higher in patients with significant fibrosis (F3) than in those with lower fibrosis stages.

Liver fibrosis represents a chronic wound repair following diverse insults. In fibrogenesis, the normal ECM deposition in the space of Disse is switched to fibrillar, contractile ECM. Thus, it is reasonable to speculate that a proteolytic degradation of the normal ECM may occur at the onset of liver fibrogenesis by matrix metalloproteinases (MMPs). MMP-2 and MMP-9 are the most impressively induced matrix metalloproteinases [32]. Furthermore, the multifunctional cytokine transforming growth factor-beta (TGF-β) plays a pivotal role in the occurrence and progression of fibrosis to cirrhosis. TGF-β enhance hepatocyte destruction and mediate hepatic stellate cell and fibroblast activation resulting in a wound healing response, including myofibroblast generation and ECM deposition [33].

Trypsin activates both MMP-2 [34] and MMP-9 [35]. In addition, the activation of pro-MMP-9 is inhibited by the human trypsin inhibitor [36]. Protease inhibitors prevent the induced hepatic fibrosis in rats through profound inhibition of TGF-β generation [37]. So, the increased ITIH4 with higher stages of fibrosis may be an attempt of the body to counteract the fibrogenic process mediated by the upregulated inflammatory cytokines and MMPs.

ITIH4 is one of the structurally related serine protease inhibitors [13]. The approval of the new direct inhibitors of HCV replication, protease inhibitors, reflects a major

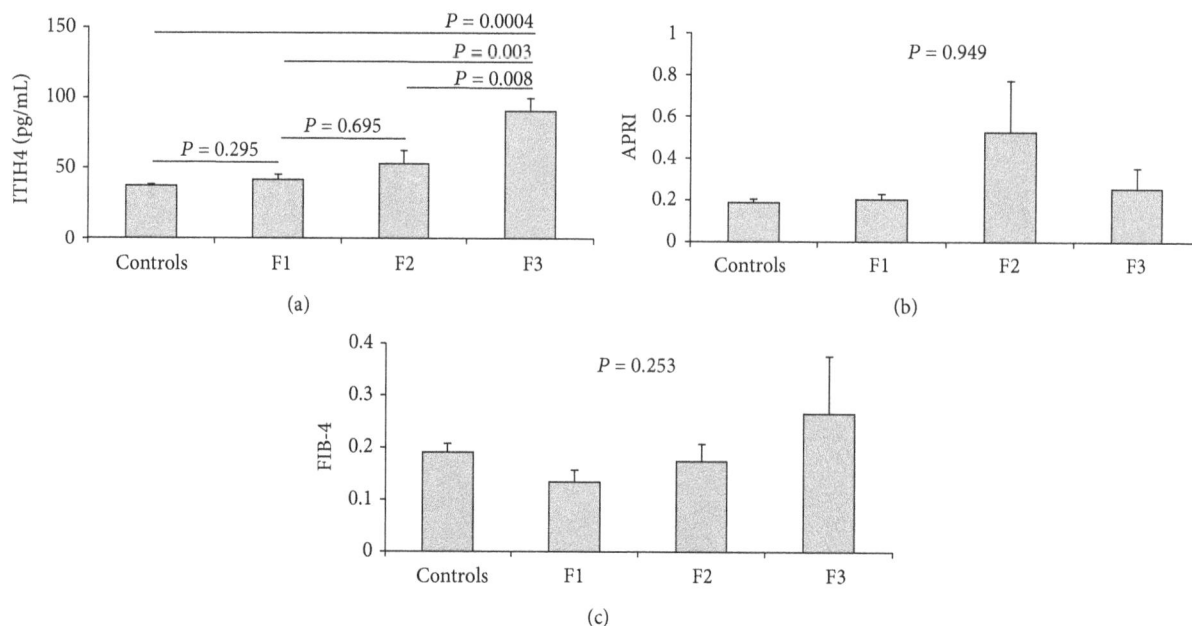

FIGURE 1: Serum fibrosis markers in the individual fibrosis stages. (a) ITIH4; (b) APRI; and (c) FIB-4.

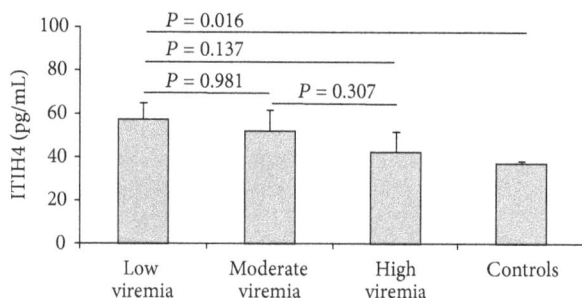

FIGURE 2: Serum ITIH4 in different levels of HCV viremia.

advance for patients infected with HCV [38]. HCV viremia is a determinant factor for the treatment customization and outcomes where low viral load was found to be associated with favourable response [39]. The main target of these direct acting antivirals is to antagonize critical viral proteins including nonstructural protein 3 (NS3) and NS3/4A serine proteases which are important for viral replication [40, 41]. This results in decreased viral load, paving the way for the action of the standard regimen of therapy (pegylated interferon/ribavirin) [42].

We found that HCV viremia was lower in patients with higher serum ITIH4 levels and increases as ITIH4 decreases with highest viremia in patients with lowest ITIH4 levels. It was reported that influenza virus is activated upon trypsin treatment [43] and protease inhibitors were found to inhibit influenza virus in vitro [44]. Furthermore, human pancreatic trypsin inhibitor was found to inhibit the NS3 protease of HCV [45]. Worth to mention, ITIH4 is predominantly expressed in the liver and pancreas [28]. Taken together, it would be logical to postulate that ITIH4 may have potential antiviral properties against HCV.

The small number of the study population represents a limitation which cannot be easily overcome in a single center study. This preliminary work needs to be confirmed in a larger population. In addition, it is worthwhile to evaluate the diagnostic performance of ITIH4 in other pediatric liver diseases with more advanced fibrosis or even cirrhosis.

5. Conclusion

In conclusion, our study demonstrated that ITIH4 serum levels were associated with higher stages of liver fibrosis and were significantly higher in patients with significant fibrosis than in those with lower fibrosis stages. The trend of higher ITIH4 levels in those with lower viral loads suggests potential antiviral properties of ITIH4 and further studies to investigate its effect on HCV replication are worthwhile.

Conflict of Interests

The authors declare that there is no conflict of interests regarding the publication of this paper.

Acknowledgment

This study was funded by the National Liver Institute, Menofiya University, Egypt, without any particular role in the study design, data collection and analysis, or the writing of the report.

References

[1] P. Valva, P. Casciato, C. Lezama et al., "Serum apoptosis markers related to liver damage in chronic hepatitis C: sFas as a marker of advanced fibrosis in children and adults while M30 of severe

steatosis only in children," *PLoS ONE*, vol. 8, no. 1, Article ID e53519, 2013.

[2] N. Mohan, R. P. Gonzalez-Peralta, T. Fujisawa et al., "Chronic hepatitis C virus infection in children," *Journal of Pediatric Gastroenterology and Nutrition*, vol. 50, no. 2, pp. 123–131, 2010.

[3] N. Yazigi and W. Balistreri, "Viral hepatitis," in *Nelson Textbook of Pediatrics*, R. M. Kliegman, R. E. Behrman, H. B. Jenson, and B. F. Stanton, Eds., vol. 350, pp. 1393–1400, Saunders, Philadelphia, Pa, USA, 19th edition, 2011.

[4] E. M. Lehman and M. L. Wilson, "Epidemic hepatitis C virus infection in Egypt: estimates of past incidence and future morbidity and mortality," *Journal of Viral Hepatitis*, vol. 16, no. 9, pp. 650–658, 2009.

[5] M. S. El-Raziky, M. El-Hawary, G. Esmat et al., "Prevalence and risk factors of asymptomatic hepatitis C virus infection in Egyptian children," *World Journal of Gastroenterology*, vol. 13, no. 12, pp. 1828–1832, 2007.

[6] A. A. Bravo, S. G. Sheth, and S. Chopra, "Liver biopsy," *The New England Journal of Medicine*, vol. 344, no. 7, pp. 495–500, 2001.

[7] P. Thampanitchawong and T. Piratvisuth, "Liver biopsy: complications and risk factors," *World Journal of Gastroenterology*, vol. 5, no. 4, pp. 301–304, 1999.

[8] N. H. Afdhal and D. Nunes, "Evaluation of liver fibrosis: a concise review," *The American Journal of Gastroenterology*, vol. 99, no. 6, pp. 1160–1174, 2004.

[9] S. M. Martínez, G. Crespo, M. Navasa, and X. Forns, "Noninvasive assessment of liver fibrosis," *Hepatology*, vol. 53, no. 1, pp. 325–335, 2011.

[10] L. Yang, K. D. Rudser, L. Higgins et al., "Novel biomarker candidates to predict hepatic fibrosis in hepatitis C identified by serum proteomics," *Digestive Diseases and Sciences*, vol. 56, no. 11, pp. 3305–3315, 2011.

[11] B. Gangadharan, R. Antrobus, R. A. Dwek, and N. Zitzmann, "Novel serum biomarker candidates for liver fibrosis in hepatitis C patients," *Clinical Chemistry*, vol. 53, no. 10, pp. 1792–1799, 2007.

[12] M. Piñeiro, M. Andrés, M. Iturralde et al., "ITIH4 (inter-alpha-trypsin inhibitor heavy chain 4) is a new acute-phase protein isolated from cattle during experimental infection," *Infection and Immunity*, vol. 72, no. 7, pp. 3777–3782, 2004.

[13] E. Fries and A. Kaczmarczyk, "Inter-α-inhibitor, hyaluronan and inflammation," *Acta Biochimica Polonica*, vol. 50, no. 3, pp. 735–742, 2003.

[14] A. Someya, N. Tanaka, and A. Okuyama, "Inhibition of influenza virus A WSN replication by a trypsin inhibitor, 6-amidino-2-naphthyl p-guanidinobenzoate," *Biochemical and Biophysical Research Communications*, vol. 169, no. 1, pp. 148–152, 1990.

[15] A. Alisi, D. Comparcola, and V. Nobili, "Treatment of chronic hepatitis C in children: is it necessary and, if so, in whom?" *Journal of Hepatology*, vol. 52, no. 4, pp. 472–474, 2010.

[16] S. L. Chen and T. R. Morgan, "The natural history of hepatitis C virus (HCV) infection," *International Journal of Medical Sciences*, vol. 3, no. 2, pp. 47–52, 2006.

[17] T. Witthöft, B. Möller, K. H. Wiedmann et al., "Safety, tolerability and efficacy of peginterferon alpha-2a and ribavirin in chronic hepatitis C in clinical practice: the German open safety trial," *Journal of Viral Hepatitis*, vol. 14, no. 11, pp. 788–796, 2007.

[18] K. S. Brown, M. J. Keogh, N. Tagiuri et al., "Severe fibrosis in hepatitis C virus- infected patients is associated with increased activity of the mannan-binding lectin (MBL)/MBL-associated

[19] K. Ishak, A. Baptista, L. Bianchi et al., "Histological grading and staging of chronic hepatitis," *Journal of Hepatology*, vol. 22, no. 6, pp. 696–699, 1995.

[20] C.-T. Wai, J. K. Greenson, R. J. Fontana et al., "A simple noninvasive index can predict both significant fibrosis and cirrhosis in patients with chronic hepatitis C," *Hepatology*, vol. 38, no. 2, pp. 518–526, 2003.

[21] S. D. Holmberg, M. Lu, L. B. Rupp et al., "Noninvasive Serum fibrosis markers for screening and staging chronic hepatitis C virus patients in a large US cohort," *Clinical Infectious Diseases*, vol. 57, no. 2, pp. 240–246, 2013.

[22] C. Camarero, N. Ramos, A. Moreno, A. Asensio, M. L. Mateos, and B. Roldan, "Hepatitis C virus infection acquired in childhood," *European Journal of Pediatrics*, vol. 167, no. 2, pp. 219–224, 2008.

[23] F. Bortolotti, P. Jara, C. Diaz et al., "Posttransfusion and community-acquired hepatitis C in childhood," *Journal of Pediatric Gastroenterology and Nutrition*, vol. 18, no. 3, pp. 279–283, 1994.

[24] J. J. Díaz, K. M. Gura, J. Roda et al., "Aspartate aminotransferase to platelet ratio index correlates with hepatic cirrhosis but not with fibrosis in pediatric patients with intestinal failure," *Journal of Pediatric Gastroenterology and Nutrition*, vol. 57, no. 3, pp. 367–371, 2013.

[25] V. de Lédinghen, B. Le Bail, L. Rebouissoux et al., "Liver stiffness measurement in children using fibroscan: feasibility study and comparison with fibrotest, aspartate transaminase to platelets ratio index, and liver biopsy," *Journal of Pediatric Gastroenterology and Nutrition*, vol. 45, no. 4, pp. 443–450, 2007.

[26] R. K. Sterling, E. Lissen, N. Clumeck et al., "Development of a simple noninvasive index to predict significant fibrosis in patients with HIV/HCV coinfection," *Hepatology*, vol. 43, no. 6, pp. 1317–1325, 2006.

[27] P. Valva, P. Casciato, J. M. D. Carrasco et al., "The role of serum biomarkers in predicting fibrosis progression in pediatric and adult hepatitis C virus chronic infection," *PLoS ONE*, vol. 6, no. 8, Article ID e23218, 2011.

[28] A. Hamm, J. Veeck, N. Bektas et al., "Frequent expression loss of Inter-α-trypsin inhibitor heavy chain (ITIH) genes in multiple human solid tumors: a systematic expression analysis," *BMC Cancer*, vol. 8, article 25, 2008.

[29] L. Zhuo, V. C. Hascall, and K. Kimata, "Inter-α-trypsin inhibitor, a covalent protein-glycosaminoglycan-protein complex," *The Journal of Biological Chemistry*, vol. 279, no. 37, pp. 38079–38082, 2004.

[30] H.-G. Wisniewski, D. Naime, J.-C. Hua, J. Vilcek, and B. N. Cronstein, "TSG-6, a glycoprotein associated with arthritis, and its ligand hyaluronan exert opposite effects in a murine model of inflammation," *Pflügers Archiv*, vol. 431, no. 6, supplement 2, pp. R225–R226, 1996.

[31] M. Yano, H. Kumada, M. Kage et al., "The long-term pathological evolution of chronic hepatitis C," *Hepatology*, vol. 23, no. 6, pp. 1334–1340, 1996.

[32] Y. P. Han, "Matrix metalloproteinases, the pros and cons, in liver fibrosis," *Journal of Gastroenterology and Hepatology*, vol. 21, supplement 3, no. 3, pp. S88–S91, 2006.

[33] S. Dooley and P. Ten Dijke, "TGF-β in progression of liver disease," *Cell and Tissue Research*, vol. 347, no. 1, pp. 245–256, 2012.

serine protease 1 (MASP-1) complex," *Clinical and Experimental Immunology*, vol. 147, no. 1, pp. 90–98, 2007.

[34] R. I. Lindstad, I. Sylte, S.-O. Mikalsen, P. O. Seglen, E. Berg, and J.-O. Winberg, "Pancreatic trypsin activates human promatrix metalloproteinase-2," *Journal of Molecular Biology*, vol. 350, no. 4, pp. 682–698, 2005.

[35] M. E. Duncan, J. P. Richardson, G. I. Murray, W. T. Melvin, and J. E. Fothergill, "Human matrix metalloproteinase-9: activation by limited trypsin treatment and generation of monoclonal antibodies specific for the activated form," *European Journal of Biochemistry*, vol. 258, no. 1, pp. 37–43, 1998.

[36] K. Hashimoto, Y. Nagao, K. Kato, Y. Mori, and A. Ito, "Human urinary trypsin inhibitor inhibits the activation of promatrix metalloproteinases and proteoglycans release in rabbit articular cartilage," *Life Sciences*, vol. 63, no. 3, pp. 205–213, 1998.

[37] M. Okuno, K. Akita, H. Moriwaki et al., "Prevention of rat hepatic fibrosis by the protease inhibitor, camostat mesilate, via reduced generation of active TGF-β," *Gastroenterology*, vol. 120, no. 7, pp. 1784–1800, 2001.

[38] G. Esmat, M. El Raziky, M. El Kassas, M. Hassany, and M. E. Gamil, "The future for the treatment of genotype 4 chronic hepatitis C," *Liver International*, vol. 32, supplement 1, pp. 146–150, 2012.

[39] H. A. El-Araby, M. M. Sira, B. E. Behairy, A. O. El-Refaie, and E. M. Ghoneim, "Interferon induction regimen for chronic hepatitis C genotype 4 in Egyptian children," *Journal of Pediatric Infectious Diseases*, vol. 5, no. 3, pp. 233–241, 2010.

[40] A. Rosenquist, B. Samuelsson, P. O. Johansson et al., "Discovery and development of simeprevir (TMC435), a HCV NS3/4A protease inhibitor," *Journal of Medicinal Chemistry*, vol. 57, no. 5, pp. 1673–1693, 2014.

[41] K. L. Berger, I. Triki, M. Cartier et al., "Baseline hepatitis C virus (HCV) NS3 polymorphisms and their impact on treatment response in clinical studies of the HCV NS3 protease inhibitor faldaprevir," *Antimicrobial Agents and Chemotherapy*, vol. 58, no. 2, pp. 698–705, 2014.

[42] B. L. Pearlman and C. Ehleben, "Hepatitis C genotype 1 virus with low viral load and rapid virologic response to peginterferon/ribavirin obviates a protease inhibitor," *Hepatology*, vol. 59, no. 1, pp. 71–77, 2014.

[43] O. P. Zhirnov, A. V. Ovcharenko, and A. G. Bukrinskaya, "Myxovirus replication in chicken embryos can be suppressed by aprotinin due to the blockage of viral glycoprotein cleavage," *Journal of General Virology*, vol. 66, part 7, pp. 1633–1638, 1985.

[44] M. Hosoya, S. Matsuyama, M. Baba, H. Suzuki, and S. Shigeta, "Effects of protease inhibitors on replication of various myxoviruses," *Antimicrobial Agents and Chemotherapy*, vol. 36, no. 7, pp. 1432–1436, 1992.

[45] N. Dimasi, F. Martin, C. Volpari et al., "Characterization of engineered hepatitis C virus NS3 protease inhibitors affinity selected from human pancreatic secretory trypsin inhibitor and minibody repertoires," *Journal of Virology*, vol. 71, no. 10, pp. 7461–7469, 1997.

Measuring the Response of Extrahepatic Symptoms and Quality of Life to Antiviral Treatment in Patients with Hepatitis C

David Isaacs,[1] Nader Abdelaziz,[1] Majella Keller,[2] Jeremy Tibble,[2] and Inam Haq[1,2]

[1] *Brighton and Sussex Medical School, Brighton BN1 9PX, UK*
[2] *Medicine, Royal Sussex County Hospital, Brighton BN2 5BE, UK*

Correspondence should be addressed to David Isaacs; bsms2165@uni.bsms.ac.uk

Academic Editor: Alessandro Antonelli

Background. HCV infection is associated with musculoskeletal manifestations such as chronic widespread pain, sicca syndrome, polyarthritis, and a reduced HRQOL. Little data is available on the effect of treatment on these manifestations. This study measured changes in extrahepatic symptoms and HRQOL before and after antiviral treatment in a large UK patient cohort. *Methods.* 118 patients completed HQLQ and rheumatological questionnaires before and after treatment with pegylated interferon-α and ribavirin, with specific regard to chronic widespread pain, sicca syndrome, and sustained virological response. *Results.* There was significant improvement in HQLQ domains of physical functioning, physical disability, social functioning, limitations and health distress due to hepatitis, and general health. There was significant deterioration in domains of positive well-being, health distress, and mental health. There was a significant decline prevalence of CWP (26.3% versus 15.3%, $P = 0.015$). Sicca syndrome prevalence fell insignificantly (12.7% versus 11%). SVR was associated positively with all HRQOL changes and significantly with CWP remission. *Conclusions.* HCV antivirals significantly improve poor HRQOL scores and CWP. Before treatment, both were common, coassociated, and unaccounted for through mixed cryoglobulinemia alone. Although a role of the hepatitis C virus in CWP cannot be deduced by these results, symptomatic improvement via antiviral treatment exists for this subset of patients.

1. Introduction

Past clinical understanding confined the burden of chronic hepatitis C infection (HCV) to later stages of hepatic impairment. Now it is known that HCV's extrahepatic manifestations (EHMs) and reduced health-related quality of life (HRQOL) often develop before hepatic impairment [1]. Diagnostically, this understanding helps uncover underlying HCV in people presenting with associated EHMs and vice versa. Prognostically, it is unclear whether EHMs independently lower HRQOL in HCV patients and whether they respond to antiviral therapy with or without a sustained virological response (SVR). Answers to these questions would help to determine whether the burden of EHMs in HCV patients merits additional management approaches beyond antiviral therapy.

HRQOL reduction in HCV is multifactorial. Poor baseline HRQOL is partly psychosocial in origin, relating to the stigma of illness, a history of illicit drug use for a large proportion of patients, and high rates of fatigue, anxiety, and depression [2, 3]. Mood-related aspects of HRQOL may even be organically mediated by HCV colonization of brain microglia and activation of brain interleukins [4]. However, HRQOL is also impaired through somatic symptoms, which may be specific to HCV pathophysiology. For example, HCV patients score worse than hepatitis B patients on somatic symptoms of the SF-36 questionnaire, and patients unaware of their HCV infection still score worse than the general population [2, 5]. Furthermore, most evidence points to an improvement in HRQOL as being associated with SVR after treatment with pegylated interferon alone or with ribavirin [2, 6–9], which was confirmed by a meta-analysis that also suggests that a minimum change of 4.2 points on the SF-36 vitality scale is needed for a significant improvement in HRQOL [3]. Several trials, however, show improvements in HRQOL independently of SVR, raising the hypothesis that viral suppression alone can achieve significant physiological changes [6, 8, 10, 11].

HCV associated EHMs create somatic symptoms that probably contribute to patients' lower HRQOL scores, although this has not been sufficiently assessed. Arthralgia and myalgia are among the common rheumatological symptoms associated with HCV, with one study displaying a prevalence of 23% and 15% for each, respectively [12]. Less common rheumatological EHMs include arthritis, vasculitis, sicca syndrome, Sjögren's syndrome, and systemic lupus erythematosus [12, 13].

Mixed cryoglobulinaemia (MC), which has been found in 1–60% of people with HCV, describes the presence of IgM immunoglobulins (rarely IgG or IgA) that form complexes with monoclonal (type II) or polyclonal (type III) rheumatoid factors (RFs) [12]. Types II and III MC are far commoner than simple cryoglobulinaemia (type I) that does not include RF complexes and is not associated with HCV. However, reported prevalence of MC depends heavily on the accuracy of laboratory techniques in cryoprecipitation at low temperatures and measuring cryoglobulin concentrations.

Deposition of MC immune complexes, alongside poor clearance and reduced complement fragments, can result in small-vessel vasculitis and study populations with idiopathic MC have high reported incidences for cutaneous, musculoskeletal, and renal manifestations. Therefore, secondary MC may play a common role in EHMs as 5–10% of HCV patients display an overt MC vasculitic triad of weakness, arthralgia, and purpura [13, 14]. Multiple tropism of the virus, particularly to lymphocytes, may account for many EHMs with or without development of MC [15]. The HCV virus seems to facilitate a state of increased autoantibody and cryoglobulin production by expanding B cells through the envelope protein E2 interacting with the CD81 receptor and increasing B-cell survival by activating the Bcl2 proto-oncogene [13, 16, 17]. A similar state may also be achieved by the virus molecular mimicry of host autoantigens [17, 18]. As of yet, no factors specific to host background, environment, or viral genotype have been associated with the emergence of EHMs [17].

Chronic pain in particular has been shown to impair HRQOL in HCV patients [19]. However, apart from a specific role for MC in some cases of arthralgia, there is no overarching evidence for a pathogenic role of the virus in most presentations of chronic pain. For example, histopathological presence of HCV in muscles of myalgia sufferers [13, 20] and an increased prevalence of HCV in fibromyalgia patients have not been consistently found [21, 22].

There have been limited studies on the role of antiviral therapy for EHMs. Antiviral therapy has some evidence for improving pain in the context of MC complicated HCV. In one study, arthralgia and myalgia improved for approximately half the patients, and in those achieving SVR fatigue and MC levels dropped significantly [23]. In another study, interferon and ribavirin therapy cleared MC in 37.8% and arthralgia in 80% of patients [24]. However, to our knowledge no other studies have yet assessed therapeutic effects on EHMs alongside measured HRQOL changes in HCV patients.

2. Methods

2.1. Aims

(1) Investigate whether HRQOL improves following antiviral therapy.

(2) Investigate whether extrahepatic outcomes improve following antiviral therapy.

(3) Determine whether an association exists between extrahepatic symptoms and HRQOL before and after treatment.

(4) Investigate whether improvement in HRQOL or extrahepatic symptoms is dependent on SVR after treatment.

2.2. Ethics. A study protocol for a cross-sectional epidemiological study into the prevalence of musculoskeletal symptoms among HCV positive adults in a Brighton cohort was proposed and granted ethics approval by the Brighton East Research Ethics Committee in January 2006 (reference. 06/Q/1907/134).

Out of a cohort of 537 HCV patients managed at the Digestive Diseases Unit at the Brighton and Sussex University Hospital Trust (BSUH), in the UK, we assessed the results of 118 patients who were not coinfected with HIV or HBV and who had completed standard antiviral treatment with pegylated interferon-α and ribavirin.

2.3. Outcomes. Participants answered the hepatitis quality of life questionnaire (HQLQ) [25] and a survey of symptoms affecting the spine, muscles, bones, and joints before treatment and six months after finishing treatment. The HQLQ is generically based on SF-36 health survey but is validated as a hepatitis-specific instrument in the measurement of HRQOL [8]. Outcome measures included presence of chronic widespread pain (CWP) according to the Manchester criteria (pain in the axial skeleton and at least two contralateral body quadrants for at least 3 months), the number of affected joints, pain intensity, and interference with daily life as scored on a visual analogue scale (VAS). The binary CWP Manchester criteria outcome was preferred over assessments of fibromyalgia, as the latter would require validation via physician led examinations (self-reports of having a diagnosis of fibromyalgia at baseline were not considered). A lack of physical examinations also excluded the presence of vasculitic rashes from our assessments. In the context of this study, patients were considered positive for sicca syndrome if they reported both mouth and eye sicca symptoms using standardized questions into xeropthalmia and xerostomia; a full assessment of Sjögren's with antiRO/SSA or other autoantibodies was not performed.

2.4. Statistics. A paired samples t-test or Wilcoxon test was used to analyze changes in HRQOL, VAS, and number of painful joints from before treatment to 6 months after treatment. An independent samples t-test or Mann-Whitney U test (nonparametric) was used to analyze the relationship

TABLE 1: Background information.

Background variable	% (n)
Age	
Mean = 46	
Gender	
Male	59 (69)
Female	41 (48)
Ethnicity	
White British	79 (90)
White Irish	3 (4)
White other	12 (14)
Other	6 (6)
In employment	59 (68)
Transmission mode	
Intravenous drugs	77.8 (49)
Blood transfusion	3.2 (2)
Homosexual sex	6.3 (4)
Heterosexual sex	1.6 (1)
Other	8 (7)
Missing	(55)
Genotype	
1	36.5 (19)
2	3.8 (2)
3	26.9 (14)
2, 3	30.8 (16)
4	1.9 (1)
Missing	(66)
SVR	
Achieved	67 (76)
Not achieved	33 (38)
No record	(4)
Arthritis	
Osteoarthritis	5 (6)
Rheumatoid	5 (6)
Unknown	5 (6)
Other	2.5 (3)
Positive for cryoglobulins	5.9 (7)
Inflammatory bowel disease	5.9 (7)

TABLE 2: Background serology.

Assay	Abnormal result N (total found)	Normal reference range	Value taken as abnormal result
Rheumatoid factor	48 (74)	<15 IU/mL	>14 IU/mL
ANA	5 (76)	Nil	>1 : 160
ENA	4 (65)	Nil	+
Mixed cryoglobulinemia	7 (82)	Nil	+
C3 low	4 (81)	0.75–1.65 g/L	<0.75 g/L
C4 low	14 (80)	0.14–0.54 g/L	<0.14 g/L

TABLE 3: HQLQ scores before and after treatment.

HQLQ domain	Mean score		Significance of change
	Before treatment	6 months after treatment	P value
Physical functioning	76.3	80.2	0.024
Role physical	60.2	73.1	0.002
Body pain	60.6	66.3	0.055
General health	50.9	59.1	>0.001
Vitality	46.1	43.9	0.233
Social functioning	62.4	70.4	0.009
Role emotional	63.8	69.3	0.350
Mental health	63.3	59.5	0.048
Health distress	63.8	52.8	0.008
Positive well-being	68.1	51.6	>0.001
Hepatitis-specific functional limitations	58.6	69.3	>0.001
Hepatitis-specific distress	17.2	46.3	>0.001

between HRQOL changes and SVR. A Pearson chi-square test was used in the number of patients with CWP, number of patients with pain for more than 3 months, or number of patients who agreed with the statement "I ache all over." Exact P values of <0.05 in the two-tailed tests were considered significant.

3. Results

3.1. Background Information. See Table 1. Our cohort reflected a relatively young population with a mean age of 46 and an overwhelming proportion with a history of intravenous drug use—due to Brighton having one of the highest prevalence of IVDU in the UK [26]. Unemployment

was also prevalent at 41%. Furthermore, 18% of patients had preexisting arthritis. Although the presence of RF was common (see Table 2), MC prevalence was low at only 5.9%, though laboratory techniques and unsatisfactory test completion rates should be taken into account.

3.2. HRQOL Outcomes. There was a statistically significant improvement in scores in the following 6 out of the 12 domains of the HQLQ: physical functioning, physical disability, social functioning, limitations due to hepatitis, health distress due to hepatitis, and general health (see Table 3 and Figure 1). There was a statistically significant deterioration in 3 of the domains (positive well-being, health distress, and mental health), and there was no significant change in the rest of the domains (body pain, role emotional, and vitality).

3.3. Rheumatological Outcomes. There were a high baseline prevalence of chronic pain symptoms and statistically significant declines after treatment in the number of patients with CWP (11% reduction, $P = 0.015$), number of patients with

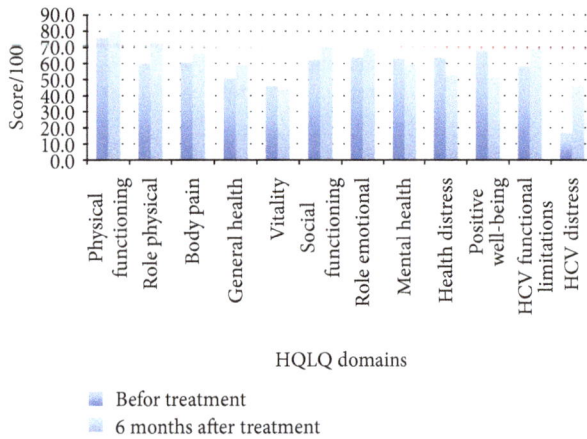

FIGURE 1: HQLQ scores before and after treatment.

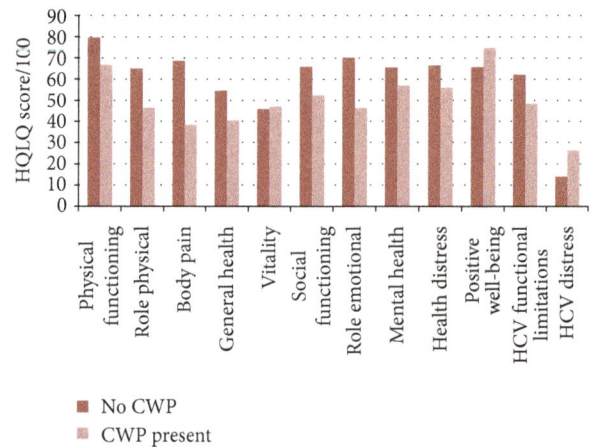

FIGURE 2: Pretreatment HQLQ scores in people with CWP versus no CWP.

pain for more than 3 months (11% reduction, $P = 0.041$), or number of patients who agreed with the statement "I ache all over" (10.1%, $P = 0.029$) (see Table 4).

Having CWP before treatment was significantly associated with worse pretreatment pain levels (5.7/10 versus 2.7/10, $P > 0.001$) and their interference with daily life as reported on VAS (5.0/10 versus 2.1/10, $P > 0.001$), though the overall VAS pain scores and the average number of painful joints did not fall significantly after treatment. Having CWP before treatment was also negatively associated with all HQLQ domains (significantly in all except vitality and health distress and hepatitis-specific distress), except for positive well-being where people with CWP scored significantly higher (75/100 versus 66/100, $P = 0.023$) (see Table 5).

A remission of CWP after treatment was significantly associated with improvements in the HQLQ domain of body pain (15.4 improvement in CWP remission versus 11.8 if it stays the same and 14.8 reduction if CWP develops, $P = 0.024$), physical function ($P = 0.043$), and nearly role emotional ($P = 0.052$) (see Figure 2). In contrast to pretreatment CWP, having CWP after treatment was only significantly associated with a worse role physical and body pain HQLQ score ($P = 0.008$, $P < 0.001$).

There were a small number of patients who matched the study's criteria for sicca syndrome, and the decline after treatment was not significant (12.7% versus 11%, $P = 0.804$).

3.4. Associations with SVR. After treatment 67% of patients achieved SVR. There were positive nonsignificant associations between SVR and changes in all HQLQ scores and significant positive associations between SVR and changes in CWP ($P = 0.038$) (see Figure 3). However, achieving SVR was not associated with the minor regression in sicca symptoms.

4. Discussion

4.1. Quality of Life. Patients in this study showed significant improvement in 6 of the 12 domains of HQLQ following treatment, which on the whole improved the total score.

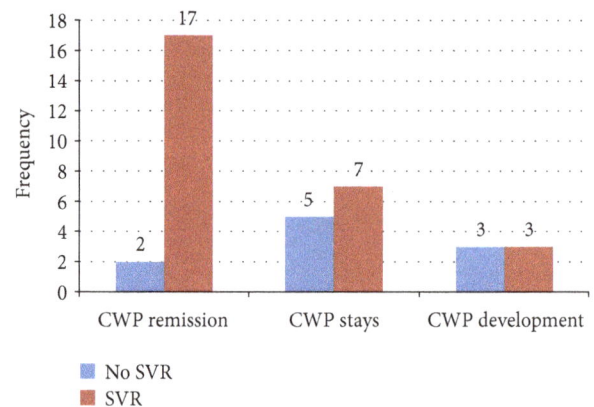

FIGURE 3: CWP progression versus SVR.

However, these improvements did not include an increase of more than 4.2 points on the vitality scale, which has been defined by Spiegel et al. as the minimally clinically important difference in HRQOL [3]. Therefore, to argue that in this case antiviral therapy has had a positive effect on HRQOL is dependent on the weighting given to different domains.

In keeping with previous studies, HRQOL improvement was seen in the domains relating to physical health [2, 6, 7]. Given the significant improvement in domains relating to general health, disease limitations, social functioning, and hepatitis-related distress, the deterioration in domains relating to mental well-being and positive well-being distress suggests a complex range of effects with antiviral treatment. This may be an exacerbation of a high baseline incidence of anxiety and depressive symptoms, which are commonly reported among HCV-infected patients [11, 27]. These baseline symptoms may be related to a patient's distress at being diagnosed with a chronic and serious illness [28], a history of illicit drug use [29], or a direct effect of the virus [30]. The exacerbation of these symptoms, on the other hand, may be caused by antiviral treatment itself, as interferon alpha is known to cause depression [27]. Our results support the hypothesis that initial impairments in physical domains are

TABLE 4: EHMs before and after treatment.

Extrahepatic symptom	Prevalence/mean score		Significance of change (P value)
	Before treatment	6 months after treatment	
CWP	26.3%	15.3%	0.015
Sicca syndrome	12.7%	11%	0.804
Average pain intensity in past month (0–10)	3.5	3.03	0.135
Interference with daily activities in past month (0–10)	2.91	2.67	0.48
Number of painful joints in past month	2.59	2.24	0.306
Pain for more than 3 months	64.4%	53.4%	0.041
"I ache all over"	23.7%	13.6%	0.029

TABLE 5: Variables associated with pretreatment CWP.

	CWP before treatment	No CWP before treatment	Statistical significance (P value)
No. of painful joints	5.19	1.67	>0.001
VAS pain rating (mean)	5.7/10	2.7/10	>0.001
VAS interference rating (mean)	5.0/10	2.1/10	>0.001
HQLQ domain			
Physical functioning	66.8	79.7	0.025
Role physical	46.5	65.1	0.025
Body pain	38.5	68.6	>0.001
General health	40.6	54.6	0.002
Vitality	47.1	45.8	NS (0.553)
Social functioning	52.4	65.9	0.028
Role emotional	46.2	70.1	0.005
Mental health	57.2	65.5	0.035
Health distress	56.1	66.5	NS (0.182)
Positive well-being	74.8	65.7	0.023
Hepatitis-specific functional limitations	48.5	62.2	0.014
Hepatitis-specific distress	26.3	14.0	NS (0.064)

more likely to be virus related than impairments in domains of mental health given that the former domains improved following treatment while the latter did not [1, 31].

4.2. Rheumatological Symptoms. Our results reflect the direction of previous findings that fewer patients experience myalgia and arthralgia following treatment [23, 24, 32]. Interestingly, however, while patients with CWP, 3-month pain and "I ache all over" reported that pain levels all fell significantly, the average VAS pain intensity and impact levels, bodily pain aspects of the HQLQ, and the number of painful joints were all low and changed little with treatment. This demonstrates that extrahepatic pain manifestations in HCV patients pool together in a subset of patients and are unaltered by treatment in the majority of cases.

An analysis comparing patients with and without CWP before treatment revealed baseline HQLQ scores to be significantly worse in 9 domains in those with CWP, though whether this was cause or effect is not ascertainable here. The discrepancy of a greater positive well-being in patients with baseline CWP represents a psychological anomaly as mental health and other psychological domains were significantly worse in this subset. CWP remission after treatment was also significantly associated with an improved body pain

and physical function score, which changed little otherwise for the whole cohort. This shows that having CWP before treatment is significantly associated with a worse HRQOL and that the bodily pain aspect may be particularly responsive to treatment in this subset, which has not been illustrated in the literature before. The clinical implications for this lie in better recognition of this subset of patients in order to discuss the potential effects of treatment for them specifically and in using appropriate additional management strategies such as analgesia or exercise.

If the observed trends in pain reflect the effects of a viral immunomodulatory process affecting a subset of patients, one would expect more patients to also undergo remission of sicca syndrome. A lack of response to treatment may be due to unknown factors and an already underwhelming sicca prevalence in the cohort relative to other studies. [33]. However, a more evident response would be expected because sicca syndrome has an established viral pathogenesis where HCV exocrine gland tropism is strongly associated with lymphocytic infiltration, sometimes in combination with rheumatoid factor and autoantibodies and resultant xerostomia and xerophthalmia [34]. Arthralgia on the other hand is more known to be associated with HCV through a mechanism of elevated autoantibodies and MC that promotes tissue injury, a biomarker which was rare in our cohort [35]. Thus, our observed improvements in pain scores may also be due to unmeasured nonvirological changes, such as nutritional status improvements, reduced alcoholic consumption, and subsequent improvements in vitamin D levels that are associated with nonspecific musculoskeletal pain [36].

4.3. SVR Discussion. Data from a meta-analysis of HRQOL studies in HCV patients has suggested that SVR is associated with improved HRQOL. In this study, there was a general trend in that direction without statistical significance, which reflects the power of the sample size. Our results suggest that antiviral therapy can improve HRQOL and pain scores in the absence of SVR, which may be due to a placebo response, which this study did not control for, or due to the immunomodulatory effects of antiviral therapy, which have not been fully described yet. For example, interferon has been found to have antiproliferative effects on MC and has been used on MC even before link with HCV was found. Furthermore, it has been suggested that this effectiveness may be irrespective of interferon's antiviral properties [37]. Conversely, other studies have shown that MC and subsequent vasculitic symptoms can persist despite SVR [38], which supports the hypothesis of there being both memory (virus-dependent) and naïve (virus-independent) autoimmune B cell expansion after HCV infection [24].

5. Limitations

The main drawback of this study is the lack of a matched control group not undergoing antiviral treatment, due to there being only a minority of such patients, of whom many have concurrent psychiatric illness, IVDU, and alcoholism. Furthermore, concomitant use of vitamin D supplementation, analgesia, and anti-inflammatories during questionnaire completion was not controlled for. Due to the small proportion of patients with the extrahepatic symptoms in this study, a larger sample may be necessary to improve the power of measuring the effects of treatment and SVR. Therefore, larger study participation with controls and longer followup are needed to validate the study's results.

6. Conclusions

Antiviral therapy with pegylated interferon-α and ribavirin can significantly improve physical and functional aspects of HRQOL as well as rheumatological CWP symptoms in HCV patients, despite no changes in vitality and deterioration in mental health and positive well-being. In our cohort, CWP prevalence is high, demonstrably related to HRQOL, and unaccounted for through cryoglobulinaemia alone. A role for the virus in CWP is purely speculative on the basis of these results, and other potential causes such as vitamin D deficiency were not measured. Of relevance to clinical practice, however, are the study's observed CWP prevalence and response in HCV patients undergoing antiviral treatment. An awareness of this finding may prompt earlier diagnosis and investigation of CWP in HCV patients and warrant chronic

pain relief as an additional indication for antiviral treatment besides existing benefits on hepatitis and HRQOL. Additional management strategies such as graded exercise and analgesia should be discussed in this subset of chronic pain sufferers for whom antivirals are deemed inappropriate.

Abbreviations

HCV: Hepatitis C virus
EHMs: Extrahepatic manifestations
CWP: Chronic widespread pain
HRQOL: Health-related quality of life
HQLQ: Hepatitis quality of life questionnaire
SVR: Sustained virological response
MC: Mixed cryoglobulinaemia
SS: Sicca syndrome.

Conflict of Interests

None of the authors declare any conflict of interests.

References

[1] M. C. Teixeira, F. Ribeiro Mde, L. C. Gayotto, A. Chamone Dde, and E. Strauss, "Worse quality of life in volunteer blood donors with hepatitis C," *Transfusion*, vol. 46, no. 2, pp. 278–283, 2006.

[2] A. Hollander, G. R. Foster, and O. Weiland, "Health-related quality of life before, during and after combination therapy with interferon and ribavirin in unselected Swedish patients with chronic hepatitis C," *Scandinavian Journal of Gastroenterology*, vol. 41, no. 5, pp. 577–585, 2006.

[3] B. M. Spiegel, Z. M. Younossi, R. D. Hays, D. Revicki, S. Robbins, and F. Kanwal, "Impact of hepatitis C on health related quality of life: a systematic review and quantitative assessment," *Hepatology*, vol. 41, no. 4, pp. 790–800, 2005.

[4] K. Weissenborn, A. B. Tryc, M. Heeren et al., "Hepatitis C virus infection and the brain," *Metabolic Brain Disease*, vol. 24, no. 1, pp. 197–210, 2009.

[5] A. J. Rodger, D. Jolley, S. C. Thompson, A. Lanigan, and N. Crofts, "The impact of diagnosis of hepatitis C virus on quality of life," *Hepatology*, vol. 30, no. 5, pp. 1299–1301, 1999.

[6] M. Wright, R. Grieve, J. Roberts, J. Main, and H. C. Thomas, "Health benefits of antiviral therapy for mild chronic hepatitis C: randomised controlled trial and economic evaluation," *Health Technology Assessment*, vol. 10, no. 21, pp. 1–113, 2006.

[7] M. P. Neary, S. Cort, M. S. Bayliss, and J. E. Ware Jr., "Sustained virologic response is associated with improved health-related quality of life in relapsed chronic hepatitis C patients," *Seminars in Liver Disease*, vol. 19, supplement 1, pp. 77–85, 1999.

[8] J. E. Ware Jr., M. S. Bayliss, M. Mannocchia, and G. L. Davis, "Health-related quality of life in chronic hepatitis C: impact of disease and treatment response," *Hepatology*, vol. 30, no. 2, pp. 550–555, 1999.

[9] J. G. McHutchison, J. E. Ware Jr., M. S. Bayliss et al., "The effects of interferon alpha-2b in combination with ribavirin on health related quality of life and work productivity," *Journal of Hepatology*, vol. 34, no. 1, pp. 140–147, 2001.

[10] M. Wright, D. Forton, J. Main et al., "Treatment of histologically mild hepatitis C virus infection with interferon and ribavirin: a multicentre randomized controlled trial," *Journal of Viral Hepatitis*, vol. 12, no. 1, pp. 58–66, 2005.

[11] H. H. Thein, P. Maruff, M. D. Krahn et al., "Improved cognitive function as a consequence of hepatitis C virus treatment," *HIV Medicine*, vol. 8, no. 8, pp. 520–528, 2007.

[12] P. Cacoub, T. Poynard, P. Ghillani et al., "Extrahepatic manifestations of chronic hepatitis C. MULTIVIRC Group. Multidepartment virus CMULTIVIRC Group. Multidepartment virus C," *Arthritis and Rheumatism*, vol. 42, no. 10, pp. 2204–2212, 1999.

[13] C. Lormeau, G. Falgarone, D. Roulot, and M.-C. Boissier, "Rheumatologic manifestations of chronic hepatitis C infection," *Joint Bone Spine*, vol. 73, no. 6, pp. 633–638, 2006.

[14] D. Sène, N. Limal, and P. Cacoub, "Hepatitis C virus-associated extrahepatic manifestations: a review," *Metabolic Brain Disease*, vol. 19, no. 3-4, pp. 357–381, 2004.

[15] A. L. Zignego, D. Macchia, M. Monti et al., "Infection of peripheral mononuclear blood cells by hepatitis C virus," *Journal of Hepatology*, vol. 15, no. 3, pp. 382–386, 1992.

[16] P. Pileri, Y. Uematsu, S. Campagnoli et al., "Binding of hepatitis C virus to CD81," *Science*, vol. 282, no. 5390, pp. 938–941, 1998.

[17] C. Ferri, A. Antonelli, M. T. Mascia et al., "HCV-related autoimmune and neoplastic disorders: the HCV syndrome," *Digestive and Liver Disease*, vol. 39, supplement 1, pp. S13–S21, 2007.

[18] F. B. Bianchi, P. Muratori, A. Granito, G. Pappas, S. Ferri, and L. Muratori, "Hepatitis C and autoreactivity," *Digestive and Liver Disease*, vol. 39, supplement 1, pp. S22–S24, 2007.

[19] K. I. Penny, A. M. Purves, B. H. Smith, W. A. Chambers, and W. C. Smith, "Relationship between the chronic pain grade and measures of physical, social and psychological well-being," *Pain*, vol. 79, no. 2-3, pp. 275–279, 1999.

[20] J. Bartolomé, E. Rodríguez-Iñigo, A. Erice, S. Vidal, I. Castillo, and V. Carreño, "Hepatitis C virus does not infect muscle, the intervertebral disk, or the meniscus in patients with chronic hepatitis C," *Journal of Medical Virology*, vol. 79, pp. 1818–1820, 2007.

[21] C. Palazzi, E. D'Amico, S. D'Angelo, A. Nucera, A. Petricca, and I. Olivieri, "Hepatitis C virus infection in Italian patients with fibromyalgia," *Clinical Rheumatology*, vol. 27, no. 1, pp. 101–103, 2008.

[22] J. Narváez, J. M. Nolla, and J. Valverde-García, "Lack of association of fibromyalgia with hepatitis C virus infection," *The Journal of Rheumatology*, vol. 32, pp. 1118–1121, 2005.

[23] P. Cacoub, V. Ratziu, R. P. Myers et al., "Impact of treatment on extra hepatic manifestations in patients with chronic hepatitis C," *Journal of Hepatology*, vol. 36, no. 6, pp. 812–818, 2002.

[24] D. Saadoun, A. Delluc, J. C. Piette, and P. Cacoub, "Treatment of hepatitis C-associated mixed cryoglobulinemia vasculitis," *Current Opinion in Rheumatology*, vol. 20, no. 1, pp. 23–28, 2008.

[25] M. S. Bayliss, B. Gandek, K. M. Bungay, D. Sugano, M.-A. Hsu, and J. E. Ware Jr., "A questionnaire to assess the generic and disease-specific health outcomes of patients with chronic hepatitis C," *Quality of Life Research*, vol. 7, no. 1, pp. 39–55, 1998.

[26] C. Griffiths, E. Romeri, A. Brock, and O. Morgan, "Geographical variations in deaths related to drug misuse in England and Wales, 1993–2006," *Health Statistics Quarterly*, no. 39, pp. 14–21, 2008.

[27] R. J. Fontana, K. B. Hussain, S. M. Schwartz, C. A. Moyer, G. L. Su, and A. S. Lok, "Emotional distress in chronic hepatitis C patients not receiving antiviral therapy," *Journal of Hepatology*, vol. 36, no. 3, pp. 401–407, 2002.

[28] J. Golden, R. M. Conroy, A. M. O'Dwyer, D. Golden, and J.-B. Hardouin, "Illness-related stigma, mood and adjustment to illness in persons with hepatitis C," *Social Science and Medicine*, vol. 63, no. 12, pp. 3188–3198, 2006.

[29] M. G. Carta, M. C. Hardoy, A. Garofalo et al., "Association of chronic hepatitis C with major depressive disorders: irrespective of interferon-alpha therapy," *Clinical Practice and Epidemiology in Mental Health*, vol. 3, article 22, 2007.

[30] D. M. Forton, H. C. Thomas, C. A. Murphy et al., "Hepatitis C and cognitive impairment in a cohort of patients with mild liver disease," *Hepatology*, vol. 35, no. 2, pp. 433–439, 2002.

[31] J. Rivera, A. de Diego, M. Trinchet, and A. García Monforte, "Fibromyalgia-associated hepatitis C virus infection," *British Journal of Rheumatology*, vol. 36, no. 9, pp. 981–985, 1997.

[32] C. Mazzaro, G. Pozzato, F. Zorat et al., "Etiologic treatment of hepatitis C virus-associated mixed cryoglobulinemia," *Digestive and Liver Disease*, vol. 39, supplement 1, pp. S102–S106, 2007.

[33] C. Jorgensen, M.-C. Legouffe, P. Perney et al., "Sicca syndrome associated with hepatitis C virus infection," *Arthritis and Rheumatism*, vol. 39, no. 7, pp. 1166–1171, 1996.

[34] M. Ramos-Casals, S. De Vita, and A. G. Tzioufas, "Hepatitis C virus, Sjögren's syndrome and B-cell lymphoma: linking infection, autoimmunity and cancer," *Autoimmunity Reviews*, vol. 4, no. 1, pp. 8–15, 2005.

[35] R. Sterling and S. Bralow, "Extrahepatic manifestations of hepatitis C virus," *Current Gastroenterology Reports*, vol. 8, no. 1, pp. 53–59, 2006.

[36] K. V. Knutsen, M. Brekke, S. Gjelstad, and P. Lagerløv, "Vitamin D status in patients with musculoskeletal pain, fatigue and headache: a cross-sectional descriptive study in a multi-ethnic general practice in Norway," *Scandinavian Journal of Primary Health Care*, vol. 28, no. 3, pp. 166–171, 2010.

[37] J.-M. Durand, P. Cacoub, F. Lunel-Fabiani et al., "Ribavirin in hepatitis C related cryoglobulinemia," *Journal of Rheumatology*, vol. 25, no. 6, pp. 1115–1117, 1998.

[38] J. W. Levine, C. Gota, B. J. Fessler, L. H. Calabrese, and S. M. Cooper, "Persistent cryoglobulinemic vasculitis following successful treatment of hepatitis C virus," *Journal of Rheumatology*, vol. 32, no. 6, pp. 1164–1167, 2005.

13

Spectrum of Histomorphologic Findings in Liver in Patients with SLE: A Review

Shrruti Grover, Archana Rastogi, Jyotsna Singh, Apurba Rajbongshi, and Chhagan Bihari

Department of Pathology, Institute of Liver and Biliary Sciences D-1, Vasant Kunj, New Delhi 110070, India

Correspondence should be addressed to Chhagan Bihari; drcbsharma@gmail.com

Academic Editor: Piero Luigi Almasio

Collagen vascular diseases (CVDs) like systemic lupus erythematosus (SLE), rheumatoid arthritis, Sjogren syndrome (SS), and scleroderma are immunologically mediated disorders that typically have multisystem involvement. Although clinically significant liver involvement is rare, liver enzyme abnormalities are common in these patients. The reported prevalence of hepatic involvement in SLE, histopathologic findings, and its significance is very variable in the existing literature. It is important to be familiar with the causes of hepatic involvement in SLE along with histomorphological features which aid in distinguishing hepatitis of SLE from other hepatic causes as they would alter the patient management and disease course. Histopathology of liver in SLE shows a wide morphological spectrum commonly due to a coexisting pathology. Drug induced hepatitis, viral etiology, and autoimmune overlap should be excluded before attributing the changes to SLE itself. Common histopathologic findings in SLE include fatty liver, portal inflammation, and vascular changes like hemangioma, congestion, nodular regenerative hyperplasia, arteritis, and abnormal vessels in portal tracts.

1. Introduction

Systemic lupus erythematosus (SLE) is a chronic autoimmune disease with features of multisystem involvement and diverse clinical and serological manifestations, mostly affecting women during the child bearing age. Hepatic involvement is usually subclinical and has been demonstrated by many studies [1]. Clinically significant hepatic dysfunction is generally considered uncommon in SLE and treatment with hepatotoxic drugs or viral hepatitis has usually been implicated as the most pertinent causes for such unusual complications [2]. Commonly recognised features include mild elevation of liver enzymes and nonspecific histological features. Liver involvement may vary from a mild asymptomatic elevation of liver transaminases to a fulminant hepatitis rarely. Liver involvement as a manifestation of underlying SLE requires cautious exclusion of hepatotoxic drugs or coincident viral hepatitis.

Hepatic involvement in SLE could be due to a wide range of factors such as drug induced damage, steatosis, viral hepatitis, vascular thrombosis, and overlaps with autoimmune hepatitis (AIH) or due to SLE itself. It is important to differentiate between the above causes of hepatic involvement as they alter the disease course and management [3]. A range of studies evaluating the causes of liver involvement in SLE have been conducted and results of histopathological features have been inconsistent. A review of histomorphological features of liver in patients with SLE is presented.

2. Methodology

We searched the literature on PubMed database with the following keywords: "SLE, liver histopathology" which showed a total of 168 studies. Out of these, all studies which evaluated the causes of liver dysfunction in SLE patients by histopathology were shortlisted. These amounted to a total of 36 studies. All studies where histopathology of liver was not available were excluded from the histological spectrum in the present review.

All the 36 studies were assessed on methodology. These included patients diagnosed with SLE according to revised criteria proposed by American College of Rheumatology. The criteria for ascertaining lupus as the primary cause of liver dysfunction were based on exclusion of all other possible

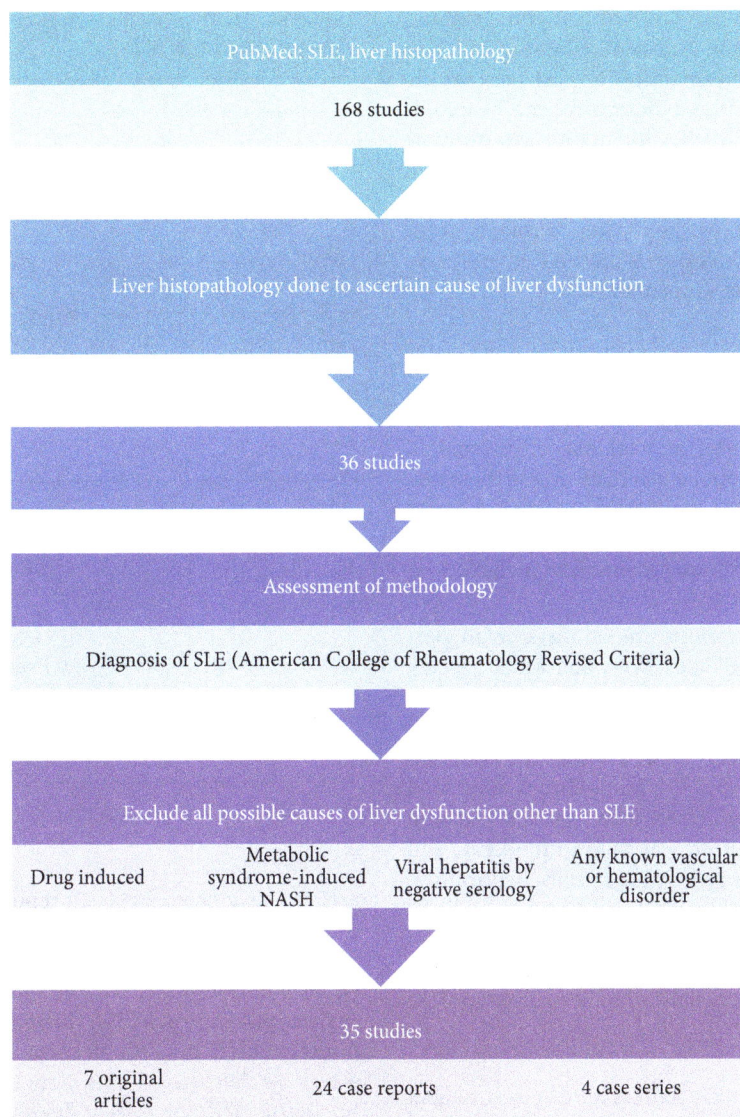

FIGURE 1: Summarized methodology.

causes of liver dysfunction such as viral hepatitis, drug induced liver damage, nonalcoholic steatohepatitis, and any known underlying vascular or haematological disorder. Viral hepatitis excluded by negative serology and drug induced toxicity was evaluated by history and histopathological features in these studies. Patients of SLE who were on drugs/steroids as a part of the treatment of underlying autoimmune disease were included, excluding patients on any other kind of drug treatment. Patients who had known association with vascular thrombosis or any haematological disorder were excluded in the present review. Patients with features of metabolic syndrome were also excluded. A radiological study reporting benign vascular lesions in SLE was also included although no histological confirmation was available in this study.

After applying the above standard the total number of studies amounted to 35 comprising 7 original articles, 24 case reports, and 4 case series. Combining all the above studies histopathological spectrum of liver in SLE was studied in 293 patients. Few cross-references in these articles were also studied and included in the review (methodology summarized in Figure 1).

3. Review

3.1. Subclinical Liver Disease.
Subclinical liver disease is a common phenomenon in SLE mostly manifesting as abnormal liver function test. The reported values of liver enzyme elevation range up to 55% [4]. Recently a study by Vaiphei et al. reported a much higher value of 81% of SLE patients showing raised transaminases [5]. A prospective study reported liver enzyme elevations in 23% out of which in 8% cases the elevations were unexplained. Liver tissue available from 14 patients revealed no significant lesions. This study suggested that subclinical liver disease is a manifestation of SLE [1].

The reported frequency of hepatic involvement in SLE ranges from 8 to 23% [4]. Clinical examination may show a palpably enlarged liver in 33% cases [5].

3.2. Biochemical Abnormalities. Biochemical abnormalities are typically mild and show transient elevation of liver enzymes. The histologic abnormalities in most patients are commonly nonprogressive. Such biochemical and histologic findings can be attributed to the underlying autoimmune condition and require no specific management. Patients with a coexisting primary liver disease show a more persistently deranged LFT and further workup using serologic tests, imaging studies, and liver biopsy is needed to precisely identify the cause of liver test abnormalities [6].

3.3. Histopathology of Liver in SLE. Pathologically, a wide variety of lesions have been described in the hepatic parenchyma of patients diagnosed with SLE. Liver histology can show steatosis, portal and lobular inflammation, hepatic granulomas, centrilobular necrosis, microabscesses, haemochromatosis, cholestasis, nonspecific reactive changes, and infrequent cirrhosis [4].

Histopathological findings are summarized in Table 1.

3.3.1. Portal Changes. The various alterations seen in portal areas include portal inflammation, abnormal vessels, interface hepatitis, chronic persistent hepatitis, nonspecific reactive hepatitis, portal tract fibrosis, and periductal fibrosis. Portal tract inflammation was a relatively common histopathological finding [4, 5, 7–9]. Vaiphei et al. studied 21 autopsy cases of SLE and portal tract inflammation was seen in 14 patients. The inflammation was mild to moderate and comprised of mainly lymphocytes, plasma cells, neutrophils, and occasional eosinophils (Figure 2). No lymphoid follicle, bile duct epithelial cell injury, plasma cell dominant infiltration, or hepatocyte rosette formation was seen in these cases [5]. Along with this interface hepatitis has been also reported by some authors [4, 5, 7].

3.3.2. Lobular Changes. Lobular changes were not as frequent as portal changes. These included lobular inflammation, steatosis, and focal necrosis [5, 8] (Figure 3). Hydropic degeneration of hepatocytes has also been described by one author in 8 of the 47 SLE cases studied [8]. Hepatocytic steatosis was a fairly common morphologic observation in many studies and it could not be conclusively attributed to lupus alone since similar changes can occur due to steroid therapy which is commonly prescribed to these patients [4, 7–10] (Figure 4). Matsumoto et al. studied 52 livers from patients with systemic lupus erythematosus and found fatty liver in a significant number of patients (38/52). They considered steatosis as a finding specific to SLE. Exposure to steroids in these patients was a significant etiologic factor in development of fatty liver [10]. There have been rare case reports of secondary amyloidosis of liver in patients of long-standing SLE [11].

3.3.3. Vascular Changes. A wide morphologic spectrum of vascular changes have been described by many authors which include hepatic congestion, abnormal vessels in portal tracts, hemangioma, peliosis hepatis, arteritis, and occasionally infarct due to arteritis. Rarely hepatic artery aneurysms [12] and spontaneous hepatic rupture due to arteritis of hepatic

TABLE 1: Spectrum of salient histomorphological findings in liver biopsy in patients of SLE.

Portal changes [4, 5, 7–10]	Portal inflammation
	Interface hepatitis
	Chronic persistent hepatitis
	Portal tract fibrosis
	Cholestasis
	Periductal fibrosis
	Cholangiolitis
Lobular changes [5, 8]	Lobular inflammation
	Focal necrosis
	Steatosis
	NAFL
	Hydropic degeneration
Fibrosis [3, 5, 7–9]	Bridging fibrosis
	Cirrhosis
Vascular changes [5, 10, 12–15, 17]	Abnormal vessels in portal tracts
	Arteritis
	Infarct due to arteritis
	Nodular regenerative hyperplasia
	Haemangioma
	Hepatic congestion
	Peliosis hepatis

arteries have been also been reported [13]. Matsumoto et al. found hepatic congestion to be the commonest (76%) in 52 livers studied, along with arteritis (22%), peliosis hepatis (11.5%), hemangioma, and nodular regenerative hyperplasia in three patients each (5%) [10]. Fatty change was a significant finding noted in 73% of cases. Their data suggested that arteritis of liver in SLE was more common than that reported previously and one patient developed hepatic infarction as a complication induced by arteritis. Congestion was linked to acute terminal illness.

Vaiphei et al. studied 21 SLE patients with no known association with chronic liver disease or vascular thrombosis or hematological disorder and found diffuse nodular regenerative hyperplasia of liver (NRHL) in a significant proportion of cases (43%) with some portal tracts showing mild-to-moderate chronic inflammation with occasional bridging fibrosis [5]. This finding of NRH was more frequent in their study than previous reported series [14, 15]. Matsumoto et al. reported numerous abnormal thin-walled vessels in intermediate- and small-sized portal tracts with no vascular occlusion or inflammation. These vascular channels were seen involving about 40% of intermediate- and small-sized portal tracts entrapping bile ducts and hepatic arteries with a variable amount of collagen in between. Etiopathogenesis for NRHL in SLE is an immune complex deposit in small vessels resulting in obliterative venopathy. Obliterative fibroinflammation of the terminal portal tract was observed in all NRHL cases in this study. The proposed pathogenesis of NRHL is a small vessel vasculitis producing hepatocytic atrophy associated with compensatory hyperplasia [16].

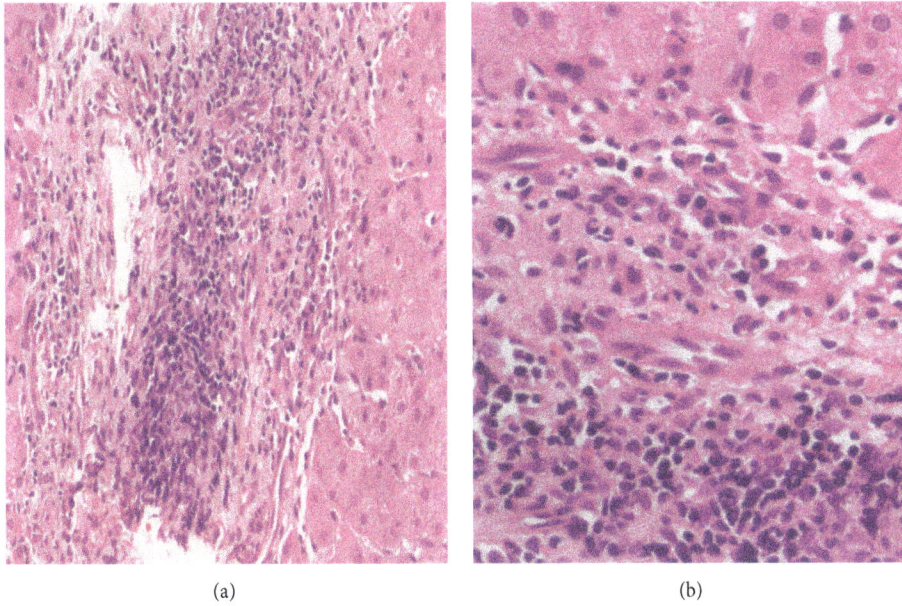

FIGURE 2: (a) Portal inflammation with lymphoid aggregate (H&E stain; 200x). (b) Portal inflammation comprising of numerous plasma cells with interface activity (H&E; 400x).

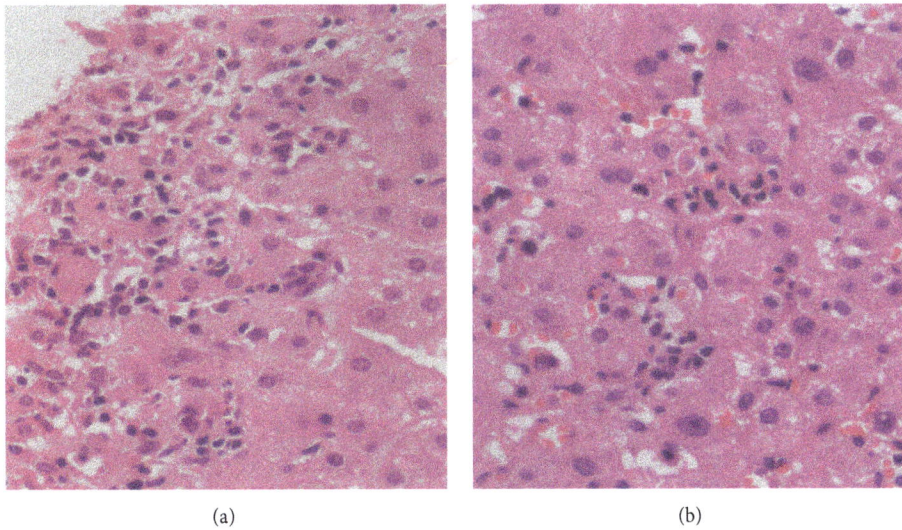

FIGURE 3: (a) Foci of confluent necrosis infiltrated by inflammatory cells (H&E; 400x). (b) Microabscesses in hepatic lobule (H&E stain; 400x).

The prevalence of liver hemangioma was 54.2% in 1 study involving 35 patients of SLE compared to 14% in general population. The above authors also reported a case of Budd-Chiari syndrome with NRH and NRH associated with hepatic hemangioma both in patients hospitalized for abdominal symptoms, suggesting that vascular liver diseases should be specifically investigated in this population, but this study lacked the histological confirmation of hemangioma in most patients as imaging modalities were used for diagnosis [17].

3.3.4. Biliary Changes. Biliary changes are not frequent in SLE. Histopathology has revealed cholestasis, cholangiolitis,

and periductal fibrosis in few cases and acute cholestatic hepatitis has been reported rarely [5, 10]. Runyon et al. demonstrated a peculiar form of cholestasis resembling a canalicular cast of bile in three of four SLE patients with cirrhosis [7]. The canalicular cast of bile is a form of cholestatic liver cell rosettes and can be found in any long-standing canalicular cholestasis. Occasional case report describes hemobilia in liver biopsy in a patient who developed acalculous cholecystitis [18].

3.3.5. Advanced Fibrosis/Cirrhosis. Portal tract fibrosis and bridging fibrosis were a common observation reported by many [5, 7, 9] with cirrhosis in few and progression to liver

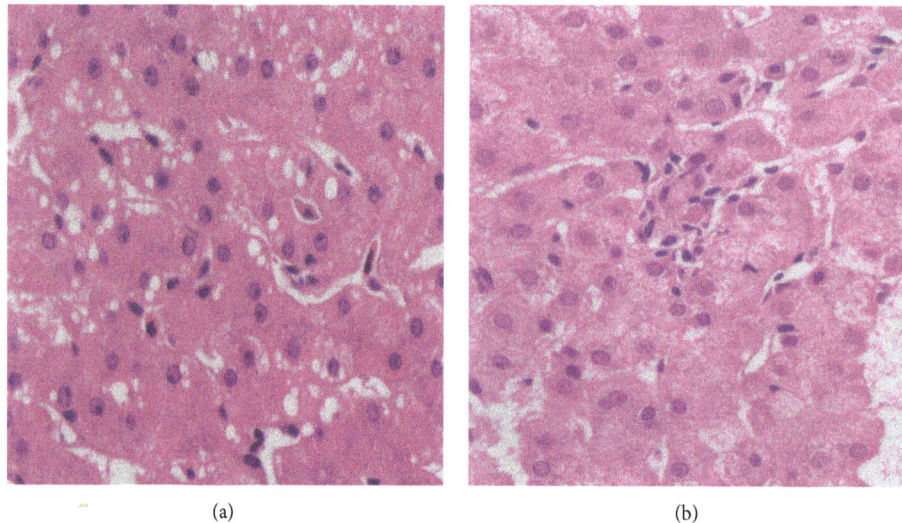

FIGURE 4: (a) Mild macrovesicular steatosis in hepatocytes (H&E stain; 400x). (b) Small focus of lobular inflammation (H&E; 400x).

failure was reported by Runyon et al. in 3 cases [7]. This was the first study to highlight that severe and fatal liver disease can occur in SLE due to liver failure. Vaiphei et al. observed portal tract fibrosis in 76% and bridging fibrosis in 42% of the cases with progression to cirrhosis in minority of cases by various authors [3, 7, 8, and 9]. Matsumoto's autopsy registry review of 1468 patients suggested an incidence of chronic hepatitis in 2.4% of SLE patients with 1.1% progressing to cirrhosis [10].

3.3.6. AIH and SLE Overlap.
Differentiating between liver involvement in CVDs and overlap syndrome with AIH could be difficult given their common clinical and serologic manifestations. Differentiating features for AIH from SLE-related liver disease are portal and periportal inflammation, piecemeal necrosis with dense lymphoid infiltrates, dominant portal tract plasma cell infiltration, hepatocyte pseudorosette formation whereas lupus-associated hepatitis shows predominantly lobular involvement with mild lobular inflammation and no piecemeal necrosis [19].

One study suggested use of antiribosomal P antibodies to distinguish between the two entities as they are not found in patients with AIH but are present in a significant proportion of patients with lupus-associated hepatitis [20].

Distinguishing the two entities is important as the diagnosis has important prognostic and therapeutic implications, where lupus-associated hepatitis has a more benign course and does not require corticosteroid therapy.

3.4. Coexistent Liver Pathologies in SLE.
Liver disease in SLE could be the result of a variety of factors including fat infiltration, drug toxicity, coexisting viral hepatitis, vascular thrombosis, and overlap with autoimmune hepatitis (AIH) or of SLE itself. It is important to exclude these coexistent pathologies affecting the liver which may occur concurrently or sequentially, as they alter the disease course and management (summarized in Table 2).

TABLE 2: Associated liver pathology in patients of SLE.

	Drug induced hepatitis
	Viral hepatitis
	Primary biliary cirrhosis
	Autoimmune hepatitis
Associated pathology [3, 7, 22–24]	Lymphoma
	Granuloma
	Liver failure
	Infections

Excessive fatty infiltration is a common finding in tissue and may be attributed either to the disease process itself or to the steroid treatment. Drug induced hepatitis is a relatively common cause of liver dysfunction in this group of patients which should therefore be excluded first before ascribing the cause of liver dysfunction as SLE. According to Gibson and Myers, a significant number of patients (14 out of 45) of SLE with elevated liver enzymes had drug induced hepatitis [4]. After excluding other nonhepatic causes 19 patients had enzyme elevation due to SLE itself. Van Hoek studied the spectrum of liver disease in SLE patients and suggested drug induced hepatitis as the most common cause of liver dysfunction [21].

A wide spectrum of primary liver diseases in systemic lupus erythematosus have been demonstrated by various authors and include viral hepatitis, autoimmune hepatitis, primary biliary cirrhosis, granulomatous hepatitis, giant cell hepatitis, chronic hepatitis with IgA or IgD deficiency, porphyria or idiopathic portal hypertension, and rarely lymphoma. Few infections like *Cryptococcus*, *Candida*, and *Listeria monocytogenes* have also been described [3, 7, 20, 22–24].

Chowdhary et al. retrospectively reviewed 40 cases of SLE to determine the presence of end-stage liver disease in patients with SLE and found that all except 6 cases had multiple causes of liver involvement other than SLE. These included drug induced ($n = 4$), viral hepatitis (hepatitis B or C and cytomegalovirus; $n = 8$), nonalcoholic fatty liver disease (NAFLD; $n = 8$), autoimmune hepatitis (AIH; $n = 6$), primary biliary cirrhosis (PBC; $n = 3$), and liver involvement from infection (2), cryptogenic cirrhosis (2), lymphoma (1), and indeterminate (6). Eight patients died. Mortality was not directly related to liver disease in any patient. They concluded that complications of portal hypertension, cirrhosis, and hepatic encephalopathy are rare manifestations of SLE unless coexistent liver disease such as NAFLD, viral hepatitis, or AIH is present [3].

There is no definite pathogenetic mechanism to explain the above histopathologic findings in SLE patients. Hepatic hemangioma is a benign vascular tumor and reported as a common finding in SLE. Hemangiomas are formed as a result of imbalance between proangiogenic and antiangiogenic factors [25]. Estrogen overactivity promotes angiogenesis and is exemplified by increased incidence of hemangiomas during pregnancy and estrogen therapy. Berzigotti et al. hypothesised that since SLE patients have increased circulating estrogen levels and angiogenic factors like vascular endothelial growth factor (VEGF), this proangiogenic state might lead to development of liver hemangiomas in SLE [17]. Nodular regenerative hyperplasia is proposed to occur due to a small vessel vasculitis leading to atrophy with compensatory hyperplasia [5].

4. Conclusion

To summarise, histopathology of liver in SLE shows a wide morphological spectrum commonly due to a coexisting pathology. Drug induced hepatitis, viral etiology, and autoimmune overlap should be excluded before attributing the changes to SLE itself. Common histopathologic findings in SLE include fatty liver, portal inflammation, and vascular changes like hemangioma, congestion, nodular regenerative hyperplasia, arteritis, and abnormal vessels in portal tracts. Progression to cirrhosis is not very common, but liver failure can occur rarely.

Conflict of Interests

The authors declare that there is no conflict of interests regarding the publication of this paper.

References

[1] H. Miller, M. B. Urowitz, D. D. Gladman, and L. M. Blendis, "The liver in systemic lupus erythematosus," *Quarterly Journal of Medicine*, vol. 53, no. 3, pp. 401–409, 1984.

[2] A. Soultati and S. Dourakis, "Hepatic manifestations of autoimmune rheumatic diseases," *Annals of Gastroenterology*, vol. 18, no. 3, pp. 309–324, 2005.

[3] V. R. Chowdhary, C. S. Crowson, J. J. Poterucha, and K. G. Moder, "Liver involvement in systemic lupus erythematosus: case review of 40 patients," *Journal of Rheumatology*, vol. 35, no. 11, pp. 2159–2164, 2008.

[4] T. Gibson and A. R. Myers, "Subclinical liver disease in systemic lupus erythematosus," *Journal of Rheumatology*, vol. 8, no. 5, pp. 752–759, 1981.

[5] K. Vaiphei, A. Bhatia, and S. K. Sinha, "Liver pathology in collagen vascular disorders highlighting the vascular changes within portal tracts," *Indian Journal of Pathology and Microbiology*, vol. 54, no. 1, pp. 25–31, 2011.

[6] C. Schlenker, T. Halterman, and K. V. Kowdley, "Rheumatologic disease and the liver," *Clinics in Liver Disease*, vol. 15, no. 1, pp. 153–164, 2011.

[7] B. A. Runyon, D. R. LaBrecque, and S. Anuras, "The spectrum of in systemic lupus erythematosus. Report of 33 histologically-proved cases and review of the literature," *The American Journal of Medicine*, vol. 69, no. 2, pp. 187–194, 1980.

[8] J. H. Wang, S. B. Wang, J. Chen, W. M. Guan, and M. H. Chen, "Clinical and immunopathological features of patients with lupus hepatitis," *Chinese Medical Journal*, vol. 126, no. 2, pp. 260–266, 2013.

[9] I. Mackay, L. I. Taft, and D. C. Cowling, "lupoid hepatitis and the hepatic lesions of systemic lupus erythematosus," *The Lancet*, vol. 273, no. 7063, pp. 65–69, 1959.

[10] T. Matsumoto, T. Yoshimine, K. Shimouchi et al., "The liver in systemic lupus erythematosus: pathologic analysis of 52 cases and review of Japanese autopsy registry data," *Human Pathology*, vol. 23, no. 10, pp. 1151–1158, 1992.

[11] A. Garcia-Tobaruela, A. Gil, P. Lavilla et al., "Hepatic amyloidosis associated with systemic lupus erythematosus," *Lupus*, vol. 4, no. 1, pp. 75–77, 1995.

[12] C. Liu, Q. B. Tang, H. Zeng, X. H. Yu, L. B. Xu, and Y. Li, "Clinical and pathological analysis of hepatic artery aneurysm in a patient with systemic lupus erythematosus: report of a case," *Surgery Today*, vol. 41, no. 11, pp. 1571–1574, 2011.

[13] PM. Levitin, D. Sweet, CM. Brunner, RE. Katholi, and WK. Bolton, "Spontaneous rupture of the liver. An unusual complication of SLE," *Arthritis Rheum*, vol. 20, no. 2, pp. 748–750, 1977.

[14] W. I. Youssef and A. S. Tavill, "Connective tissue diseases and the liver," *Journal of Clinical Gastroenterology*, vol. 35, no. 4, pp. 345–349, 2002.

[15] F. P. Ruiz, F. J. O. Martinez, A. C. Z. Mendoza, L. R. del Arbol, and A. M. Caparros, "Nodular regenerative hyperplasia of the liver in rheumatic diseases: report of seven cases and review of the literature," *Seminars in Arthritis and Rheumatism*, vol. 21, no. 1, pp. 47–54, 1991.

[16] I. R. Wanless, L. C. Solt, and P. Kortan, "Nodular regenerative hyperplasia of the liver associated with macroglobulinemia: a clue to the pathogenesis," *The American Journal of Medicine*, vol. 70, no. 6, pp. 1203–1209, 1981.

[17] A. Berzigotti, M. Frigato, E. Manfredini et al., "Liver hemangioma and vascular liver diseases in patients with systemic lupus erythematosus," *The World Journal of Gastroenterology*, vol. 17, no. 40, pp. 4503–4508, 2011.

[18] A. J. Rhoton, J. H. Gilliam, and K. R. Geisinger, "Hemobilia in systemic lupus erythematosus," *Southern Medical Journal*, vol. 86, no. 9, pp. 1049–1051, 1993.

[19] R. Kaw, C. Gota, A. Bennett, D. Barnes, and L. Calabrese, "Lupus-related hepatitis: complication of lupus or autoimmune association? Case report and review of the literature," *Digestive Diseases and Sciences*, vol. 51, no. 4, pp. 813–818, 2006.

[20] H. Ohira, J. Takiguchi, T. Rai et al., "High frequency of anti-ribosomal P antibody in patients with systemic lupus erythematosus-associated hepatitis," *Hepatology Research*, vol. 28, no. 3, pp. 137–139, 2004.

[21] B. van Hoek, "The spectrum of liver disease in systemic lupus erythematosus," *Netherlands Journal of Medicine*, vol. 48, no. 6, pp. 244–253, 1996.

[22] A. Cairns and R. F. T. McMahon, "Giant cell hepatitis associated with systemic lupus erythematosus," *Journal of Clinical Pathology*, vol. 49, no. 2, pp. 183–184, 1996.

[23] T. Kumada, T. Enari, S. Kobayashi et al., "Four cases of adult *Listeria monocytogenes* infection in the last 5 years—hepatic necrotic foci in the adult septic case," *Kansenshogaku Zasshi*, vol. 63, no. 5, pp. 534–540, 1989.

[24] M. Kimura, S. Udagawa, A. Shoji et al., "Pulmonary aspergillosis due to Aspergillus terreus combined with staphylococcal pneumonia and hepatic candidiasis," *Mycopathologia*, vol. 111, no. 1, pp. 47–53, 1990.

[25] M. González Folch, "Erythema nodosum," *Revista Médica de Chile*, vol. 106, no. 11, pp. 915–922, 1978.

14

Hepatitis Viruses in Heamodialysis Patients: An Added Insult to Injury?

Kranthi Kosaraju,[1] **Sameer Singh Faujdar,**[1] **Aashima Singh,**[1] **and Ravindra Prabhu**[2]

[1] Department of Microbiology, Kasturba Medical College and Hospital, Manipal University, Madhav Nagar, Manipal 576104, Karnataka, India
[2] Department of Nephrology, Kasturba Medical College and Hospital, Manipal University, Madhav Nagar, Manipal 576104, Karnataka, India

Correspondence should be addressed to Kranthi Kosaraju; medkranthi@gmail.com

Academic Editor: Piero Luigi Almasio

Hepatitis B (HBV) and hepatitis C (HCV) viruses are the most important causes of chronic liver disease in patients with end stage renal disease on hemodialysis. The prevalence of hepatitis infection among hemodialysis patients is high and varies between countries and between dialysis units within a single country. This case-control study was undertaken to estimate the occurrence of HBV and HCV infections in patients undergoing hemodialysis in our tertiary care center. All patients receving hemodialysis at our centre with HCV or HBV infection were included in the study. The total number of patients admitted for hemodialysis during the study period was 1710. Among these, 26 patients were positive for HBV, 19 were positive for HCV, and 2 were positive for both HCV and HBV. Mean age of the infected cases in our study was 48.63 years. Mean duration of dialysis for infected cases was 4.8 years while that of the noninfected controls was 3.18 years. The mean dialysis interval was twice a week. Interventions to reduce the occurrence of these infections are of utmost need to reduce the risk of long-term complications among hemodialysis patients.

1. Introduction

Hepatitis B virus (HBV) and hepatitis C virus (HCV) infections cause morbidity and mortality in haemodialysis patients. Prolonged vascular exposure and multiple blood transfusions increase the risk of acquiring these blood-borne infections in these patients. Contaminated devices, equipments, and supplies, environmental surfaces, and attending personnel may also play a crucial role in the nosocomial transmission of these infections. Infections with hepatitis viruses in haemodialysis patients are further promoted by the significant immune status dysfunction developing due to irreversible renal compromise [1–3].

Furthermore, hepatitis viral infections in haemodialysis patients cause liver disease in renal failure patients undergoing replacement therapy. They also pose a significant problem in the management of these cases as patients with renal failure cannot clear the viruses effectively. Patients with coinfections with these viruses develop severe clinical presentations and resistance to interferon treatment [3].

There are very limited data available on the occurrence of such infections in haemodialysis patients from this part of the country. The present study aimed to investigate the occurrence of HBV and HCV infections in haemodialysis patients and the risk factors associated with such infections.

2. Materials and Methods

This study was conducted as a retrospective case-control study involving the haemodialysis patients at a dialysis centre of a tertiary care hospital. All the patients who underwent haemodialysis from January 2004 to June 2012 were included in the study.

Patients receiving haemodialysis were considered as a "case" for the study if their serum tested positive for either HBV or HCV. In contrast, the patients receiving haemodialysis were considered as a "control" if their serum tested negative for all the three viruses. For every case, one age- and gender-matched control receiving haemodialysis was selected.

Patients' medical records were reviewed to obtain details like age, gender, clinical diagnosis, and duration and frequency of dialysis, history of blood transfusions, and past surgeries and these details were recorded in a preformed questionnaire for all cases and controls. Further, the results of serological tests (HBsAg, Anti-HCV antibodies), renal function tests (serum urea and creatinine), and liver function tests were recorded for both groups. The results of biochemical parameters were correlated with serological findings.

Duration of dialysis, frequency of dialysis, and the results of biochemical parameters were compared for infected cases and non-infected controls and were analyzed statistically using nonparametric tests and chi-square tests.

3. Results

The present retrospective study was conducted for a period of 102 months, that is, from January 2004 to June 2012. A total of 180 patients were diagnosed to have chronic kidney disease and were on maintenance haemodialysis during the study period. Also, our dialysis unit caters to approximately 15 in-patients per month referred from other departments or hospitals for haemodialysis. Therefore, the total number of patients who received haemodialysis at our centre during the study period was 1710.

Among these patients, 45/1710 cases (2.63%) were found to be infected with either HBV or HCV and were included as cases for our study.

Out of 45 cases studied, 26/1710 (1.52%) tested positive for HBsAg and 19/1710 (1.11%) tested positive for Anti-HCV antibodies. Out of 26 cases infected with HBV, 22 (84.6%) were males and 4 (15.4%) were females. Among HCV positive cases, 18 (94.7%) were males and 1 (5.2%) was female. Among the cases, dual infection with HBV and HCV was seen in two patients, 1 male and 1 female.

Mean age of the infected cases in our study was 48.63 years. HBV infection was seen most commonly in the age group of 50–60 yrs, whereas HCV was commonest in the age group of 30–40 years.

Mean duration of dialysis for infected cases was 4.8 years while that of the non-infected controls was 3.18 years. There was a statistically significant (P = 0.008) difference between the cases and controls with respect to duration of dialysis (Mann-Whitney U test since mean was less than 2 standard deviations, non-parametric tests were used). When comparing frequency of dialysis between cases and controls, as it was a categorical variable, chi-square test was applied and there was no statistically significant (P value = 0.228) correlation of the frequency of dialysis between cases and controls.

With respect to liver function tests, a significant elevation of AST (aspartate aminotransferase) and ALT (alanine transaminase) values among infected cases (P value = 0.001) was observed in this study.

Most of the patients (80%) on haemodialysis in our study were anaemic with haemoglobin concentration <10 g% as shown in Figure 1. The comparison of haemoglobin values among cases and controls is depicted in Figure 2. With respect to renal function tests in cases and controls, mean

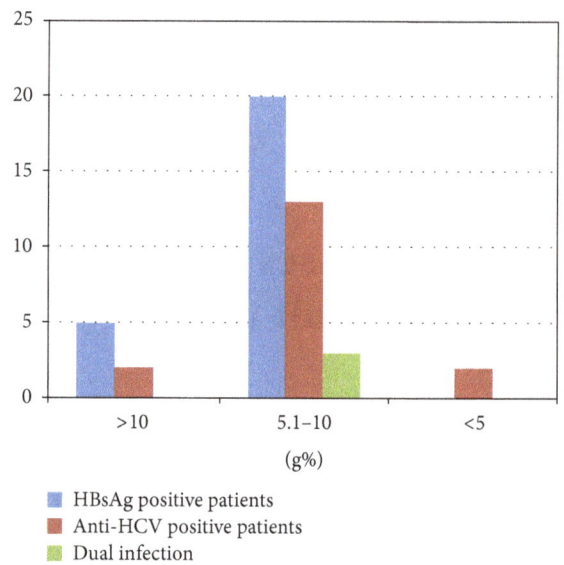

FIGURE 1: Hemoglobin values in cases infected with HBV and HCV.

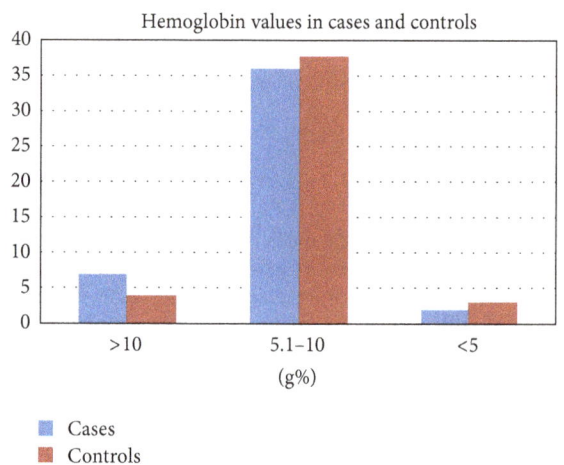

FIGURE 2: Comparison of hemoglobin values among cases and controls (n = 45).

value of blood urea for cases was 99.85 and for controls was 103.1, and mean value of creatinine was 22.3 for cases and 8.65 for controls, respectively. No statistically significant difference was observed between both groups with respect to serum levels of urea (P value = 0.6), creatinine (P value = 0.228), and haemoglobin (P value = 0.6).

Risk factors for acquiring HBV and HCV infections were studied for both groups. Among the infected cases, multiple blood transfusions were seen only in 3 cases (2 positive for HBsAg and 1 for HCV). Among the three, one case with positive Anti-HCV underwent multiple blood transfusions and in the remaining two cases, blood transfusion was received only twice. The history of undergoing surgeries was obtained in nine cases. Among the 9 cases, HBV infection was seen in 4, HCV in 4, and dual infection was seen in one case. Twelve cases were diabetic, with HBV infection in 6, HCV in 5 cases, and dual infection in 1 case (Figure 3).

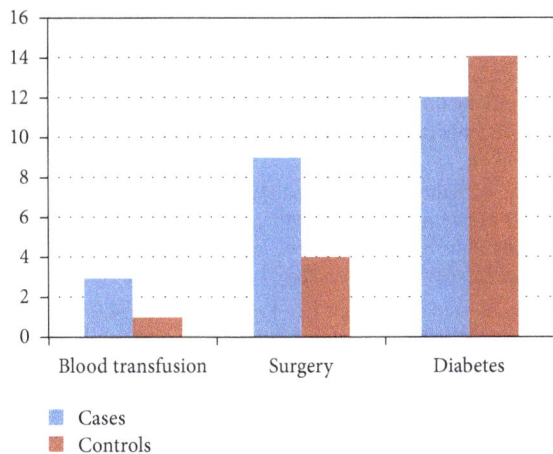

FIGURE 3: Risk factors among cases and controls.

With respect to similar risk factors in the control group, 14 control patients had diabetes and 4 of them had history of undergoing surgery in the past. Only 1 control patient had history of undergoing blood transfusion (Figure 3).

4. Discussion

Patients diagnosed with chronic renal failure (CRF) on maintenance haemodialysis pose a higher risk for acquiring HBV or HCV infections due to frequent use of blood and blood products and multiple invasive procedures performed in these patients [1]. The literature review points to the fact that viral hepatitis is a serious threat for haemodialysis patients as 1.9% of all deaths among this population were related to the consequence of viral hepatitis [4].

The results from our study demonstrate that the occurrence of HBV and HCV infections in haemodialysis patients is 1.52% and 1.11%, respectively, which is lower than the rates reported from different studies all over the world and India [5–8]. An Indian study has reported the occurrence of HBV in haemodialysis to vary from 3.4% to 42%, much higher than that seen in our study [9]. The lower rates of infection in our study might be due to decreased transfusion requirements owing to the availability of erythropoietin and better screening of blood and blood products for blood-borne infections. Introduction of vaccination for HBV, isolation of hepatitis B virus (HBV) positive patients, and regular surveillance for HBV infection at our centre could also have contributed for the lesser rates of infection.

Occurrence of HCV infection was much less than HBV in our study which was in accordance with a study conducted in Spain which reported lesser prevalence rates for HCV infection in haemodialysis (HD) patients [10]. Another study showed a significant decline of hepatitis C infection among end-stage renal disease patients in Central Brazil, highlighting the importance of public health strategies such as screening for anti-HCV in blood banks and infection control measures for control and prevention of hepatitis C in the haemodialysis environment [11].

Since both of these viruses share a common mode of transmission, we looked for the occurrence of coinfections among the cases studied. Among the cases, dual infection with HBV and HCV was seen in two patients, 1 male and 1 female (2/45 = 4.4%). Study from the same centre on the occurrence of coinfections in the general population reported lower rates (1.68%) of dual infections [12]. Studies from other centres in India have reported a varying prevalence of coinfections with HBV and HIV (9–40%) and for HCV and HIV (2–8%) [13].

The higher occurrence in our study may be due to the study population being restricted to haemodialysis patients and also due to the lesser sample size in the current study. Another factor contributing to the higher rates is the enhanced risk of coinfections among chronic renal failure patients on haemodialysis due to multiple transfusions and invasive procedure performed in these patients [14]. However, dual infection with HBV and HCV in our study which was 4.4%, similar to the study conducted in Hyderabad [3].

The present study highlights the duration of dialysis as an important risk factor for infection among haemodialysis patients. This observation was in agreement with previous reports in Palestine, Moldavia, and other studies from different regions of the world [15–17]. Duration of dialysis is an important risk factor for acquiring infections as it is related to nosocomial transmission and dissemination of the infections in the dialysis units [1].

On comparison of AST and ALT values among cases and controls, it was found that cases had higher mean value. This can be explained on the basis of destruction of hepatocytes caused by the immune reaction of body responding to the hepatitis viruses leading to excessive release of the aminotransferases. These findings were in accordance with the studies conducted in Karachi and Jenin district and Gaza strip in Palestine [1, 18].

In our study, when compared with the control group, 67% of the patients on haemodialysis with HBV/HCV were found to have higher hemoglobin levels. This interesting finding was supported by few studies and was attributed to the increase in RBC counts after infection with hepatitis viruses and also to increased erythropoietin production after hepatic stimulation by chronic infection with hepatitis virus. However, the exact cause for the same is not yet established [19–22].

5. Conclusion

A study from our centre brings to light that HBV and HCV infections, though less common, continue to remain as an important causes of infection in haemodialysis patients. The risk of exposure increases with the number of dialysis sessions and is maximum in patients on maintenance haemodialysis. Interventions to reduce the occurrence of these infections are of utmost need to reduce the risk of long-term complications.

References

[1] J. Q. Abumwais and O. F. Idris, "Prevalence of hepatitis C, hepatitis B, and HIV infection among haemodialysis patients

in Jenin District (Palestine)," *Iranian Journal of Virology*, vol. 4, no. 2, pp. 38–44, 2010.

[2] P. Bhaumik and K. Debnath, "Prevalence of hepatitis B and C among haemodialysis patients of Tripura, India," *Euroasian Journal of Hepato-Gastroenterology*, vol. 2, no. 1, pp. 10–13, 2012.

[3] G. A. Reddy, K. V. Dakshinamurthy, P. Neelaprasad, T. Gangadhar, and V. Lakshmi, "Prevalence of HBV and HCV dual infection in patients on haemodialysis," *Indian Journal of Medical Microbiology*, vol. 23, no. 1, pp. 41–43, 2005.

[4] A. Aghakhani, M. Banifazl, A. Eslamifar, F. Ahmadi, and A. Ramezani, "Viral hepatitis and HIV infection in hemodialysis patients," *Hepatitis Monthly*, vol. 12, no. 7, pp. 463–464, 2012.

[5] A. E. O. Otedo, S. O. Mc'Ligeyo, F. A. Okoth, and J. K. Kayima, "Seroprevalence of hepatitis B and C in maintenance dialysis in a public hospital in a developing country," *South African Medical Journal*, vol. 93, no. 5, pp. 380–384, 2003.

[6] S. U. Busek, E. H. Babá, H. A. Tavares Filho et al., "Hepatitis C and hepatitis B virus infection in different hemodialysis units in Belo Horizonte, Minas Gerais, Brazil," *Memorias do Instituto Oswaldo Cruz*, vol. 97, no. 6, pp. 775–778, 2002.

[7] S. K. Agarwal, S. C. Dash, and M. Irshad, "Hepatitis C virus infection during haemodialysis in India," *Journal of Association of Physicians of India*, vol. 47, no. 12, pp. 1139–1143, 1999.

[8] A. Chowdhury, A. Santra, R. Chakravorty et al., "Community-based epidemiology of hepatitis B virus infection in West Bengal, India: prevalence of hepatitis B e antigen-negative infection and associated viral variants," *Journal of Gastroenterology and Hepatology*, vol. 20, no. 11, pp. 1712–1720, 2005.

[9] D. Saha and S. K. Agarwal, "Hepatitis and HIV infection during haemodialysis," *Journal of the Indian Medical Association*, vol. 99, no. 4, pp. 194–199, 2001.

[10] M. Espinosa, A. Martín-Malo, R. Ojeda et al., "Marked reduction in the prevalence of hepatitis C virus infection in hemodialysis patients: causes and consequences," *American Journal of Kidney Diseases*, vol. 43, no. 4, pp. 685–689, 2004.

[11] M. A. S. Carneiro, S. A. Teles, M. A. Dias et al., "Decline of hepatitis C infection in hemodialysis patients in Central Brazil: a ten years of surveillance," *Memorias do Instituto Oswaldo Cruz*, vol. 100, no. 4, pp. 345–349, 2005.

[12] K. Kosaraju, S. Padukone, and I. Bairy, "Co-infection with hepatitis viruses among HIV-infected individuals at a tertiary care centre in South India," *Tropical Doctor*, vol. 41, no. 3, pp. 170–171, 2011.

[13] J. Tourret, I. Tostivint, S. T. du Montcel et al., "Outcome and prognosis factors in HIV-infected haemodialysis patients," *Clinical Journal of the American Society of Nephrology*, vol. 1, no. 6, pp. 1241–1247, 2006.

[14] M. Chandra, M. N. Khaja, M. M. Hussain et al., "Prevalence of hepatitis B and hepatitis C viral infections in Indian patients with chronic renal failure," *Intervirology*, vol. 47, no. 6, pp. 374–376, 2004.

[15] M. J. Zahedi, S. D. Moghaddam, S. M. Alavian, and M. Dalili, "Seroprevalence of hepatitis viruses B, C, D and HIV infection among hemodialysis patients in Kerman Province, South-East Iran," *Hepatitis Monthly*, vol. 12, no. 5, pp. 339–343, 2012.

[16] A. Covic, L. Iancu, C. Apetrei et al., "Hepatitis virus infection in haemodialysis patients from Moldavia," *Nephrology Dialysis Transplantation*, vol. 14, no. 1, pp. 40–45, 1999.

[17] D. N. Irish, C. Blake, J. Christophers et al., "Identification of hepatitis C virus seroconversion resulting from nosocomial transmission on a haemodialysis unit: implications for infection control and laboratory screening," *Journal of Medical Virology*, vol. 59, no. 2, pp. 135–140, 1999.

[18] A. E. Y. El-Ottol, A. A. Elmanama, and B. M. Ayesh, "Prevalence and risk factors of hepatitis B and C viruses among haemodialysis patients in Gaza strip, Palestine," *Virology Journal*, vol. 7, p. 210, 2010.

[19] A. A. A. Sabry, K. F. El-Dahshan, K. M. Mahmoud, and A. A. El-Husseini, "Effect of HCV infection on hematocrit and hemoglobin level in Egyptian hemodialysis patients," *International Urology and Nephrology*, vol. 41, no. 1, pp. 189–193, 2009.

[20] K. A. Alsaran, A. A. Sabry, A. H. Alghareeb, and G. Al Sadoon, "Effect of hepatitis C virus on hemoglobin and hematocrit levels in Saudi hemodialysis patients," *Renal Failure*, vol. 31, no. 5, pp. 349–354, 2009.

[21] Y. L. Lin, C. W. Lin, C. H. Lee, I. C. Lai, H. H. Chen, and T. W. Chen, "Chronic hepatitis ameliorates anaemia in haemodialysis patients," *Nephrology*, vol. 13, no. 4, pp. 289–293, 2008.

[22] M. Radovic, W. Jelkmann, L. Djukanovic, and V. Ostric, "Serum erythropoietin and interleukin-6 levels in hemodialysis patients with hepatitis virus infection," *Journal of Interferon and Cytokine Research*, vol. 19, no. 4, pp. 369–373, 1999.

15

MHC Class I Presented T Cell Epitopes as Potential Antigens for Therapeutic Vaccine against HBV Chronic Infection

Joseph D. Comber,[1] Aykan Karabudak,[1] Vivekananda Shetty,[2]
James S. Testa,[3] Xiaofang Huang,[1] and Ramila Philip[1]

[1] *Immunotope, Inc., Doylestown, PA 18902, USA*
[2] *Baylor College of Medicine, Houston, TX 77030, USA*
[3] *Celldex Therapeutics, Hampton, NJ 08827, USA*

Correspondence should be addressed to Ramila Philip; rphilip@immunotope.com

Academic Editor: Piero Luigi Almasio

Approximately 370 million people worldwide are chronically infected with hepatitis B virus (HBV). Despite the success of the prophylactic HBV vaccine, no therapeutic vaccine or other immunotherapy modality is available for treatment of chronically infected individuals. Clearance of HBV depends on robust, sustained CD8+ T activity; however, the limited numbers of therapeutic vaccines tested have not induced such a response. Most of these vaccines have relied on peptide prediction algorithms to identify MHC-I epitopes or characterization of T cell responses during acute infection. Here, we took an immunoproteomic approach to characterize MHC-I restricted epitopes from cells chronically infected with HBV and therefore more likely to represent the true targets of CD8+ T cells during chronic infection. In this study, we identified eight novel MHC-I restricted epitopes derived from a broad range of HBV proteins that were capable of activating CD8+ T cells. Furthermore, five of the eight epitopes were able to bind HLA-A2 and A24 alleles and activated HBV specific T cell responses. These epitopes also have potential as new tools to characterize T cell immunity in chronic HBV infection and may serve as candidate antigens for a therapeutic vaccine against HBV infection.

1. Introduction

Hepatitis B virus (HBV) is a member of the Hepadnaviridae family of viruses which also includes woodchuck hepatitis virus (WHV) and duck hepatitis B virus. These viruses are primarily hepatotropic with infections characterized by fever, fatigue, muscle aches, and yellowing of the eyes and/or skin. The severity of these symptoms can vary with a proportion of cases being asymptomatic [1]. More than 2.5 billion people worldwide have been infected by HBV, but, for the vast majority of adults encountering the virus (>90%), the infection is acute and readily cleared by the immune system [2, 3]. For the remaining 5–10% of adults, and for neonates and unvaccinated children, HBV establishes a chronic infection. Approximately 370 million people worldwide are chronically infected and over 500,000 people die each year due to complications from HBV [1, 4]. These complications include liver cirrhosis, liver failure, and/or hepatocellular carcinoma

(HCC) and it is estimated that up to 40% of chronically infected patients will develop at least one of these complications [5].

The primary determinant of whether hepatitis B virus is cleared or establishes a chronic infection is the robustness of the immune response, in particular the CD8+ T cell response [6–9]. Data from both animal models and infected patients indicate that strong innate immune responses are crucial in controlling initial HBV replication and for subsequently activating the adaptive T cell response (reviewed in [2, 3]). In patients that resolve acute infections, there are greater numbers of IFN-γ secreting CD4+ and CD8+ T cells [10] with a broader range of epitope recognition [11, 12] than in chronically infected patients [3, 13]. Although individuals that initially fail to mount vigorous T cell responses develop chronic infection, data indicate that virus specific T cells are still capable of a broad, effective T cell response. Rehermann et al. demonstrated that a small number of chronically infected individuals mount robust CTL responses against HBV either spontaneously or in response to IFN-α treatment [14]. These T cells are directed against multiple proteins indicating that chronically infected patients can also mount a broad response to viral antigens. These data suggest that therapeutic interventions designed to stimulate robust and multiepitope specific responses may be sufficient to resolve chronic HBV infections. Yet, despite an effective prophylactic vaccine, there are currently no therapies capable of eliminating HBV from chronically infected individuals. A number of anti-HBV therapeutic vaccines have been tested including traditional prophylactic vaccines, antigen/antibody complexes [15], lipopeptide [16], DNA [17], and recombinant virus [18] based strategies with limited success. Thus, there is a critical need for more targeted therapeutic vaccines capable of inducing robust, sustained T cell responses capable of permanent clearance of virus.

Therapeutic peptide based vaccines are an attractive method for inducing CD4$^+$ and CD8$^+$ T cell responses in chronically infected individuals. Formulating a vaccine with multiple epitopes presented by the chronically infected cells that are capable of activating polyclonal T cell responses may have the ability to eradicate the infected cells in chronically infected patients. Peptide antigens for the early stage clinical studies were identified by motif prediction algorithms and selected by screening CTLs from acute and chronically HBV infected patients [19]. However, the T cell epitopes presented by HBV infected cells have not been reported or used in a clinical study. Here we took an immunoproteomic approach to identify MHC class I peptides presented by chronically HBV infected cells. This approach has distinct advantages over traditional vaccine design algorithms as it identifies antigens naturally processed and presented by infected, but not healthy, cells. Using this approach we identified 8 naturally processed HLA-A2 restricted epitopes capable of stimulating robust CD8$^+$ T cell responses. Interestingly a subset of these epitopes is also capable of binding HLA-A24 molecules and stimulates both HLA-A2 and HLA-A24 restricted T cell responses.

2. Materials and Methods

2.1. Mice.
Four- to eight-week-old female HLA-A2 transgenic (CB6F1-Tg(HLA-A*0201/H2-K^b)A*0201) or HLA-A24 transgenic (CB6F1-Tg(HLA-A*2402/H2-K^b)A24.01) mice were obtained from Taconic and housed at Lampire Biologicals (Pipersville, PA). All animal experiments were conducted in adherence to the Guide for Care and use of Laboratory Animals of the NIH. Experimental protocols were approved by the Institutional Animal Care and Use Committee of Lampire Biologicals.

2.2. Cells, Viruses, and Plasmids.
The HLA-A2 and A24 positive liver hepatocellular carcinoma cell line HepG2 and its hepatitis B infected derivatives HepDE19 and HepG2.2.15 were cultured in Dulbecco's Modified Eagle Medium/Ham's F-12 50/50 Mix (Mediatech Inc, Manassas VA). 293-T cells

were maintained in Dulbecco's Modified Eagle Medium and T2 cells were maintained in RPMI-1640 (Mediatech Inc). All media were supplemented with 10% fetal bovine serum (Atlanta Biologicals, Flowery Branch, GA), L-glutamine (300 mg/mL), 1x nonessential amino acids, 0.5 mM sodium pyruvate, and 1x penicillin/streptomycin (Mediatech Inc). Cells were maintained at 37°C and 5% CO_2.

Adenovirus containing the HBV genome (Ad-HBV) was a kind gift of Dr. Anand Mehta (Drexel University). 293T-HLA.A2$^+$ cells were seeded into 6-well plates and infected with AdHBV virus. 48–72 hours later, the cells were harvested and used in downstream applications.

2.3. Isolation, Purification, and Fractionation of MHC Class I Bound Peptides.
Hepatitis B virus specific MHC class I restricted peptides were isolated as previously described [20]. Briefly, 1×10^9 HepDE19 cells were lysed (150 mM NaCl, 10 mM Na_2HPO_4, 1 mM EDTA, 1%NP40) and peptide/MHC complexes (p/MHC) were immunoprecipitated using protein A/G beads (UltraLink Immobilized Protein A/G, Pierce, Rockford, IL) coated with W6/32, a monoclonal antibody that recognizes pan-MHC class I molecules. Antibody coated beads were incubated with cell lysate for 2 hours with rocking and then separated from the lysate by centrifugation (1000 rpm/5 min). The p/MHC complexes were eluted from the beads using 0.1% trifluoroacetic acid and the peptides were dissociated from the MHC molecules by heating at 85°C for 15 minutes. The mixture was cooled and the peptides separated using an Amicon Ultra-3 kDA filter (Millipore, Billerica, MA). The resulting peptide mixture was then fractionated using a C-18 reversed phase (RP) column on an offline 3000 HPLC (Dionex).

2.4. Mass Spectrometry Analysis.
Mass spectrometry experiments were carried out using Orbitrap instruments (Thermo Electron, San Jose, CA) interfaced with nano ultimate high-performance liquid chromatography (HPLC; Dionex). RP-HPLC-purified peptide fractions were injected individually into the LC-MS/MS system to identify the sequences [20, 21] of the peptides. The peptides were concentrated using a 300 μm ID $\times$ 5 mm C18 RP trap column (Dionex) and separated using a 75 μm ID $\times$ 15 cm C18 RP analytical column (Dionex), equilibrated in 4% ACN/0.1% FA at 250 nL/minute flow rate. Mobile phase A was 2% ACN and 0.1% FA in water, whereas mobile phase B was 0.1% FA and 90% ACN in water. Peptides were separated with a gradient of 4%–50% B in 60 minutes and 50%–80% in 90 minutes and eluted directly into the mass spectrometer. Peptides were analyzed using a data-dependent method. The acquired spectra data were searched against HBV protein database using Proteome Discoverer 1.3 (Thermo) to interpret data and derive peptide sequences. The database search parameters were enzyme-no enzyme, threshold-100, peptide tolerance-20 ppm, and fragment ion tolerance-0.8 Da. The search results were filtered with XCorr according to individual peptide charge status (+1 : 1.6, +2 : 1.8, and +3 : 2.0) and the results were also verified manually to confirm the correct peptide sequence.

HBV infected cells
↓
Immunoprecipitation of
peptide/MHC-I complexes
↓
Elution of peptides
↓
HPLC fractionation and
LC-MS/MS analysis
↓
Database search: peptide/protein identification
↓
Validation using synthetic analogs
by LC-MS/MS and *in vitro* CTL
generation
↓
In vitro and *in vivo* CTL experiments

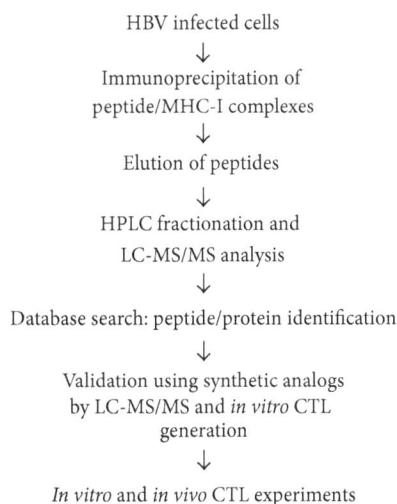

FIGURE 1: Immunoproteomics method work flow for the identification and characterization of HBV specific T cell epitopes.

2.5. Peptide Validation by Synthetic Peptides.

Synthetic peptides for validating the peptides identified in this study were obtained from GenScript Corporation and China peptides Co., Ltd. The synthetic peptides were subjected to LC-MS/MS analysis under identical experimental conditions as described above, and their sequences were confirmed based on their MS/MS data. Candidate peptide sequences were confirmed by comparison of MS/MS spectra with synthetic analogues.

2.6. Generation of Epitope Specific CTLs In Vitro.

Peptide specific CTLs were generated as previously described [20–23]. Briefly, PBMCs were isolated from heparinized blood of healthy HLA-A2$^+$ donors (Research Blood Components, LLC, Boston MA) using lymphocyte separation medium (Corning, Corning, NY) and cultured in 6-well plates overnight in RPMI-1640. The next day, the nonadherent cells were harvested and saved and the adherent cells were pulsed with MHC class I restricted synthetic peptides (50 μg) + β2 microglobulin (1.5 μg) in order to selectively expand epitope specific CD8$^+$ T lymphocytes (CTLs). After a two-hour incubation, the nonadherent cells were resuspended in a cytokine rich medium of RPMI-1640 supplemented with IL-7 (5 ng/mL), GM-CSF (25 ng/mL), IL-4 (50 ng/mL), and keyhole limpet hemocyanin (5 ug/mL KLH; Sigma-Aldrich). The nonadherent cells were added back into the 6-well plates to a final volume of 5 mL/well and cultured at 37°C at 5% CO_2. T cells in culture were restimulated 12–14 days after initial stimulation with autologous PBMCs depleted of CD4$^+$ and CD8$^+$ T cells and pulsed with synthetic peptides (10 ug/mL) and β2-microglobulin (1.5 ug/mL). Restimulated cells were cultured in RPMI-1640 supplemented with IL-15 (5 ng/mL), GM-CSF (12.5 ng/mL), and IL-2 (10U/mL) for 7 days. Restimulation was performed a total of three times prior to CTL functional assays. Unless otherwise specified, all cytokines and growth factors were purchased from eBiosciences (San Diego, CA).

2.7. Generation of Epitope Specific CTLs In Vivo.

All transgenic mouse manipulations (i.e., injections and spleen harvests) were carried out at Lampire Biologicals. HLA-A2$^+$ and HLA-A24$^+$ transgenic mice were injected with PBS alone or 10 ug of synthetic peptides in PBS or a 50:50 emulsion with Montanide ISV 51 (Seppic Inc, Fairfield, NJ). Mice were injected at two sites: subcutaneously (s.c.) on the flank and intradermally (i.d.) near the base of the tail. Mice received a total of three injections, at 10 days intervals. A week after the third injection, mice were euthanized and the spleens were harvested for use in T cell functional assays.

2.8. ELISpot Assays.

96-well PVDF-membrane plates (Millipore) were coated with IFN-gamma capture antibody overnight at 4°C. On the day of the assay, the plates were blocked for 2 hours in RPMI-1640 complete medium and washed prior to use in the ELISpot assay. *In vitro* generated CTLs were assayed 7 days after the final restimulation. Peptide specific CTLs were harvested, counted, and cultured overnight with appropriate antigen presenting cells that were unpulsed or pulsed with synthetic peptides (T2 or HepG2 cells) or antigen presenting cells that are productively infected with HBV (HepDE19, HepG2.2.15, and 293/T/A2 Ad-HBV infected cells). The next day the assay was developed according to the manufacturer's instructions (BD Biosciences, San Jose, CA). *In vivo* generated CTLs were assayed 7 days after the final peptide injection. Spleens were harvested and homogenized into a single cell suspension. After lysis of RBCs, the cells were extensively washed, counted, and cultured overnight with HepG2 cells unpulsed or pulsed with synthetic peptides or HepDE19 cells. The next day the assay was developed according to the manufacturer's instructions (BD Biosciences). For both ELISpot assays, spots were quantified using the ELISpot Reader System (AID, San Diego, CA).

2.9. MAGPIX Cytokine Detection.

Cytokine secretion from activated CD8$^+$ T cells was measured using a customized MILLIPLEX magnetic bead assay according to manufacturer's instructions (Millipore). Briefly, supernatants were harvested from CD8$^+$ T cells stimulated with various targets and cleared of cellular debris by a brief centrifugation. 25 μL of samples, standards, and controls was added to a 96-well plate containing assay buffer (1:1 dilution). Next, magnetic beads coated with antibodies against the cytokines being analyzed were added to each well. The plate was then sealed and incubated on a plate shaker overnight at 4°C. The next day, the plate was washed twice with wash buffer and biotinylated detection antibodies were added. The plate was sealed again and rocked for 1 hour at RT followed by the addition of streptavidin-PE for additional 30 minutes. The plate was washed twice with wash buffer, loaded with sheath fluid, and read on the MAGPIX system. Data was analyzed with Milliplex Analyst software according to manufacturer's instructions (Luminex, Austin, TX).

2.10. Flow Cytometry Analysis.

To detect epitope specific, cytotoxic CD8$^+$ T cells (CD8$^+$CD107a$^+$), splenocytes derived

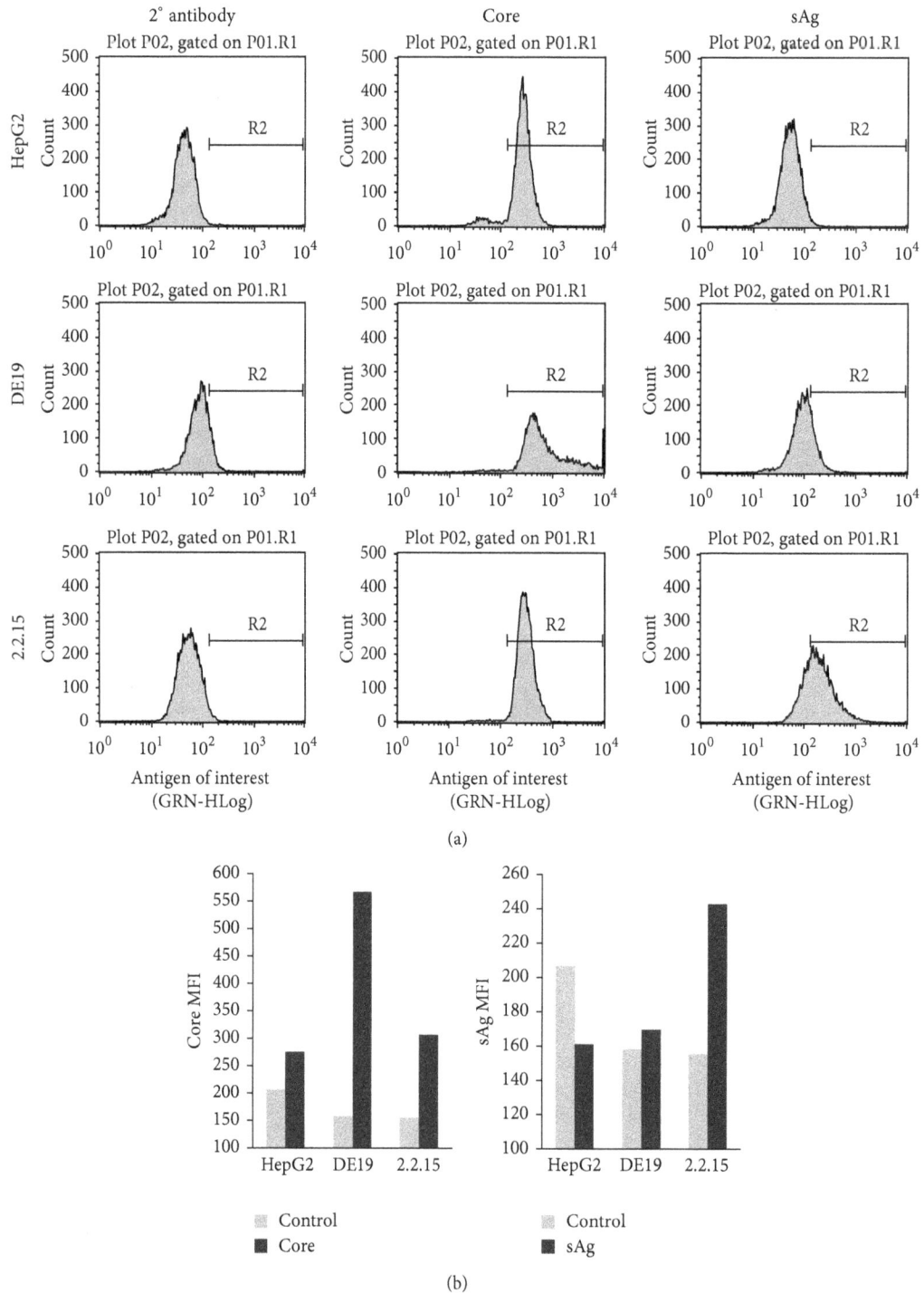

FIGURE 2: HBV protein expression in infected cell lines. (a) HepG2, DE19 (lacks sAg), and 2.2.15 (complete HBV genome) were harvested, fixed and permeabilized, and stained with HBV specific antibodies directed against core or sAg. (b) Median fluorescent intensity (MFI) derived from the flow plots shown in (a).

from peptide primed mice were cultured with HepG2 cells left unpulsed or pulsed with specific peptides or with HepDE19 cells for six hours in the presence of anti-CD107a-PE (BD Biosciences). After six hours, cells were washed and CD8$^+$ T cells were detected by addition of anti-CD8α-FITC (eBiosciences). For verification of infectivity, HepG2, HepDE19, HepG2.2.15, or 293T/A2/HBV cells were washed, fixed, and permeabilized

with the Cytofix/Cytoperm kit according to manufacturer's instructions (BD Biosciences). Cells were incubated with antibodies against HBV core (Abcam, Cambridge, MA) or HBV sAg (Santa Cruz Biotechnology, Dallas, TX) for 30 minutes at RT. Following extensive washes with permeabilization wash buffer, cells were incubated with anti-mouse IgG FITC conjugated secondary antibody (BD Biosciences)

TABLE 1: HBV specific MHC class I restricted peptides identified by immunoproteomics. The LC-MS/MS selection criteria for peptides are as follows: Charge 1: Xcorr > 1.6; Charge 2: Xcorr > 1.8; Charge 3: Xcorr > 2.0. The HLA binding scores were calculated using the SYFPEITHI prediction program [28].

Peptide sequence	Protein	Accession ID	HLA motif	m/z	Charge	Xcorr	HLA binding score
GGPNLDNIL	Large E	Q8QSF2	A2	457	2	1.88	13
LTFGRETVLEN	Precore/core (C)	Q6UFV9	A2	640	2	2.18	19
LTTVPAASLLA	Large E	Q9YKJ7	A2	530	2	2.12	20
ILRSFIPLL	Surface (S)	Q6WYY8	A2/24	537	2	1.81	A2: 28; A24: 12
FLKQQYMNL	Polymerase (P)	I0DE20	A2/24	1185	1	1.92	A2: 20; A24: 9
FLSKQYMDL	Polymerase (P)	L7QBE1	A2/A24	573	2	1.80	A2: 21; A24: 11
TVSTKLCKI	Polymerase (P)	Q8B4E6	A2/A24	497	2	1.92	A2: 19; A24: 14
FLGGPPVCL	Surface (S)	Q0EED2	A2/A24	452	2	2.05	A2: 26; A24: 11

for 20 minutes at RT. Cells were washed extensively and resuspended in PBS/0.1% BSA before acquiring. All flow cytometry events were acquired on the Guava easyCyte 8HT (Millipore). Data was analyzed using InSight software on the guavaSoft 2.6 platform (Millipore).

3. Results

3.1. Identification of MHC Class I Presented Epitopes from Hepatitis B Virus Infected Cells by Nano LC/MS/MS Methods. T cell therapeutic vaccines are an attractive treatment option for individuals chronically infected with hepatitis B virus. In order for a therapeutic vaccine to induce sustained T cell responses, it must include antigens that are naturally processed and presented by the infected cells. Therefore, we set out to identify naturally processed and presented HBV specific MHC class I restricted epitopes using an immunoproteomics approach. In this approach, peptides associated with MHC class I molecules are isolated from the infected cells and identified using mass spectrometry analysis [20–27] (Figure 1). Peptide/MHC complexes were isolated from cells chronically expressing HBV antigens (HepDE19 and HepG2.2.15) and cells infected with an adenovirus encoding for the HBV genome (293T/A2-AdHBV). Using multiple cell types was essential because it allowed for identification of epitopes from the complete genome (e.g., HepDE19 do not express surface Ag (sAg)) (Figure 2). Using stringent mass spectra search criteria, we identified eight novel MHC-I peptide epitopes with high confidence: three HLA-A2 restricted peptides (GGP; LTF; LTT) and five peptides (ILR; FLK; FLS; TVS; FLG) that show promiscuity to binding both HLA-A2 and HLA-A24 (Table 1). The HLA binding affinities of the peptides calculated using the SYFPEITHI algorithm ([28] accessed via http://www.syfpeithi.de/) showed variable binding scores (Table 1). We then confirmed the sequence identity of these epitopes using synthetic analogs. The MS/MS spectra of the synthetic epitopes matched the spectra of the experimentally identified epitopes nearly identically (Figure 3). In addition to these novel epitopes, we identified 19 MHC-I restricted peptides derived from HBV that have been previously described by motif prediction method with low mass spec Xcorr search criteria that do not meet our established standards for high abundance and

confidence and therefore were not included in our assays (see Table 1 in Supplementary Materials available online at http://dx.doi.org/10.1155/2014/860562).

3.2. Epitopes Identified by Immunoproteomics Analysis Activate HBV Specific CTLs In Vitro. After confirming the sequence of the experimentally identified epitopes, we determined if these epitopes could activate CD8$^+$ T cells. To do so, we generated epitope specific CTLs from PBMCs isolated from healthy HLA-A2$^+$ donors using the synthetic peptide versions. Epitope specific CD8$^+$ T cells were activated (as measured by IFN-gamma ELISpot) when cultured with T2s pulsed with peptide (Figure 4(a)) and with HepDE19 or 293-T/A2-AdHBV cell lines (Figure 4(b)). Importantly, these responses were specific as only background CD8$^+$ T cell activation was observed when the cells were cultured with normal liver, uninfected HepG2, or uninfected 293T/A2 cells (Figure 4(b)). Furthermore, the CTL responses did not correlate with their HLA binding affinities (Table 1).

3.3. Epitopes Identified by Immunoproteomics Analysis Activate HBV Specific CTLs In Vivo. After establishing that epitopes could specifically induce CD8$^+$ T cell activation *in vitro*, we next sought to determine if the experimentally identified peptides could also stimulate CD8$^+$ T cells *in vivo*. Because a subset of our peptides (ILR; FLK; FLS; TVS; FLG) had the motif to bind both HLA-A2 and HLA-A24 molecules, we assessed CD8$^+$ T cell activation of these peptides in both HLA contexts. Synthetic versions of these peptides were injected into HLA-A2$^+$ or HLA-A24$^+$ transgenic mice with or without Montanide ISV-51 adjuvant, three times in total. One week after the third injection, splenocytes were harvested and cultured with HepG2 cells pulsed individually with peptides alone or HBV infected cells in an IFN-gamma ELISPot assay. As shown in Figure 5(a), CD8$^+$ T cells generated *in vivo* specifically recognized peptide loaded HepG2 cells as well as HBV infected HepDE19 cells. In addition, CD8$^+$ T cells generated *in vivo* also upregulated a classical marker of degranulation (CD107a) [29, 30] after stimulation with both peptide pulsed HepG2s and HBV chronically infected cell line HepDE19 (Figure 5(b)). Interestingly, the peptides induced IFN-gamma secretion and CD107a upregulation independent of the HLA molecule tested which indicates that

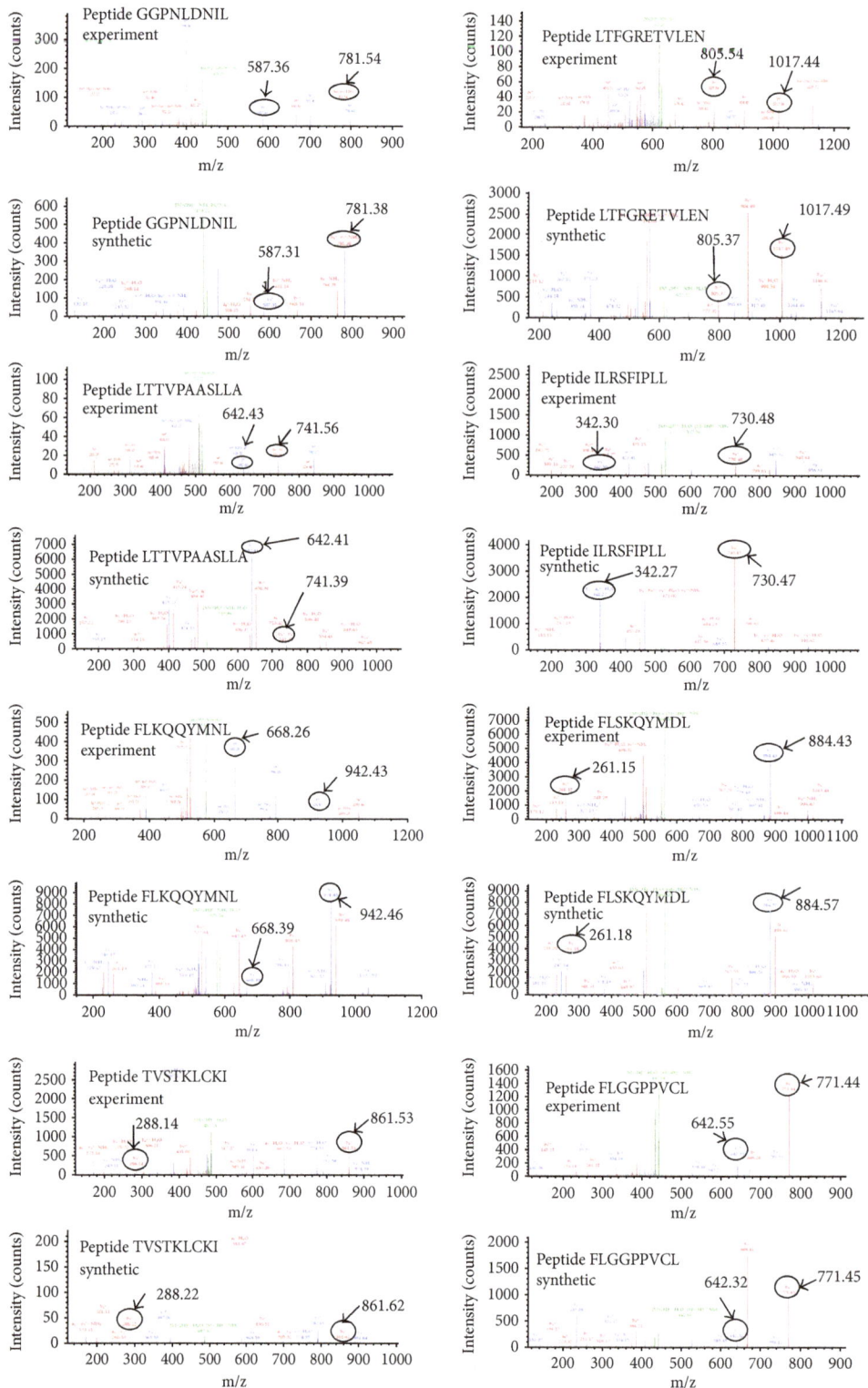

FIGURE 3: Validation of naturally presented MHC peptides from HBV infected cells. Mass spectrometry (MS/MS) spectra of the experimentally identified peptides (top spectra) versus their synthetic analogs (bottom spectra). Fragment masses that match are denoted.

these HLA-A2 and HLA-A24 double binding peptides are capable of activating both HLA-A2 and HLA-A24 specific T cell responses.

Because degranulation is associated with delivery of perforin and granzyme to target cells, we next checked the levels

of granzyme B being secreted by the peptide activated CD8+ T cells. Supernatants were collected from the stimulated cells and the levels of granzyme B were detected using Milliplex magnetic bead technology [31, 32]. CD8+ T cells from both HLA-A2 and HLA-A24 immunized mice secreted high levels

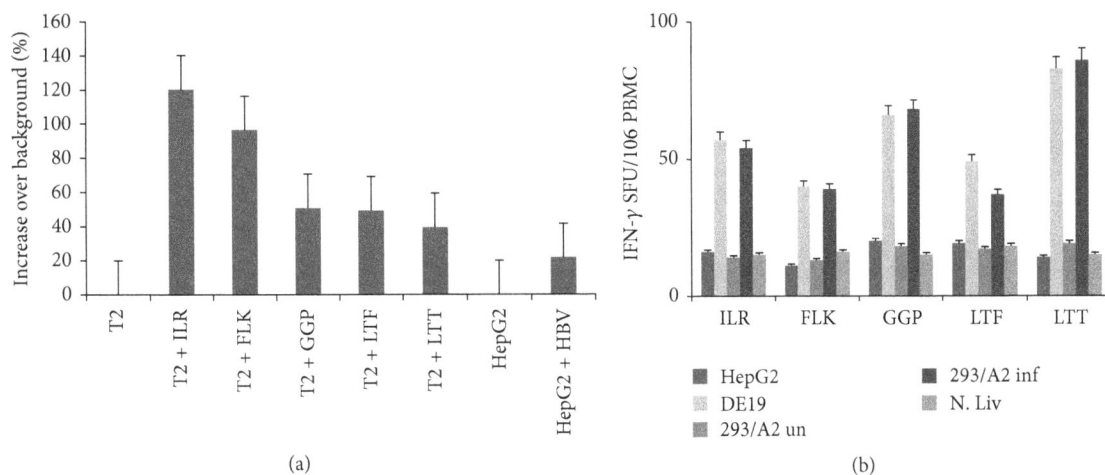

(a)

(b)

FIGURE 4: HBV specific peptides stimulate CD8$^+$ T cell activation *in vitro*. (a) HLA-A2 restricted CTLs directed against the identified peptides (peptides are represented as first 3 residues of the sequence) were generated using peripheral blood from healthy donors. PBMCs containing the epitope specific CTLs were harvested, washed, and cultured with the peptide pulsed or HBV expressing cells overnight in an IFN-gamma ELISpot assay. Data is represented as % increase over background. (b) PBMCs containing epitope specific CTLs were harvested, washed, and cultured with uninfected or HBV expressing cells overnight in an IFN-gamma ELISpot assay. Normal liver cells served as a negative, nonspecific control.

of granzyme-B in response to peptide stimulation and HBV chronically infected HepDE19 cell stimulation compared to their naïve counterparts indicating the activation of a specific cytotoxic response (Figure 6).

4. Discussion

The peptides described in this report are newly identified epitopes and, to our knowledge, have not been reported elsewhere. Importantly, these peptides were derived from multiple viral proteins, thereby potentially increasing the targets for T cells and inducing the broad response needed for chronic viral clearance. Two peptides (GGP and LTT) are derived from the large E protein, one (LTF) is derived from the core protein, two (ILR and FLG) are derived from surface protein, and three (FLK; FLS; TVS) are derived from the polymerase protein. The diversity of our identified peptides is similar to that of the response induced during a natural infection (reviewed in [3]). Previous studies in HLA-A2 restricted models have identified immunodominant epitopes from core protein (HBc18-27; [11, 19]), envelope and polymerase proteins (HBe 348–357, HBp455-463; [19]), and X protein (HBx4-10; [33]). Although we were able to detect a few of these peptides in our analysis (including the clinically well studied HBcAg 18–27 epitope, FLPSDFFPSV), the scores (Xcorr values) obtained from MS/MS analysis did not meet standard abundance and confidence cutoff criteria for inclusion in our assays (Supplementary Table 1). A few potential explanations exist to clarify this observation. First, although a subset of these peptides was shown to induce T cell activation in patients acutely infected with HBV [19], T cell responses generated during acute HBV infections may very well differ from those necessary to clear virus during a chronic infection due to alterations in MHC peptide repertoire on chronically

infected cells. Differences in epitope specificity between acute and chronic phases of infection have been observed in other models of chronic infections, for example, LCMV [34, 35] and HIV-1 [36]. Secondly, the low confidence epitopes identified may not be presented at very high levels on the surface of the chronically infected cells, which would lead to a low representation in the MS/MS analysis. Interestingly, several recent reports have demonstrated that low level antigen presentation preferentially favors the expansion of naïve but not memory CD8$^+$ T cells [37–39], which may explain the transient (not sustained) increases in these epitopes specific CD8$^+$ T cell responses in previous clinical trials. Together these data indicate that low scoring peptides may not be the right target for inclusion in therapeutic vaccines and the most relevant targets should be identified by analyzing chronically infected cells.

In order to identify epitopes that are naturally processed and presented by chronically infected cells, we utilized an immunoproteomic approach. Using this approach, we identified eight novel MHC class I restricted epitopes that are derived from four different proteins of the HBV genome. We first confirmed that the identified peptides were able to induce CD8$^+$ T cell activation by measuring IFN-gamma production in an ELISpot assay. Importantly, the T cells were able to recognize the naturally processed and presented epitope appearing on a variety of HBV infected cells regardless of their HLA binding affinities (Table 1). Interestingly, five out of eight peptides that we have characterized contained the appropriate motifs to bind both the HLA-A2 and HLA-A24 supertypes (http://www.hiv.lanl.gov/content/immunology/motif_scan/supertype.html). HLA-A2 supertype is prevalent in >40% of the world population and HLA-A24 supertype is prevalent in >50% of HBV endemic population

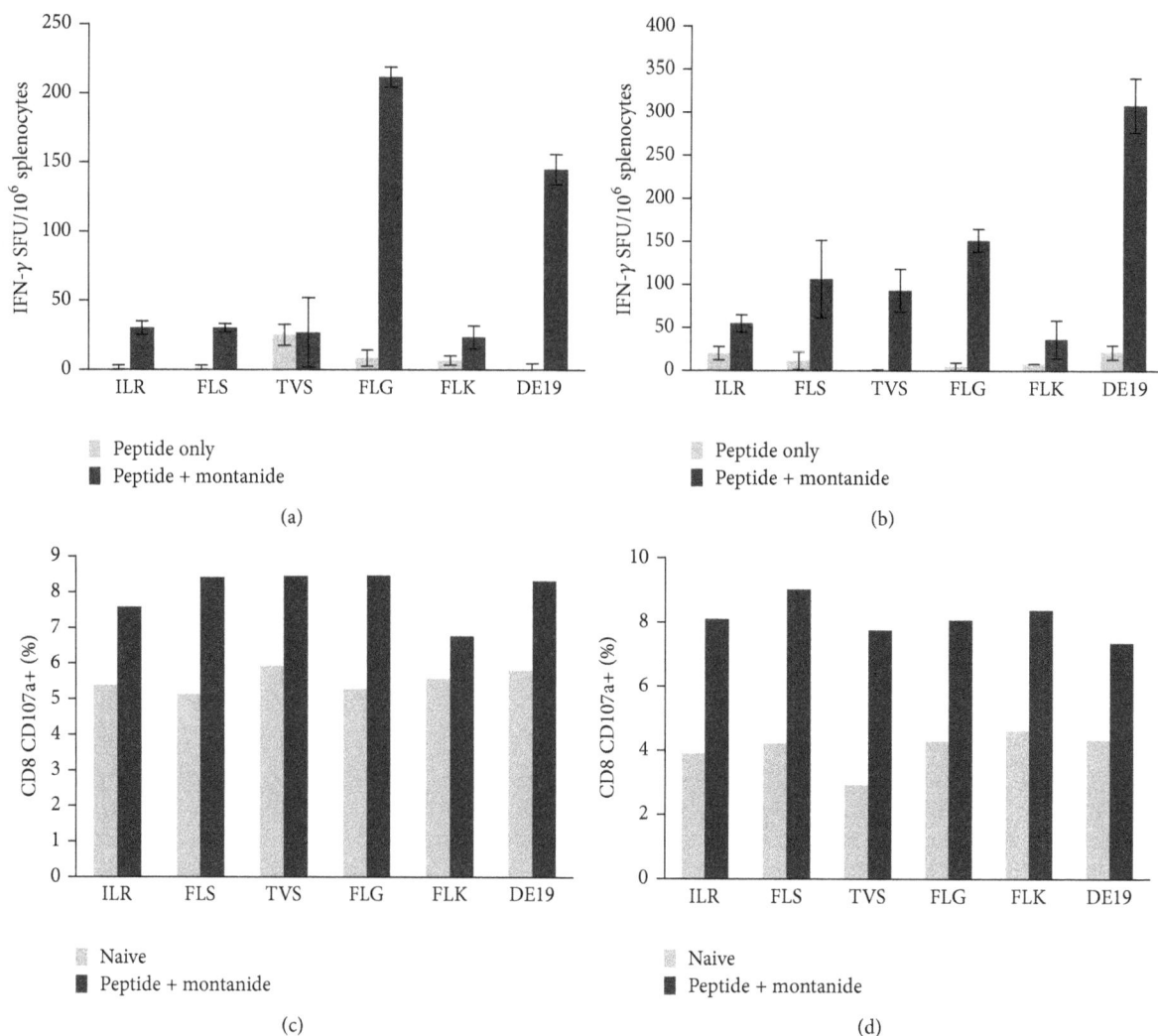

FIGURE 5: HBV specific peptides are able to activate CD8$^+$ T cells *in vivo* in both an HLA-A2 and HLA-A24 restricted fashion. HLA-A2 (a) or HLA-A24 (b) transgenic mice were primed and boosted with peptides as previously described. Spleens were harvested, homogenized into single cell suspensions, and cultured with peptide pulsed (peptides are represented as first 3 residues of the sequence) HepG2 cells or HBV expressing cells overnight in an IFN-gamma ELISpot assay. T cell activation was also measured by examining CD107a upregulation on HLA-A2 (c) or HLA-A24 (d) CD8$^+$ T cells. Splenocytes were cultured for 6 hours with peptide pulsed or HBV expressing cells in the presence of anti-CD107a and subsequently stained for CD8$^+$ expression. Data is presented as the percent of cells in culture that are CD8$^+$ CD107a$^+$.

(http://www.allelefrequencies.net/). Indeed, *in vivo* experiments using mice transgenic for the HLA-A2 or HLA-A24 molecule demonstrated that these peptides can induce T cell activation (as measured by IFN-gamma secretion) and cytolytic activity (as measured by CD107a upregulation and granzyme B secretion) in both A2 and A24 restricted manner.

Thus far, the large majority of epitope discovery for HBV has relied on peptide motif prediction software that estimates how well peptides bind to MHC class I molecules. Strong binders are selected and verified by using synthetic versions to stimulate T cells of both uninfected and infected individuals. However, peptides predicted to bind to the class I molecule may not accurately represent the epitopes presented on the surface of naturally infected cells *in vivo*, nor is a positive binding score a guarantee that T cells will be activated (unpublished observations). As such, differences

in epitope identification approaches will undoubtedly lead to different immunodominant hierarchies being established. For example, Gehring et al. [40] demonstrated that, relative to other immunodominant epitopes (i.e., HBc18-27), T cell specific responses against polymerase epitopes are low. In contrast, our data indicates that, for the epitopes identified by the immunoproteomic approach, the polymerase specific T cells respond just as robustly (in terms of IFN-gamma secretion and granzyme B secretion) as those specific for core and envelope peptides.

Clearance of viral infections such as hepatitis B virus and hepatitis C virus is driven by rapid and robust CD4$^+$ and CD8$^+$ T cell responses. Not surprisingly, individuals who become chronically infected do not mount these vigorous responses [2, 3, 9, 41, 42]. Therefore, any therapeutic intervention to stimulate viral clearance in chronically infected patients must activate a robust, sustained T cell

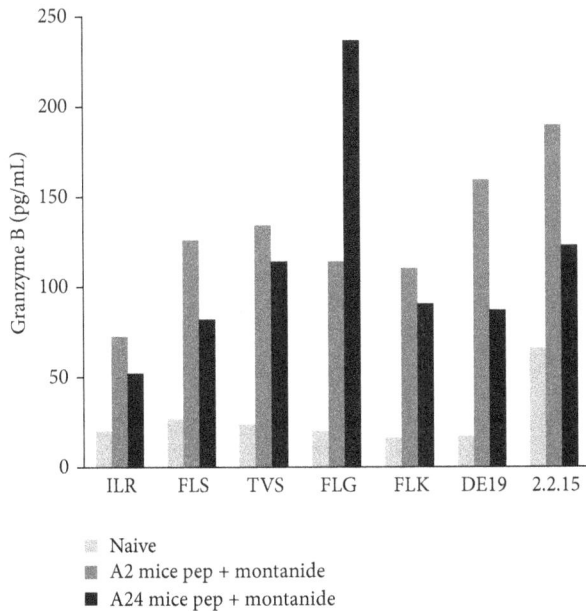

FIGURE 6: HBV peptide specific CD8$^+$ T cells activated *in vivo* secrete cytotoxic effector molecules. In an assay that mirrored the setup described in Figure 5, splenocytes were cultured with peptide pulsed (peptides are represented as first 3 residues of the sequence) or HBV expressing cells overnight. Supernatant was harvested and used in the Milliplex magnetic bead assay to detect granzyme B secretion in response to specific stimulation. Splenocytes from PBS primed, naïve mice were used as a negative control.

response directed at a diverse range of epitopes processed and presented by the chronically infected cell. A number of therapeutic vaccines for HBV have been studied in animal and human models. Although these therapeutic vaccine formulations have stimulated T cells [16–18, 43–45], sustained responses were not achieved [17, 46] and it is unclear from these studies if the T cell responses induced are capable of clearing virus from chronically infected patients. The lack of clinical responses may be due to the fact that the T cell responses induced by these therapies may not accurately reflect the epitopes that are presented by the chronically infected cells. Therefore, formulating an effective therapeutic vaccine for chronic infections should include those epitopes that are naturally processed and presented by the chronically infected cells.

Currently, there is no effective therapeutic vaccine or other immunotherapy to treat chronic HBV infected individuals. The large majority of epitope discovery by motif analysis for hepatitis B virus has been done in HLA-A2 restricted systems. Although HLA-A2 allele represents >40% of the world population, the HLA-A24 allele is more prevalent in HBV endemic population. There are no reliable algorithms for predicting HLA-A2 and A24 binding peptides. However, to design a more universal therapeutic vaccine, multiple HLA restricted epitopes need to be identified. Using an immuno-proteomic approach, it is possible to purify multiple HLA alleles from the same HBV infected cell lysate and subject the isolated peptides to MS/MS analysis without a significant

increase in workload or difficulty. Additionally, this approach can identify epitopes that can bind to more than one HLA allele. In our study, we identified naturally presented HBV specific T cell epitopes with double HLA binding properties, which have the potential to form the basis for a therapeutic vaccine appropriate for the HBV endemic population. Five of the identified peptides reported here share motifs that allow binding to HLA-A2 and HLA-A24 and activation of CD8$^+$ T cells in both settings. Including epitopes that bind to single, distinct HLA alleles and epitopes that bind to multiple HLA alleles in a vaccine formulation may overcome HLA differences between patient populations, increase the breadth of the T cell response, and prevent escape due to antigen downregulation. These (and other) novel MHC class I binding epitopes can readily be incorporated into therapeutic vaccine formulations and tested in preclinical experiments prior to being tested in human clinical trials.

5. Conclusions

Our finding of novel HLA-A2 and A24-associated peptides from HBV infected cells and demonstration of HBV specific CTL responses broadens the applicability of the immuno-proteomics methodology and provides candidate antigens for the development of immunotherapeutic vaccines for the treatment of chronic HBV infection. The data presented in this paper is preliminary and extensive preclinical data is needed to develop these antigens into a therapeutic vaccine.

Conflict of Interests

The authors declare that there is no conflict of interests regarding the publication of this paper.

References

[1] A. S. F. Lok and B. J. McMahon, "Chronic hepatitis B," *Hepatology*, vol. 34, no. 6, pp. 1225–1241, 2001.

[2] B. Rehermann and M. Nascimbeni, "Immunology of hepatitis B virus and hepatitis C virus infection," *Nature Reviews Immunology*, vol. 5, no. 3, pp. 215–229, 2005.

[3] A. Bertoletti and A. J. Gehring, "The immune response during hepatitis B virus infection," *Journal of General Virology*, vol. 87, part 6, pp. 1439–1449, 2006.

[4] C. W. Shepard, E. P. Simard, L. Finelli, A. E. Fiore, and B. P. Bell, "Hepatitis B virus infection: epidemiology and vaccination," *Epidemiologic Reviews*, vol. 28, no. 1, pp. 112–125, 2006.

[5] D. Lavanchy, "Hepatitis B virus epidemiology, disease burden, treatment, arid current and emerging prevention and control measures," *Journal of Viral Hepatitis*, vol. 11, no. 2, pp. 97–107, 2004.

[6] L. G. Guidotti, T. Ishikawa, M. V. Hobbs, B. Matzke, R. Schreiber, and F. V. Chisari, "Intracellular inactivation of the hepatitis B virus by cytotoxic T lymphocytes," *Immunity*, vol. 4, no. 1, pp. 25–36, 1996.

[7] L. G. Guidotti, R. Rochford, J. Chung, M. Shapiro, R. Purcell, and F. V. Chisari, "Viral clearance without destruction of infected cells during acute HBV infection," *Science*, vol. 284, no. 5415, pp. 825–829, 1999.

[8] R. Thimme, S. Wieland, C. Steiger et al., "CD8$^+$ T cells mediate viral clearance and disease pathogenesis during acute hepatitis B virus infection," *Journal of Virology*, vol. 77, no. 1, pp. 68–76, 2003.

[9] J. J. Chang and S. R. Lewin, "Immunopathogenesis of hepatitis B virus infection," *Immunology and Cell Biology*, vol. 85, no. 1, pp. 16–23, 2007.

[10] G. J. M. Webster, S. Reignat, M. K. Maini et al., "Incubation phase of acute hepatitis B in man: dynamic of cellular immune mechanisms," *Hepatology*, vol. 32, no. 5, pp. 1117–1124, 2000.

[11] C. Ferrari, A. Penna, A. Bertoletti et al., "Cellular immune response to hepatitis B virus-encoded antigens in acute and chronic hepatitis B virus infection," *Journal of Immunology*, vol. 145, no. 10, pp. 3442–3449, 1990.

[12] B. Rehermann, P. Fowler, J. Sidney et al., "The cytotoxic T lymphocyte response to multiple hepatitis B virus polymerase epitopes during and after acute viral hepatitis," *Journal of Experimental Medicine*, vol. 181, no. 3, pp. 1047–1058, 1995.

[13] C. P. Desmond, A. Bartholomeusz, S. Gaudieri, P. A. Revill, and S. R. Lewin, "A systematic review of T-cell epitopes in hepatitis B virus: identification, genotypic variation and relevance to antiviral therapeutics," *Antiviral Therapy*, vol. 13, no. 2, pp. 161–175, 2008.

[14] B. Rehermann, D. Lau, J. H. Hoofnagle, and F. V. Chisari, "Cytotoxic T lymphocyte responsiveness after resolution of chronic hepatitis B virus infection," *The Journal of Clinical Investigation*, vol. 97, no. 7, pp. 1655–1665, 1996.

[15] D.-Z. Xu, K. Zhao, L.-M. Guo et al., "A randomized controlled phase IIb trial of antigen-antibody immunogenic complex therapeutic vaccine in chronic hepatitis B patients," *PLoS ONE*, vol. 3, no. 7, Article ID e2565, 2008.

[16] B. D. Livingston, C. Crimi, H. Grey et al., "The hepatitis B virus-specific CTL responses induced in humans by lipopeptide vaccination are comparable to those elicited by acute viral infection," *Journal of Immunology*, vol. 159, no. 3, pp. 1383–1392, 1997.

[17] M. Mancini-Bourgine, H. Fontaine, D. Scott-Algara, S. Pol, C. Bréchot, and M.-L. Michel, "Induction or expansion of T-cell responses by a hepatitis B DNA vaccine administered to chronic HBV carriers," *Hepatology*, vol. 40, no. 4, pp. 874–882, 2004.

[18] P. Pancholi, D.-H. Lee, Q. Liu et al., "DNA prime/canarypox boost-based immunotherapy of chronic hepatitis B virus infection in a chimpanzee," *Hepatology*, vol. 33, no. 2, pp. 448–454, 2001.

[19] A. Sette, A. Vitiello, B. Reherman et al., "The relationship between class I binding affinity and immunogenicity of potential cytotoxic T cell epitopes," *Journal of Immunology*, vol. 153, no. 12, pp. 5586–5592, 1994.

[20] J. S. Testa, V. Shetty, J. Hafner et al., "MHC class I-presented T cell epitopes identified by immunoproteomics analysis are targets for a cross reactive influenza-specific T cell response," *PLoS ONE*, vol. 7, no. 11, Article ID e48484, 2012.

[21] J. S. Testa, V. Shetty, G. Sinnathamby et al., "Conserved MHC class I-presented dengue virus epitopes identified by immunoproteomics analysis are targets for cross-serotype reactive T-cell response," *The Journal of Infectious Diseases*, vol. 205, no. 4, pp. 647–655, 2012.

[22] V. Shetty, Z. Nickens, J. Testa, J. Hafner, G. Sinnathamby, and R. Philip, "Quantitative immunoproteomics analysis reveals novel MHC class I presented peptides in cisplatin-resistant ovarian cancer cells," *Journal of Proteomics*, vol. 75, no. 11, pp. 3270–3290, 2012.

[23] V. Shetty, G. Sinnathamby, Z. Nickens et al., "MHC class I-presented lung cancer-associated tumor antigens identified by immunoproteomics analysis are targets for cancer-specific T cell response," *Journal of Proteomics*, vol. 74, no. 5, pp. 728–743, 2011.

[24] K. T. Hogan, M. A. Coppola, C. L. Gatlin et al., "Identification of a shared epitope recognized by melanoma-specific, HLA-A3-restricted cytotoxic T lymphocytes," *Immunology Letters*, vol. 90, no. 2-3, pp. 131–135, 2003.

[25] S. Feyerabend, S. Stevanovic, C. Gouttefangeas et al., "Novel multi-peptide vaccination in Hla-A2+ hormone sensitive patients with biochemical relapse of prostate cancer," *Prostate*, vol. 69, no. 9, pp. 917–927, 2009.

[26] O. E. Hawkins, R. S. Vangundy, A. M. Eckerd et al., "Identification of breast cancer peptide epitopes presented by HLA-A*0201," *Journal of Proteome Research*, vol. 7, no. 4, pp. 1445–1457, 2008.

[27] K. T. Hogan, M. A. Coppola, C. L. Gatlin et al., "Identification of novel and widely expressed cancer/testis gene isoforms that elicit spontaneous cytotoxic T-lymphocyte reactivity to melanoma," *Cancer Research*, vol. 64, no. 3, pp. 1157–1163, 2004.

[28] H.-G. Rammensee, J. Bachmann, N. P. N. Emmerich, O. A. Bachor, and S. Stevanović, "SYFPEITHI: database for MHC ligands and peptide motifs," *Immunogenetics*, vol. 50, no. 3-4, pp. 213–219, 1999.

[29] M. R. Betts, J. M. Brenchley, D. A. Price et al., "Sensitive and viable identification of antigen-specific CD8$^+$ T cells by a flow cytometric assay for degranulation," *Journal of Immunological Methods*, vol. 281, no. 1-2, pp. 65–78, 2003.

[30] E. A. Mittendorf, C. E. Storrer, C. D. Shriver, S. Ponniah, and G. E. Peoples, "Evaluation of the CD107 cytotoxicity assay for the detection of cytolytic CD8$^+$ cells recognizing HER2/neu vaccine peptides," *Breast Cancer Research and Treatment*, vol. 92, no. 1, pp. 85–93, 2005.

[31] A. Parmigiani, M. L. Alcaide, R. Freguja et al., "Impaired antibody response to influenza vaccine in HIV-infected and uninfected aging women is associated with immune activation and inflammation," *PLoS ONE*, vol. 8, no. 11, Article ID e79816, 2013.

[32] J. K. Nieminen, M. Niemi, T. Sipponen et al., "Dendritic cells from Crohn's disease patients show aberrant STAT1 and STAT3 signaling," *PLoS ONE*, vol. 8, no. 8, Article ID e70738, 2013.

[33] S. Malmassari, Y. C. Lone, M. Zhang, C. Transy, and M.-L. Michel, "In vivo hierarchy of immunodominant and subdominant HLA-A*0201- restricted T-cell epitopes of HBx antigen of hepatitis B virus," *Microbes and Infection*, vol. 7, no. 4, pp. 626–634, 2005.

[34] E. J. Wherry, J. N. Blattman, K. Murali-Krishna, R. Van Der Most, and R. Ahmed, "Viral persistence alters CD8 T-cell immunodominance and tissue distribution and results in distinct stages of functional impairment," *Journal of Virology*, vol. 77, no. 8, pp. 4911–4927, 2003.

[35] R. G. van der Most, K. Murali-Krishna, J. G. Lanier et al., "Changing immunodominance patterns in antiviral CD8 T-cell responses after loss of epitope presentation or chronic antigenic stimulation," *Virology*, vol. 315, no. 1, pp. 93–102, 2003.

[36] P. J. R. Goulder, M. A. Altfeld, E. S. Rosenberg et al., "Substantial differences in specificity of HIV-specific cytotoxic T cells in acute and chronic HIV infection," *Journal of Experimental Medicine*, vol. 193, no. 2, pp. 181–193, 2001.

[37] E. R. Jellison, M. J. Turner, D. A. Blair et al., "Distinct mechanisms mediate naive and memory CD8 T-cell tolerance,"

Proceedings of the National Academy of Sciences of the United States of America, vol. 109, no. 52, pp. 21438–21443, 2012.

[38] M. D. Martin, S. A. Condotta, J. T. Harty, and V. P. Badovinac, "Population dynamics of naive and memory CD8 T cell responses after antigen stimulations in vivo," *Journal of Immunology*, vol. 188, no. 3, pp. 1255–1265, 2012.

[39] E. R. Mehlhop-Williams and M. J. Bevan, "Memory CD8$^+$ T cells exhibit increased antigen threshold requirements for recall proliferation," *The Journal of Experimental Medicine*, vol. 211, no. 2, pp. 345–356, 2014.

[40] A. J. Gehring, D. Sun, P. T. F. Kennedy et al., "The level of viral antigen presented by hepatocytes influences CD8 T-cell function," *Journal of Virology*, vol. 81, no. 6, pp. 2940–2949, 2007.

[41] F. Lechner, D. K. Wong, P. R. Dunbar et al., "Analysis of successful immune responses in persons infected with hepatitis C virus," *The Journal of Experimental Medicine*, vol. 191, no. 9, pp. 1499–1512, 2000.

[42] N. H. Shoukry, A. G. Cawthon, and C. M. Walker, "Cell-mediated immunity and the outcome of hepatitis C virus infection," *Annual Review of Microbiology*, vol. 58, pp. 391–424, 2004.

[43] A. Vitiello, G. Ishioka, H. M. Grey et al., "Development of a lipopeptide-based therapeutic vaccine to treat chronic HBV infection. I. Induction of a primary cytotoxic T lymphocyte response in humans," *The Journal of Clinical Investigation*, vol. 95, no. 1, pp. 341–349, 1995.

[44] R. Schirmbeck, P. Riedl, N. Fissolo, F. A. Lemonnier, A. Bertoletti, and J. Reimann, "Translation from cryptic reading frames of DNA vaccines generates an extended repertoire of immunogenic, MHC class I-restricted epitopes," *Journal of Immunology*, vol. 174, no. 8, pp. 4647–4656, 2005.

[45] P. Buchmann, C. Dembek, L. Kuklick et al., "A novel therapeutic hepatitis B vaccine induces cellular and humoral immune responses and breaks tolerance in hepatitis B virus (HBV) transgenic mice," *Vaccine*, vol. 31, no. 8, pp. 1197–1203, 2013.

[46] S. Pol, B. Nalpas, F. Driss et al., "Efficacy and limitations of a specific immunotherapy in chronic hepatitis B," *Journal of Hepatology*, vol. 34, no. 6, pp. 917–921, 2001.

16

Hepatitis B Awareness among Medical Students and Their Vaccination Status at Syrian Private University

Nazir Ibrahim[1] and Amr Idris[2]

[1] *Internal Medicine and Gastroenterology Departments, Syrian Private University, P.O. Box 36822, Damascus, Syria*
[2] *Internal Medicine Department, Syrian Private University, Mazzeh Street, P.O. Box 36822, Damascus, Syria*

Correspondence should be addressed to Amr Idris; amr-idris@hotmail.com

Academic Editor: Piero Luigi Almasio

Background. Hepatitis B virus (HBV) is a potentially life-threating infection and a well-recognized occupational hazard for health-care workers including medical students. *Methods.* A cross-sectional study was conducted at Syrian Private University (SPU), Faculty of Medicine, to assess the knowledge and awareness about hepatitis B, the status of hepatitis B vaccination, and the reasons for not getting vaccinated among the first- and the fifth-year medical students. *Results.* The present study demonstrates surprising results and raises issues about the high number of medical students that are not vaccinated or not sure about their vaccination status, which puts them at a higher risk of being infected in the future. Another important issue is the medical students' overall knowledge about this life-threating infection. The students have not been totally educated about the gravity of the situation which requires the need of further HBV education. It is highly recommended that SPU provides the HBV vaccine to all nonvaccinated students attending the faculty of medicine at no cost to encourage them to take the HBV vaccine and to reform some of its educational curriculum to effectively limit the hazardous effects of this disease and elaborate on the serious health consequences of HBV.

1. Introduction

Hepatitis B infection is a disease of the liver caused by the hepatitis B virus (HBV), which has a partially double-stranded circular DNA and belongs to the family Hepadnaviridae [1, 2]. Hepatitis B is a major public health concern worldwide. Approximately 30% of the world's population has been infected with HBV [3–5], and more than 350 million are chronically infected with HBV and carry high risk for cirrhosis and liver cancer [6]. At least one million people die annually from HBV related chronic liver disease [7].

HBV is transmitted by body fluids, such as blood and serum, and can exhibit vertical transmission from mother to child. Sexual transmission, vertical transmission, and unsafe injections, including intravenous drug use, are the most common routes of infection for HBV [8–12]. Household contact and occupational health-care exposure to blood products and hemodialysis are other risk factors [13–20]. Health-care workers (HCWs) are reported to have the highest occupational risk for HBV infection [21]. There are 35 million

HCWs worldwide, and percutaneous injuries have been estimated to result in approximately 66,000 hepatitis B viral infections per year [21]. Data from the United States in the 1990s showed that unvaccinated HCWs had serologic evidence of past or current HBV infection three to five times greater than the general population [22]. In Syria, there is no specific national strategy or guidelines for preventing hepatitis B infection in health-care settings [23].

A survey of the medical students showed that 30% of reported needle stick injuries occurred in the operation room [22].

The clinical manifestations and natural history of HBV infection vary with age. Clinical acute hepatitis B is more frequent in adults than children, and the probability of becoming a chronic carrier of hepatitis B is greater in children than adults: 80–90% of people perinatally infected compared to <5% of infections occurring in adults [24]. People with chronic hepatitis B have a 15% to 25% risk of dying prematurely from HBV related complications [25].

Acute hepatitis B infection is an illness that begins with prodromal symptoms like anorexia, chills, headache, nausea, vomiting, and malaise. Development of jaundice may then occur but is noted in only 30% of all patients with acute infection. Acute hepatitis B is often unrecognized in children younger than five years old.

Chronic infection with the HBV may be either asymptomatic or associated with chronic inflammation of the liver. After 10 years of chronic infection, about 20% of the patients with hepatitis B have progressed to cirrhosis and about 5% have developed HCC [26]. Chronically infected HBV patients have a 15–25% risk of dying prematurely due to HBV-related cirrhosis and HCC [27]. Hepatitis B is estimated to be the cause of 30% of cirrhosis and 53% of HCC worldwide [28]. Also of note, hepatitis B virus has been linked to membranous glomerulonephritis [29]. Given HBV and its ability to affect multiple organ systems including the liver and kidney, chronic infection is of particular concern.

Prevention is the only safe strategy against high prevalence of viral hepatitis. Having enough knowledge and proper attitudes toward this infection is cornerstones of preventing transmission. Medical students have a very important role in preventing the disease by improving the disease knowledge among themselves and the patients they treat. Safe and effective HBV vaccines have been available since 1982. The implementations of mass immunization programs have been recommended by the World Health Organization since 1991. Since its global expanded coverage, the incidence of HBV infection and liver cancer among infants, children, and adolescents has dramatically decreased. Prevention is focused on vaccination of population groups most at risk. Included in these at risk groups are persons working in the health care field. Since the early 1990's, Syria was among the first countries in the Middle East to use the second generation HBV vaccine as an integral part of the national infant immunization programs. However, in Syria, the universal vaccination of adolescents does not have the same implementation success as compared to infant vaccinations. At the Syrian medical universities including SPU, there is no requirement for the students to be hepatitis B vaccinated or to check the hepatitis B immunity status to be admitted to the medical faculty or begin training at the teaching hospitals. However, there is no information provided that the government has established the goal of eliminating hepatitis B or set a strategy that focuses exclusively or primarily on the prevention and control of viral hepatitis [23].

The aims of this study were to assess the knowledge and awareness of HBV infection and estimate the number of first- and fifth-year medical students covered by hepatitis B vaccination.

2. Subjects and Methods

A cross-sectional study was conducted by Internal Medicine and Gastroenterology Departments at the Syrian Private University, Damascus, Syria, in February 2014. The study targeted the first- and the fifth-year medical students at the Syrian Private University, Faculty of Medicine. The total

TABLE 1: Descriptive characteristics of the subjects included in the analyses.

Characteristics	Number of subjects (%)
Group years	
First year	64 (50%)
Fifth year	64 (50%)
Sex	
Male	80 (62.5%)
Female	48 (37.5%)

number of students enrolled at the time of the study at Syrian Private University in their first medical school year was 120 students and 80 students in their fifth medical school year. The invitation to complete the survey was sent to all the first-year medical students. The overall response was 64 students from the first-year students. Afterward, a proportionate stratified sampling was taken from the fifth-year medical students. Therefore, the overall response from both the first- and fifth-year medial students was 128.

This study was conducted to assess the students' knowledge and awareness about hepatitis B and to assess the number of students covered by hepatitis B vaccine. All students were interviewed using a structured self-completed questionnaire consisting of 20 questions. The questionnaire consisted of five sections: (1) demographic and academic characteristics; (2) HBV knowledge; (3) HBV prevention; (4) personal HBV-related health history; (5) perception of HBV vaccine and vaccination status. The language of instruction at Syrian Private University is English. Therefore, the questionnaire was given in English. All the subjects were interviewed, questions were explained and translated for all the students included in the study; and anonymity was assured. Before the distribution of the questionnaire, the objectives of the study were explained to participants, and they were informed that their participation was voluntary.

2.1. Statistical Analysis Used. Data was coded, entered, and analyzed using the Statistical Package for Social Science (SPSS) version 20.0 (SPSS, Chicago, IL, USA).

Ethical approval of this study was received from the Institutional Ethical Review Board of the Faculty of Medicine, Syrian Private University, Damascus, Syria.

3. Results

The demographic characteristics of the study sample are shown in Table 1 and Figure 1. A total of 128 students responded to the questionnaire, 80 (62.5%) males and 48 (37.5%) females. The age of the participants ranged from 17 to 25 years (mean: 21.4). All of the students were from the Faculty of Medicine and were Arabic and English speakers (100%).

The study revealed the weakness of general knowledge about hepatitis B among the junior medical students compared to those in the fifth year. As documented in Table 2, the survey showed that, out of 128 participants who completed

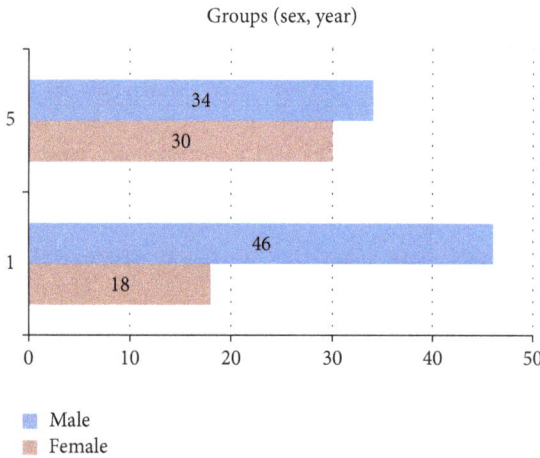

FIGURE 1: Age groups of the study sample in the first- and fifth-year medicine students.

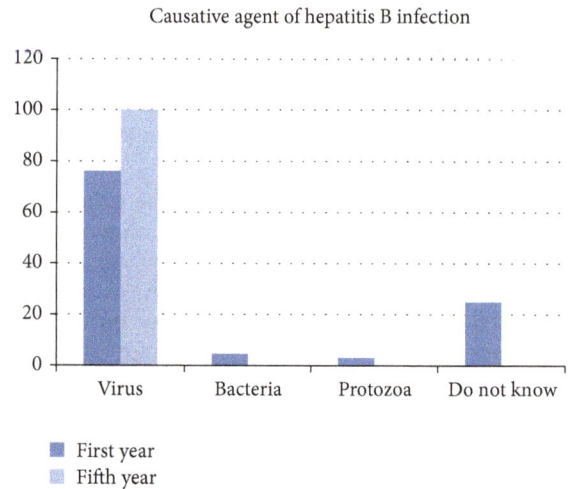

FIGURE 2: Student's knowledge about the causative agent of hepatitis B infection.

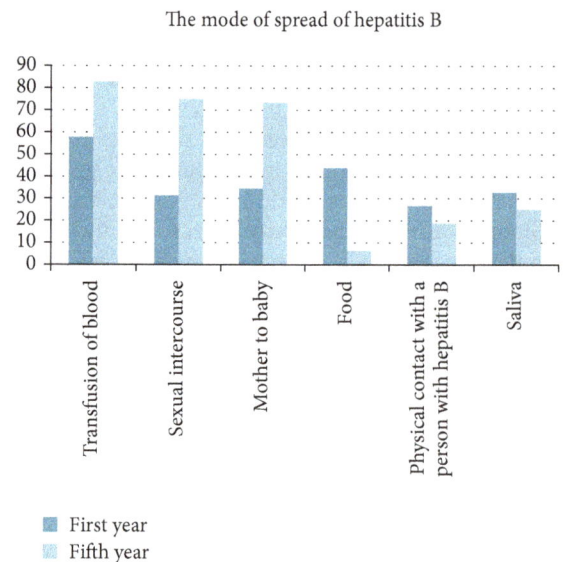

FIGURE 3: Student's knowledge about the risk factors of hepatitis B infection.

the survey, around 92% of subjects are aware of hepatitis B infection, yet unaware of the symptoms, which is significantly associated with the academic level of the students ($P = 0.000$).

The symptoms were well understood by only 37 (57.81%) and 52 (81.25%) of the first- and fifth-year medical students, respectively. In addition, 89.07% of the students did not know that chronic HBV infection is often asymptomatic and only 35.15% of all the students knew that chronic HBV infection confers a high risk of cirrhosis, liver cancer, kidney disease, and its consequences. Understanding of the symptoms and the disease consequences is significantly associated with the medical year of the students ($P = 0.000$).

A remarkable difference is found between the students' knowledge of HBV concerning the causative agent and nature ($P = 0.000$), in which the cause of HBV was known to only 43 (67.18%) and 64 (100%) of the first-year and fifth-year students, respectively (Figure 2).

Their knowledge about the mode of transmission was also lacking with 52 (40.62%) students unaware that contaminated blood, contaminated needles, unprotected sex with an infected person, and birth to an infected mother are all modes of HBV transmission ($P = 0.000$). Only 25 (39.06%) first-year students and 49 (76.56%) of the fifth-year students are aware of all the modes of HBV transmission (Figure 3). Among 64 first-year students, only one student was aware about all risk factors including piercings, tattoos, transfusion of blood, and dental visits. This number is compared to 33 of the fifth-year students ($P = 0.000$) (Figure 4).

Furthermore, out of the 128 subjects, only 43.75% of the students had taken the hepatitis B vaccine and 26.56% do not know their vaccination status. Of the first-year students, only 20 (31.25%) received the vaccine, compared to 36 (56.25%) of the fifth-year students ($P = 0.000$) (Figure 5). When asked about the reasons of not taking the hepatitis B vaccine, the answers varied between "never thought of vaccination" (23.5%), "lack of motivation" (34.2%), "afraid of needles" (8%), "lack of belief" (8%), and "no need felt" (26.3%), (Figure 6).

Only 16.4% of all the students have gone through the test of HBV infection. Moreover, 12.5% of the individuals did not know that receiving the hepatitis B vaccine and avoiding the reuse of needles are two of the most efficient ways to prevent HBV transmission. 50% of the first-year students are aware that doctors and medical students are more prone of getting hepatitis B via cross-infection while 92.18% of the fifth-year students are aware ($P = 0.000$).

4. Discussion

This study showed that the first-year medical students have poor knowledge and lack of awareness about hepatitis B, its routes of transmission, risk factors, and modes of preventions compared to the fifth-year medical students. Similarly, most

TABLE 2: Hepatitis B knowledge questions and correct responses in percentage.

Question	Correct responses (%)	First year ($n = 64$)	Fifth year ($n = 64$)
Have you heard of hepatitis B?	Yes: 92% No: 8%	Yes: 89.06% No: 10.94%	Yes: 96.87% No: 3.13%
Is most Chronic hepatitis b infection (A) symptomatic, (B) asymptomatic?	(A) Symptomatic: 89.07% (B) Asymptomatic: 10.93%	(A) Symptomatic: 84.38% (B) Asymptomatic: 15.62%	(A) Symptomatic: 93.75% (B) Asymptomatic: 6.25%
Are doctors and medical students more prone of getting hepatitis B via cross-infection?	Yes: 71.09% No: 28.91%	Yes: 50% No: 50%	Yes: 92.18% No: 7.82%
Does hepatitis B vaccination protect against the infection?	Yes: 89.84% No: 10.16%	Yes: 90.62% No: 9.38%	Yes: 89.06% No: 10.94%
Have you received hepatitis B vaccine before in Syria or outside Syria?	Yes: 43.75% No: 29.69% Do not know: 26.56%	Yes: 31.25% No: 18.75% Do not know: 50%	Yes: 56.25% No: 40.62% Do not know: 3.13%
What is ideal age of vaccination?	(A) Infancy: 55.46% (B) Youth: 32.03% (C) Adulthood: 12.5%	(A) Infancy: 51.56% (B) Youth: 42.18% (C) Adulthood: 4.68%	(A) Infancy: 59.37% (B) Youth: 21.87% (C) Adulthood: 20.31%
What is the reason behind not being vaccinated?	(A) Lack of motivation: 34.20% (B) No need felt: 26.30% (C) Never thought of vaccination: 23.50% (D) Lack of belief: 8% (E) Fear of injection: 8%	(A) 16.6% (B) 33.33% (C) 25% (D) 16.6% (E) 8.33%	(A) 42.3% (B) 23.07% (C) 23.07% (D) 3.84% (E) 7.69%
Should hepatitis patients be allowed to work?	Yes: 47.65% No: 32.03% Do not Know: 20.31%	Yes: 29.68% No: 46.87% Do not know: 23.43%	Yes: 65.63% No: 17.18% Do not know: 17.18%
What is the causative agent of hepatitis B?	(A) Virus: 83.6% (B) Bacteria: 2.34% (C) Protozoa: 1.56% (D) Do not know: 12.53%	(A) Virus: 67.18% (B) Bacteria: 4.68% (C) Protozoa: 3.12% (D) Do not know: 25%	(A) Virus: 100% (B) Bacteria: 0% (C) Protozoa: 0% (D) Do not know: 0%
What is the mode of spread of hepatitis B?	(A) Transfusion of blood: 70.3% (B) Sexual intercourse: 53.12% (C) Mother to her baby: 53.9% (D) Food: 25% (E) Physical contact with a person with hepatitis B: 22.65% (F) Saliva: 28.9%	(A) 57.81% (B) 31.25% (C) 34.37% (D) 43.75% (E) 26.56% (F) 32.81%	(A) 82.81% (B) 75% (C) 73.43% (D) 6.25% (E) 18.75% (F) 25%
What are the risk factors that may be the cause of hepatitis B?	(A) Smoking: 10.15% (B) Alcohol: 30.46% (C) Piercing and tattoo: 62.5% (D) Blood transfusion: 72.65% (E) Dental visits: 57% (F) Eating from contaminated food: 33.59% (G) Drinking from contaminated drinks: 25%	(A) 17.18% (B) 45.31% (C) 45.31% (D) 51.56% (E) 40.6% (F) 62.5% (G) 46.87%	(A) 3.12% (B) 15.62% (C) 79.68% (D) 93.75% (E) 73.43% (F) 4.68% (G) 3.12%
Do hepatitis B infections cause the following singes and symptoms?	(A) Fever: 19.5% (B) Loss of appetite: 13.28% (C) Nausea: 11.7% (D) Vomiting: 10.15% (E) Jaundice: 22.66% (F) All of the above: 69.53%	(A) 28.12% (B) 17.18% (C) 17.18% (D) 14.06% (E) 32.81% (F) 57.81%	(A) 10.93% (B) 9.37% (C) 6.25% (D) 6.25% (E) 12.5% (F) 81.25%

TABLE 2: Continued.

Question	Correct responses (%)	First year ($n = 64$)	Fifth year ($n = 64$)
What does chronic hepatitis B infection lead to?	(A) Liver disease: 48.44% (B) Cirrhosis: 45.31% (C) Kidney disease: 4.69% (D) Liver cancer: 27.34% (E) All of the above: 35.15% (F) None of the above: 2.34%	(A) 57.81% (B) 51.56% (C) 7.81% (D) 18.75% (E) 15.62% (F) 4.68%	(A) 39.06% (B) 39.06% (C) 1.56% (D) 35.93% (E) 54.68% (F) 0%
Is hepatitis B infection preventable or not?	Ye: 87.5% No: 12.5%	Yes: 92.18% No: 7.82%	Yes: 82.81% No: 17.19%
Have you ever been tested for hepatitis B?	Yes: 16.4% No: 83.6%	Yes: 21.87% No: 78.13%	Yes: 26.56% No: 73.44%
Have you ever been diagnosed with any liver disease before?	Yes: 15.63% No: 84.37%	Yes: 23.44% No: 76.56%	Yes: 7.82% No: 92.18%

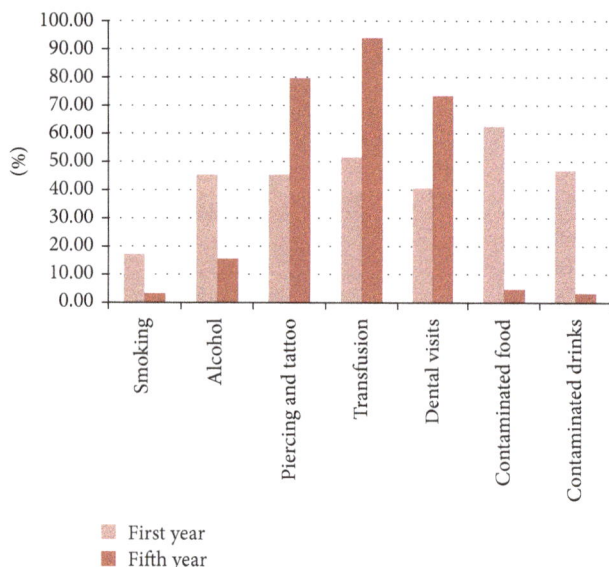

FIGURE 4: Student's knowledge about routes of transmission of hepatitis B Virus.

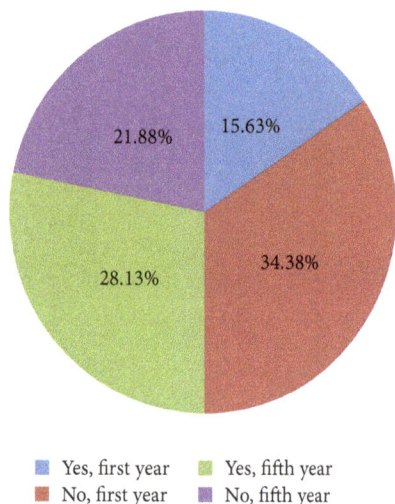

FIGURE 6: The reason behind not being vaccinated against hepatitis B Virus.

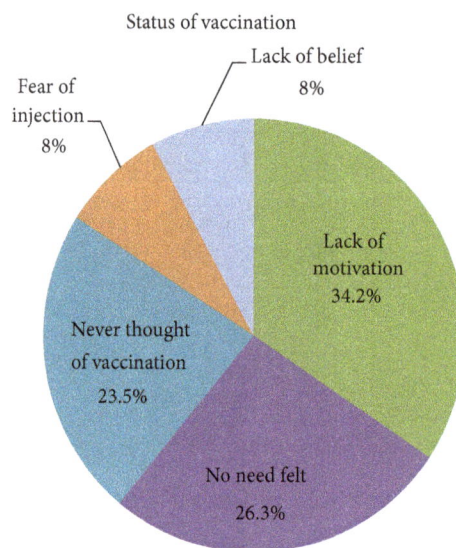

FIGURE 5: Number of students who received the hepatitis B vaccine.

of the first-year students 63 (98.44%) were not vaccinated against hepatitis B, which makes them vulnerable to the disease. Interestingly, the main reason for not being vaccinated is the lack of motivation (34.2%). However, the survey also shows that most of the students (92%) were aware of hepatitis.

The present study demonstrates surprising results and raises issues about the high number of medical students that are not vaccinated or not sure about their vaccination status. According to a recent study on medical students by Al-Ghamdi, anti-HBs levels were significantly low in many students after their primary immunization. Therefore, testing medical students for anti-HBs levels may be warranted as they represent a high-risk population [30]. Another important issue also rises about the medical students' knowledge about this life-threating infection and the need of further HBV education. Therefore, it is highly recommended that the SPU makes reforms to its educational curriculum to promote awareness among the medical students. One important realization from this study is that education is necessary. As students play an important role in dissemination of knowledge and raising awareness among their communities, more educational efforts should be exerted on the students themselves for the importance of viral hepatitis, and SPU must participate more in national/regional/international meetings about hepatitis in order to contribute to the prevention of viral hepatitis. Furthermore, educational initiatives should also be focused toward avoiding infection and seeking care in case of exposure to infected body fluids.

Another suggestion for a new initiative could be providing free HBV vaccines to all the nonvaccinated students attending medical faculty to encourage universal vaccinations for all students upon their entry. Future studies may be directed at measuring the hepatitis B antibody titers and evaluating the response to the hepatitis B vaccine among the medical students.

Conflict of Interests

The authors declare that there is no conflict of interests regarding the publication of this paper.

Acknowledgment

The authors are very grateful to the students who participated in the study and helped collect the data.

References

[1] W. F. Carman and H. C. Thomas, "Genetic variation in hepatitis B virus," *Gastroenterology*, vol. 102, no. 2, pp. 711–719, 1992.

[2] N. Gitlin, "Hepatitis B: diagnosis, prevention, and treatment," *Clinical Chemistry*, vol. 43, no. 8, pp. 1500–1506, 1997.

[3] A. J. Zuckerman, "More than third of world's population has been infected with hepatitis B virus," *British Medical Journal*, vol. 318, no. 7192, article 1213, 1999.

[4] World Health Organization, "The world health report 1996. Fighing disease. Fostering development," Executive Summary, World Health Organization, Geneva, Switzerland, 1996.

[5] M. J. Alter, "Epidemiology and prevention of hepatitis B," *Seminars in Liver Disease*, vol. 23, no. 1, pp. 39–46, 2003.

[6] D. Lavanchy, "Hepatitis B virus epidemiology, disease burden, treatment, arid current and emerging prevention and control measures," *Journal of Viral Hepatitis*, vol. 11, no. 2, pp. 97–107, 2004.

[7] Z. Sun, L. Ming, X. Zhu, and J. Lu, "Prevention and control of hepatitis B in China," *Journal of Medical Virology*, vol. 67, no. 3, pp. 447–450, 2002.

[8] M. J. Alter, J. Ahtone, I. Weisfuse, K. Starko, T. D. Vacalis, and J. E. Maynard, "Hepatitis B virus transmission between heterosexuals," *The Journal of the American Medical Association*, vol. 256, no. 10, pp. 1307–1310, 1986.

[9] L. A. Kingsley, C. R. Rinaldo Jr., D. W. Lyter, R. O. Valdiserri, S. H. Belle, and M. Ho, "Sexual transmission efficiency of hepatitis B virus and human immunodeficiency virus among homosexual men," *The Journal of the American Medical Association*, vol. 264, no. 2, pp. 230–234, 1990.

[10] R. P. Beasley, C. Trepo, C. E. Stevens II, and W. Szmuness, "The e antigen and vertical transmission of hepatitis B surface antigen," *The American Journal of Epidemiology*, vol. 105, no. 2, pp. 94–98, 1977.

[11] A. Kane, J. Lloyd, M. Zaffran, L. Simonsen, and M. Kane, "Transmission of hepatitis B, hepatitis C and human immunodeficiency viruses through unsafe injections in the developing world: model-based regional estimates," *Bulletin of the World Health Organization*, vol. 77, no. 10, pp. 801–807, 1999.

[12] B. Broers, C. Junet, M. Bourquin, J.-J. Déglon, L. Perrin, and B. Hirschel, "Prevalence and incidence rate of HIV, hepatitis B and C among drug users on methadone maintenance treatment in Geneva between 1988 and 1995," *AIDS*, vol. 12, no. 15, pp. 2059–2066, 1998.

[13] A. Vegnente, R. Iorio, S. Guida, and L. Cimmino, "Chronicity rate of hepatitis B virus infection in the families of 60 hepatitis B surface antigen positive chronic carrier children: role of horizontal transmission," *European Journal of Pediatrics*, vol. 151, no. 3, pp. 188–191, 1992.

[14] J. L. Lauer, N. A. VanDrunen, J. W. Washburn, and H. H. Balfour Jr., "Transmission of hepatitis B virus in clinical laboratory areas," *Journal of Infectious Diseases*, vol. 140, no. 4, pp. 513–516, 1979.

[15] D. J. Hu, M. A. Kane, and D. L. Heymann, "Transmission of HIV, hepatitis B virus, and other bloodborne pathogens in health care settings: a review of risk factors and guidelines for prevention," *Bulletin of the World Health Organization*, vol. 69, no. 5, pp. 623–630, 1991.

[16] J. F. Fernandes, R. F. S. Braz, F. A. V. Neto, M. A. Silva, N. F. Costa, and A. M. Ferreira, "Prevalence of serologic markers of hepatitis B virus in hospital personnel," *Revista de Saúde Pública*, vol. 33, no. 2, pp. 122–128, 1999.

[17] M. Colombo, S. Oldani, M. F. Donato et al., "A multicenter, prospective study of posttransfusion hepatitis in Milan," *Hepatology*, vol. 7, no. 4, pp. 709–712, 1987.

[18] R. Saxena, V. Thakur, B. Sood, R. C. Guptan, S. Gururaja, and S. K. Sarin, "Transfusion-associated hepatitis in a tertiary referral hospital in India. A prospective study," *Vox Sanguinis*, vol. 77, no. 1, pp. 6–10, 1999.

[19] S. V. Williams, J. C. Huff, E. J. Feinglass, M. B. Gregg, M. H. Hatch, and J. M. Matsen, "Epidemic viral hepatitis, type B, in hospital personnel," *The American Journal of Medicine*, vol. 57, no. 6, pp. 904–911, 1974.

[20] V. A. Mioli, E. Balestra, L. Bibiano et al., "Epidemiology of viral hepatitis in dialysis centers: a national survey," *Nephron*, vol. 61, no. 3, pp. 278–283, 1992.

[21] A. Prüss-Üstün, E. Rapiti, and Y. Hutin, "Estimation of the global burden of disease attributable to contaminated sharps injuries among health-care workers," *The American Journal of Industrial Medicine*, vol. 48, no. 6, pp. 482–490, 2005.

[22] J. L. Gerberding, "Incidence and prevalence of human immunodeficiency virus, hepatitis B virus, hepatitis C virus, and cytomegalovirus among health care personnel at risk for blood exposure: final report from a longitudinal study," *Journal of Infectious Diseases*, vol. 170, no. 6, pp. 1410–1417, 1994.

[23] World Health Organization, "Global policy report on the prevention and control of viral hepatitis in WHO Member States," Tech. Rep., World Health Organization, Geneva, Switzerland, 2013.

[24] B. J. McMahon, W. L. M. Alward, D. B. Hall et al., "Acute hepatitis B virus infection: relation of age to the clinical

expression of disease and subsequent development of the carrier state," *Journal of Infectious Diseases*, vol. 151, no. 4, pp. 599–603, 1985.

[25] K. C. Hyams, "Risks of chronicity following acute hepatitis B virus infection: a review," *Clinical Infectious Diseases*, vol. 20, no. 4, pp. 992–1000, 1995.

[26] K. Ikeda, S. Saitoh, Y. Suzuki et al., "Disease progression and hepatocellular carcinogenesis in patients with chronic viral hepatitis: a prospective observation of 2215 patients," *Journal of Hepatology*, vol. 28, no. 6, pp. 930–938, 1998.

[27] R. P. Beasley and L. Y. Hwang, "Overview of the epidemiology of hepatocellular carcinoma," in *Viral Hepatitis and Liver Disease: Proceedings of the International Symposium on Viral Hepatitis and Liver Disease: Contemporary Issues and Future Prospects*, F. B. Hollinger, S. M. Lemon, and H. S. Margolis, Eds., pp. 532–535, Williams & Wilkins, Baltimore, Md, USA, 1991.

[28] J. F. Perz, G. L. Armstrong, L. A. Farrington, Y. J. F. Hutin, and B. P. Bell, "The contributions of hepatitis B virus and hepatitis C virus infections to cirrhosis and primary liver cancer world-wide," *Journal of Hepatology*, vol. 45, no. 4, pp. 529–538, 2006.

[29] *Hepatitis B Vaccine*, Hepatitis B Foundation, Doylestown, Pa, USA, 2009.

[30] S. S. Al Ghamdi, H. I. Fallatah, D. M. Fetyani, J. A. Al-Mughales, and A. T. Gelaidan, "Long-term efficacy of the hepatitis B Vaccine in a high-risk group," *Journal of Medical Virology*, vol. 85, no. 9, pp. 1518–1522, 2013.

17

Occult Hepatitis B: Clinical Viewpoint and Management

Mehdi Zobeiri

Internal Medicine Department, Imam Reza Hospital, Kermanshah University of Medical Sciences, Kermanshah, Iran

Correspondence should be addressed to Mehdi Zobeiri; mehdizobeiri@yahoo.com

Academic Editor: Yoichi Hiasa

Occult HBV infection (OBI) is defined as HBV DNA detection in serum or in the liver by sensitive diagnostic tests in HBsAg-negative patients with or without serologic markers of previous viral exposure. OBI seems to be higher among subjects at high risk for HBV infection and with liver disease. OBI can be both a source of virus contamination in blood and organ donations and the reservoir for full blown hepatitis after reactivation. HBV reactivation depends on viral and host factors but these associations have not been analyzed thoroughly. In OBI, it would be best to prevent HBV reactivation which inhibits the development of hepatitis and subsequent mortality. In diverse cases with insufficient data to recommend routine prophylaxis, early identification of virologic reactivation is essential to start antiviral therapy. For retrieving articles regarding OBI, various databases, including OVID, PubMed, Scopus, and ScienceDirect, were used.

1. Introduction

Hepatitis B virus (HBV) infection is a major global health problem with about 350–400 million chronically infected individuals [1]. HBV infection can induce a wide spectrum of clinical features, ranging from an inactive carrier state to fulminate hepatitis, cirrhosis, or hepatocellular carcinoma [2]. According to European Association for the Study of the Liver (EASL), about one-third of the world's populations have serological evidence of past or present HBV infection [3]. Many of these individuals may unknowingly carry the virus for several years after recovery from acute hepatitis B without showing any clinical or biochemical evidence of liver disease, and serological markers can identify different clinical states of viral persistence [4, 5]. HBV infection is usually diagnosed when circulating hepatitis B surface antigen (HBsAg) is detected. Chronic infection is characterized by persistence of this antigen and presence of HBV DNA in serum and resolved HBV infection when patients show seropositivity for –HBc and HBs antibodies.

Occult hepatitis B infection (OBI) is defined as the existence of low-level HBV DNA in the serum (<200 IU/mL), cells of the lymphatic (immune) system, and/or hepatic tissue in patients with serological markers of previous infection (anti-HBc and/or anti-HBs positive) and the absence of serum HBsAg. More than 20 percent of patients had no serologic markers because the antibody titer may become undetectable over time, leaving HBV DNA as the only marker of the infection. Thus depending on the HBV antibodies (anti-HBc and/or anti-HBs), OBI may be seropositive or seronegative [2, 3].

2. Diagnosis

The gold standard for diagnosis of OBI became possible by highly sensitive and specific molecular biology techniques like HBV nucleic acid amplification testing (NAT), a PCR technique with detection limits of <10 copies HBV DNA per reaction [3]. Samples for analysis include specimens from the liver and blood but diagnosis of OBI most commonly is based on the analysis of serum samples, because liver specimens are only available in a minority of cases and standardized assays for use in liver tissue are not yet available [3]. If highly sensitive HBV DNA testing is not feasible, anti-HBc should be used as a less than ideal surrogate marker for identifying potential seropositive OBI individuals in cases of blood, tissue, or organ donation, and when immune suppressive therapy has to be administered [6]. In this context, it has to be stressed that not all anti-HBc-positive individuals are found to be HBV DNA positive and that anti-HBc tests may provide false positive results [7].

OBI is more often detected in patients positive for anti-HBc but negative for anti-HBs, presumably because these patients lack the neutralizing effect of anti-HBs [8]. Most frequently, seropositive occult HBV infection follows resolution of acute hepatitis and continues indefinitely after clearance of HBsAg and biochemical improvement in liver function; it can also occur after years of chronic HBsAg-positive infection [9, 10]. OBI must be differentiated from S-escape mutants infection, in which undetectable HBsAg is present in spite of the episomal, free HBV genomes at intrahepatic level as in overt infection. These cases (so-called false occult HBV) result from HBV strains with key mutations in pre-S region which is not recognized by commercially available kits, even when the most sensitive ones are used [11].

False OBI has been reported in up to 40% of patients with OBI [3, 11–13]. In the HBsAg assays, the use of multivalent anti-HBs antibodies is recommended for detection of false OBI [3].

3. Pathogenesis of HBV Persistence

OBI is mostly due to the indefinitely intrahepatic persistence of the viral genome of wild-type HBV (without any mutations in the precore and core promoter regions) [14]. Strong suppression of viral replication and gene expression by antiviral cytotoxic T cells is responsible for the very low or undetectable levels of serum HBV DNA in OBI [15]. Conversion of viral genome to a covalently closed circular DNA (cccDNA), which is formed in the nuclei of infected hepatocytes within the first 24 h following virus inoculation and forming of a minichromosome after binding to proteins, is the molecular basis of persistence [11, 16].

The stability and long-term persistence of viral cccDNA molecules, together with the long half-life of hepatocytes, imply that HBV infection, once it has occurred, may possibly continue for life [17].

The cccDNA correlation with serum HBV DNA is poor, especially among HBeAg-negative individuals [18].

Clinical utility of intrahepatic cccDNA assay is very limited due to the invasiveness of liver biopsy but a more realistic approach is the quantitative measurement of serum HBsAg, which correlates well with intrahepatic cccDNA levels in both HBeAg-positive and -negative patients [18].

cccDNA is the main template for the transcription of viral mRNAs and has been shown to persist in hepatocytes even with successful cellular and humoral control of the infection indicated by HBsAg/anti-HBs seroconversion. With the impairment of host defense systems, cccDNA can evade host immunity and actively replicate again [19]. The majority of healthy individuals, positive for anti-HBc, which had been assumed to denote a past history of transient HBV infection, were latently infected with the episomal form of HBV accompanied by ongoing viral replication and few nucleotide mutations in the precore and core regions [20].

4. Clinical Impact of OBI

OBI is a complex entity that comprises many conditions and different situations [20]. OBI may be involved in several clinical contexts as follows: reactivation of the infection and consequent development of the HBV- related liver disease; transmission of the "occult" virus mainly through blood transfusion and orthotopic liver transplantation (OLT) with consequent hepatitis B in the recipient; the effect on occurrence and progression of the CLD; and the role in hepatocarcinogenesis [21].

In OBI, HBV reactivation can be induced by treatment of cancers and autoimmune diseases [22, 23]. Development of a classic hepatitis B that often has a severe clinical course is possible if suppression of viral replication discontinued as in several conditions including HIV infection, hematological malignancies, patients undergoing chemotherapy, transplantation (bone marrow, liver, or kidney), and treatment with potent immunosuppressive drugs like rituximab (anti-CD20), alemtuzumab (anti-CD52), or infliximab (antitumor necrosis factor) [20].

Different reports suggest that OBI could be responsible for the acceleration of chronic hepatitis C virus (HCV) progression and interfere with treatment response [24, 25].

OBI is found in up to 30% of serum samples and 50% of liver biopsies of patients with chronic hepatitis C and 20% and 30% in subjects with cryptogenic liver disease [26, 27].

OBI may favor or accelerate the progression toward cirrhosis, associated with the most severe forms of liver disease in HCV-infected patients. Preliminary evidence suggests a possible involvement in faster progression of posttransplant liver disease in HCV-positive patients with OBI in donor or recipient [28].

HCV has been suspected to strongly suppress HBV replication up to the point where it determines OBI development in coinfected individuals. However, more recent studies have brought into question the interplay between HCV and HBV and when the in vitro cotransfection experiments were conducted, no interference between the two viruses was noted [29].

OBI is the major cause of posttransfusion hepatitis B in western countries and in countries like India and Taiwan, with higher risk of transmission than for HCV or HIV [30–32].

Hepatitis B after OLT with OBI in donor is a well-known cause of de novo hepatitis in the HBV-negative recipient but appears to have very low rates of occurrence in cases of kidney, heart, and bone marrow transplantation as a consequence of the fact that hepatocyte is a reservoir of HBV cccDNA [11].

Anti-HBV prophylaxis (with hepatitis B immunoglobulin, lamivudine, or their combination) appears to be very effective in preventing de novo HBV hepatitis in the recipients but not to avoid HBV reinfection [33].

Recently, a meta-analysis showed an increased risk of HCC associated with OBI with an odds ratio of 2.9 (95% CI: 1.6–4.1) in retrospective and prospective studies [34]. It is generally believed that OBI maintains most of the pro-oncogenic properties and can contribute to hepatocellular transformation through the same direct and indirect mechanisms that subtend HCC development in overt HBV infection [21].

Aflatoxin B 1 has synergistic hepatocarcinogenesis with chronic HBV infection. Aflatoxin B 1 exposure is common in the area of high prevalence for chronic HBV infection. This effect increased the risk of HCC more than 8-fold compared to HBV infection alone [35]. OBI must be investigated in the following clinical situations: (1) solid organ, hematopoietic stem cell transplantation, and blood transfusion; (2) cryptogenic chronic hepatitis and hepatocellular carcinoma unrelated to HCV, atypical alcoholic hepatitis; (3) immunosuppresive therapy; (4) haemodialysis; (5) chronic hepatitis C especially those with flare in liver enzymes [36].

Consequently, it is important to detect high-risk groups for occult HBV infection [16, 37–39].

Clinicians must be aware of these clinical events and establish a standard strategy to prevent HBV reactivation [40].

5. Epidemiology

OBI was reported for the first time more than 30 years ago in the context of blood transfusion of anti-HBc-positive donor as the only marker of HBV infection [41]. No standardized assays evaluating the analysis of occult HBV on liver specimens [16]. Thus OBI prevalence is generally underestimated [21].

Prevalence in different areas and individuals categories, with lack of standardization of laboratory techniques and differences in selection criteria of subjects, does not allow meaningful comparisons [11].

However, OBI prevalence seems to be higher among subjects at high risk for HBV infection and with liver disease than among individuals at low risk of infection and without liver disease [42].

The prevalence of OBI is estimated to be 4–25% in anti-HBc-positive patients [43].

OBI is more prevalent in certain groups such as HCV and HIV populations. Many studies have found a higher OBI prevalence in subjects with than those without chronic liver disease. There is a wide variation in prevalence of OBI in different case series in patients with cryptogenic chronic hepatitis, HCC, and in HCV-or HIV-infected individuals [44].

This variability depends on the difference in endemicity of HBV infection, utilized assays in the studies, and studied populations in different parts of the world [11].

6. HBV Reactivation

Two decades ego, OBI and resolved or past hepatitis B were not recognized to be at risk of HBV reactivation when receiving conventional systemic chemotherapy [45]. But now patients with OBI represent an important group with a high risk for reactivation, especially in endemic areas in the same way as HBsAg-positive patients [46]. Definition of HBV reactivation among patients with OBI has been reported as the reappearance of HBsAg or HBV-DNA in the blood [47].

With resolved hepatitis, HBV reactivation usually begins later than 4 months [48].

Because of the low risk of HBV reactivation in patients with resolved infection with anti-HBs titer >10 IU/L, close followup of LFTs was thought to be sufficient in immunosuppressive treatment groups [49, 50]; although serial HBV-DNA monitoring is a reasonable strategy.

7. Risk Factor of HBV Reactivation

Certain host and viral factors are associated with the risk of HBV reactivation in patients with OBI. Host factors include intensity of immunosuppression especially with rituximab plus steroid and hematopoietic stem cell transplantation, and viral factors include absence of anti-HBs before chemotherapy, decrease in anti-HBs during chemotherapy, detectable HBV DNA in the serum, HBV genotype B, and mutations in the precore and core promoters [51, 52].

The degree of immunosuppression in the frequency and severity of HBV reactivation is highlighted by reports of severe reactivation following aggressive forms of chemotherapy or immune suppression like in lymphoma than in those with solid tumors [53].

This can be attributed to the fact that hematological disease itself induces a greater degree of immunosuppression or that chemotherapy is stronger in cases of hematological malignancies [54].

Several reports highlight the increasing incidence of reverse seroconversion in anti-HBs-positive patients after chemotherapy regiments containing anti-CD20 (rituximab) and or autologous hematopoietic stem cell transplantation for hematological malignances ++ with diverse outcomes [51, 55–58].

High percentage of subclinical reactivation of HBV in HBsAg negative after-solid organ transplant, without clinical hepatitis reported [59, 60].

The risk of occult HBV transmission from donors who are HBsAg-negative and anti- HBc-positive is very low after kidney, heart, or bone marrow but higher (17–90%) in orthotopic liver transplantation especially if the recipient is negative for all HBV serum markers [41, 61].

HBV-related hepatitis following solid organ transplantation from anti-HBc positive donors to healthy recipient usually has a benign course and is often less severe when compared to hepatitis B that develops as a result of HBV reactivation in anti-HBc positive recipient [40].

Persistence of the virus in the hepatocyte nuclei as cccDNA in those with serological evidence of resolved infection is considered mostly to be important risk factor in patients with HBV reactivation following systemic chemotherapy [3].

Quantification of HBV core-related antigen (HBcrAg) which has been reported to be correlated with the amount of cccDNA in the liver would be expected to represent a predictive marker for HBV reactivation [62].

Different non-A genotypes (especially B genotypes) and precore and core promoter mutations, which are prevalent in B and C genotypes of Asians, have been reported to be associated with the reactivation of HBV in the setting of systemic chemotherapy [63].

Reactivation of the patient's HBV infection differs according to the replication status prior to systemic chemotherapy as well as to the degree of immunosuppression. The risk of HBV reactivation in the HBsAg-negative patients was 2.7% versus 48% in HBsAg-positive patients [64].

According to recommendations neither patients with serological evidence of resolved HBV infection needed pre-chemotherapy assessment of viral load, nor any of them were candidates for preemptive nucleoside analogue treatment [49].

8. Preventive Measure

At least one-third of patients die from HBV reactivation despite treatment with lamivudine. It would probably be best to administer preventive treatment for HBV reactivation as this would inhibit the development of hepatitis and mortality with the aim of inhibiting the replication of HBV [65].

In OBI, exact risk of HBV reactivation depends on viral and host factors but associations with HBV reactivation have not been analyzed thoroughly [66].

Initiating antiviral treatment after hepatitis onset may be insufficient to control HBV reactivation and fulminant hepatitis and mortality following HBV reactivation is higher than acute hepatitis B [66].

Antiviral prophylaxis should be continued for ≥6 months after stopping chemotherapy and for certain immunosuppressive therapies, such as rituximab; it may be better to maintain the prophylaxis until restoration of host immunity [67]. There is insufficient evidence to recommend routine prophylaxis, but treatment is recommended for patients with risk factors and in other cases, followup and early treatment should be recommended in case of reactivation [65]. All patients who receive chemotherapy and immunotherapy should be tested for serologic markers of HBV infection, including HBsAg, anti-HBc, and anti-HBs before any chemotherapy or immunosuppressive therapy, and monitored for several months or years after stopping treatment because antibody titers may be reduced by the immunosuppressive therapy [40]. Antiviral drugs should be initiated to OBI, especially in the absence of anti-HBs which are potentially at greater risk for HBV reactivation prior to chemotherapy and continued for ≥6 months after stopping immunosuppressive treatment [68, 69]. The appearances of HBsAg and HBV DNA in up to 50% of anti-HBc positive patients undergoing bone marrow transplantation have been reported. The serial determination of anti-HBs in the serum of these bone marrow recipients has shown a steady decline to undetectable levels by 1–3 years after transplantation. Decreased titers of anti-HBs have been reported to be closely associated with HBV reactivation and with the loss of anti-HBs, HBV DNA increases and HBsAg reappears [70, 71]. Prophylaxis with antiviral agents prevents reactivation of OBI in most of transplant cases with HBsAg-negative and anti-HBc-positive donors and it is not known if prior hepatitis B immunization with an optimal anti-HBs response can modulate or abort the infection [40].

Current data are insufficient to recommend routine prophylaxis and antiviral therapy to prevent HBV reactivation for HBVDNA and HBsAg-negative but anti-HBc and/or anti-HBs positive patients, except in intense chemotherapy like rituximab. Thus early identification of virologic reactivation is essential to start antiviral therapy and prevent the occurrence of hepatitis B [19, 51, 65]. Serial HBV-DNA monitoring (monthly during and after chemotherapy for at least 1 year) is a reasonable strategy recommended by the latest Japanese guidelines; in this regard multicenter clinical trial in Japan is now continued [72]. With HBV-DNA NAT antiviral therapy begins when the result is >30 IU/mL and with a highly sensitive HBsAg assay (low limit of detection <0.1 ng/mL) antiviral therapy begin when the test becomes positive [20]. Although in blood transfusion the risk of transmission is insignificant when anti-HBs is present in the blood, caution is recommended when immunodeficient patients receive anti-HBc-positive and anti-HBs-positive donations [40]. The use of HBV-DNA NAT and multivalent anti-HBs antibodies in the HBsAg assays is recommended for detection of true and false OBI, respectively, and to minimize the risk of HBV transmission through transfusion [40]. This is important because almost 50% of transfused blood in Western Europe is given to immunodeficient patients [73].

9. Conclusions

For detection of OBI -HBV DNA nucleic acid testing should be implemented even if anti-HBc and anti-HBs were negative especially in endemic area and in suspected high-risk cases (populations at high risk of parenterally transmitted infections) with probable previous exposure before blood and organ donation, transplantation, and chemotherapy and in hemodialysis and cryptogenic chronic hepatitis. The use of multivalent anti-HBs antibodies in the HBsAg detection kits is strongly recommended. All patients receiving chemo- and immunotherapy should be tested at least once for anti-HBc antibodies before starting therapy and monitored periodically for ALT elevations. If ALT elevations occurred, the diagnosis of HBV reactivation must be established with further testing before initiation of antiviral prophylaxis. Optimal duration of prophylaxis in different risk populations should be clarified or even individualized in the future.

References

[1] D. Lavanchy, "Hepatitis B virus epidemiology, disease burden, treatment, arid current and emerging prevention and control measures," *Journal of Viral Hepatitis*, vol. 11, no. 2, pp. 97–107, 2004.

[2] M. Torbenson and D. L. Thomas, "Occult hepatitis B," *Lancet Infectious Diseases*, vol. 2, no. 8, pp. 479–486, 2002.

[3] G. Raimondo, J. P. Allain, M. R. Brunetto et al., "Statements from the Taormina expert meeting on occult hepatitis B virus infection," *Journal of Hepatology*, vol. 49, no. 4, pp. 652–657, 2008.

[4] H. Yotsuyanagi, K. Yasuda, S. Iino et al., "Persistent viremia after recovery from self-limited acute hepatitis B," *Hepatology*, vol. 27, no. 5, pp. 1377–1382, 1998.

[5] S. Urbani, F. Fagnoni, G. Missale, and M. Franchini, "The role of anti-core antibody response in the detection of occult hepatitis B virus infection," *Clinical Chemistry and Laboratory Medicine*, vol. 48, no. 1, pp. 23–29, 2010.

[6] W. H. Gerlich, D. Glebe, and C. G. Schüttler, "Deficiencies in the standardization and sensitivity of diagnostic tests for hepatitis B virus," *Journal of Viral Hepatitis*, vol. 14, no. 1, pp. 16–21, 2007.

[7] L. Comanor and P. Holland, "Hepatitis B virus blood screening: unfinished agendas," *Vox Sanguinis*, vol. 91, no. 1, pp. 1–12, 2006.

[8] C. Bréchot, V. Thiers, D. Kremsdorf, B. Nalpas, S. Pol, and P. Paterlini-Bréchot, "Persistent hepatitis B virus infection in subjects without hepatitis B surface antigen: clinically significant or purely "occult"?" *Hepatology*, vol. 34, no. 1, pp. 194–203, 2001.

[9] P. M. Mulrooney-Cousins and T. I. Michalak, "Persistent occult hepatitis B virus infection: experimental findings and clinical implications," *World Journal of Gastroenterology*, vol. 13, no. 43, pp. 5682–5686, 2007.

[10] T. I. Huo, J. C. Wu, P. C. Lee et al., "Sero-clearance of hepatitis B surface antigen in chronic carriers does not necessarily imply a good prognosis," *Hepatology*, vol. 28, no. 1, pp. 231–236, 1998.

[11] G. Raimondo, T. Pollicino, I. Cacciola, and G. Squadrito, "Occult hepatitis B virus infection," *Journal of Hepatology*, vol. 46, no. 1, pp. 160–170, 2007.

[12] D. Jeantet, I. Chemin, B. Mandrand et al., "Cloning and expression of surface antigens from occult chronic hepatitis B virus infections and their recognition by commercial detection assays," *Journal of Medical Virology*, vol. 73, no. 4, pp. 508–515, 2004.

[13] S. H. Ahn, Y. N. Park, J. Y. Park et al., "Long-term clinical and histological outcomes in patients with spontaneous hepatitis B surface antigen seroclearance," *Journal of Hepatology*, vol. 42, no. 2, pp. 188–194, 2005.

[14] R. A. De la Fuente, M. L. Gutiérrez, J. Garcia-Samaniego, C. Fernández-Rodriguez, J. L. Lledó, and G. Castellano, "Pathogenesis of occult chronic hepatitis B virus infection," *World Journal of Gastroenterology*, vol. 17, no. 12, pp. 1543–1548, 2011.

[15] M. Bes, V. Vargas, M. Piron et al., "T cell responses and viral variability in blood donation candidates with occult hepatitis B infection," *Journal of Hepatology*, vol. 56, pp. 765–774, 2012.

[16] S. Ocana, M. L. Casas, I. Buhigas, and J. L. Lledo, "Diagnostic strategy for occult hepatitis B virus infection," *World Journal of Gastroenterology*, vol. 17, no. 12, pp. 1553–1557, 2011.

[17] F. Zoulim, "New insight on hepatitis B virus persistence from the study of intrahepatic viral cccDNA," *Journal of Hepatology*, vol. 42, no. 3, pp. 302–308, 2005.

[18] M. Levrero, T. Pollicino, J. Petersen, L. Belloni, G. Raimondo, and M. Dandri, "Control of cccDNA function in hepatitis B virus infection," *Journal of Hepatology*, vol. 51, no. 3, pp. 581–592, 2009.

[19] C. J. Liu, P. J. Chen, D. S. Chen, and J. H. Kao, "Hepatitis B virus reactivation in patients receiving cancer chemotherapy: natural history, pathogenesis, and management," *Hepatology International*, 2011.

[20] J. L. Lledó, C. Fernández, M. L. Gutiérrez, and S. Ocaña, "Management of occult hepatitis B virus infection: an update for the clinician," *World Journal of Gastroenterology*, vol. 17, no. 12, pp. 1563–1568, 2011.

[21] G. Raimondo, G. Caccamo, R. Filomia, and T. Pollicino, "Occult HBV infection," *Seminars in Immunopathology*, vol. 35, no. 1, pp. 39–52, 2013.

[22] Y. Ide, Y. Ito, S. Takahashi et al., "Hepatitis B virus reactivation in adjuvant chemotherapy for breast cancer," *Breast Cancer*, 2010.

[23] T. Matsumoto, H. Marusawa, M. Dogaki, Y. Suginoshita, and T. Inokuma, "Adalimumab-induced lethal hepatitis B virus reactivation in an HBsAg-negative patient with clinically resolved hepatitis B virus infection," *Liver International*, vol. 30, no. 8, pp. 1241–1242, 2010.

[24] M. Levast, S. Larrat, M. A. Thelu et al., "Prevalence and impact of occult hepatitis B infection in chronic hepatitis C patients treated with pegylated interferon and ribavirin," *Journal of Medical Virology*, vol. 82, no. 5, pp. 747–754, 2010.

[25] N. J. Shire, S. D. Rouster, S. D. Stanford et al., "The prevalence and significance of occult hepatitis B virus in a prospective cohort of HIV-infected patients," *Journal of Acquired Immune Deficiency Syndromes*, vol. 44, no. 3, pp. 309–314, 2007.

[26] A. S. F. Lok and B. J. McMahon, "Chronic hepatitis B," *Hepatology*, vol. 45, no. 2, pp. 507–539, 2007.

[27] D. K. Wong, F. Y. Huang, C. L. Lai et al., "Occult hepatitis B infection and HBV repli-cative activity in patients with cryptogenic cause of hepatocellular carcinoma," *Hepatology*, vol. 54, pp. 829–836, 2011.

[28] P. Toniutto, R. Minisini, C. Fabris et al., "Occult hepatitis B virus infection in liver transplant recipients with recurrent hepatitis C: relationship with donor age and fibrosis progression," *Clinical Transplantation*, vol. 23, no. 2, pp. 184–190, 2009.

[29] P. Bellecave, J. Gouttenoire, M. Gajer et al., "Hepatitis B and C virus coinfection: a novel model system reveals the absence of direct viral interference," *Hepatology*, vol. 50, no. 1, pp. 46–55, 2009.

[30] F. A. M. Regan, P. Hewitt, J. A. J. Barbara, and M. Contreras, "Prospective investigation of transfusion transmitted infection in recipients of over 20,000 units of blood," *British Medical Journal*, vol. 320, no. 7232, pp. 403–406, 2000.

[31] J. P. Allain, "Occult hepatitis B virus infection: implications in transfusion," *Vox Sanguinis*, vol. 86, no. 2, pp. 83–91, 2004.

[32] C. J. Liu, S. C. Lo, J. H. Kao et al., "Transmission of occult hepatitis B virus by transfusion to adult and pediatric recipients in Taiwan," *Journal of Hepatology*, vol. 44, no. 1, pp. 39–46, 2006.

[33] E. Cholongitas, G. V. Papatheodoridis, and A. K. Burroughs, "Liver grafts from anti-hepatitis B core positive donors: a systematic review," *Journal of Hepatology*, vol. 52, no. 2, pp. 272–279, 2010.

[34] Y. Shi, Y. H. Wu, W. Wu et al., "Association between occult hepatitis B infection and the risk of hepatocellular carcinoma: a meta-analysis," *Liver International*, vol. 32, pp. 231–240, 2012.

[35] H. B. El-Serag, "Epidemiology of viral hepatitis and hepatocellular carcinoma," *Gastroenterology*, vol. 142, pp. 1264–1273, 2012.

[36] H. S. Selim, H. A. Abou-Donia, H. A. Taha, G. I. El Azab, and A. F. Bakry, "Role of occult hepatitis B virus in chronic hepatitis C patients with flare of liver enzymes," *European Journal of Internal Medicine*, vol. 22, no. 2, pp. 187–190, 2011.

[37] J. R. Larrubia, "Occult hepatitis B virus infection: a complex entity with relevant clinical implications," *World Journal of Gastroenterology*, vol. 17, no. 12, pp. 1529–1530, 2011.

[38] K. Shetty, M. Hussain, L. Nei, K. R. Reddy, and A. S. F. Lok, "Prevalence and significance of occult hepatitis B in a liver transplant population with chronic hepatitis C," *Liver Transplantation*, vol. 14, no. 4, pp. 534–540, 2008.

[39] O. Ceneli, Z. N. Ozkurt, K. Acar et al., "Hepatitis B-related events in autologous hematopoietic stem cell transplantation recipients," *World Journal of Gastroenterology*, vol. 16, pp. 1765–1771, 2010.

[40] J. -R. Larrubia, J. L. Lledó, C. Fernández, M. L. Gutiérrez, and S. Ocaña, "Management of occult hepatitis B virus infection: an update for the clinician," *World Journal of Gastroenterology*, vol. 17, no. 12, pp. 1563–1568, 2011.

[41] E. Tabor, J. H. Hoofnagle, and L. A. Smallwood, "Studies of donors who transmit posttransfusion hepatitis," *Transfusion*, vol. 19, no. 6, pp. 725–731, 1979.

[42] G. Raimondo, G. Navarra, S. Mondello et al., "Occult hepatitis B virus in liver tissue of individuals without hepatic disease," *Journal of Hepatology*, vol. 48, no. 5, pp. 743–746, 2008.

[43] C. J. Liu, D. S. Chen, and P. J. Chen, "Epidemiology of HBV infection in Asian blood donors: emphasis on occult HBV infection and the role of NAT," *Journal of Clinical Virology*, vol. 36, no. 1, pp. S33–S44, 2006.

[44] L. Covolo, T. Pollicino, G. Raimondo, and F. Donato, "Occult hepatitis B virus and the risk for chronic liver disease: a meta-analysis," *Dog Liver Disease*, vol. 45, no. 3, pp. 238–244, 2013.

[45] A. S. F. Lok, R. H. S. Liang, E. K. W. Chiu, K. L. Wong, T. K. Chan, and D. Todd, "Reactivation of hepatitis B virus replication in patients receiving cytotoxic therapy: report of a prospective study," *Gastroenterology*, vol. 100, no. 1, pp. 182–188, 1991.

[46] S. P. Georgiadou, K. Zachou, E. Rigopoulou et al., "Occult hepatitis B virus infection in Greek patients with chronic hepatitis C and in patients with diverse nonviral hepatic diseases," *Journal of Viral Hepatitis*, vol. 11, no. 4, pp. 358–365, 2004.

[47] C. K. Hui, W. W. W. Cheung, H. Y. Zhang et al., "Kinetics and risk of de novo hepatitis B infection in HBsAg-negative patients undergoing cytotoxic chemotherapy," *Gastroenterology*, vol. 131, no. 1, pp. 59–68, 2006.

[48] G. Lalazar, D. Rund, and D. Shouval, "Screening, prevention and treatment of viral hepatitis B reactivation in patients with haematological malignancies," *British Journal of Haematology*, vol. 136, no. 5, pp. 699–712, 2007.

[49] Y. F. Liaw, N. Leung, J. H. Kao et al., "Asian-Pacific consensus statement on the management of chronic hepatitis B: a 2008 update," *Hepatology International*, vol. 2, pp. 263–283, 2008.

[50] European Association for the Study of the Liver, "EASL Clinical Practice Guidelines: management of chronic hepatitis B," *Journal of Hepatology*, vol. 50, no. 2, pp. 227–242, 2009.

[51] S. Kusumoto, Y. Tanaka, R. Ueda, and M. Mizokami, "Reactivation of hepatitis B virus following rituximab-plus-steroid combination chemotherapy," *Journal of Gastroenterology*, vol. 46, no. 1, pp. 9–16, 2011.

[52] T. Umemura, E. Tanaka, K. Kiyosawa et al., "Mortality secondary to fulminant hepatic failure in patients with prior resolution of hepatitis B virus infection in Japan," *Clinical Infectious Diseases*, vol. 47, no. 5, pp. e52–e56, 2008.

[53] J. H. Hoofnagle, "Reactivation of hepatitis B," *Hepatology*, vol. 49, supplement 5, pp. S156–S165, 2009.

[54] W. Yeo, P. K. Chan, S. Zhong et al., "Frequency of hepatitis B virus reactivation in cancer patients undergoing cytotoxic chemotherapy: a prospective study of 626 patients with identification of risk factors," *Journal of Medical Virology*, vol. 62, pp. 299–307, 2000.

[55] P. Papamichalis, A. Alexiou, M. Boulbou, G. N. Dalekos, and E. I. Rigopoulou, "Reactivation of resolved hepatitis B virus infection after immunosuppression: is it time to adopt preemptive therapy?" *Clinics and Research in Hepatology and Gastroenterology*, vol. 36, no. 1, pp. 84–93, 2012.

[56] M. Watanabe, A. Shibuya, Y. Tsunoda et al., "Re-appearance of hepatitis B virus following therapy with rituximab for lymphoma is not rare in Japanese patients with past hepatitis B virus infection," *Liver International*, vol. 31, no. 3, pp. 340–347, 2011.

[57] J. E. Uhm, K. Kim, T. K. Lim et al., "Changes in serologic markers of hepatitis B following autologous hematopoietic stem cell transplantation," *Biology of Blood and Marrow Transplantation*, vol. 13, no. 4, pp. 463–468, 2007.

[58] T. Sera, Y. Hiasa, K. Michitaka et al., "Anti-HBs-positive liver failure due to hepatitis B virus reactivation induced by Rituximab," *Internal Medicine*, vol. 45, no. 11, pp. 721–724, 2006.

[59] A. Knöll, M. Pietrzyk, M. Loss, W. A. Goetz, and W. Jilg, "Solid-organ transplantation in HBsAg-negative patients with antibodies to HBV core antigen: Low risk of HBV reactivation," *Transplantation*, vol. 79, no. 11, pp. 1631–1633, 2005.

[60] M. F. Abdelmalek, T. M. Pasha, N. N. Zein, D. H. Persing, R. H. Wiesner, and D. D. Douglas, "Subclinical reactivation of hepatitis B virus in liver transplant recipients with past exposure," *Liver Transplantation*, vol. 9, no. 12, pp. 1253–1257, 2003.

[61] R. A. de la Fuente, M. L. Gutiérrez, J. Garcia-Samaniego, C. Fernández-Rodriguez, J. L. Lledó, and G. Castellano, "Pathogenesis of occult chronic hepatitis B virus infection," *World Journal of Gastroenterology*, vol. 17, no. 12, pp. 1543–1548, 2011.

[62] N. Shinkai, Y. Tanaka, E. Orito et al., "Measurement of hepatitis B virus core-related antigen as predicting factor for relapse after cessation of lamivudine therapy for chronic hepatitis B virus infection," *Hepatology Research*, vol. 36, no. 4, pp. 272–276, 2006.

[63] P. Borentain, P. Colson, D. Coso et al., "Clinical and virological factors associated with hepatitis B virus reactivation in HBsAg-negative and anti-HBc antibodies-positive patients undergoing chemotherapy and/or autologous stem cell transplantation for cancer," *Journal of Viral Hepatitis*, vol. 17, no. 11, pp. 807–815, 2010.

[64] R. Loomba, A. Rowley, R. Wesley et al., "Systematic review: the effect of preventive lamivudine on hepatitis B reactivation during chemotherapy," *Annals of Internal Medicine*, vol. 148, no. 7, pp. 519–528, 2008.

[65] M. L. Manzano-Alonso and G. Castellano-Tortajada, "Reactivation of hepatitis B virus infection after cytotoxic chemotherapy or immunosuppressive therapy," *World Journal of Gastroenterology*, vol. 17, no. 12, pp. 1531–1537, 2011.

[66] W. Yeo, P. K. S. Chan, W. M. Ho et al., "Lamivudine for the prevention of hepatitis B virus reactivation in hepatitis B s-antigen seropositive cancer patients undergoing cytotoxic chemotherapy," *Journal of Clinical Oncology*, vol. 22, no. 5, pp. 927–934, 2004.

[67] W. Yeo and P. J. Johnson, "Diagnosis, prevention and management of hepatitis B virus reactivation during anticancer therapy," *Hepatology*, vol. 43, no. 2, pp. 209–220, 2006.

[68] F. B. Hollinger and G. Sood, "Occult hepatitis B virus infection: a covert operation," *Journal of Viral Hepatitis*, vol. 17, no. 1, pp. 1–15, 2010.

[69] A. S. F. Lok and B. J. McMahon, "Chronic hepatitis B: update 2009," *Hepatology*, vol. 50, no. 3, pp. 661–662, 2009.

[70] M. L. Manzano-Alonso and G. Castellano-Tortajada, "Reactivation of hepatitis B virus infection after cytotoxic chemotherapy or immunosuppressive therapy," *World Journal of Gastroenterology*, vol. 17, no. 12, pp. 1531–1537, 2011.

[71] E. B. Kim, D. S. Kim, S. J. Park, Y. Park, K. H. Rho, and S. J. Kim, "Hepatitis B virus reactivation in a surface antigen-negative and antibodypositive patient after rituximab plus

CHOP chemotherapy," *Cancer Research and Treatment*, vol. 40, pp. 36–38, 2008.

[72] H. Tsubouchi, H. Kumada, K. Kiyosawa et al., "Prevention of immunosuppressive therapy or chemotherapy-induced reactivation of hepatitis B virus infection—Joint report of the Intractable Liver Diseases Study Group of Japan and the Japanese Study Group of the Standard Antiviral Therapy for Viral Hepatitis," *Acta Hepatologica Japonica*, vol. 50, no. 1, pp. 38–42, 2009.

[73] D. Candotti and J. P. Allain, "Transfusion-transmitted hepatitis B virus infection," *Journal of Hepatology*, vol. 51, no. 4, pp. 798–809, 2009.

18

Involvement of Differential Relationship between HCV Replication and Hepatic PRR Signaling Gene Expression in Responsiveness to IFN-Based Therapy

Nobukazu Yuki,[1] Shinji Matsumoto,[2] Michio Kato,[3] and Toshikazu Yamaguchi[2]

[1] Department of Gastroenterology, Osaka National Hospital, Hoenzaka 2-1-14, Chuo-ku, Osaka 540-0006, Japan
[2] BML, Inc., Kawagoe 350-1101, Japan
[3] Department of Gastroenterology, Minamiwakayama National Hospital, Tanabe 646-8558, Japan

Correspondence should be addressed to Nobukazu Yuki; yuki@onh.go.jp

Academic Editor: Man-Fung Yuen

Aim. To gain an insight into the effect of HCV replication-associated interference with the IFN system on hepatic mRNA expression involved in IFN production. *Methods.* Relative mRNA expression of TLR3/RIG-I signaling genes involved in IFN-β production was correlated with positive- and negative-strand HCV RNAs in pretreatment liver tissues responsive and nonresponsive to peginterferon and ribavirin for chronic hepatitis C genotype 1. Treatment response was analyzed for per protocol population at weeks 12 ($n = 45$) and 24 ($n = 40$) and at 24 weeks aftertreatment ($n = 38$). *Results.* HCV replication had no relation to the expression of TLR3, RIG-I, TRIF, IPS-1, IRF3, and IFN-β mRNAs in responders. In striking contrast, positive- and/or negative-strand HCV showed positive correlations with TLR3, RIG-I, TRIF, IPS-1, and IRF3 mRNAs in week-12 nonresponders; with RIG-I, TRIF, IPS-1, and IRF3 mRNAs in week-24 nonresponders; and with TLR3, RIG-I, and IRF3 mRNAs in posttreatment nonresponders. Thus mRNA expression of TLR3/RIG-I signaling genes was increased in relation to viral replication in nonresponders. *Conclusions.* The findings in IFN nonresponders may imply a host feedback response to severe impairment of the IFN system associated with HCV replication.

1. Introduction

Upon recognition of hepatitis C virus (HCV) infection by Toll-like receptor 3 (TLR3) and retinoic-acid inducible gene I (RIG-I), the innate immune response is promptly activated in hepatocytes. The two pattern recognition receptors (PRRs) recruit their respective adaptors, Toll/interleukin-1 receptor-domain containing adaptor inducing interferon (IFN)-β (TRIF) and IFN-β promoter stimulator-1 (IPS-1), that relay the signal to downstream IFN regulatory factor-3 (IRF3), leading to the induction of IFN-β, known as the "front line" of host antiviral defenses in the liver [1, 2].

HCV has evolved highly successful multiple mechanisms for counteracting host antiviral responses. HCV NS3/4A serine protease in infected cells cleaves TRIF and IPS-1 and thereby disrupts the signal for IFN-β induction [3–5]. HCV interferes with various aspects of the downstream IFN action [6]. For example, HCV disrupts JAK-Stat signaling by NS5A

and inhibits protein kinase R by NS5A and E2 proteins. Recent studies demonstrated that interference of HCV proteins with IFN production and its action depends on the levels of HCV propagation [7, 8].

Under the circumstances, we hypothesized that HCV replication-associated interference with the host IFN system may cause changes in hepatic gene expression involved in IFN production at the mRNA levels and that, if so, this host feedback response may occur in different fashion according to responsiveness to IFN-based therapy as interference with the host IFN system is considered to be more severe in nonresponders. To gain an insight into this hypothesis, we measured hepatic mRNA expression involved in IFN-β production, and the results were correlated with copy numbers of liver positive- and negative-strand HCV RNAs using pretreatment liver tissues responsive to IFN-based treatment and liver tissues that were nonresponsive to the treatment.

TABLE 1: Patient characteristics regarding virologic response to PEG-IFN and ribavirin.

Characteristics	Response at week 12		Response at week 24		Posttreatment response	
	Yes	No	Yes	No	Yes	No
No.	14	31	26	14	22	16
Sex, M/F (% men)	10/4 (71)	19/12 (61)	17/9 (65)	9/5 (64)	16/6 (73)	9/7 (56)
Age	52 ± 11	59 ± 10	55 ± 11	59 ± 10	52 ± 10[a]	61 ± 8
Previous IFN therapy, n (%)	3 (21)	15 (48)	7 (27)	7 (50)	5 (23)[a]	9 (56)
ALT (IU/L)	85 ± 63	77 ± 41	83 ± 55	68 ± 31	89 ± 57	60 ± 29
Serum HCV RNA (log IU/mL)	6.1 ± 0.6	6.2 ± 0.4	6.2 ± 0.5	6.2 ± 0.3	6.2 ± 0.5	6.2 ± 0.3
Liver inflammatory score	7.0 ± 2.1	7.0 ± 2.5	7.0 ± 2.1	6.7 ± 2.9	7.1 ± 2.3	6.6 ± 2.7
Liver fibrosis score	1.7 ± 1.2	2.2 ± 1.1	1.9 ± 1.2	2.2 ± 1.1	1.8 ± 1.2	2.4 ± 1.0

Variables are presented as mean ± SD.
[a]Statistically significant difference $P < 0.05$ between responders and nonresponders.

2. Patients and Methods

2.1. Liver Tissues Responsive and Nonresponsive to IFN-Based Treatment. Liver tissues were obtained from 45 patients with chronic hepatitis C genotype 1 before 48-week treatment with weight-based doses of PEG-IFN-α 2b (PEG-Intron; MSD K.K., Tokyo, Japan) and ribavirin (Rebetol; MSD K.K.) [9]. A portion of the liver biopsy specimen was immediately frozen and stored at $-80°C$ for real-time PCR. Slow virologic responders showing HCV RNA clearance after week 12 were assigned to 72-week extended treatment. Treatment response was analyzed for per protocol population at week 12 ($n = 45$), week 24 ($n = 40$), and 24 weeks aftertreatment ($n = 38$). Table 1 summarizes the study cohort regarding achievement of complete early virologic response (cEVR) (serum HCV RNA clearance at week 12), virologic response at week 24 (VR24) (HCV RNA clearance at week 24), and sustained virologic response (SVR) (HCV RNA clearance at 24 weeks aftertreatment). The SVR group was younger and tended to be more treatment-naïve than the non-SVR group. Otherwise, no difference was seen in gender, serum alanine aminotransferase (ALT), serum HCV RNA, and liver histology. The study was approved by the local research ethics committee in accordance with the 1975 Declaration of Helsinki, and all patients provided written informed consent.

2.2. Hepatic mRNA Quantitation. Relative mRNA expression of TLR3, RIG-I, TRIF, IPS-1, IRF3, and IFN-β was determined by real-time PCR [9]. Total hepatic RNA was extracted using the TRIzol Reagent (Invitrogen, Carlsbad, CA). One μg of RNA was denatured at 65°C for 5 min and reverse transcribed in a 20 μL reaction mixture containing 4 μL of 5× reverse-transcription (RT) buffer (Invitrogen), 0.2 μmol of DTT, 100 U of Superscript II (Invitrogen), 20 U of RNasin (Promega, Madison, WI), 10 nmol of each dNTP, and 100 pmol of random hexamers. The RT reaction was performed for 10 min at 25°C, 120 min at 42°C, and then 15 min at 70°C. Primers and probes for target and reference genes studied were purchased from Applied Biosystems (Foster City, CA) (TaqMan Gene Expression Assays Hs00152933_m1 [TLR3], Hs00184937_m1 [RIG-I], Hs00706140_s1 [TRIF], Hs00325038_m1 [IPS-1], Hs00155574_m1 [IRF3],

Hs0027188_s1 [IFN-β], and 4310884E [GAPDH]). The cDNA product was diluted 1 : 2.5, and 5 μL was amplified in a 20 μL reaction mixture containing 10 μL of 2× TaqMan Universal PCR Master Mix and 1 μL of 20× gene-specific primers and probe mixture (Applied Biosystems). PCR cycling was performed as follows: 50°C for 2 min, 95°C for 10 min, followed by 40 cycles of 95°C for 15 s and 60°C for 1 min, in an ABI PRISM 7900 Sequence Detection System (Applied Biosystems). Duplicate cycle threshold (Ct) values were analyzed by using the comparative Ct ($\Delta\Delta$Ct) method. The relative amount of target mRNA ($2^{-\Delta\Delta Ct}$) was obtained by normalization to an endogenous GAPDH reference and expressed relative to the amount from normal liver tissue derived from an HCV-uninfected individual who had received hepatectomy for a metastatic liver tumor.

2.3. Virologic and Histologic Evaluation. HCV replication was evaluated by serum HCV RNA levels (COBAS AMPLICOR HCV MONITOR Test v.2.0, Roche Diagnostics K.K., Tokyo, Japan) and copy numbers of liver positive- and negative-strand HCV RNAs as measured by strand-specific real-time PCR [10]. Liver histology was assessed using the Knodell score [11].

2.4. Statistical Analysis. Data on continuous variables were presented as mean ± SD. An arbitrary value of 0 was attributed to the liver tissues negative by PCR to detect host mRNAs and viral RNAs. The range of serum HCV RNA quantitation was from 3.7 to 6.7 log IU/mL. For statistics, an arbitrary value of 7 log IU/mL was attributed to HCV RNA levels of >6.7 log IU/mL. Group comparisons were performed by nonparametric tests (Wilcoxon and Mann-Whitney) for continuous variables and by Fisher's exact test for binary variables. Spearman rank order correlations were used to study the relationship between the variables. A value of $P < 0.05$ (two-tailed) was considered to indicate significance.

3. Results

The relationship of hepatic PRR signaling gene expression with hepatic and circulating HCV loads was analyzed regarding responsiveness to PEG-IFN and ribavirin. In liver tissues

TABLE 2: Correlations between HCV replication (liver positive- and negative-strand HCV RNAs and circulating HCV RNA) and hepatic PRR signaling gene expression regarding virologic response at week 24.

Hepatic gene expression		Responders at week 24 ($n = 26$)			Nonresponders at week 24 ($n = 14$)		
		Liver HCV RNA		Serum HCV RNA	Liver HCV RNA		Serum HCV RNA
		+Strand	−Strand		+Strand	−Strand	
TLR3 mRNA	r	0.149	0.173	0.100	0.407	0.442	0.066
	P	0.469	0.398	0.626	0.149	0.114	0.823
RIG-I mRNA	r	0.217	0.324	−0.070	**0.797**	**0.744**	0.513
	P	0.288	0.107	0.735	**<0.001**	**0.002**	0.060
TRIF mRNA	r	0.014	0.091	−0.254	**0.659**	**0.620**	0.280
	P	0.946	0.659	0.211	**0.010**	**0.018**	0.333
IPS-1 mRNA	r	0.012	0.100	−0.217	**0.563**	**0.538**	0.209
	P	0.952	0.627	0.288	**0.036**	**0.047**	0.473
IRF3 mRNA	r	0.023	−0.005	−0.312	**0.647**	0.521	0.189
	P	0.911	0.981	0.121	**0.012**	0.056	0.517
IFN-β mRNA	r	−0.154	−0.222	−0.174	0.433	0.411	−0.022
	P	0.453	0.275	0.394	0.122	0.144	0.940

showing cEVR, none of the mRNA expressions studied (TLR3, RIG-I, TRIF, IPS-1, IRF3, and IFN-β) showed a relationship with liver positive- and negative-strand HCV RNAs and circulating HCV RNA (see Supplementary Figure 1 in Supplementary Material available online at http://dx.doi.org/10.1155/2013/917261). In contrast, mRNA expression of the PRR signaling genes involved in IFN-β production was uniformly increased in parallel with HCV loads in liver tissues nonresponsive at week 12. Liver positive- and/or negative-strand HCV RNA(s) showed positive correlations with the mRNA levels of TLR3 ($r = 0.396$, $P = 0.028$ and $r = 0.303$, $P = 0.097$), RIG-I ($r = 0.595$, $P < 0.001$ and $r = 0.682$, $P < 0.001$), TRIF ($r = 0.256$, $P = 0.165$ and $r = 0.414$, $P = 0.021$), IPS-1 ($r = 0.304$, $P = 0.096$ and $r = 0.358$, $P = 0.048$), and IRF3 ($r = 0.397$, $P = 0.027$ and $r = 0.384$, $P = 0.033$, resp.). However, the correlations of IFN-β mRNA with positive- and negative-strand HCV RNAs did not reach a significant level ($r = 0.309$, $P = 0.090$ and $r = 0.275$, $P = 0.134$, resp.). Unexpectedly, these figures in nonresponders were not seen when HCV propagation was assessed by circulating HCV loads. No relationship was found between serum HCV RNA levels and any mRNA expression in liver tissues (Figure 1). Supplementary Figure 2 represents the interrelationship of liver positive- and negative-strand HCV RNAs and serum HCV RNA in the study cohort. Liver positive- and negative-strand HCV RNAs were closely correlated ($r = 0.801$, $P < 0.001$), whereas there were significant but weak correlations between serum HCV RNA and liver positive- and negative-strand HCV RNAs ($r = 0.474$, $P = 0.001$ and $r = 0.476$, $P = 0.001$, resp.).

The relationship between hepatic gene expression and HCV loads was further investigated with regard to treatment responsiveness at later time points. Like liver tissues showing cEVR, none of the mRNA expression levels showed a relationship with hepatic HCV loads when liver tissues showing VR24 and SVR were analyzed. On the other hand, the expression of a certain set of the PRR signaling genes, albeit not all, showed significant correlations with hepatic HCV loads in nonresponders. Positive- and/or negative-strand HCV RNA(s) were positively correlated with mRNA expression of RIG-I ($r = 0.797$, $P < 0.001$ and $r = 0.744$, $P = 0.002$), TRIF ($r = 0.659$, $P = 0.010$ and $r = 0.620$, $P = 0.018$), IPS-1 ($r = 0.563$, $P = 0.036$ and $r = 0.538$, $P = 0.047$), and IRF3 ($r = 0.647$, $P = 0.012$ and $r = 0.521$, $P = 0.056$, resp.) in liver tissues nonresponsive at week 24 (Table 2). When liver tissues not attaining SVR were analyzed, positive- and/or negative-strand HCV RNA(s) were positively correlated with mRNA expression of TLR3 ($r = 0.632$, $P = 0.009$ and $r = 0.632$, $P = 0.009$), RIG-I ($r = 0.760$, $P < 0.001$ and $r = 0.693$, $P = 0.003$), and IRF3 ($r = 0.545$, $P = 0.029$ and $r = 0.426$, $P = 0.099$, resp.) (Table 3). Again, the relationship of circulating HCV RNA with hepatic mRNA expression was not evident, regardless of treatment responsiveness. A significant relationship was seen only between serum HCV RNA and RIG-I mRNA expression in liver tissues without SVR ($r = 0.511$, $P = 0.043$).

4. Discussion

Previous studies showed that HCV proteins produced in infected cells impair the PRR signaling involved in IFN-β production via cleavage of TRIF and IPS-1 [3–5] and further impair downstream IFN action in various ways [6]. It has also been demonstrated that impairment of the host antiviral response by HCV depends on HCV propagation. The cleavage of IPS-1 by HCV NS3/4A serine protease is more extensive in the liver with high levels of HCV propagation [7, 8]. Hepatic mRNA expression of downstream IFN-stimulated genes (ISGs) is negatively correlated with hepatic HCV loads, indicating HCV replication-related impairment of antiviral signaling involved in ISG expression [8]. How hepatic HCV propagation is related to the expression of various PRR signaling genes involved in IFN-β production has not been fully clarified.

Of the PRR signaling genes, some are known ISGs (TLR3, and RIG-I), while others (TRIF, IPS-1 and IRF3) are not. We

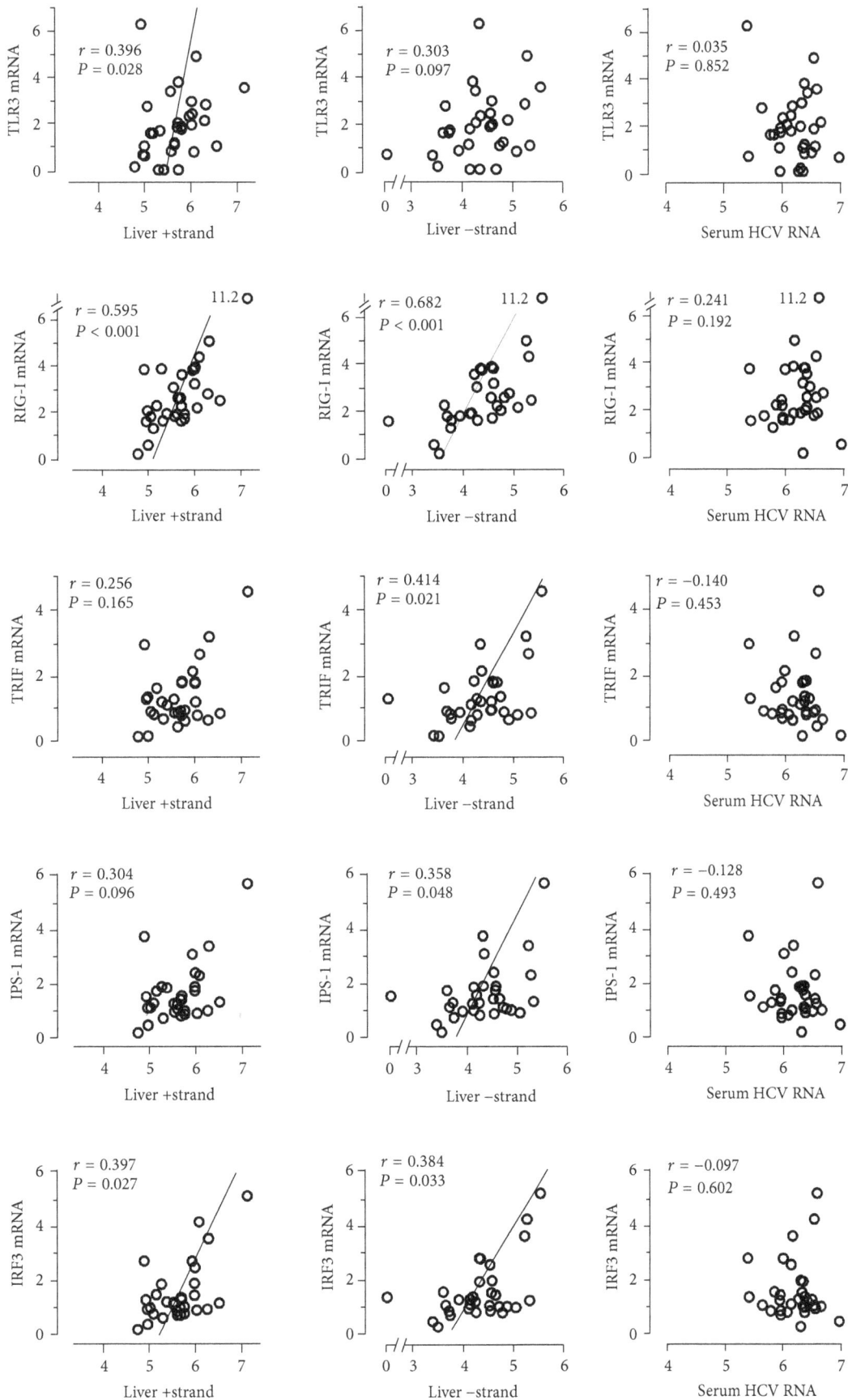

(a)

FIGURE 1: Continued.

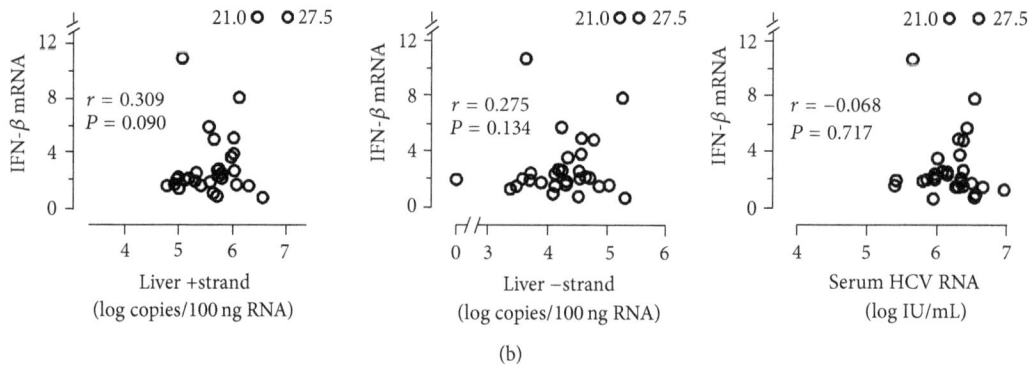

(b)

FIGURE 1: Relationship between HCV replication and hepatic PRR signaling gene expression in 31 patients nonresponsive at week 12. HCV replication was assessed by liver positive- and negative-strand HCV RNAs and circulating HCV RNA.

TABLE 3: Correlations between HCV replication (liver positive- and negative-strand HCV RNAs and circulating HCV RNA) and hepatic PRR signaling gene expression regarding posttreatment virologic response.

Hepatic gene expression		Patients with SVR (n = 22)			Patients without SVR (n = 16)		
		Liver HCV RNA		Serum HCV RNA	Liver HCV RNA		Serum HCV RNA
		+Strand	−Strand		+Strand	−Strand	
TLR3 mRNA	r	0.021	0.132	0.068	**0.632**	**0.632**	0.214
	P	0.925	0.557	0.763	**0.009**	**0.009**	0.427
RIG-I mRNA	r	0.192	0.243	−0.176	**0.760**	**0.693**	**0.511**
	P	0.392	0.277	0.432	**<0.001**	**0.003**	**0.043**
TRIF mRNA	r	0.109	0.200	−0.214	0.465	0.485	−0.029
	P	0.631	0.373	0.339	0.069	0.057	0.914
IPS-1 mRNA	r	0.072	0.131	−0.260	0.389	0.365	0.159
	P	0.750	0.562	0.243	0.137	0.165	0.556
IRF3 mRNA	r	0.056	0.023	−0.380	**0.545**	0.426	0.175
	P	0.803	0.918	0.081	**0.029**	0.099	0.516
IFN-β mRNA	r	0.034	−0.078	−0.107	0.158	0.112	−0.267
	P	0.882	0.730	0.634	0.560	0.680	0.318

found that pretreatment hepatic mRNA expression of these genes uniformly increased in parallel with hepatic HCV loads in patients not attaining early antiviral response to PEG-IFN and ribavirin. In striking contrast, these increases were absent in responders. In IFN nonresponders, HCV replication-related increase in the mRNA expression of the PRR signaling genes was not accompanied with that in IFN-β mRNA expression. The mechanism underlying these findings remains unclear. Thus far, impairment of IFN production and its action has not been well studied regarding responsiveness to exogenous IFN. Our results may imply differential impairment of the host antiviral response by HCV propagation in liver tissues responsive and nonresponsive to exogenous IFN. HCV propagation may cause more severe impairment in IFN nonresponders compared with responders and, in turn, work host feedback systems to upregulate the PRR signaling gene expression involved in IFN production at the mRNA level. Further studies are needed to address these unresolved issues.

Unlike hepatic HCV loads, circulating HCV loads showed much less evident correlations with the PRR signaling gene expression in IFN nonresponders. This discrepancy may imply that circulating HCV loads do not correctly reflect

HCV loads in liver tissues, which are the key compartments in which viral propagation occurs, and the HCV proteins produced interfere with IFN production and its action. Circulating HCV loads can be modified by various factors after release of HCV particles from hepatocytes, including the degree of immune clearance. Indeed, liver positive- and negative-strand HCV RNAs were closely correlated in our study cohort, whereas serum HCV RNA was weakly correlated with liver positive- and negative-strand HCV RNAs.

5. Conclusions

Hepatic mRNA expression of the PRR signaling genes involved in IFN production showed differential relationship with hepatic HCV loads in responders and nonresponders to IFN-based treatment. In liver tissues of nonresponders, the expression of various PRR signaling genes was uniformly increased at the mRNA levels in parallel with HCV loads. These figures were absent in liver tissues of responders. Given that interference of HCV proteins with IFN production and its action depends on the levels of HCV replication; the findings in nonresponders may reflect a host feedback response to severe HCV replication-associated impairment of the IFN system.

Conflict of Interests

The authors declare that they have no conflict of interests.

References

[1] M. Gale Jr. and E. M. Foy, "Evasion of intracellular host defence by hepatitis C virus," *Nature*, vol. 436, no. 7053, pp. 939–945, 2005.

[2] E. C. Freundt and M. J. Lenardo, "Interfering with interferons: hepatitis C virus counters innate immunity," *Proceedings of the National Academy of Sciences of the United States of America*, vol. 102, no. 49, pp. 17539–17540, 2005.

[3] E. Meylan, J. Curran, K. Hofmann et al., "Cardif is an adaptor protein in the RIG-I antiviral pathway and is targeted by hepatitis C virus," *Nature*, vol. 437, no. 7062, pp. 1167–1172, 2005.

[4] K. Li, E. Foy, J. C. Ferreon et al., "Immune evasion by hepatitis C virus NS3/4A protease-mediated cleavage of the Toll-like receptor 3 adaptor protein TRIF," *Proceedings of the National Academy of Sciences of the United States of America*, vol. 102, no. 8, pp. 2992–2997, 2005.

[5] X. D. Li, L. Sun, R. B. Seth, G. Pineda, and Z. J. Chen, "Hepatitis C virus protease NS3/4A cleaves mitochondrial antiviral signaling protein off the mitochondria to evade innate immunity," *Proceedings of the National Academy of Sciences of the United States of America*, vol. 102, no. 49, pp. 17717–17722, 2005.

[6] M. G. Katze, Y. He, and M. Gale Jr., "Viruses and interferon: a fight for supremacy," *Nature Reviews Immunology*, vol. 2, no. 9, pp. 675–687, 2002.

[7] P. Bellecave, M. Sarasin-Filipowicz, O. Donzé et al., "Cleavage of mitochondrial antiviral signaling protein in the liver of patients with chronic hepatitis C correlates with a reduced activation of the endogenous interferon system," *Hepatology*, vol. 51, no. 4, pp. 1127–1136, 2010.

[8] L. Jouan, L. Chatel-Chaix, P. Melanon et al., "Targeted impairment of innate antiviral responses in the liver of chronic hepatitis C patients," *Journal of Hepatology*, vol. 56, no. 1, pp. 70–77, 2012.

[9] N. Yuki, S. Matsumoto, M. Kato, and T. Yamaguchi, "Hepatic Toll-like receptor 3 expression in chronic hepatitis C genotype 1 correlates with treatment response to peginterferon plus ribavirin," *Journal of Viral Hepatitis*, vol. 17, no. 2, pp. 130–138, 2010.

[10] N. Yuki, S. Matsumoto, K. Tadokoro, K. Mochizuki, M. Kato, and T. Yamaguchi, "Significance of liver negative-strand HCV RNA quantitation in chronic hepatitis C," *Journal of Hepatology*, vol. 44, no. 2, pp. 302–309, 2006.

[11] R. G. Knodell, K. G. Ishak, W. C. Black et al., "Formulation and application of a numerical scoring system for assessing histological activity in asymptomatic chronic active hepatitis," *Hepatology*, vol. 1, no. 5, pp. 431–435, 1981.

19

Parvovirus B19 Associated Hepatitis

Chhagan Bihari,[1] Archana Rastogi,[1] Priyanka Saxena,[2] Devraj Rangegowda,[3] Ashok Chowdhury,[3] Nalini Gupta,[1] and Shiv Kumar Sarin[3]

[1] *Department of Pathology, Institute of Liver and Biliary Sciences, D-1, Vasant Kunj, New Delhi 110070, India*
[2] *Department of Hematology, Institute of Liver and Biliary Sciences, D-1, Vasant Kunj, New Delhi 110070, India*
[3] *Department of Hepatology, Institute of Liver and Biliary Sciences, D-1, Vasant Kunj, New Delhi 110070, India*

Correspondence should be addressed to Chhagan Bihari; drcbsharma@gmail.com

Academic Editor: Piero Luigi Almasio

Parvovirus B19 infection can present with myriads of clinical diseases and syndromes; liver manifestations and hepatitis are examples of them. Parvovirus B19 hepatitis associated aplastic anemia and its coinfection with other hepatotropic viruses are relatively underrecognized, and there is sufficient evidence in the literature suggesting that B19 infections can cause a spectrum of liver diseases from elevation of transaminases to acute hepatitis to fulminant liver failure and even chronic hepatitis. It can also cause fatal macrophage activation syndrome and fibrosing cholestatic hepatitis. Parvovirus B19 is an erythrovirus that can only be replicate in pronormoblasts and hepatocytes, and other cells which have globosides and glycosphingolipids in their membrane can also be affected by direct virus injury due to nonstructural protein 1 persistence and indirectly by immune mediated injury. The virus infection is suspected in bone marrow aspiration in cases with sudden drop of hemoglobin and onset of transient aplastic anemia in immunosuppressed or immunocompetent patients and is confirmed either by IgM and IgG positive serology, PCR analysis, and in situ hybridization in biopsy specimens or by application of both. There is no specific treatment for parvovirus B19 related liver diseases, but triple therapy regimen may be effective consisting of immunoglobulin, dehydrohydrocortisone, and cyclosporine.

1. Background

Parvoviridae family includes many pathogenic animal viruses including adeno-associated viruses which appear to infect humans without causing clinical manifestations. Most parvoviruses depend upon the help from host cells or other viruses to replicate, whereas only few (autonomous) parvoviruses propagate in actively dividing cells. Parvovirus B19 (B19) is the type member of the erythrovirus genus which propagates primarily in erythroid progenitor cells [1].

B19 can infect erythroid precursors, hepatocytes, and other cells that possess globosides and glycosphingolipids in their cell membrane, but it can only replicate in the erythroid precursors and few other cells including fetal liver, isolated stem and bone marrow cells, and megakaryocytic leukemia cell lines maintained with erythropoietin [2, 3].

Infection of parvovirus B19 is globally prevalent with infection being very common among children. The virus spreads primarily through respiratory droplets, and secondary infection is by household contacts. It can also be transmitted as nosocomial infections and by blood products. B19 is resistant to heat inactivation and organic detergent, because of their stable genomic structure and absence of lipid envelope [1].

B19 is an etiologic agent of erythema infectiosum (fifth disease), fever/rash illness of childhood, whereas, in adults, the commonest manifestation is clinically significant arthropathy [1–3]. Both of these clinical diseases are thought to be due to immune complex deposition in skin and in the joints, respectively [3–5]. Systemic manifestation of B19 infection includes multisystem involvement and viral hemophagocytic syndrome [2]. Ever expanding spectrum of clinical disease has been attributed to human B19 infection with adult seroprevalence rate of around 50% [1].

The clinical diseases caused by B19 are categorized into two broad groups—common and uncommon. Common

TABLE 1: Common clinical manifestations of parvovirus B19.

Diseases	Group of patients
Fifth disease	Children
Arthropathy	Adults
Transient aplastic crisis	Patients with increased erythroid proliferation (underlying hemolytic disease)
Persistent anemia	Patients with immunocompromised or immunodeficient status
Hydrops fetalis	Fetus

TABLE 2: Uncommon clinical diseases associated with parvovirus B19.

Clinical disease	References
Hepatitis	[6]
Myocarditis	[7]
Necrotizing vasculitis	[8]
Kawasaki's disease	[9]
Henoch-Schönlein purpura	[10]
Giant-cell arteritis	[11]
Gloves-and-socks syndrome	[12]
Chronic fatigue syndrome	[13]
Meningitis	[14]
Encephalitis	[14]
Ophthalmitis	[14]

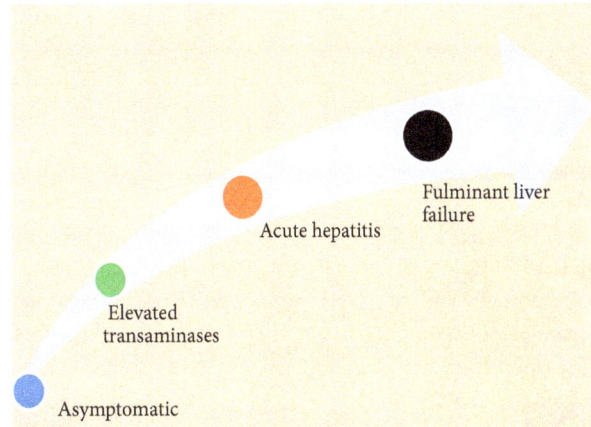

FIGURE 1: Diagrammatic representation of spectrum of liver diseases associated with parvovirus B19 infection according to the severity.

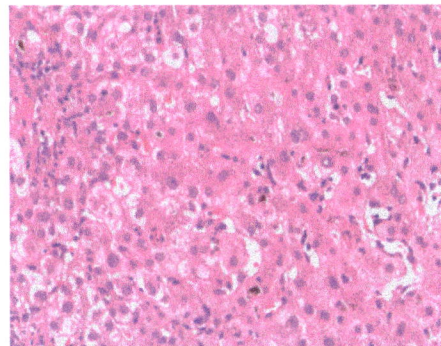

FIGURE 2: Liver biopsy showing features of acute cholestatic hepatitis (H&E, 200x). The patient was a case of thalassemia trait, and parvovirus B19 IgM serology was positive.

clinical diseases are the ones listed in Table 1 [1], and the uncommon clinical manifestations associated with B19 are enlisted in Table 2 [6–14].

Acute hepatitis and fulminant liver failure may be caused by B19; however, this incidence is very rare [2], with only a few cases reported in the literature with clinical manifestation of hepatitis as a result of B19 infection. We undertook this facet of B19 infection for the discussion and reviewed various liver related conditions along with diagnosis, pathogenesis, and treatment of B19 induced hepatitis.

2. Parvovirus B19 and Hepatitis

Liver diseases caused by B19 infection range from elevation of transaminases to acute hepatitis to fulminant liver failure and even chronic hepatitis (Figure 1). According to a study by Mihály et al., parvovirus B 19 related hepatitis may occur in 4.1% of patients infected by this virus [15]. Around 50 cases of B19 related hepatitis have been reported in the literature till date which is summarized in Table 3 [16–53]. Spectrum of liver diseases has been reported in all age groups from neonates to elderly.

2.1. Parvovirus B19 Acute Hepatitis and Fulminant Hepatic Failure. Presentation as acute hepatitis or fulminant liver failure has been mostly reported in the paediatric age groups; however, the same has also been reported in adults. In adults, parvovirus B19 hepatitis course is found to be less severe than in children [16–22] and can be manifested in immunocompetent or immunodeficient patients with or without underlying hemolytic abnormalities [25]. Most of the time, B19 acute hepatitis shows complete and spontaneous remission, particularly in adults [25]. Fulminant hepatic failure induced as a result of acute B19 infection remains a rare clinical entity. And these may be underreported also due to infrequent testing and lack of awareness [25, 26]. Liver biopsy in affected patients displays cellular and canalicular cholestasis, apoptosis (Figure 2), and variable amounts of necrosis depending upon immune status of the host and the severity of liver involvement [19].

2.2. Parvovirus B19 and Chronic Hepatitis. B19 can also cause chronic hepatitis. In a case by Mogensen et al., chronic hepatitis due to B19 was reported in a patient with lymphopenia [23]. Pongratz et al. found that the persistence of B19 and occurrence of chronic hepatitis directly correlate with the extent of liver involvement [27]. Wang et al. described B19 persistence in the chronic hepatitis B (CHBV) and chronic hepatitis C (CHCV) infected patients and concluded that the persistence of B19 virus infection does not cause any significant worsening of liver functions in the HBV and HCV

TABLE 3: List of reported cases of parvovirus B19 hepatitis.

Author	Cases	Associated condition	References
Martínez González et al. (2012)	One (acute hepatitis)		[16]
Sun and Zhang (2012)	One (FHF)	Aplastic anemia	[17]
Larsen (2011)	One (acute hepatitis)		[18]
Hatakka et al. (2011)	One (acute hepatitis)		[19]
Yang et al. (2012)	One (acute hepatitis)	DLBCL	[20]
Sun et al. (2011)	Two (acute hepatiti)		[21]
Al Nahdi et al. (2010)	One (recurrent acute hepatitis)		[22]
Mogensen et al. (2010)	One (chronic hepatitis)	Lymphopenia	[23]
Wang et al. (2009)	One (chronic hepatitis)		[24]
Krygier et al. (2009)	One (acute hepatitis)		[25]
Kim et al. (2009)	One (acute hepatitis)		[26]
Pongratz et al. (2009)	One (acute hepatitis)		[27]
Cao et al. (2009)	One (fulminant hepatic failure)		[28]
Kishore and Sen (2009)	One (fulminant hepatic failure)	Coexistent A and E	[29]
Al-Abdwani et al. (2008)	One (acute hepatitis)	Aplastic anemia	[30]
Giørtz-Carlsen et al. (2007)	One (acute hepatitis)		[31]
Özçay et al. (2006)	One (fulminant hepatic failure)	Pure red cell aplasia	[32]
Aydin et al. (2006)	One (acute hepatitis)		[33]
Toshihiro et al. (2003)	One (acute hepatitis)		[34]
Chehal et al. (2002)	One (acute hepatitis)		[35]
Dame et al. (2002)	One (acute hepatitis)	Aplastic anemia	[36]
Díaz and Collazos (2000)	One (acute hepatitis)		[37]
Lee et al. (2000)	One (acute hepatitis)	Post-renal-transplant immunosuppression	[38]
Pinho et al. (2001)	One (acute hepatitis)		[39]
Shan et al. (2001)	One (FCH)	Post-renal-transplant immunosuppression	[40]
Alliot et al. (2001)	One (acute hepatitis)	HIV	[41]
Karetnyi et al. (1999)	One (fulminant hepatic failure)		[42]
Drago et al. (1999)	One (acute hepatitis)		[43]
Sokal et al. (1998)	One (fulminant hepatic failure)		[44]
Hillingsø et al. (1998)	One (acute hepatitis)		[45]
Hillingsø et al. (1998)	One (acute hepatitis)		[46]
Longo et al. (1998)	One (acute hepatitis)	Still's disease	[47]
Pardi et al. (1998)	Two (acute hepatitis)	Post-Liver-transplant aplastic anemia	[48]
Weinberg et al. (1996)	One (acute hepatitis)		[49]
Naides et al. (1996)	One (acute hepatitis)		[50]
Yoto et al. (1996)	One (acute hepatitis)		[51]
Langnas et al. (1995)	Six (2 acute hepatitis, 4 fulminant hepatitis)	Aplastic anemia	[52]
Pouchot et al. (1993)	One (acute hepatitis)		[53]

affected patients [24]. A study by Toan et al. on 463 hepatitis B positive Vietnamese patients showed that 99/463 patients (21.4%) were positive for B19 DNA which was significantly higher than those of healthy controls. They also concluded that in HBV/B19 coinfection the probability of progression to more severe hepatitis is significantly higher [54].

The association of B19 with chronic hepatitis B and C has also been described by Hsu et al. They found that B19 serology for IgM and IgG was positive in 35.2% and 85%. 2% of the cases of chronic hepatitis B with B19 DNA were detected in 37% of the cases of chronic hepatitis B. In cases of chronic hepatitis C, IgM and IgG antibodies for B19 were

positive in 15.7% and 70.6%, and B19 DNA was detected in 23.5% of HCV cases. Distinctive subtypes of B19 were detected in chronic hepatitis B and C, TW-3 in chronic hepatitis B and TW-9 in cases of chronic hepatitis C infection. Liver dysfunction was not associated with B19 coexistence in the chronic hepatitis cases. The study also revealed that a significant proportion of coinfection occurs in chronic hepatitis cases with B19 infection [55]. It is important to note that although liver functions are not much affected by the coinfection of B19 [24, 55], large cohort studies are required to explore the pathological course of B19 in association with chronic hepatitis and their clinical outcomes.

2.3. Parvovirus B19 and Fibrosing Cholestatic Hepatitis. There was a single case report of fibrosing cholestatic hepatitis (FCH) due to B19 infection in a patient with renal allograft for IgA nephropathy. During the postoperative period, the patient developed features of acute liver failure. All viral markers were negative except for HBV and B19 DNA. The patient was given lamivudine therapy; however, his condition got deteriorated, and the patient subsequently died. The postmortem liver tissue revealed FCH. On immunohistochemical examination, the biopsy was negative for HBsAg and HBcAg, while the PCR showed strong positivity in liver tissue for B19 infection, and it was considered that B19 was the cause of FCH [40].

2.4. Parvovirus B19 Coinfection with Other Hepatotropic Viruses. B19 coinfection with other hepatotropic viruses can lead to severe acute fulminant hepatic failure (FHF) with severe outcome as compared to isolated B19 or other hepatotropic virus associated FHF. Dwivedi et al. in their study of 48 patients with FHF, divided them into three groups as those associated with (i) B19 infection alone, (ii) one or more other hepatotropic viral infection in the absence of B19 infection, and (iii) B19 coinfection with other hepatotropic viruses. They found that FHF caused by B19 and coinfection with other hepatitis viruses had severe jaundice, high bilirubin, high alanine aminotransferase or aspartate aminotransferase activity, and unfavorable outcome resulting in death of most of these patients, compared with those with isolated B19 or other hepatitis viruses infection [56]. It was hypothesized that B19 possibly may cause injury to hepatocytes independently or by producing synergistic effect when present along with other hepatitis viruses.

2.5. Parvovirus B19 and Hepatitis Associated Aplastic Anemia (HAAA). Hepatitis associated aplastic anemia (HAAA) is a distinct variant of acquired aplastic anemia (AA), in which an acute attack of hepatitis culminates in marrow failure and pancytopenia [57]. Several hepatitis viruses such as hepatitis A, B, C, E, and G have been anticipated to be associated with this set of symptoms. Besides the hepatitis viruses, other viruses have also been implicated as causative agent of AA which include B19, *Cytomegalovirus*, Epstein Barr virus, echovirus 3, GB virus-C, transfusion transmitted virus (TTV), SEN virus, and non-A-E hepatitis virus (unknown viruses). B19, an underrecognized hepatotropic virus, is documented as an offending agent of acute hepatitis, FHF, and HAAA in immunocompromised patients [58]. There have been reports of B19 related HAAA in post-liver-transplant immunocompromised patients [48, 52]. The myelotoxic effect in B19 or other viral infections is thought to be due to increased circulating cytotoxic CD8$^+$ T cells and IFN-γ secretion by these cells. Similarly, high circulating CD8$^+$ T cells cause the altered and defective monocyte and macrophage differentiation, decreased level of circulating IL-1, and increased secretion of TNF-α, IFN-γ, and IL-2 receptors which causes onlooker damage of hepatocytes and subsequently occurrence of acute hepatitis [59, 60].

2.6. Parvovirus B19 Hepatitis in Underlying Hematological Diseases. In patients with hemolytic anemia, B19 infection can cause an abrupt cessation of red cell production which is exacerbated in case of acute infection or in compensated states and provokes severe anemia. Anemic crisis in hereditary spherocytosis and in sickle cell disease has long been recognized. The bone marrow in patients with transient aplastic crisis is characterized by an absence of maturing erythroid precursors and presence of giant pronormoblasts. Thrombocytopenia and pancytopenia have also been reported in patients with acute B19 infection [2]. Transient aplastic crisis (TAC) is a self-limiting condition, and normal individuals usually recover as the neutralizing antibodies are produced, while in immunocompromised patients, neutralizing antibody cannot be produced, and this can lead to persistent pure red aplasia [1]. Zaki et al. found that the incidence of B19 infection is significantly higher among children with hematological disorders, including hemolytic anemias, lymphomas, and leukemias on chemotherapy [61]. B19 has a tropism for the immature proliferating pronormoblasts and is essentially an erythrovirus. Globoside, a neutral glycolipid that acts as a cellular receptor and nonstructural protein of parvovirus, is responsible for the apoptotic death of erythroid progenitors, and some other cells such as megakaryocytes may be lysed by restricted expression of viral proteins in the absence of viral propagation [62]. Thus, the high propensity of B19 in hematological disease at times can also cause acute hepatitis [63].

2.7. Parvovirus B19 Hepatitis and Hemophagocytosis Lymphohistiocytosis (HLH). Hemophagocytic lymphohistiocytosis (HLH) is a hyperinflammatory condition clinically characterized by fever, splenomegaly, jaundice, and phagocytosis of erythrocytes, leukocytes, platelets, and their precursors by macrophages in bone marrow and other tissues [64]. Among viruses, Epstein-Barr virus, *Cytomegalovirus*, human herpesvirus 6, and parvovirus B19 have been implicated to cause virus associated HLH (VAHLH) [65]. B19 related HLH is not so uncommon and can occur both in immunocompetent and immunocompromised hosts [66]. The hallmark of HLH pathogenesis is T cell activation leading to stimulation of macrophages which thereby initiates hemophagocytosis. Thus, CD8$^+$ and CD4$^+$ T cells activation triggers marked cytokine production of TNF-α, a key factor in histiocytic activation [67]. As described above, activated T cells and released cytokines may also lead to hepatocyte damage and ultimately hepatitis.

3. Diagnosis

3.1. Hematological Tests. In patients with evidence of clinically significant anemia or transient aplastic crisis (TAC), a complete blood count with reticulocyte count aids in suspecting B19 infection with the following possible scenarios: (1) patients infected with parvovirus B19 will have a low reticulocyte count (0-1%) and (2) in an aplastic crisis, hemoglobin levels will drop below the patient's baseline by at least 2 g/dL [68]. Bone marrow examination in these patients

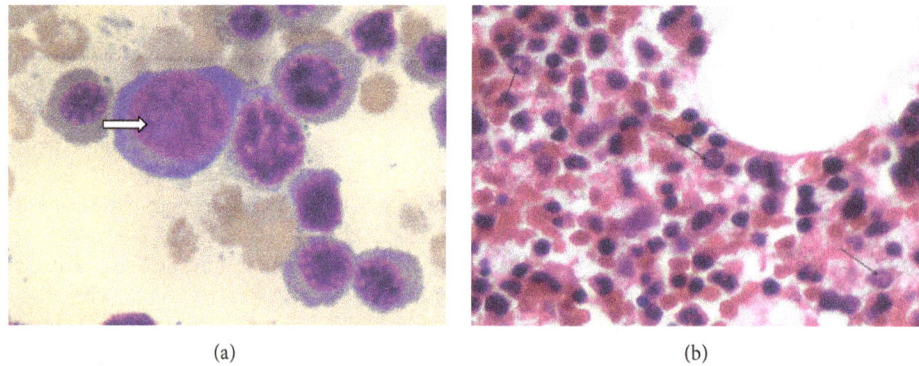

FIGURE 3: (a) Parvovirus B19 inclusion in Pronormoblast in bone marrow aspirate (Geimsa, 1000x), in same case as described above. (b) Clearing of nuclei in pronormoblasts, due to Parvovirus B19 inclusion (HE, 400x); an adult case of hereditary spherocytosis with acute hepatitis and sudden drop of haemoglobin, Parvovirus IgM serology positive.

reveals absence of maturing red cell with prominence of pronormoblast having cytoplasmic blebs and intranuclear inclusions (Figure 3(a)). Bone marrow biopsy examination shows nuclear clearing due to viral inclusions present in them [69] (Figure 3(b)).

3.2. Serology. Parvovirus serology (anti-parvovirus B19 immunoglobulin M (IgM) and immunoglobulin G (IgG) antibodies) can be determined using enzyme-linked immunoassay (ELISA), radioimmunoassay, or immunofluorescence. Results of IgM testing are maybe difficult to interpret; however, reliable results can be obtained by using automated instruments dedicated for serological testing. Generally, IgM antibodies are detectable 3 days after infection, and IgG antibodies can be detected after 2 weeks at the time of recovery of hematopoiesis. IgM antibodies once formed remain detectable for months, while IgG can be detected for lifetime. In immunodeficient patients, inability to clear the virus leads to chronic B19 infection and leads to pure red cell aplasia (PRAC). In contrast to TAC, PRAC is characterized by very low or absent antibody levels, and they are diagnosed best by polymerase chain reaction (PCR) [70]. Pregnant women exposed to parvovirus B19 should get IgG and IgM serology done as soon as possible, as infection risk for fetus remains due [71].

3.3. Polymerase Chain Reaction (PCR). PCR testing for parvovirus B19 is routinely available with high sensitivity level. Low levels of B19 DNA can be detected for more than 4 months in serum after acute infection and for years in other tissues. PCR can also be used to diagnose chronic infection by detecting viral DNA present in the blood or other tissues/fluids. However, the interpretation pertaining to pregnant women is uncertain [72].

3.4. Immunohistochemistry. Parvovirus B19 monoclonal antibody R92F6 against VP1/VP2 capsid protein antigen can also be detected in liver tissue and in bone marrow biopsy by immunohistochemistry [39].

3.5. Other Potential Diagnostic Methods. Enzyme-linked immunosorbent spot assay (ELISPOT) is a method to measure the qualitative and quantitative immune response in humans and animals. This method identifies and enumerates cytokine-producing cells at the single cell level. By having appropriate conditions, the ELISPOT assay allows visualization of the secretory product of individual activated or responding cells [27]. Each spot that develops in the assay represents a single reactive cell. This ELISPOT technique can be used to detect $CD4^+$ T cells specific for B19 viral proteins in cases of persistent infection [27].

The diagnosis of acute or chronic infection should be made on the basis of standard DNA hybridization or quantitative (real-time) PCR in combination with serologic assays for B19-specific IgG, IgM, or both [73].

4. Pathogenesis

The mechanism by which parvovirus B19 infection may result in hepatic injury is exactly not clear. Hepatic cell damage related to direct viral invasion is one possibility. Alternatively, injury may result as an indirect consequence of the immune response directed against the virus.

4.1. Direct Cytopathic Effect. B19 is a single-stranded DNA virus and has a genome length of 5.4 kb with hairpin structures at each extremity. Two major open reading frames (ORFs) extend through the entire genome of virus. A nonstructural protein (NS1) is found on the N-terminal region of the genome, and its molecular weight is 70 to 77 kDa. NS1 is thought to be essential for viral DNA replication and also for the regulation of viral promoters. NS1 contains a consensus sequence for ATP- or GTP-binding, which is associated with ATPase and DNA helicase activities. NS1 is also known to be cytotoxic for erythroid cells and is possibly related to the pathogenesis of B19 virus infection [74]. B19 can replicate only in the erythroid precursors and few other cells including fetal liver, isolated stem and bone marrow cells, and megakaryocytic leukemia cell lines maintained with erythropoietin.

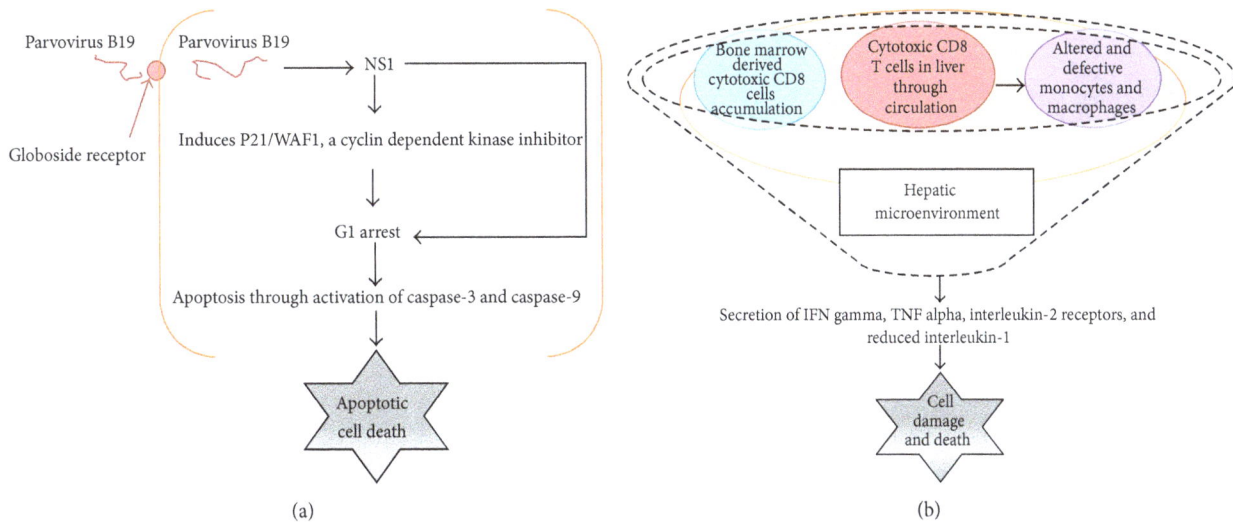

FIGURE 4: Schematic presentation of direct and indirect hepatocellular injury in parvovirus B19 infection.

Hepatocytes express globoside and glycosphingolipids, the putative receptors for B19 virus. B19 virus enters hepatocytes through globoside and establishes a restricted infection with the production of NS1 without the production of viral progeny [75]. NS1 expression plays a critical role in G1 arrest induced by B19 virus. Furthermore, NS1 expression also significantly increases p21/WAF1 expression, a cyclin dependent kinase inhibitor that induces G1 arrest. Ultimately, the G1 arrested hepatocytes undergo apoptosis by activation of caspase-3 and caspase-9 [74, 76]. Diagrammatic summary is depicted in Figure 4(a).

4.2. Indirect Immunological Effect. The hepatotoxic effect caused by parvovirus B19 infection is thought to be due to increased circulating CD8$^+$ cytotoxic T cells and IFN-γ and TNF-α secretion by these cells [58]. Similarly, high circulating CD8$^+$ T cells cause the altered and defective monocyte and macrophage differentiation, decreased level of circulating IL-1, and increased secretion of TNF-α, IFN-γ, and IL-2 receptors which causes damage of hepatocytes and subsequently leading to acute hepatitis [58–60]. Diagrammatic summary is depicted in Figure 4(b).

5. Treatment

There are no specific treatment guidelines for infection caused by B19 virus, and most of the symptoms and elevation of liver enzymes presented during infection stage resolve without any treatment. In case of acute and fulminant hepatitis, combination therapy consisting of an intravenous infusion of immunoglobulin and dehydrohydrocortisone and subcutaneous injections of granulocyte colony-stimulating factor for three months has been tried [17]. For HAAA and HLH, an immunosuppressive therapy comprising antithymocyte Globulin (ATG), cyclosporine, and steroids has proven

to be effective [58]. Aplastic crises and PRAC are transiently responsive to erythropoietin, growth factors, granulocyte colony-stimulating factor, granulocyte macrophage colony stimulating factor, interleukin-3, and androgens [77]. Nonresponsive HAAA should be treated by allogenic bone marrow (BM) transplantation from HLA matched siblings [78].

6. Conclusion

There are sufficient lines of evidence in the literature that state that Parvovirus B19 infection can be associated with the development of acute hepatitis, FHF, HAAA, hepatitis with HLH, chronic hepatitis, and rarely FCH. There is a significant rate of coexistence of B19 with chronic hepatitis B and C as suggested by the literature. This area needs to be further explored and validated through large cohort studies. Infection with parvovirus B19 should be considered in the differential diagnosis in both immunocompromised and immunocompetent patients presenting with acute hepatitis of unknown etiology particularly in cases of underlying hemolytic diseases and immunodeficient host with aplastic anemia. The parvovirus B19 infection can be detected by positive IgM serology and by PCR in infected tissues. Parvovirus B19 can cause hepatitis due to direct cytopathic and indirect immunological injury through CD8$^+$ cytotoxic T cells. A combination of an intravenous infusion of immunoglobulin, dehydrohydrocortisone and cyclosporine and subcutaneous injections of granulocyte colony-stimulating factor for three months has proved to be an effective therapy for parvovirus B19 hepatitis and HAAA.

Conflict of Interests

The authors declare that they have no conflict of interests.

References

[1] N. S. Young and K. E. Brown, "Mechanisms of disease: parvovirus B19," *The New England Journal of Medicine*, vol. 350, no. 6, pp. 586–597, 2004.

[2] K. E. Brown and N. S. Young, "The simian parvoviruses," *Reviews in Medical Virology*, vol. 7, pp. 211–218, 1997.

[3] T. L. Moore, "Parvovirus-associated arthritis," *Current Opinion in Rheumatology*, vol. 12, no. 4, pp. 289–294, 2000.

[4] T. Chorba, P. Coccia, and R. C. Holman, "The role of parvovirus B19 in aplastic crisis and erythema infectiosum (fifth disease)," *Journal of Infectious Diseases*, vol. 154, no. 3, pp. 383–393, 1986.

[5] Z. He, H. Zhuang, X. Wang et al., "Retrospective analysis of non-A-E hepatitis: possible role of hepatitis B and C virus infection," *Journal of Medical Virology*, vol. 69, no. 1, pp. 59–65, 2003.

[6] S. Arista, S. De Grazia, V. Di Marco, R. Di Stefano, and A. Craxi, "Parvovirus B19 and "cryptogenic" chronic hepatitis," *Journal of Hepatology*, vol. 38, no. 3, pp. 375–376, 2003.

[7] M. Beghetti, A. Gervaix, C. A. Haenggeli, M. Berner, and P. C. Rimensberger, "Myocarditis associated with parvovirus B19 infection in two siblings with merosin-deficient congenital muscular dystrophy," *European Journal of Pediatrics*, vol. 159, no. 1-2, pp. 135–136, 2000.

[8] T. H. Finkel, T. J. Török, P. J. Ferguson et al., "Chronic parvovirus B19 infection and systemic necrotising vasculitis: opportunistic infection or aetiological agent?" *The Lancet*, vol. 343, no. 8908, pp. 1255–1258, 1994.

[9] G. Nigro, M. Zerbini, A. Krzysztofiak et al., "Active or recent parvovirus B19 infection in children with Kawasaki disease," *The Lancet*, vol. 343, no. 8908, pp. 1260–1261, 1994.

[10] P. J. Ferguson, F. T. Saulsbury, S. F. Dowell, T. J. Török, D. D. Erdman, and L. J. Anderson, "Prevalence of human parvovirus B19 infection in children with Henoch-Schönlein purpura," *Arthritis and Rheumatism*, vol. 39, no. 5, pp. 880–881, 1996.

[11] S. E. Gabriel, M. Espy, D. D. Erdman, J. Bjornsson, T. F. Smith, and G. G. Hunder, "The role of parvovirus B19 in the pathogenesis of giant cell arteritis: a preliminary evaluation," *Arthritis and Rheumatism*, vol. 42, pp. 1255–1258, 1999.

[12] S. B. Smith, L. F. Libow, D. M. Elston, R. A. Bernert, and K. E. Warschaw, "Gloves and socks syndrome: early and late histopathologic features," *Journal of the American Academy of Dermatology*, vol. 47, no. 5, pp. 749–754, 2002.

[13] S. Kim Jacobson, J. S. Daly, G. M. Thorne, and K. McIntosh, "Chronic parvovirus B19 infection resulting in chronic fatigue syndrome: case history and review," *Clinical Infectious Diseases*, vol. 24, no. 6, pp. 1048–1051, 1997.

[14] J. R. Kerr, F. Barah, M. L. Chiswick et al., "Evidence for the role of demyelination, HLA-DR alleles, and cytokines in the pathogenesis of parvovirus B19 meningoencephalitis and its sequelae," *Journal of Neurology Neurosurgery and Psychiatry*, vol. 73, no. 6, pp. 739–746, 2002.

[15] I. Mihály, A. Trethon, Z. Arányi et al., "Observations on human parvovirus B19 infection diagnosed in 2011," *Orvosi Hetilap*, vol. 153, no. 49, pp. 1948–1957, 2012.

[16] J. Martínez González, C. Senosiain Lalastra, F. Mesonero Gismero, and V. Moreira Vicente, "An exceptional cause of acute hepatitis in an adult: parvovirus B19," *Journal of Gastroenterology and Hepatology*, vol. 35, no. 10, pp. 697–699, 2012.

[17] L. Sun and J.-C. Zhang, "Acute fulminant hepatitis with bone marrow failure in an adult due to parvovirus B19 infection," *Hepatology*, vol. 55, no. 1, pp. 329–330, 2012.

[18] L. Larsen, "Parvovirus B19-akut hepatitis hos immunkompetent patient," *Ugeskrift for Laeger*, vol. 173, no. 43, pp. 2719–2720, 2011.

[19] A. Hatakka, J. Klein, R. He, J. Piper, E. Tam, and A. Walkty, "Acute hepatitis as a manifestation of parvovirus B19 infection," *Journal of Clinical Microbiology*, vol. 49, no. 9, pp. 3422–3424, 2011.

[20] S.-H. Yang, L.-W. Lin, Y.-J. Fang, A.-L. Cheng, and S.-H. Kuo, "Parvovirus B19 infection-related acute hepatitis after rituximab-containing regimen for treatment of diffuse large B-cell lymphoma," *Annals of Hematology*, vol. 91, no. 2, pp. 291–294, 2012.

[21] L. Sun, J.-C. Zhang, and Z.-S. Jia, "Association of parvovirus B19 infection with acute icteric hepatitis in adults," *Scandinavian Journal of Infectious Diseases*, vol. 43, no. 6-7, pp. 547–549, 2011.

[22] N. Al Nahdi, H. Wiesinger, H. Sutherland, and E. M. Yoshida, "Recurrent idiopathic acute hepatitis-associated aplastic anemia/pancytopenia fourteen years after initial episode," *Annals of Hepatology*, vol. 9, no. 4, pp. 468–470, 2010.

[23] T. H. Mogensen, J. M. B. Jensen, S. Hamilton-Dutoit, and C. S. Larsen, "Chronic hepatitis caused by persistent parvovirus B19 infection," *BMC Infectious Diseases*, vol. 10, article 246, 2010.

[24] C. Wang, A. Heim, V. Schlaphoff et al., "Intrahepatic long-term persistence of parvovirus B19 and its role in chronic viral hepatitis," *Journal of Medical Virology*, vol. 81, no. 12, pp. 2079–2088, 2009.

[25] D. S. Krygier, U. P. Steinbrecher, M. Petric et al., "Parvovirus B19 induced hepatic failure in an adult requiring liver transplantation," *World Journal of Gastroenterology*, vol. 15, no. 32, pp. 4067–4069, 2009.

[26] B. J. Kim, K. H. Yoo, K. Li, and M. N. Kim, "Parvovirus B19 infection associated with acute hepatitis in infant," *Pediatric Infectious Disease Journal*, vol. 28, no. 7, article 667, 2009.

[27] G. Pongratz, J. Lindner, S. Modrow, S. Schimanski, J. Schölmerich, and M. Fleck, "Persistent parvovirus B19 infection detected by specific CD4+ T-cell responses in a patient with hepatitis and polyarthritis," *Journal of Internal Medicine*, vol. 266, no. 3, pp. 296–301, 2009.

[28] Y.-H. Cao, G.-Y. Zhang, and G.-C. Zhang, "Successful treatment with high-dose intravenous immunoglobulin for parvovirus B19 infection associated with acute fulminant hepatitis in a chinese child," *Clinical Pediatrics*, vol. 48, no. 6, pp. 674–676, 2009.

[29] J. Kishore and M. Sen, "Parvovirus B19-induced thrombocytopenia and anemia in a child with fatal fulminant hepatic failure coinfected with hepatitis A and E viruses," *Journal of Tropical Pediatrics*, vol. 55, no. 5, pp. 335–337, 2009.

[30] R. M. Al-Abdwani, F. A. Khamis, A. Balkhair, M. Sacharia, and Y. A. Wali, "A child with human parvovirus B19 infection induced aplastic anemia and acute hepatitis: effectiveness of immunosuppressive therapy," *Pediatric Hematology and Oncology*, vol. 25, no. 7, pp. 699–703, 2008.

[31] B. Giørtz-Carlsen, S. Rittig, and T. Thelle, "Neurological symptoms and acute hepatitis associated with parvovirus B19," *Ugeskrift for Laeger*, vol. 169, no. 47, pp. 4075–4077, 2007.

[32] F. Özçay, Y. E. Bikmaz, O. Canan, and N. Özbek, "Hepatitis A and parvovirus B19 infections in an infant with fulminant hepatic failure," *Turkish Journal of Gastroenterology*, vol. 17, no. 2, pp. 148–150, 2006.

[33] M. Aydin, Y. Bulut, G. Poyrazoglu, M. Turgut, and A. Seyrek, "Detection of human parvovirus B19 in children with acute hepatitis," *Annals of Tropical Paediatrics*, vol. 26, no. 1, pp. 25–28, 2006.

[34] M. Toshihiro, Y. Takikawa, Y. Fukuda, S.-I. Sato, R. Endou, and K. Suzuki, "A case of acute hepatitis associated with Parvovirus B19," *Japanese Journal of Gastroenterology*, vol. 100, no. 11, pp. 1312–1316, 2003.

[35] A. Chehal, A. I. Sharara, H. A. Haidar, J. Haidar, and A. Bazarbachi, "Acute viral hepatitis A and parvovirus B19 infections complicated by pure red cell aplasia and autoimmune hemolytic anemia," *Journal of Hepatology*, vol. 37, no. 1, pp. 163–165, 2002.

[36] C. Dame, C. Hasan, U. Bode, and A. M. Eis-Hübinger, "Acute liver disease and aplastic anemia associated with the persistence of B19 DNA in liver and bone marrow," *Pediatric Pathology and Molecular Medicine*, vol. 21, no. 1, pp. 25–29, 2002.

[37] F. Díaz and J. Collazos, "Hepatic dysfunction due to parvovirus B19 infection," *Journal of Infection and Chemotherapy*, vol. 6, no. 1, pp. 63–64, 2000.

[38] P. C. Lee, C. J. Hung, H. Y. Lei, T. T. Chang, J. R. Wang, and M. S. Jan, "Parvovirus B19-related hepatitis in an immunosuppressed kidney transplant," *Nephrology Dialysis Transplantation*, vol. 15, pp. 1486–1488, 2000.

[39] J. R. R. Pinho, V. A. F. Alves, A. F. Vieira et al., "Detection of human parvovirus B19 in a patient with hepatitis," *Brazilian Journal of Medical and Biological Research*, vol. 34, no. 9, pp. 1131–1138, 2001.

[40] Y.-S. Shan, P.-C. Lee, J.-R. Wang, H.-P. Tsai, C.-M. Sung, and Y.-T. Jin, "Fibrosing cholestatic hepatitis possibly related to persistent parvovirus B19 infection in a renal transplant recipient," *Nephrology Dialysis Transplantation*, vol. 16, no. 12, pp. 2420–2422, 2001.

[41] C. Alliot, M. Barrios, J. Taib, and M. Brunel, "Parvovirus B19 infection in an HIV-infected patient with febrile pancytopenia and acute hepatitis," *European Journal of Clinical Microbiology and Infectious Diseases*, vol. 20, no. 1, pp. 43–45, 2001.

[42] Y. V. Karetnyi, P. R. Beck, R. S. Markin, A. N. Langnas, and S. J. Naides, "Human parvovirus B19 infection in acute fulminant liver failure," *Archives of Virology*, vol. 144, no. 9, pp. 1713–1724, 1999.

[43] F. Drago, M. Semino, P. Rampini, and A. Rebora, "Parvovirus B19 infection associated with acute hepatitis and a purpuric exanthem," *British Journal of Dermatology*, vol. 141, no. 1, pp. 160–161, 1999.

[44] E. M. Sokal, M. Melchior, C. Cornu et al., "Acute parvovirus B19 infection associated with fulminant hepatitis of favourable prognosis in young children," *The Lancet*, vol. 352, no. 9142, pp. 1739–1741, 1998.

[45] J. G. Hillingsø, I. P. Jensen, and L. Tom-Petersen, "Parvovirus B19 as causative agent of acute hepatitis in adults," *Ugeskrift for Laeger*, vol. 160, no. 44, pp. 6355–6356, 1998.

[46] J. G. Hillingsø, I. P. Jensen, and L. Tom-Petersen, "Parvovirus B19 and acute hepatitis in adults," *The Lancet*, vol. 351, no. 9107, pp. 955–956, 1998.

[47] G. Longo, M. Luppi, M. Bertesi, L. Ferrara, G. Torelli, and G. Emilia, "Still's disease, severe thrombocytopenia, and acute hepatitis associated with acute parvovirus B19 infection," *Clinical Infectious Diseases*, vol. 26, no. 4, pp. 994–995, 1998.

[48] D. S. Pardi, Y. Romero, L. E. Mertz, and D. D. Douglas, "Hepatitis-associated aplastic anemia and acute parvovirus B19 infection: a report of two cases and a review of the literature," *The American Journal of Gastroenterology*, vol. 93, no. 3, pp. 468–470, 1998.

[49] J. M. Weinberg, J. T. Wolfe, A. L. Frattali, V. P. Werth, S. J. Naides, and E. M. Spiers, "Parvovirus B19 infection associated

with acute hepatitis, arthralgias, and rash," *Journal of Clinical Rheumatology*, vol. 2, no. 2, pp. 85–88, 1996.

[50] S. J. Naides, Y. V. Karetnyi, L. L. W. Cooling et al., "Human parvovirus B19 infection and hepatitis," *The Lancet*, vol. 347, no. 9014, pp. 1563–1564, 1996.

[51] Y. Yoto, T. Kudoh, K. Haseyama, N. Suzuki, and S. Chiba, "Human parvovirus B19 infection associated with acute hepatitis," *The Lancet*, vol. 347, no. 9005, pp. 868–869, 1996.

[52] A. N. Langnas, R. S. Markin, M. S. Cattral, and S. J. Naides, "Parvovirus B19 as a possible causative agent of fulminant liver failure and associated aplastic anemia," *Hepatology*, vol. 22, no. 6, pp. 1661–1665, 1995.

[53] J. Pouchot, H. Ouakil, M. L. Debin, and P. Vinceneux, "Adult Still's disease associated with acute human parvovirus B19 infection," *The Lancet*, vol. 341, no. 8855, pp. 1280–1281, 1993.

[54] N. L. Toan, L. H. Song, P. G. Kremsner et al., "Co-infection of human parvovirus B19 in Vietnamese patients with hepatitis B virus infection," *Journal of Hepatology*, vol. 45, no. 3, pp. 361–369, 2006.

[55] T.-C. Hsu, T.-Y. Chen, M.-C. Lin, B.-S. Tzang, and G. J. Tsay, "Human parvovirus B19 infection in patients with chronic hepatitis B or hepatitis C infection," *Journal of Gastroenterology and Hepatology*, vol. 20, no. 5, pp. 733–738, 2005.

[56] M. Dwivedi, H. Manocha, S. Tiwari, G. Tripathi, and T. N. Dhole, "Coinfection of parvovirus b19 with other hepatitis viruses leading to fulminant hepatitis of unfavorable outcome in children," *The Pediatric Infectious Disease Journal*, vol. 28, no. 7, pp. 649–650, 2009.

[57] Y. Osugi, H. Yagasaki, M. Sako et al., "Antithymocyte globulin and cyclosporine for treatment of 44 children with hepatitis associated aplastic anemia," *Haematologica*, vol. 92, no. 12, pp. 1687–1690, 2007.

[58] B. Rauff, M. Idrees, S. A. R. Shah et al., "Hepatitis associated aplastic anemia: a review," *Virology Journal*, vol. 8, article 87, 2011.

[59] R. Andreesen, W. Brugger, C. Thomssen, A. Rehm, B. Speck, and G. W. Lohr, "Defective monocyte-to-macrophage maturation in patients with aplastic anemia," *Blood*, vol. 74, no. 6, pp. 2150–2156, 1989.

[60] T. Muta, Y. Tanaka, E. Takeshita et al., "Recurrence of hepatitis-associated aplastic anemia after a 10-year Interval," *Internal Medicine*, vol. 47, no. 19, pp. 1733–1737, 2008.

[61] M. E. S. Zaki, S. A. Hassan, T. Seleim, and R. A. Lateef, "Parvovirus B19 infection in children with a variety of hematological disorders," *Hematology*, vol. 11, no. 4, pp. 261–266, 2006.

[62] S. Serke, T. F. Schwarz, H. Baurmann et al., "Productive infection of in vitro generated haemopoietic progenitor cells from normal human adult peripheral blood with parvovirus B19: studies by morphology, immunocytochemistry, flow-cytometry and DNA-hybridization," *British Journal of Haematology*, vol. 79, no. 1, pp. 6–13, 1991.

[63] T. Kudoh, Y. Yoto, N. Suzuki et al., "Human parvovirus B19-induced aplastic crisis in iron deficiency anemia," *Acta Paediatrica Japonica*, vol. 36, no. 4, pp. 448–449, 1994.

[64] G. Janka, "Hemophagocytic lymphohistiocytosis: when the immune system runs amok," *Klinische Padiatrie*, vol. 221, no. 5, pp. 278–285, 2009.

[65] M. P. Hoang, D. B. Dawson, Z. R. Rogers, R. H. Scheuermann, and B. B. Rogers, "Polymerase chain reaction amplification of archival material for Epstein-Barr virus, cytomegalovirus, human herpesvirus 6, and parvovirus B19 in children with bone

marrow hemophagocytosis," *Human Pathology*, vol. 29, no. 10, pp. 1074–1077, 1998.

[66] K. Shirono and H. Tsuda, "Parvovirus B19-associated haemophagocytic syndrome in healthy adults," *British Journal of Haematology*, vol. 89, no. 4, pp. 923–926, 1995.

[67] I.-J. Su, C.-H. Wang, A.-L. Cheng, and R.-L. Chen, "Hemophagocytic syndrome in Epstein-Barr virus-associated T-lymphoproliferative disorders: disease spectrum, pathogenesis, and management," *Leukemia and Lymphoma*, vol. 19, no. 5-6, pp. 401–406, 1995.

[68] M. M. Mustafa and K. L. McClain, "Diverse hematologic effects of parvovirus B19 infection," *Pediatric Clinics of North America*, vol. 43, no. 3, pp. 809–821, 1996.

[69] K. Smith-Whitley, H. Zhao, R. L. Hodinka et al., "Epidemiology of human parvovirus B19 in children with sickle cell disease," *Blood*, vol. 103, no. 2, pp. 422–427, 2004.

[70] The American Academy of Pediatrics Committee on Infectious Diseases, "Parvovirus B19," in *Red Book: Report of the Committee on Infectious Diseases*, L. K. Pickering, C. J. Baker, D. W. Kimberlin, and S. S. Long, Eds., pp. 491–493, The American Academy of Peiatrics, Elk Grove Village, Ill, USA, 28th edition, 2009.

[71] C. K. Fairley, J. S. Smoleniec, O. E. Caul, and E. Miller, "Observational study of effect of intrauterine transfusions on outcome of fetal hydrops after parvovirus B19 infection," *The Lancet*, vol. 346, no. 8986, pp. 1335–1337, 1995.

[72] M. Söderlund-Venermo, K. Hokynar, J. Nieminen, H. Rautakorpi, and K. Hedman, "Persistence of human parvovirus B19 in human tissues," *Pathologie Biologie*, vol. 50, no. 5, pp. 307–316, 2002.

[73] G. L. Mandell, J. E. Bennet, and R. Dolin, *Mandell, Douglas and Bennett's Principals and Practice of Infectious Diseases*, vol. 2, Churchill Livingstone, Philadelphia, Pa, USA, 6th edition, 2005.

[74] E. Morita, A. Nakashima, H. Asao, H. Sato, and K. Sugamura, "Human parvovirus B19 nonstructural protein (NS1) induces cell cycle arrest at G1 phase," *Journal of Virology*, vol. 77, no. 5, pp. 2915–2921, 2003.

[75] L. L. W. Cooling, T. A. W. Koerner, and S. J. Naides, "Multiple glycosphingolipids determine the tissue tropism of parvovirus B19," *Journal of Infectious Diseases*, vol. 172, no. 5, pp. 1198–1205, 1995.

[76] B. D. Poole, Y. V. Karetnyi, and S. J. Naides, "Parvovirus B19-induced apoptosis of hepatocytes," *Journal of Virology*, vol. 78, no. 14, pp. 7775–7783, 2004.

[77] N. S. Young and J. Maciejewski, "The pathophysiology of acquired aplastic anemia," *The New England Journal of Medicine*, vol. 336, no. 19, pp. 1365–1372, 1997.

[78] K. Doney, W. Leisenring, R. Storb, and F. R. Appelbaum, "Primary treatment of acquired aplastic anemia: outcomes with bone marrow transplantation and immunosuppressive therapy," *Annals of Internal Medicine*, vol. 126, no. 2, pp. 107–115, 1997.

Transforming Growth Factor-β1 Gene Polymorphism (T29C) in Egyptian Patients with Hepatitis B Virus Infection: A Preliminary Study

Roba M. Talaat,[1] Mahmoud F. Dondeti,[1] Soha Z. El-Shenawy,[2] and Omaima A. Khamiss[3]

[1] *Molecular Biology Department, Genetic Engineering and Biotechnology Research Institute (GEBRI), University of Sadat City, Sadat City 22857, Egypt*

[2] *Biochemistry Department, National Liver Institute (NLI), Menoufiya University, Shebeen El-Kom, Menoufiya 32511, Egypt*

[3] *Animal Biotechnology Department, Genetic Engineering and Biotechnology Research Institute (GEBRI), University of Sadat City, Sadat City 22857, Egypt*

Correspondence should be addressed to Roba M. Talaat; robamtalaat@yahoo.com

Academic Editor: Piero Luigi Almasio

The interindividual variations in the capacity of transforming growth factor-β1 (TGF-β1) production have been ascribed to genetic polymorphisms in TGF-β1 gene. As pathogenesis of HBV has a genetic background, this preliminary study was designed to assess the impact of TGF-β1 (T29C) on the susceptibility of Egyptians to HBV infection. Genotyping was performed using single stranded polymorphism-polymerase chain reaction (SSP-PCR) in 65 Egyptian hepatitis B patients and 50 healthy controls. TGF-β1 plasma levels were measured using Enzyme-linked immunosorbent assay (ELISA). The frequency of CC genotype was significantly higher ($P < 0.05$) in HBV patients compared to controls. On the contrary, TC genotype did not show significant difference in both groups. TT genotype was significantly higher ($P < 0.01$) in controls than HBV patients. Our current preliminary data revealed that the frequency of the genotypes in the controls were within Hardy-Weinberg equilibrium (HWE) while the patients group was out of HWE ($P < 0.01$). TGF-β1 was significantly ($r = -0.684$; $P < 0.001$) deceased in the sera of patients as compared to normal subjects. Depending on our preliminary work, CC genotype may act as a host genetic factor in the susceptibility to HBV infection in Egyptians. Taken together, the current data pointed to the importance of polymorphism of TGF-β1 gene (T29C) in HBV infection.

1. Introduction

Hepatitis B virus infection (HBV) is a worldwide problem and it is still the main factor of developing chronic HBV, cirrhosis, and hepatocellular carcinoma (HCC), especially in developing countries [1]. There are about 400 million carriers of HBV infection worldwide and over 1 million deaths occur each year as a consequence of fulminant hepatic failure, cirrhosis, and hepatocellular carcinoma [2]. Moreover, 5–10% of infected individuals cannot clear the infection, which leads to a chronic carrier state with or without liver disease chronic [3]. The interaction of the host immune response with HBV, the impact of this interaction on the clinical outcome, and the factors of viral persistence are not yet fully understood. Host genetic factors have been reported to be critical factors which affect the natural history of liver diseases [4].

Transforming growth factor-β1 (TGF-β1) is a multifunctional cytokine that regulates cell growth, proliferation, and differentiation [5]. It is produced by several cell types, including monocytes, macrophages, endothelial cells, and vascular smooth muscle cell [6, 7] and it is also produced from a variety of liver cell populations including HSCs, hepatocytes, and LSECs in addition to platelets and infiltrating mononuclear cells [8, 9]. TGF-β1 is key molecule in many physiological processes in the liver since it induces apoptosis and reduces hepatocytes proliferation besides its essential role in hepatic fibrogenesis. Host genetic factors play a critical role in developing fibrosis whereas many genes are reported to be associated with liver fibrosis and cirrhosis including TGF-β1 [10]. In addition, TGF-β1 has potential impact on the immune response since it has immunosuppressive effects like its inhibitory effect on T-cells proliferation via IL-2 down-regulation [11]. TGF-β1 gene is located on chromosome 19q13.1–13.3 with 7 exons and 6 introns [12, 13]. Several polymorphisms in both coding and non-coding regions of the TGF-β1 gene have been reported and found to affect TGF-β1 protein expression [14]. There is a functional single nucleotide polymorphism (SNP) at the 29th nucleotide (T29C), 868 nt relative to the transcription start site, (rs1982073 merged into rs1800470) in exon 1 with transition from T to C resulting in amino change in the region encoding the signal sequence from Leucine to Proline at the 10th amino acid [14–16]. This transition disrupts the structure [17, 18] and results in increased levels of TGF-β1 protein and mRNA in individuals with C allele with a 2.8-fold increase in TGF-β1 secretion compared with T allele in vitro [16, 19–21]. Additionally, the substitutions of amino acid residue might affect the function of the signal peptide, possibly by influencing intracellular trafficking or export efficiency of the TGF-β1 protein [20]. It was also reported that C allele of 29T/C is associated with increased TGF-β1 serum levels, thereby the T29C polymorphism maybe influence the development and severity of TGF-β1-related diseases and it has been associated with susceptibility to several diseases [7, 20, 22, 23]. Thus, this preliminary study was tailored to investigate the role of TGF-β1 gene (T29C) in HBV infection in Egyptians. No such study has been conducted to investigate the association between SNP in TGF-β1 gene (T29C) and HBV infection in Egypt.

2. Materials and Methods

2.1. Patients and Controls. Sixty five patients with chronic HBV infection were recruited from the National Liver Institute, Menoufiya University, Egypt, were enrolled in this study. The males over numbered the females (53 men and 12 women) with mean age of 44.93 ± 11.57 years (range: 68–22). The demographic and biochemical characteristics are presented in Table 1. Fifty healthy controls with no history of previous liver disease, normal liver function tests, and negative HBV and HCV serology were enrolled in the study. Patients with HCV or other viral infections or any liver diseases were excluded from the study. All investigations were performed in accordance with the Menoufiya University, Health and Human Ethical Clearance Committee guidelines for Clinical Researches. Local Ethics Committee approved the study protocol and informed consents were got from all subjects.

2.2. Viral Assessment. Hepatitis B surface antigen (HBsAg) was tested using a commercial kit (Sorin Biomedica, Milan, Italy) while HBV-DNA in HBV-positive patients was tested by polymerase chain reaction (PCR), (Roche Diagnostics Corp., Indianapolis, IN). HCV antibodies were tested by using enzyme-linked immunosorbent assay (ELISA) (Murex Biotech Ltd., Dartford, UK) All patients were positive for HBsAg, HBV-DNA, and negative for HCV antibodies. Alanine aminotransferase (ALT), aspartate aminotransferase (AST) (bioMérieux S.A, Marcy l'Etoile, France), direct and indirect bilirubin (Roche Diagnostics Corp., Indianapolis, IN), and albumin (Human Gesellschaft Fur Biochemica Und

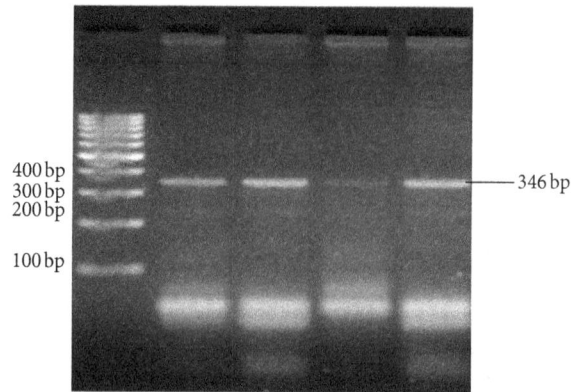

FIGURE 1: TGF-β1 (T29C) PCR products of two samples. Sample 1 in lane (2 and 3) TC genotype; sample 2 in lane (4 and 5) CC genotype and lane (1) 100 bp ladder.

Diagnostica Mbh, Wiesbaden, Germany) were all measured according to their respective kits' manufacturers' instructions.

2.3. DNA Isolation. Blood samples were collected by withdrawal of 5 mL venous blood from each individual involved in this study into sterile vacutainer tubes containing EDTA.K$_3$, and then the tubes were centrifuged at 1500 rpm for 10 minutes. Plasma was separated, aliquoted, and stored at $-80°$C for cytokine secretion analysis. Genomic DNA was extracted from whole blood-EDTA samples by Wizard Genomic DNA Purification Kit (Promega Corporation, Madison, USA) according to manufacturer's instructions.

2.4. Genotyping. TGF-β1 T29C was genotyped by single stranded polymorphism-polymerase chain reaction (SSP-PCR) [24] using the following primers: T allele specific primer 5-CTCCGGGCTGCGGCTGCTGCT-3, C allele specific primer 5-CTC CGG GCT GCG GCT GCT GCC-3, and reverse common primer 5-GTT GTG GGT TTC CAC CAT TAG-3 [15]. The PCR reaction was performed in two tubes in which each tube contains forward primer specific to one allele in addition to generic primer. The final total volume for each PCR reaction was 25μL. PCR reaction ingredients were DreamTaq Green Master Mix 2x (Fermentas, Thermo Fisher Scientific Inc.), 10 P moles of each primer (Metabion, Martinsried, Deutschland) and 0.1μg DNA. The PCR cycling was the following; one cycle of $94°$C for 5 minutes followed by 35 cycles of $96°$C for 30 seconds, $59°$C for 30 seconds, $72°$C for 55 seconds, and a final extension step of 5 minutes. PCR reaction was performed in Biometra thermal cycler (Biometra GmbH, Germany). The PCR products were visualized on 2% agarose gel and estimated in comparison to 100 bp DNA ladder (Fermentas, Thermo Fisher Scientific Inc.). The size of PCR product for TGF-β1 T29C primers was 346 bp for T or C allele (Figure 1).

2.5. Measurement of Plasma TGF-β1. TGF-β1 plasma levels were measured in HBV patients and normal controls by sandwich enzyme linked immunosorbent assay (ELISA)

TABLE 1: Demographic and biochemical characteristics of HBV patients and healthy controls.

Parameter	Control group ($N = 65$)	HBV group ($N = 50$)	P	Correlation with disease
Demographic data				
Age (mean ± SD)	44.92 ± 11.76	32.11 ± 14.89	NS	$r = 0.437$ $P < 0.001$
Gender (Male ♂: Female ♀)	53/12 (81.5/18.5%)	14/36 (28%/72%)	$P < 0.001$	$r = 0.523$ $P < 0.001$
Laboratory investigations (mean ± SD)				
AST (IU/L)	41.59 ± 3.47	22.18 ± 1.05	$P < 0.001$	$r = 0.473$ $P < 0.001$
ALT (IU/L)	44.49 ± 5.61	16.74 ± 0.86	$P < 0.01$	$r = 0.455$ $P < 0.001$
Albumin (g/L)	3.37 ± 0.12	4.35 ± 0.07	$P < 0.01$	$r = -0.625$ $P < 0.001$
Total bilirubin (mg/dL)	1.03 ± 0.08	0.70 ± 0.04	$P < 0.05$	$r = 0.381$ $P < 0.01$
Direct bilirubin (mg/dL)	0.25 ± 0.06	0.12 ± 0.03	$P < 0.05$	$r = 0.198$ NS
Creatinine (mg/dL)	1.11 ± 0.06	0.89 ± 0.03	$P < 0.01$	$r = 0.332$ $P < 0.01$
Urea (mg/dL)	33.16 ± 2.26	29.85 ± 1.41	$P < 0.01$	$r = 0.130$ NS
HBV DNA (IU/L)	—	1003076.02 ± 914392.11	—	$r = 0.168$ $P < 0.05$

All data are presented as mean ± SD. Alanine aminotransferase (ALT); Aspartate aminotransferase (AST).

(R&D System, Inc., Minneapolis, USA) according to manufacturer's instructions. The ELISA reader-controlling software (Softmax, Molecular Devices Corp., USA) readily processed the digital data of raw absorbance value into a standard curve from which cytokine concentrations of unknown samples can be derived directly and expressed as pg/mL.

2.6. Statistical Analysis. The statistical analyses were performed by SPSS statistical package version 19 (SPSS, IBM Corporation, USA). Comparisons were made using independent *t*-test and results were presented as mean ± SD. Chi-squared tests were performed to examine the differences in the allele frequency and genotype distribution between different groups. Odds ratios (with 95% CI) were calculated to measure the relative risks in both control and HBV patients. All P values were two-tailed, and P values <0.05 were considered to be statistically significant.

3. Results

3.1. Association between TGF-β1 Gene (T29C) Polymorphism and Hepatitis B Infection. TGF-β1 T29C genotypes and allele frequencies in controls and patients are shown in (Table 2). The frequency of TGF-β1 (T29C) genotypes in the controls were within Hardy-Weinberg equilibrium (HWE) while they were out of HWE ($P < 0.01$) in the patients group. Genotyping of TGF-β1 T29C showed a significant decrease ($P < 0.01$) in the distribution of TT genotype in controls in comparison to HBV patients (44.4% versus 16.9%, for control and HBV, resp.). While CC genotype was not detected in the

control group while it appeared in the patient group with a percentage of 15.4%. On the contrary, the frequency of TC genotype was insignificantly different in normal controls compared with HBV patients. C allele was significantly ($P < 0.01$) more frequent in HBV patients more than controls groups while distribution of T allele did not show significant difference between both groups (92.6%, 84.6% for T allele versus 55.6%, 83.1% for C allele in control and HBV, resp.).

3.2. Plasma Levels of TGF-β1 in HBV and Normal Controls and Its Differential Expression according to TGF-β1 T29C. Mean plasma levels were significantly lower ($P < 0.001$) in HBV patients than controls (63.48 ± 7.59 pg/mL versus 12151.76 ± 2124.90 pg/mL). Hepatitis B was significantly correlated with a reduction in TGF-β1 plasma levels ($r = -0.684$; $P < 0.001$). The comparisons between concentration of plasma TGF-β1 levels with different genotypes in both controls and HBV patients are shown in (Table 3). The reduction in TGF-β1 secretion levels, observed in HBV patients compared to normal controls, were relevant to TGF-β1 T29C genotypes. Thus, CC genotype was responsible for the significant decrease of TGF-β1 level between both groups while TT genotype was relevant to high TGF-β1 serum level.

4. Discussion

Genetic susceptibility to chronic HBV infection and other infectious diseases may reside in the variability in host recognition, cytokine, or antigen presenting and processing genes [25]. Since genetic interactions are complex, it is unlikely

TABLE 2: Genotype and allelic frequencies of the TGF-β1 T29C in patients with hepatitis B and healthy controls.

SNP	HBV group ($N = 65$)	Control group ($N = 50$)	P	OR (95% CI)
		Genotype frequency (N, %)		
T/T	11 (16.9%)	12 (44.4%)	$P < 0.01$	0.2546 (0.0938–0.6910)
T/C	44 (67.7%)	15 (55.6%)	NS	1.6762 (0.6680–4.2062)
C/C	10 (15.4%)	0 (0.0%)	$P < 0.05$	10.4054 (0.5878–184.1951)
TCCC	54 (83.1%)	15 (55.6%)	$P < 0.05$	3.2000 (1.1697–8.7541)
		Allele frequency		
T	66 (84.6%)	39 (92.6%)	NS	0.3966 (0.1994–0.7889)
C	64 (83.1%)	15 (55.6%)	$P < 0.01$	2.5212 (1.2676–5.0147)

TABLE 3: Comparison between mean serum concentrations of TGF-β1 according to TGF-β1 T29C in hepatitis B patients and healthy controls.

Genotype (Control, HBV)	Control group ($N = 65$)	HBV group ($N = 27$)	P
T/T (11, 12)	11577.47 ± 3111.76	83.89 ± 21.15	$P < 0.001$
T/C (44, 15)	1289.61 ± 2919.49	63.72 ± 9.46	$P < 0.001$
C/C (10, 0)	—	39.94 ± 10.21	$P < 0.001$

that a single allelic variant is responsible for HBV resistance or susceptibility [26]. The ongoing study of the distributions and functions of the implicated allele polymorphisms will not only provide insight into the pathogenesis of HBV infection, but may also provide a novel rationale for new methods of diagnosis and therapeutic strategies [27]. The aim of studying such polymorphisms and their association with diseases is to enhance the understanding of the etiology and pathology of human disease, and to identify potential markers of susceptibility, severity, and clinical outcome, and to identify potential markers for responders versus nonresponders in therapeutic trials, and to identify targets for therapeutic intervention, in addition to identify novel strategies to prevent disease or to improve existing preventions such as vaccines [28]. The majority of the human genetic studies associated with HBV infection have focused on HLA associations [29, 30]. There are many studies of host genetic factors especially cytokine genes that influence the immune response mounted against HBV infection [31]. In addition, Cytokine gene polymorphisms have been reported to be associated with liver disease severity in patients with viral hepatitis [10, 25] besides their impact on the cytokines production capacity [32–34]; therefore, heterogeneity of the candidate gene in HBV-infected patients serves as a probable biomarker for influence the disease phenotypes.

Several polymorphisms located in genes that code pro- and anti-inflammatory molecules have been reported to be associated with HBV infection. Moreover, more light was shed on TGF-β1 since it is a central regulator in immuno-inflammatory mechanisms. Therefore, this preliminary was conducted to investigate the role of polymorphisms in TGF-β1 gene and HBV infection among Egyptians. In the present preliminary study TGF-β1 T29C was studied in 65 Egyptian hepatitis B patients and 50 healthy controls. The common T29C transition in TGF-β1, resulting in a Leu10Pro substitution in the signal peptide sequence, is a good candidate

locus because it has been associated with higher levels of circulating TGF-β1 [16, 22] especially the presence of the C allele in exon 1 results in increasing the production of TGF-β1 [7, 16, 19, 35, 36]. Interestingly, Gewaltig et al., reported that the presence of C allele at TGF-β1 (T29C) either C/C or C/T genotype, was associated with higher stage of fibrosis in HCV-infected patients [10].

Our preliminary results showed that TT genotype, which was more frequent in controls than HBV patients, was associated with higher significant levels of serum TGF-β1. Additionally, the plasma levels were significantly higher in the controls more than the patients and this is contradictory to previous results which showed that T allele was associated with lower level of TGF-β1 [15, 20, 22, 37] and C allele was associated with higher TGF-β1 levels [38, 39]. On the other hand, our preliminary results were consistent with other studies of [40, 41] in which TGF-β1 serum levels were lower in the subjects with the CC homozygote than in those with the TT homozygote at T29C of TGF-β1 gene. According to our preliminary study and previous studies, there is momentous discrepancy in the revealed results but this can be attributed to the differential genetic background of investigated populations and the different ethnicity of studied populations. In addition, there are other studies which have failed to reveal any association between serum TGF-β1 levels and SNP at TGF-β1 (T29C) [41, 42]. In conclusion, our preliminary results may suggest the protective role of TT genotype against HBV infection and this will need to be confirmed further in a large study. On the other hand, CC genotype was hardly detected in controls and this may indicate the involvement of this genotype in the susceptibility of HBV infection and consequences.

There is shortcoming in the current study that it depended on one group of cases in addition to the number of subjects enrolled in the study and this made the elucidation of some results a hard and onerous task as we cannot confirm the relationship between the current findings and the progression of the infection, so the study had to include other categories of the disease as groups of cirrhotic and HBV patients with HCC. Studying genetic polymorphisms in TGF-β1 gene will clear the precise role of TGF-β1 in the pathogenesis of HBV infection and its role in the susceptibility to HBV infection as TGF-β1 has a deep impact on the immune response. Therefore, we are performing genotyping of TGF-β1 gene in large number of patients and studying many SNPs as TGF-β1-800G/A, TGF-β1-509C/T, TGF-β1+869T/C, and TGF-β1+915G/C to study the relation between TGF-β1 gene polymorphism and HBV infection and to confirm the current preliminary results.

Conflict of Interests

The authors declare that there is no conflict of interests.

Acknowledgments

This work is a part of a grant from the Egyptian Academy of Scientific Research and Technology (ASRT), Egypt. The sponsors did not participate in the study design, the collection, analysis and interpretation of data, the paper drafting, and the decision to submit the paper for publication.

References

[1] M. J. Sonneveld, V. Rijckborst, C. A. B. Boucher, B. E. Hansen, and H. L. A. Janssen, "Prediction of sustained response to peginterferon alfa-2b for hepatitis B e antigen-positive chronic hepatitis B using on-treatment hepatitis B surface antigen decline," *Hepatology*, vol. 52, no. 4, pp. 1251–1257, 2010.

[2] M. C. Kew, "Epidemiology of chronic hepatitis B virus infection, hepatocellular carcinoma, and hepatitis B virus-induced hepatocellular carcinoma," *Pathologie Biologie*, vol. 58, no. 4, pp. 273–277, 2010.

[3] G. Fattovich, "Natural history and prognosis of hepatitis B," *Seminars in Liver Disease*, vol. 23, no. 1, pp. 47–58, 2003.

[4] R. Bataller, K. E. North, and D. A. Brenner, "Genetic polymorphisms and the progression of liver fibrosis: a critical appraisal," *Hepatology*, vol. 37, no. 3, pp. 493–503, 2003.

[5] J. Massague, "TGFbeta in cancer," *Cell*, vol. 134, no. 2, pp. 215–230, 2008.

[6] W. A. Border and N. A. Noble, "Transforming growth factor β in tissue fibrosis," *The New England Journal of Medicine*, vol. 331, no. 19, pp. 1286–1292, 1994.

[7] B. Li, A. Khanna, V. Sharma, T. Singh, M. Suthanthiran, and P. August, "TGF-β1 DNA polymorphisms, protein levels, and blood pressure," *Hypertension*, vol. 33, no. 1, pp. 271–275, 1999.

[8] P. Bedossa and V. Paradis, "Transforming growth factor-β (TGF-β): a key-role in liver fibrogenesis," *Journal of Hepatology*, vol. 22, supplement 2, pp. 37–42, 1995.

[9] A. M. Gressner, "Cytokines and cellular crosstalk involved in the activation of fat-storing cells," *Journal of Hepatology*, vol. 22, supplement 2, pp. 28–36, 1995.

[10] J. Gewaltig, K. Mangasser-Stephan, C. Gartung, S. Biesterfeld, and A. M. Gressner, "Association of polymorphisms of the transforming growth factor-β1 gene with the rate of progression of HCV-induced liver fibrosis," *Clinica Chimica Acta*, vol. 316, no. 1-2, pp. 83–94, 2002.

[11] J. H. Kehrl, L. M. Wakefield, A. B. Roberts et al., "Production of transforming growth factor β by human T lymphocytes and its potential role in the regulation of T cell growth," *Journal of Experimental Medicine*, vol. 163, no. 5, pp. 1037–1050, 1986.

[12] D. Fujii, J. E. Brissenden, R. Derynck, and U. Francke, "Transforming growth factor β gene maps to human chromosome 19 long arm and to mouse chromosome 7," *Somatic Cell and Molecular Genetics*, vol. 12, no. 3, pp. 281–288, 1986.

[13] R. Derynck, L. Rhee, E. Y. Chen, and A. van Tilburg, "Intron-exon structure of the human transforming growth factor-β precursor gene," *Nucleic Acids Research*, vol. 15, no. 7, pp. 3188–3189, 1987.

[14] Y. Watanabe, A. Kinoshita, T. Yamada et al., "A catalog of 106 single-nucleotide polymorphisms (SNPs) and 11 other types of variations in genes for transforming growth factor-β1 (TGF-β1) and its signaling pathway," *Journal of Human Genetics*, vol. 47, no. 9, pp. 478–483, 2002.

[15] Y. Yamada, A. Miyauchi, J. Goto et al., "Association of a polymorphism of the transforming growth factor-β1 gene with genetic susceptibility to osteoporosis in postmenopausal Japanese women," *Journal of Bone and Mineral Research*, vol. 13, no. 10, pp. 1569–1576, 1998.

[16] D. J. Grainger, K. Heathcote, M. Chiano et al., "Genetic control of the circulating concentration of transforming growth factor type β1," *Human Molecular Genetics*, vol. 8, no. 1, pp. 93–97, 1999.

[17] L. L. Randall and S. J. S. Hardy, "Unity in function in the absence of consensus in sequence: role of leader peptides in export," *Science*, vol. 243, no. 4895, pp. 1156–1159, 1989.

[18] F. Cambien, S. Ricard, A. Troesch et al., "Polymorphisms of the transforming growth factor-β1 gene in relation to myocardial infarction and blood pressure: the Etude Cas-Temoin de l'Infarctus du Myocarde (ECTIM) study," *Hypertension*, vol. 28, no. 5, pp. 881–887, 1996.

[19] M. Suthanthiran, B. Li, J. O. Song et al., "Transforming growth factor-β1 hyperexpression in African-American hypertensives: a novel mediator of hypertension and/or target organ damage," *Proceedings of the National Academy of Sciences of the United States of America*, vol. 97, no. 7, pp. 3479–3484, 2000.

[20] A. M. Dunning, P. D. Ellis, S. McBride et al., "A transforming growth factorβ1 signal peptide variant increases secretion in vitro and is associated with increased incidence of invasive breast cancer," *Cancer Research*, vol. 63, no. 10, pp. 2610–2615, 2003.

[21] J. Kirshner, M. F. Jobling, M. J. Pajares et al., "Inhibition of transforming growth factor-β1 signaling attenuates ataxia telangiectasia mutated activity in response to genotoxic stress," *Cancer Research*, vol. 66, no. 22, pp. 10861–10869, 2006.

[22] M. Yokota, S. Ichihara, T.-L. Lin, N. Nakashima, and Y. Yamada, "Association of a T29 → C polymorphism of the transforming growth factor-β1 gene with genetic susceptibility to myocardial infarction in japanese," *Circulation*, vol. 101, no. 24, pp. 2783–2787, 2000.

[23] L. Le Marchand, C. A. Haiman, D. van den Berg, L. R. Wilkens, L. N. Kolonel, and B. E. Henderson, "T29C polymorphism in the transforming growth factor β1 gene and postmenopausal breast cancer risk: the multiethnic cohort study," *Cancer Epidemiology Biomarkers and Prevention*, vol. 13, no. 3, pp. 412–415, 2004.

[24] K. Welsh and M. Bunce, "Molecular typing for the MHC with PCR SSP," *Reviews in Immunogenetics*, vol. 1, no. 2, pp. 157–176, 1999.

[25] E. E. Powell, C. J. Edwards-Smith, J. L. Hay et al., "Host genetic factors influence disease progression in chronic hepatitis C," *Hepatology*, vol. 31, no. 4, pp. 828–833, 2000.

[26] P. D. Griffiths, "Interactions between viral and human genes," *Reviews in Medical Virology*, vol. 12, no. 4, pp. 197–199, 2002.

[27] M. Dean, M. Carrington, and S. J. O'Brien, "Balanced polymorphism selected by genetic versus infectious human disease," *Annual Review of Genomics and Human Genetics*, vol. 3, pp. 263–292, 2002.

[28] J. Bidwell, L. Keen, G. Gallagher et al., "Cytokine gene polymorphism in human disease: on-line databases," *Genes and Immunity*, vol. 1, no. 1, pp. 3–19, 1999.

[29] M. Thursz, "Genetic susceptibility in chronic viral hepatitis," *Antiviral Research*, vol. 52, no. 2, pp. 113–116, 2001.

[30] A. Almarri and J. R. Batchelor, "HLA and hepatitis B infection," *The Lancet*, vol. 344, no. 8931, pp. 1194–1195, 1994.

[31] Z. Ben-Ari, E. Mor, O. Papo et al., "Cytokine gene polymorphisms in patients infected with hepatitis B virus," *American Journal of Gastroenterology*, vol. 98, no. 1, pp. 144–150, 2003.

[32] R. G. J. Westendorp, J. A. M. Langermans, T. W. J. Huizinga et al., "Genetic influence on cytokine production and fatal meningococcal disease," *The Lancet*, vol. 349, no. 9046, pp. 170–173, 1997.

[33] J. L. Bidwell, N. A. P. Wood, H. R. Morse, O. O. Olomolaiye, L. J. Keen, and G. J. Laundy, "Human cytokine gene nucleotide sequence alignments," *European Journal of Immunogenetics*, vol. 26, no. 2-3, pp. 135–223, 1999.

[34] S. J. H. van Deventer, "Cytokine and cytokine receptor polymorphisms in infectious disease," *Intensive Care Medicine*, vol. 26, supplement 1, pp. S98–S102, 2000.

[35] J. C. Celedón, C. Lange, B. A. Raby et al., "The transforming growth factor-β1 (TGFB1) gene is associated with Chronic Obstructive Pulmonary Disease (COPD)," *Human Molecular Genetics*, vol. 13, no. 15, pp. 1649–1656, 2004.

[36] E. S. Silverman, L. J. Palmer, V. Subramaniam et al., "Transforming growth factor-β1 promoter polymorphism C-509T is associated with asthma," *American Journal of Respiratory and Critical Care Medicine*, vol. 169, no. 2, pp. 214–219, 2004.

[37] L. Wu, J. Chau, R. P. Young et al., "Transforming growth factor-β1 genotype and susceptibility to chronic obstructive pulmonary disease," *Thorax*, vol. 59, no. 2, pp. 126–129, 2004.

[38] Y. Yamada, "Association of polymorphisms of the transforming growth factor-β1 gene with genetic susceptibility to osteoporosis," *Pharmacogenetics*, vol. 11, no. 9, pp. 765–771, 2001.

[39] A. M. González-Zuloeta Ladd, A. Arias-Vásquez, C. Siemes et al., "Transforming-growth factor β1 Leu10Pro polymorphism and breast cancer morbidity," *European Journal of Cancer*, vol. 43, no. 2, pp. 371–374, 2007.

[40] P. D. Arkwright, S. Laurie, M. Super et al., "TGF-β1 genotype and accelerated decline in lung function of patients with cystic fibrosis," *Thorax*, vol. 55, no. 6, pp. 459–462, 2000.

[41] V. Hinke, T. Seck, C. Clanget, C. Scheidt-Nave, R. Ziegler, and J. Pfeilschifter, "Association of transforming growth factor-β1 (TGFβ1) T29 $\rightarrow$ C gene polymorphism with bone mineral density (BMD), changes in BMD, and serum concentrations of TGF-β1 in a population-based sample of postmenopausal German women," *Calcified Tissue International*, vol. 69, no. 6, pp. 315–320, 2001.

[42] X. Li, Z.-C. Yue, Y.-Y. Zhang et al., "Elevated serum level and gene polymorphisms of TGF-β1 in gastric cancer," *Journal of Clinical Laboratory Analysis*, vol. 22, no. 3, pp. 164–171, 2008.

21

Prevalence of *Hepatitis E Virus* among Adults in South-West of Iran

Fatemeh Farshadpour,[1,2] **Reza Taherkhani,**[1,3] **and Manoochehr Makvandi**[4]

[1]*Department of Microbiology and Parasitology, School of Medicine, Bushehr University of Medical Sciences, Bushehr 7514633341, Iran*
[2]*Persian Gulf Tropical Medicine Research Center, Bushehr University of Medical Sciences, Bushehr 7514633341, Iran*
[3]*Persian Gulf Biomedical Research Center, Bushehr University of Medical Sciences, Bushehr 7514633341, Iran*
[4]*Health Research Institute, Infectious and Tropical Disease Research Center, Ahvaz Jundishapur University of Medical Sciences, Ahvaz 6135715794, Iran*

Correspondence should be addressed to Reza Taherkhani; taherkhanireza2005@yahoo.com

Academic Editor: Piero Luigi Almasio

Background. Knowledge regarding prevalence of HEV in general population can be an indicator of the public health and hygiene. Therefore, this study was conducted to evaluate the prevalence of HEV among adults in South-West of Iran. *Methods.* Blood samples were taken from 510 participants, 206 (40.4%) males and 304 (59.6%) females from February to July 2014. Detection of anti-HEV IgG and IgM antibodies was carried out by ELISA test. *Results.* The overall anti-HEV IgG and IgM prevalence rates were 46.1% and 1.4%, respectively. Anti-HEV IgG and IgM seropositivity were not statistically associated with gender and race/ethnicity. Meanwhile, there were significant differences between the age groups regarding HEV IgG and IgM seropositivity. HEV IgG seroprevalence increased with age from 14.3% in subjects aged 18–30 years to 71.4% in persons over 71 years old, and considerably individuals aged 61 to 70 years had the highest HEV prevalence (90.9%). Also, 5.7% in the age group 18–30 years and 2.2% in the age group 31–40 years were positive for anti-HEV IgM antibodies and the highest rate was observed in subjects aged 18–30 years. *Conclusion.* In conclusion, high HEV IgG seroprevalence of 46.1% was observed among adults in South-West of Iran.

1. Introduction

Hepatitis E virus (HEV) is a nonenveloped, single stranded RNA virus which belongs to the Hepeviridae family [1]. HEV is a causative agent for acute hepatitis in one-third of the world's population and fulminant hepatitis in pregnant women [2]. The virion is relatively resistant to environmental conditions and remains infectious even in rough situation such as sewage [3]. Therefore the major route of HEV transmission is the ingestion of the fecal contaminated water; however, HEV can be spread zoonotically and by blood transfusion especially in industrialized countries [4]. Although there is an inclusive debate on the parental route of transmission, available evidence seems to prove the ability of the virus to cause congenital infections [5].

HEV infection is a significant public health concern especially in developing countries, where large outbreaks as a result of poor sanitation and lack of sewage infrastructures

have been reported [6]. There is also a growing support for the claims that seroprevalence of HEV infection in industrialized countries is increasing [6].

The clinical symptoms of HEV infection resemble other hepatotropic viruses which cause hepatitis [7]. Patients with chronic liver disease, travelers to endemic areas, and people working with animals like pigs, cows, sheep, and goats are at high risk of HEV infection [5, 8–10]. Pregnant women infected in third semester develop fulminant hepatic failure particularly in the endemic areas of HEV infection [11, 12].

Iran is an endemic country for hepatitis E infection [7, 13], but HEV prevalence has not been determined among general population in all parts of this country. Most conducted studies in Iran have reported the HEV prevalence in specific groups and studies on HEV prevalence in general populations are limited. HEV prevalence information in general population can be a better indicator of the public health and hygiene.

TABLE 1: Prevalence of anti-HEV IgG antibody according to gender, race, and age groups in adult population of Ahvaz city, Iran.

	Number of all participants (%): 510 (100%)	Number of anti-HEV IgG positive subjects (%): 235 (46.1%)	Number of anti-HEV IgG negative subjects (%): 275 (53.9%)	P value
Gender				0.106
Male	206 (40.4%)	86 (41.7%)	120 (58.3%)	
Female	304 (59.6%)	149 (49%)	155 (51%)	
Race				0.168
Arab	274 (53.7%)	134 (48.9%)	140 (51.1%)	
Farsi	236 (46.3%)	101 (42.8%)	135 (57.2%)	
Age groups (years)				<0.001
18–30	70 (13.7%)	10 (14.3%)	60 (85.7%)	
31–40	135 (26.5%)	25 (18.5%)	110 (81.5%)	
41–50	135 (26.5%)	55 (40.7%)	80 (59.3)	
51–60	80 (15.7%)	70 (87.5%)	10 (12.5%)	
60–71	55 (10.8%)	50 (90.9%)	5 (9.1%)	
>71	35 (6.9%)	25 (71.4%)	10 (28.6%)	

Ahvaz is a large city in the South-West of Iran with a population of about 1.18 million inhabitants that consists of two ethnic groups: Arab and Farsi. Ahvaz is located in the banks of the Karun River, which is the main river in this area. No data is available so far on the prevalence of HEV among general population of Ahvaz city; therefore this study was conducted to determine the prevalence of HEV among adults in South-West of Iran.

2. Material and Methods

This cross-sectional study was approved by the Ethical Committee of Ahvaz Jundishapur University of Medical Science with research Project number 91112. To estimate the prevalence of anti-HEV IgG and IgM antibodies in the general population of Ahvaz city, 510 blood samples from the adult population of Ahvaz city were collected randomly using the multistage cluster sampling method from February to July 2014. Ahvaz is a large city in the South-West of Iran that consists of 8 districts and has 94 public health centers. In the first stage, 4 public health centers were selected randomly from each district. In the next stage, the family registry code was used to randomly select 16 households within each public health center. From each family, one subject was selected randomly. The trained interviewers visited the subjects in their homes and completed a questionnaire containing information of age, gender, and race/ethnicity for each individual. In addition, the informed consent was obtained from all participants. The subjects who refused to participate in the study were replaced with the next random participants. Blood samples were taken from participants. The serum samples were tested in duplicate for anti-HEV IgG and IgM antibodies by using DIA.PRO HEV Ab ELISA kit and HEV IgM ELISA kit (DIA.PRO, Italy) according to the manufacturer's instructions.

Statistical analyses were performed using SPSS 17 Package program (SPSS Inc., Chicago, IL, USA) and P values of less

than 0.05 were considered statistically significant. Data were analyzed and compared by descriptive statistics and Chi-square test or Fisher's exact test. All data were presented as frequencies or percentage.

3. Results

Out of 510 study subjects, 206 (40.4%) were male and 304 (59.6%) were female. The average age of participants was varying from 18 to 81 years while the mean age ± SD was 45.89 ± 14.63 years. The subjects were classified into six age groups: 18–30, 31–40, 41–50, 51–60, 61–70, and over 71 years. 70 (13.7%) subjects were between 18 and 30 years old, while 135 (26.5%) were between 31 and 40 years old, 135 (26.5%) were between 41 and 50 years old, 80 (15.7%) were between 51 and 60 years old, 55 (10.8%) were between 61 and 70 years old, and 35 (6.9%) were older than 71 years. Based on race/ethnicity, 53.7% (274) of cases were Arab and 46.3% (236) were Farsi. General characteristics of all participants are summarized in Table 1. Of the 510 subjects, 235 (46.1%) are shown to be positive for anti-HEV IgG antibody by DIA.PRO HEV Ab ELISA kit, while 275 (53.9%) were negative. The overall anti-HEV IgG prevalence rate was 46.1%.

With regard to gender and race, 86/206 (41.7%) in the male group and 149/304 (49%) in the female group were positive for anti-HEV IgG antibodies. 134/274 (48.9%) in the Arab group and 101/236 (42.8%) in the Farsi group are shown to be positive for anti-HEV IgG antibody. However, the seroprevalence was higher among Arab and female groups; HEV seropositivity was not statistically associated with gender ($P = 0.106$) and race ($P = 0.168$). Meanwhile, there was statistical difference in anti-HEV IgG seroprevalence rate between the subjects grouped according to age ($P < 0.001$), so that seroprevalence of HEV increased with age from 14.3% (10/70) in subjects aged 18–30 years to 71.4% (25/35) in persons over 71 years old, with a peak among 61–70 year-olds

TABLE 2: Prevalence of anti-HEV IgM antibody according to gender, race, and age groups in adult population of Ahvaz city, Iran.

	Number of all participants (%): 510 (100%)	Number of anti-HEV IgM positive subjects (%): 7 (1.4%)	Number of anti-HEV IgM negative subjects (%): 503 (98.6%)	P value
Gender				0.448
Male	206 (40.4%)	4 (1.9%)	202 (98.1%)	
Female	304 (59.6%)	3 (1%)	301 (99%)	
Race				0.130
Arab	274 (53.7%)	6 (2.2%)	268 (97.8%)	
Farsi	236 (46.3%)	1 (0.4%)	235 (99.6%)	
Age groups (years)				0.012
18–30	70 (13.7%)	4 (5.7%)	66 (94.3%)	
31–40	135 (26.5%)	3 (2.2%)	132 (97.8%)	
41–50	135 (26.5%)	0	135 (100%)	
51–60	80 (15.7%)	0	80 (100%)	
60–71	55 (10.8%)	0	55 (100%)	
>71	35 (6.9%)	0	35 (100%)	

(90.9%, 50/55). The highest rate of anti-HEV seroprevalence was seen in subjects aged 61–70 years (Table 1).

When we evaluated anti-HEV IgM antibody seroprevalence rate in the gender and race groups, no significant differences were observed between the subjects regarding gender (1% in females and 1.9% in males, $P = 0.448$) and race (2.2% in Arab and 0.4% in Farsi, $P = 0.130$).

However, with regard to age, 4/70 (5.7%) in the age group 18–30 years and 3/135 (2.2%) in the age group 31–40 years were positive for anti-HEV IgM antibodies. There was a significant difference between the age groups regarding HEV seropositivity ($P = 0.012$). The highest rate of anti-HEV seroprevalence was observed in subjects aged 18–30 years (Table 2). Overall, 7 blood samples (1.4%) are shown to be positive for HEV-specific-IgM antibodies, while 503 samples (98.6%) were negative.

4. Discussion

Hepatitis E infection is a worldwide public health concern, which causes large outbreaks of acute hepatitis in developing countries especially Asia, Middle East, and Africa and also sporadic cases of the infection in developed countries such as South America and Europe [9]. Although HEV is mainly transmitted via the fecal-oral route especially contaminated water in endemic areas, transmission via the blood transfusion has also been suggested according to the high prevalence of anti-HEV IgG among blood donors [4, 13, 14].

Epidemiological studies in different parts of the world show the wide variation in HEV prevalence patterns, though the HEV seroprevalence rates are higher among less developed countries [15]. High prevalence rates are often reported from South Asia, Egypt in the Middle East, and the Far East except Japan, and low rates are often found in Europe and the Americas [16]. Iran is an endemic country for hepatitis E infection [7, 13], since HEV seroprevalence in general population is above 5% [7]. Previous studies have reported various HEV prevalence rates in different regions of Iran. Ataei et al. in 2005 reported HEV seroprevalence rate of 3.8% among general population in Isfahan Province, Iran [17]. Assarehzadegan et al. in 2005 reported HEV prevalence rate of 11.5% among blood donors in Khuzestan Province [15]. In Mohebbi et al. study, HEV prevalence was 9.3% in general population of Tehran [18]. In another study by Nazer et al., the prevalence of HEV was reported to be 7.8% in Khorramabad city in 2009 [19].

Regarding HEV prevalence among the general population of other countries, the overall HEV prevalence rate was reported to be 22.5% among general population in Bangladesh by Labrique et al. [20], about 3.20% in French blood donors by Boutrouille et al. [21], 13% in the general population in England by Ijaz et al. [22], 1.9% in the general population in Netherlands [23], and 5.3% in the general population of Japan [24].

In the present study we investigated the HEV seroprevalence among adult population in Ahvaz city and found that anti-HEV IgG and IgM seroprevalence were 46.1% and 1.4%, respectively. The result of the current study is considerably higher than that reported among adults in other parts of Iran [16]: 9.3% in Nahavand [25], 8.1% in Isfahan [17], 7.8% in Western Iran [26], 7.3% in sari [27], and 7.9–15% in Tehran [28]; it is also higher than that reported among adult population of some other countries: 3.9% in United Kingdom [16], 16.8% in Germany [29], 7.3% in Spain [30], about 20% in Korea [31], 23% in Thailand [32], 39–42% in USA [33], and 5.9% in Turkey [16]; however, it is lower than that reported among rural population older than four years in Egypt (51–78%) [16, 34], pregnant women in Nile Delta, Egypt (84%) [16, 35], general population older than 11 years in central Malaysia (50–67%) [16], tribes population (50–100%) and adult population (16–77%) in Andaman Islands, India [16], and homeless children in Cochabamba city, Bolivia (66%) [16].

However, a part of this difference may be due to differences in the used ELISA detection kits, the time of sampling, and the demographics and size of studied population. Overall, our results compared with the previous studies from Iran indicate that the geographic distribution of HEV infection is different even within a specific country, which most likely reflects different levels of exposure to infection over time due to different living conditions in different regions and fecal-oral transmission of HEV. In the current study, the HEV seroprevalence rate significantly increased with age from 14.3% in people aged below 31 years to 90.9% in persons aged 61–70 years. Improvement of public health and hygiene results in decreased exposure to the virus over time. However, exposure to HEV increases with age. This is consistent with most studies which reported a significant association between age and higher anti-HEV positive values, since the prevalence of the disease increases with age [26, 29, 31, 36]. Similarly high seroprevalence was found among adult population older than 60 years in China (70–80%), adult population older than 80 years in Bangladesh (67%), and adult population older than 80 years in Hong Kong (52–60%) [16]. Similar to the results of previous studies [5, 13, 17, 29, 37], our results show that the presence of anti-HEV IgG and IgM antibodies is not associated with gender; also we did not find any association between race/ethnicity and HEV seropositivity.

Our data showed that the anti-HEV IgG prevalence rate among adult population in Ahvaz is 46.1%, the highest rate reported in different parts of Iran. The implication is that Ahvaz city is a highly endemic area for HEV and the main route of HEV transmission in this city is most likely Karun River. Evidence for this claim is that the drinking water source of the city is supplied from Karun River and this river is commonly used for swimming, fishing, and other household needs by inhabitants. Moreover, the city sewage is discharged in the river. Since the major transmission route of HEV is most often the fecal contaminated drinking water and also this virus is relatively resistant to environmental conditions and remains infectious in sewage, the river can be considered as the water source for HEV infection. However more studies are required to confirm this hypothesis. Therefore, type E hepatitis is more common among adult population of Ahvaz city compared with other parts of Iran and this finding should be considered in the differential diagnosis of hepatitis infections and also prediction of possible outbreaks.

5. Conclusion

In conclusion, high anti-HEV IgG seroprevalence of 46.1% was observed among the adults population living in Ahvaz city of Iran. Determination of HEV prevalence in different regions can be used for the purpose of HEV epidemiology by developing a prevalence map on the base of HEV geographical distribution. In addition to epidemiological purposes, HEV prevalence information is important in evaluating the public health and hygiene and in identifying the major route of HEV transmission in Iran. However, further studies are required to evaluate these topics.

Conflict of Interests

There is no conflict of interests to declare.

Authors' Contribution

Reza Taherkhani takes responsibility for the accuracy of the data. Fatemeh Farshadpour and Reza Taherkhani contributed equally to the design and performance of the study. Fatemeh Farshadpour and Manoochehr Makvandi drafted the paper. All authors have read and approved the final paper.

Acknowledgments

The authors would like to thank the Deputy Research and Affairs of Ahvaz Jundishapur University of Medical Science for financial support to meet all expenses and essential equipment for this study. The study was supported financially by Grant no. 91112 provided by the Infectious and Tropical Diseases Research Center of Ahvaz Jundishapur University of Medical Sciences, Ahvaz, Iran.

References

[1] R. H. Purcell and S. U. Emerson, "Hepatitis E: an emerging awareness of an old disease," Journal of Hepatology, vol. 48, no. 3, pp. 494–503, 2008.

[2] F.-C. Zhu, J. Zhang, X.-F. Zhang et al., "Efficacy and safety of a recombinant hepatitis e vaccine in healthy adults: a large-scale, randomised, double-blind placebo-controlled, phase 3 trial," The Lancet, vol. 376, no. 9744, pp. 895–902, 2010.

[3] E. H. Teshale, D. J. Hu, and S. D. Holmberg, "The two faces of hepatitis E virus," Clinical Infectious Diseases, vol. 51, no. 3, pp. 328–334, 2010.

[4] X.-F. Cheng, Y.-F. Wen, M. Zhu et al., "Serological and molecular study of hepatitis E virus among illegal blood donors," World Journal of Gastroenterology, vol. 18, no. 9, pp. 986–990, 2012.

[5] A. Kaufmann, A. Kenfak-Foguena, C. André et al., "Hepatitis E virus seroprevalence among blood donors in Southwest Switzerland," PLoS ONE, vol. 6, no. 6, Article ID e21150, 2011.

[6] J. H. Hoofnagle, K. E. Nelson, and R. H. Purcell, "Hepatitis E," The New England Journal of Medicine, vol. 367, no. 13, pp. 1237–1244, 2012.

[7] S. Sepanlou, H. Rezvan, S. Amini-Kafiabad, M. R. Dayhim, and S. Merat, "A population-based seroepidemiological study on hepatitis E virus in Iran," Middle East Journal of Digestive Diseases, vol. 2, no. 2, pp. 97–103, 2010.

[8] L. Wang and H. Zhuang, "Hepatitis E: an overview and recent advances in vaccine research," World Journal of Gastroenterology, vol. 10, no. 15, pp. 2157–2162, 2004.

[9] R. Taherkhani, M. Makvandi, and F. Farshadpour, "Development of enzyme-linked immunosorbent assays using 2 truncated ORF2 proteins for detection of IgG antibodies against hepatitis e virus," Annals of Laboratory Medicine, vol. 34, no. 2, pp. 118–126, 2014.

[10] S. U. Emerson and R. H. Purcell, "Running like water—the omnipresence of hepatitis E," The New England Journal of Medicine, vol. 351, no. 23, pp. 2367–2368, 2004.

[11] L. Xing, J. C. Wang, T. C. Li et al., "Spatial configuration of hepatitis E virus antigenic domain," Journal of Virology, vol. 85, no. 2, pp. 1117–1124, 2011.

[12] R. Taherkhani, F. Farshadpour, and M. Makvandi, "Design and production of a multiepitope construct derived from *hepatitis E virus* capsid protein," *Journal of Medical Virology*, vol. 87, no. 7, pp. 1225–1234, 2015.

[13] H. Ehteram, A. Ramezani, A. Eslamifar et al., "Seroprevalence of Hepatitis E Virus infection among volunteer blood donors in central province of Iran in 2012," *Iranian Journal of Microbiology*, vol. 5, no. 2, pp. 172–176, 2013.

[14] F. Farshadpour, R. Taherkhani, M. Makvandi, H. R. Memari, and A. R. Samarbafzadeh, "Codon-optimized expression and purification of truncated ORF2 protein of hepatitis E virus in *Escherichia coli*," *Jundishapur Journal of Microbiology*, vol. 7, no. 7, Article ID e11261, 2014.

[15] M. A. Assarehzadegan, G. Shakerinejad, A. Amini, and S. A. R. Rezaee, "Seroprevalence of hepatitis E virus in blood donors in Khuzestan Province, Southwest Iran," *International Journal of Infectious Diseases*, vol. 12, no. 4, pp. 387–390, 2008.

[16] J. Echevarría, "Light and darkness: prevalence of hepatitis E virus infection among the general population," *Scientifica*, vol. 2014, Article ID 481016, 14 pages, 2014.

[17] B. Ataei, Z. Nokhodian, A. A. Javadi et al., "Hepatitis E virus in Isfahan Province: a population-based study," *International Journal of Infectious Diseases*, vol. 13, no. 1, pp. 67–71, 2009.

[18] S. R. Mohebbi, M. Rostami Nejad, S. M. E. Tahaei et al., "Seroepidemiology of hepatitis A and E virus infections in Tehran, Iran: a population based study," *Transactions of the Royal Society of Tropical Medicine and Hygiene*, vol. 106, no. 9, pp. 528–531, 2012.

[19] M. Nazer, E. Rafiei Alavi, and J. Hashemy, "Serologic prevalence of hepatitis E in Khoramabad City, Iran, 2009," *The Journal of Shahid Sadoughi University of Medical Sciences*, vol. 18, no. 5, pp. 451–460, 2010.

[20] A. B. Labrique, K. Zaman, Z. Hossain et al., "Population seroprevalence of hepatitis E virus antibodies in rural Bangladesh," *The American Journal of Tropical Medicine and Hygiene*, vol. 81, no. 5, pp. 875–881, 2009.

[21] A. Boutrouille, L. Bakkali-Kassimi, C. Crucière, and N. Pavio, "Prevalence of anti-hepatitis E virus antibodies in French blood donors," *Journal of Clinical Microbiology*, vol. 45, no. 6, pp. 2009–2010, 2007.

[22] S. Ijaz, A. J. Vyse, D. Morgan, R. G. Pebody, R. S. Tedder, and D. Brown, "Indigenous hepatitis E virus infection in England: more common than it seems," *Journal of Clinical Virology*, vol. 44, no. 4, pp. 272–276, 2009.

[23] L. Verhoef, M. Koopmans, E. Duizer, J. Bakker, J. Reimerink, and W. Van Pelt, "Seroprevalence of hepatitis e antibodies and risk profile of HEV seropositivity in the Netherlands, 2006-2007," *Epidemiology and Infection*, vol. 140, no. 10, pp. 1838–1847, 2012.

[24] M. Takahashi, K. Tamura, Y. Hoshino et al., "A nationwide survey of hepatitis E virus infection in the general population of Japan," *Journal of Medical Virology*, vol. 82, no. 2, pp. 271–281, 2010.

[25] M. Taremi, A. H. Mohammad Alizadeh, A. Ardalan, S. Ansari, and M. R. Zali, "Seroprevalence of hepatitis E in Nahavand, Islamic Republic of Iran: a population-based study," *Eastern Mediterranean Health Journal*, vol. 14, no. 1, pp. 157–162, 2008.

[26] R. Raoofi, M. R. Nazer, and Y. Pournia, "Seroepidemiology of hepatitis E virus in Western Iran," *Brazilian Journal of Infectious Diseases*, vol. 16, no. 3, pp. 302–303, 2012.

[27] M. J. Saffar, R. Farhadi, A. Ajami, A. R. Khalilian, F. Babamahmodi, and H. Saffar, "Seroepidemiology of hepatitis E virus infection in 2-25-year-olds in Sari district, Islamic Republic of Iran," *Eastern Mediterranean Health Journal*, vol. 15, no. 1, pp. 136–142, 2009.

[28] S. R. Mohebbi, M. R. Nejad, S. M. E. Tahaei et al., "Seroepidemiology of hepatitis A and E virus infections in Tehran, Iran: a population based study," *Transactions of the Royal Society of Tropical Medicine and Hygiene*, vol. 106, no. 9, pp. 528–531, 2012.

[29] M. S. Faber, J. J. Wenzel, W. Jilg, M. Thamm, M. Höhle, and K. Stark, "Hepatitis E virus seroprevalence among adults, Germany," *Emerging Infectious Diseases*, vol. 18, no. 10, pp. 1654–1657, 2012.

[30] M. Buti, À. Domínguez, P. Plans et al., "Community-based seroepidemiological survey of hepatitis E virus infection in Catalonia, Spain," *Clinical and Vaccine Immunology*, vol. 13, no. 12, pp. 1328–1332, 2006.

[31] H. K. Park, S.-H. Jeong, J.-W. Kim et al., "Seroprevalence of anti-hepatitis E virus (HEV) in a Korean population: comparison of two commercial anti-HEV assays," *BMC Infectious Diseases*, vol. 12, no. 1, article 142, 2012.

[32] S. Hinjoy, K. E. Nelson, R. V. Gibbons et al., "A cross-sectional study of hepatitis E virus infection in healthy people directly exposed and unexposed to pigs in a rural community in Northern Thailand," *Zoonoses and Public Health*, vol. 60, no. 8, pp. 555–562, 2013.

[33] M. H. Kuniholm, R. H. Pureell, G. M. McQuillan, R. E. Engle, A. Wasley, and K. E. Nelson, "Epidemiology of hepatitis E virus in the United States: results from the third national health and nutrition examination survey, 1988–1994," *Journal of Infectious Diseases*, vol. 200, no. 1, pp. 48–56, 2009.

[34] A. D. Fix, M. Abdel-Hamid, R. H. Purcell et al., "Prevalence of antibodies to hepatitis E in two rural Egyptian communities," *American Journal of Tropical Medicine and Hygiene*, vol. 62, no. 4, pp. 519–523, 2000.

[35] S. K. Stoszek, M. Abdel-Hamid, D. A. Saleh et al., "High prevalence of hepatitis E antibodies in pregnant Egyptian women," *Transactions of the Royal Society of Tropical Medicine and Hygiene*, vol. 100, no. 2, pp. 95–101, 2006.

[36] E. Tadesse, L. Metwally, and E. Alaa, "High prevalence of anti-hepatitis E virus among Egyptian blood donors," *Journal of General and Molecular Virology*, vol. 5, no. 1, pp. 9–13, 2013.

[37] S. Aminiafshar, M. Alimagham, L. Gachkar et al., "Anti hepatitis E virus seropositivity in a group of blood donors," *Iranian Journal of Public Health*, vol. 33, no. 4, pp. 53–56, 2004.

22

Prediction of Sustained Virological Response to Telaprevir-Based Triple Therapy Using Viral Response within 2 Weeks

Hideyuki Tamai, Ryo Shimizu, Naoki Shingaki, Yoshiyuki Mori, Shuya Maeshima, Junya Nuta, Yoshimasa Maeda, Kosaku Moribata, Yosuke Muraki, Hisanobu Deguchi, Izumi Inoue, Takao Maekita, Mikitaka Iguchi, Jun Kato, and Masao Ichinose

Second Department of Internal Medicine, Wakayama Medical University, 811-1 Kimiidera, Wakayama, Wakayama Prefecture 641-0012, Japan

Correspondence should be addressed to Hideyuki Tamai; tamahide@wakayama-med.ac.jp

Academic Editor: Piero Luigi Almasio

The aim of the present study was to predict sustained virological response (SVR) to telaprevir with pegylated interferon (PEG-IFN) and ribavirin using viral response within 2 weeks after therapy initiation. Thirty-six patients with genotype 1 hepatitis C virus (HCV) and high viral load were treated by telaprevir-based triple therapy. SVR was achieved in 72% (26/36) of patients. Significant differences between the SVR group and non-SVR group were noted regarding response to prior PEG-IFN plus ribavirin, interleukin (IL)28B polymorphism, amino acid substitution at core 70, cirrhosis, hyaluronic acid level, and HCV-RNA reduction within 2 weeks. Setting 4.56 logIU/mL as the cut-off value for HCV-RNA reduction at 2 weeks, the sensitivity, specificity, positive predictive value, negative predictive value, and accuracy for predicting SVR were 77%, 86%, 95%, 50%, and 79%, respectively, and for neither the IL28B minor allele nor core 70 mutant were 80%, 71%, 91%, 50%, and 78%, respectively. In conclusion, evaluation of viral reduction at 2 weeks or the combination of IL28B polymorphism and amino acid substitution at core 70 are useful for predicting SVR to telaprevir with PEG-IFN and ribavirin therapy.

1. Introduction

To date, although pegylated interferon (PEG-IFN) and ribavirin combination therapy has been standard care for patients with hepatitis C virus (HCV) infection, the sustained virological response (SVR) rate in patients with genotype 1 and high viral load is only approximately 40–50% [1]. Recently, some direct antiviral agents (DAAs) against HCV have been developed. The first-generation nonstructural 3/4A protease inhibitor, telaprevir, became available for clinical use in November 2011 in Japan. Triple therapy with telaprevir, PEG-IFN, and ribavirin has significantly improved SVR rates to around 70% [2]. However, compared with PEG-IFN plus ribavirin therapy, triple therapy can produce some severe adverse reactions, including serious skin disorders, exacerbation of anemia, and renal dysfunction [3–5]. Furthermore, the safety of telaprevir-based triple therapy

in elderly or cirrhotic patients has not been established. However, as elderly and/or cirrhotic patients are at high risk of developing hepatocellular carcinoma, antiviral therapy should be commenced as soon as possible for these patients [1]. Therefore, the prediction of efficacy and assessment of tolerability for each individual who might receive telaprevir-based triple therapy are crucial for deciding the optimal treatment strategy. If therapeutic efficacy can be accurately predicted before or in the very early stages of treatment, risky and unnecessary treatment can be avoided.

Regarding pretreatment predictors for efficacy in telaprevir-based triple therapy, interleukin (IL)28B single nucleotide polymorphism (SNP), amino acid substitution at core 70, and response to previous therapy have been reported as useful predictors [6–8]. The Japanese guidelines for the management of hepatitis C virus infection [1] recommend that analysis of IL28B SNP and amino acid substitution at core 70 should be performed to enable selection of the optimum therapy regimen; telaprevir-based triple therapy is not recommended in patients with both the IL28B minor allele and mutant type of amino acid substitution at core 70. However, neither the test for the IL28B SNP nor the test for amino acid substitution at core 70 has been approved by the Japan National Medical Insurance System.

Extended rapid virological response (RVR), defined as serum HCV-RNA undetectable at both treatment week 4 and week 12, is also known to be one of the significant predictors of SVR to telaprevir-based triple therapy [9, 10]. However, the best time point has not been elucidated for predicting SVR using viral response. The aim of the present study was to evaluate whether SVR to telaprevir-based triple therapy can be more accurately predicted on the basis of super rapid virological response within 2 weeks of therapy initiation than RVR and whether the predictability for SVR by virological response within 2 weeks is comparable with that by the combination of IL28B SNP and amino acid substitution at core 70.

2. Methods

2.1. Patients. A total of 36 consecutive patients with genotype 1 high viral load (more than 5.0 logIU/mL) were enrolled from March 2012 to June 2013 in our hospital. Exclusion criteria were (1) pregnant women, women who may have been pregnant, lactating women, men whose partners were pregnant, or men whose partners hoped to become pregnant; (2) patients who used shosaikoto (a Kampo medicine); (3) intractable heart disease; (4) renal failure or renal dysfunction with creatinine clearance <50 mL/min; (5) patients with uncontrollable psychoneurotic disorders; (6) hemoglobin (Hb) level <11 g/dL; (7) platelet count <60,000/mm^3; (8) white blood cell count <1500/mm^3 (or granulocyte count <1000/mm^3); and (9) hepatic failure or all types of cancer. The potential benefits and risks of the present study were explained to all patients before obtaining written informed consent. The protocol was approved by the Ethics Committee of Wakayama Medical University (no. 1081) and conformed to the Helsinki Declaration.

2.2. Treatment Regimens. Telaprevir (Telavic; Mitsubishi Tanabe Pharma, Osaka Japan), PEG-IFN-alpha-2b (Peg-Intron; MSD, Tokyo, Japan), and ribavirin (Rebetol; MSD) were used. PEG-IFN-alpha-2b at 1.5 μg/kg was administered subcutaneously once per week for 24 weeks; ribavirin was given orally for 24 weeks (1000 mg/day for patients weighing more than 80 kg, 800 mg/day for patients weighing between 80 and 60 kg, and 600 mg/day for patients weighing less than 60 kg); and telaprevir was given orally at a dose of 750 mg every 8 hours after meals for 12 weeks from the start of therapy.

However, in a clinical trial of telaprevir-based triple therapy in Japan, elderly patients or patients with cytopenia due to cirrhosis were not included, and grade 3 anemia occurred more frequently in the telaprevir group than in the group who did not receive telaprevir [2]. The Japanese guidelines for

the management of HCV infection recommend reduced doses of the combination therapy of PEG-IFN and ribavirin for compensated cirrhosis [1]. A pilot study of telaprevir-based triple therapy for elderly patients suggested that triple therapy with telaprevir 1500 mg seems safe and efficacious for elderly Japanese patients [11]. In addition, Sezaki et al. [12] also reported that, compared with telaprevir 2250 mg, telaprevir 1500 mg/day was associated with lower rates of anemia and similar antiviral efficacy, especially among elderly Japanese patients. Therefore, for safety, reduced doses of telaprevir (1500 mg), PEG-IFN-alpha-2b (1.0 μg/kg), and ribavirin (200 mg less than the recommended dose) were initially administered in the present study for patients with any of the following: (1) age ≥65 years; (2) white blood cell count <2000/mm^3; (3) platelet count <130,000/mm^3; (4) Hb level <13 g/dL; (5) comorbid disorder such as heart disease, cerebrovascular disease, thyroid disease, psychiatric disease, autoimmune disease, or uncontrolled diabetes; or (6) low body weight (<40 kg).

During treatment, reduction in the telaprevir dose was not permitted. The doses of PEG-IFN-alpha-2b and ribavirin were reduced or discontinued based on the following criteria. (1) If the Hb fell below 10 g/dL, the dose of ribavirin was reduced by 200 mg from the starting dose, and if the Hb fell below 8.5 g/dL, the ribavirin was discontinued; (2) if the granulocyte count fell below 500/mm^3 or the platelet count fell below 30,000/mm^3, the PEG-IFN was discontinued; and (3) if deemed necessary by the attending physician because of adverse events, the telaprevir, PEG-IFN, and ribavirin were all discontinued. The dose of PEG-IFN or ribavirin was increased back to the starting dose if the cytopenia improved. If there was no improvement in hematological parameters within 4 weeks, the therapy was discontinued. Although granulocyte colony-stimulating factor was used as supplementary treatment for granulocytopenia less than 500/mm^3, erythropoietin was not used for anemia.

2.3. Laboratory Tests and Ultrasound. In all patients, laboratory tests and ultrasound examination were performed before therapy began. Fatty liver was defined as positive hepatorenal contrast on ultrasound B mode imaging. The amount of HCV-RNA was measured using quantitative real-time polymerase chain reaction (RT-PCR) (COBAS TaqMan HCV test version 1.0; Roche Diagnostics, Branchburg, NJ, USA). High viral load was defined as more than 5.0 logIU/mL using quantitative RT-PCR. HCV genotype was determined according to Simmonds' classification [13]. The amount of HCV-RNA (AccuGene m-HCV, Abbott Japan, Tokyo, Japan) and HCV core antigen levels (ARCHITECT HCV; Abbott Japan, Tokyo, Japan) were measured simultaneously at three time points: the day of therapy initiation and at weeks 1 and 2. Serum levels of hyaluronic acid and type IV collagen 7S were measured for the assessment of liver fibrosis on the day of therapy initiation. Amino acid 70 and 91 substitutions in the HCV core region [14] were also measured on the day of therapy initiation. At core 70, arginine was defined as the wild type and glutamine or histidine as mutant types. At core 91, leucine was defined as the wild type and methionine as the mutant type.

During therapy, quantitative HCV-RNA (COBAS TaqMan HCV test; Roche Diagnostics), biochemical analyses including blood counts, serum alanine aminotransferase (ALT), and aspartate aminotransferase (AST), were performed every 4 weeks up to 24 weeks after the end of therapy. After treatment, the SNP of IL28B (rs8099917) that was reported as a pretreatment predictor for the efficacy of PEG-IFN plus ribavirin therapy in Japanese patients [15] was additionally evaluated, after obtaining written informed consent for genome analysis from each patient. Homozygosity for the major allele (T/T) was defined as the IL28B major type, and heterozygosity (T/G) or homozygosity for the minor allele (G/G) was defined as the IL28B minor type.

2.4. Assessment of Effectiveness. During IFN therapy, rapid virological response (RVR) was defined as undetectable HCV-RNA using quantitative RT-PCR (COBAS TaqMan PCR assay; Roche Diagnostics) at week 4 after therapy initiation. SVR was defined as follows: the HCV-RNA measured using the TaqMan PCR assay was negative at the end of therapy and remained negative for 24 weeks after the end of therapy. No response was defined as detectable HCV-RNA at week 24 from treatment initiation or at the end of treatment. Relapse was defined as HCV-RNA-negative at the end of therapy but positive at 24 weeks after the end of therapy. The viral response within two weeks after therapy initiation was assessed by viral level and viral reduction from baseline viral load at each time point.

2.5. Assessment of Safety and Tolerability. Patients were assessed for safety and tolerability during treatment by their attending physicians, who monitored adverse events and laboratory abnormalities, such as blood cell counts, every week up to week 12 and monthly thereafter. The incidence and reasons for therapy discontinuation due to adverse effects were analyzed.

2.6. Statistical Analysis. Adherence to each medication (telaprevir, PEG-IFN-alpha-2b, and ribavirin) was assessed separately and was calculated based on the recommended doses. Therapeutic effectiveness was evaluated using intention-to-treat (ITT) analysis. Predictive factors for SVR were analyzed using a per protocol (PP) analysis that excluded patients who had discontinued therapy due to adverse events within 4 weeks. The Mann-Whitney U test was used to analyze continuous variables. Fisher's exact test or the chi-square test was used to analyze categorical variables. Each optimal cut-off value for continuous variables of SVR-predicting factors was decided by the Youden index method on the basis of the receiver operating characteristic (ROC) curve. The SVR predictability of significant SVR-contributing factors was evaluated by measuring the area under the curve (AUC). The sensitivity, specificity, positive predictive value (PPV), negative predictive value (NPV) for SVR, and accuracy were calculated for week 1, week 2, and RVR. Values of $P < 0.05$ were considered significant. The statistical software used was SPSS Ver. 21.0J for Windows (SPSS, Inc., Tokyo, Japan).

TABLE 1: Baseline characteristics of the study patients.

	$n = 36$
Age (years)	61.5 (29–72)
Sex (male/female)	19/17
Height (cm)	159.3 (143.1–177.0)
Weight (kg)	62.1 (39.6–81.5)
BMI	24.2 (17.1–35.0)
Genotype (1a/1b)	1/35
Baseline HCV-RNA (LogIU/mL; TaqMan)	6.7 (4.8–7.5)
Response to prior PEG-IFN and ribavirin (NR/Relapse/Naive)	4/18/14
Fatty liver	6
Cirrhosis	18
Diabetes mellitus	7
IL28B, rs8099917 (TT/GT/GG)	24/11/1
Core 70 (wild/mutant/ND)	18/17/1
Core 91 (wild/mutant/ND)	26/9/1
WBC (/mm^3)	4785 (2700–9300)
Hb (g/dL)	14.6 (11.6–18.6)
Platelets (/mm^3)	16.5 (6.6–28.0)
ALT (IU/L)	46.0 (14–507)
γ-GT (IU/L)	35.5 (10–306)
Type VI collagen 7S (ng/mL)	4.4 (3.1–10.5)
Hyaluronic acid (ng/mL)	98.0 (12.3–839.0)
AFP (ng/mL)	4.5 (1.3–174.6)
Reduced dose regimen	30
Telaprevir adherence (%)	66.7 (0.6–100)
PEG-IFN adherence (%)	66.8 (5.5–100)
Ribavirin adherence (%)	66.7 (2.4–100)

Values are expressed as median (range). BMI, body mass index; HCV, hepatitis C virus; IL, interleukin; ND, not determined; WBC, white blood cells; Hb, hemoglobin; ALT, alanine aminotransferase; γ-GT, γ-glutamyl transferase; AFP, alpha-fetoprotein; PEG-IFN, pegylated interferon.

3. Results

3.1. Patients' Baseline Characteristics. The patients' baseline characteristics are summarized in Table 1. The patients were composed of 19 males and 17 females. Their median age was 61.5 years and the range was 29 to 72 years; 24 (67%) patients were <65 years old, and 12 (33%) were ≥65 years old. Four (11%) patients had experienced no response to prior PEG-IFN and ribavirin therapy. Thirty (81%) patients were treated by the reduced dose regimen.

3.2. Safety and Tolerability. Of the 36 patients, therapy was discontinued in 3 (8%) patients due to adverse events. The discontinuation rate was 0% (0/24) in patients <65 years old and 25% (3/12) in patients ≥65 years old, showing significant difference between groups ($P = 0.046$). Eighteen (49%) patients were clinically diagnosed with liver cirrhosis using the morphologic appearance of cirrhosis with portal

TABLE 2: Comparison of pretreatment factors between patients with and without sustained virological response.

Factors	SVR ($n = 26$)	Non-SVR ($n = 7$)	P
Age (years)	61	60	0.914
Sex (male/female)	13/13	5/2	0.413
Height (cm)	159.6	159.5	0.880
Weight (kg)	62.6	59.9	0.949
BMI	24.4	25.0	0.780
Baseline HCV-RNA (logIU/mL; TaqMan)	6.7	6.5	0.399
Baseline HCV-RNA (logIU/mL; AccuGene)	6.1	5.6	0.215
Baseline HCV core Ag (fmol/L)	4477.4	1524.4	0.330
No response to prior PEG-IFN and ribavirin	1	3	0.023
Fatty liver	6	0	0.301
Cirrhosis	9	6	0.030
Diabetes mellitus	4	1	1.000
IL28B (major/minor)	20/6	1/6	0.005
Core 70 (wild/mutant)	17/8	1/6	0.027
Core 91 (wild/mutant)	18/7	5/2	1.000
WBC (/mm3)	4995	4410	0.450
Hb (g/dL)	14.5	14.5	0.747
Platelets (/mm^3)	16.9	12.2	0.099
ALT (IU/L)	49.5	43.0	0.714
γ-GT (IU/L)	33.5	49.0	0.199
Type VI collagen 7S (ng/mL)	4.4	8.1	0.054
Hyaluronic acid (ng/mL)	72.7	367.0	0.048
AFP (ng/mL)	4.1	11.2	0.067
Reduced dose regimen	20	7	0.301

Values are expressed as median. SVR, sustained virological response; BMI, body mass index; HCV, hepatitis C virus; Ag, antigen; IL, interleukin; WBC, white blood cells; Hb, hemoglobin; ALT, alanine aminotransferase; γ-GT, γ-glutamyl transferase; AFP, alpha-fetoprotein.

hypertension, as evidenced by portosystemic shunt or hypersplenism on imaging, laboratory tests, and/or liver histology. The discontinuation rate was 17% (3/18) in cirrhotic patients and 0% (0/18) in noncirrhotic patients, with no significant difference between groups ($P = 0.229$). The discontinuation rate was 33% (3/9) in elderly cirrhotic patients and 0% (0/27) in the other patients, showing significant difference between groups ($P = 0.012$). Reasons for therapy discontinuation were psychiatric disorder in 2 patients and severe nausea in 1 patient. All of the patients who required discontinuation of therapy stopped the therapy within 4 weeks after therapy initiation.

3.3. Therapeutic Efficacy. Overall, SVR was achieved in 72% (26/36) of the study patients, relapse occurred in 8% (3/36), and no response was observed in 19% (7/36) patients. In the 30 patients who received the reduced dose regimen, SVR was achieved in 67% (20/30) of the patients, relapse occurred in 10% (3/30), and no response was observed in 23% (7/30) patients. On the other hand, the SVR rate in the 6 patients who were able to use the recommended dose regimen was 100% (6/6). With respect to patient age, the SVR rate was 79% (19/24) in patients <65 years old and 58% (7/12) in patients ≥65 years old, showing no significant difference between groups ($P = 0.247$). The SVR rate was 50% (9/18) in cirrhotic

patients and 94% (17/18) in noncirrhotic patients, showing no significant difference between groups ($P = 0.072$). However, the SVR rate was 44% (4/9) in elderly cirrhotic patients and 89% (24/27) in the other patients, showing significant difference between groups ($P = 0.013$).

3.4. Contributing Factors for SVR and Predictability of SVR. The results of univariate analysis of pretreatment factors contributing to SVR are shown in Table 2. Significant differences between the SVR group and the non-SVR group were noted regarding response to prior PEG-IFN plus ribavirin, IL28B SNP, core 70 amino acid substitution, and hyaluronic acid level. In addition, the results of univariate analysis of on-treatment factors contributing to SVR are shown in Table 3. Significant differences were noted in HCV-RNA level at week 4, RVR, and reduction of HCV-RNA within 4 weeks. However, no significant difference was noted in level and reduction of HCV core antigen at any time point, or adherence to treatment regimen. The comparison of significant predicting factors for SVR according to the AUC is shown in Table 4. The AUC of the reduction of HCV-RNA at 2 weeks was the highest. The sensitivity, specificity, PPV, NPV, and accuracy for predicting SVR according to the significant factors associated with SVR are summarized in Table 5.

TABLE 3: Comparison of on-treatment factors between patients with and without sustained virological response.

Factors	SVR ($n = 26$)	Non-SVR ($n = 7$)	P
HCV-RNA level at week 1 (logIU/mL)	1.3	2.4	0.399
HCV-RNA level at week 2 (logIU/mL)	1.1	1.8	0.199
HCV-RNA level at week 4 (logIU/mL)	0	1.2	0.039
RVR	20	2	0.027
Reduction of HCV-RNA at week 1 (log)	4.5	3.4	0.003
Reduction of HCV-RNA at week 2 (log)	5.1	4.2	0.003
Reduction of HCV-RNA at week 4 (log)	6.6	5.4	0.010
HCV core Ag level at week 1 (fmol/L)	4.9	7.0	0.949
HCV core Ag level at week 2 (fmol/L)	0.8	2.4	0.399
Reduction of HCV core Ag at week 1	4476.5	1517.5	0.399
Reduction of HCV core Ag at week 2	4477.4	1524.1	0.330
Telaprevir adherence (%)	66.7	66.7	0.949
PEG-IFN adherence (%)	68.4	68.5	0.846
Ribavirin adherence (%)	70.9	75.0	0.682

Values are expressed as median. SVR, sustained virological response; HCV, hepatitis C virus; RVR, rapid virological response; Ag, antigen; PEG-IFN, pegylated interferon.

TABLE 4: Area under the receiver operating characteristic curve according to significant predicting factors for sustained virological response.

Factors	AUC	P	95% CI
Non-NR to prior PEG-IFN and ribavirin	0.695	0.118	0.441–0.949
IL28B major	0.813	0.012	0.632–0.994
Core 70 wild	0.769	0.032	0.577–0.960
Cirrhosis	0.755	0.041	0.563–0.948
Hyaluronic acid level	0.747	0.048	0.515–0.979
Reduction of HCV-RNA at week 1	0.849	0.005	0.682–1.000
Reduction of HCV-RNA at week 2	0.857	0.004	0.716–0.999
Reduction of HCV-RNA at week 4	0.813	0.012	0.663–0.963
RVR	0.742	0.053	0.524–0.905

AUC, area under the receiver operating characteristic curve; CI, confidence interval; NR, no response; PEG-IFN, pegylated interferon; IL, interleukin; HCV, hepatitis C virus; RVR, rapid virological response.

TABLE 5: Predictive values according to significant factors related to sustained virological response.

Significant predictive factors	Sensitivity	Specificity	PPV	NPV	Accuracy
Non-NR to prior PEG-IFN and ribavirin	96% (25/26)	43% (3/7)	86% (25/29)	75% (3/4)	85% (28/33)
IL28B major	77% (20/26)	86% (6/7)	95% (20/21)	50% (6/12)	79% (26/33)
Core 70 wild	60% (15/25)	86% (6/7)	94% (15/16)	38% (6/16)	66% (21/32)
No cirrhosis	65% (17/26)	86% (6/7)	94% (17/18)	40% (6/15)	70% (23/33)
Hyaluronic acid level (<346 ng/mL)	92% (24/26)	57% (4/7)	89% (24/27)	67% (4/6)	85% (28/33)
Reduction of HCV-RNA at week 1 (>4.36 logIU/mL)	73% (19/26)	86% (6/7)	95% (19/20)	46% (6/13)	76% (25/33)
Reduction of HCV-RNA at week 2 (>4.56 logIU/mL)	77% (20/26)	86% (6/7)	95% (20/21)	50% (6/12)	79% (26/33)
Reduction of HCV-RNA at week 4 (>6.40 logIU/mL)	65% (17/26)	100% (7/7)	100% (17/17)	44% (7/16)	73% (24/33)
RVR	77% (20/26)	71% (5/7)	91% (20/22)	45% (5/11)	76% (25/33)
Neither the IL28B minor nor core 70 mutant	80% (20/25)	71% (5/7)	91% (20/22)	50% (5/10)	78% (25/32)

PPV, positive predictive value; NPV, negative predictive value; NR, no response; PEG-IFN, pegylated interferon; IL, interleukin; HCV, hepatitis C virus; RVR, rapid virological response.

TABLE 6: Comparison of pretreatment factors between patients with and without 2-week virological response.

Factors	Week 2 response (≥4.56-log reduction) (n = 21)	Non-week-2-response (<4.56-log reduction) (n = 12)	P
Age (years)	58	62	0.618
Sex (male/female)	13/8	5/7	0.300
Height (cm)	162.8	158.3	0.291
Weight (kg)	65.8	57.5	0.175
BMI	24.7	22.0	0.593
Baseline HCV-RNA (LogIU/mL; TaqMan)	6.8	6.2	0.013
Baseline HCV-RNA (LogIU/mL; AccuGene)	6.2	5.5	0.005
Baseline HCV core Ag (fmol/L)	6134.9	1485.3	0.003
No response to prior PEG-IFN and ribavirin	1	3	0.125
Fatty liver	6	0	0.065
Cirrhosis	7	8	0.083
Diabetes mellitus	3	2	1.000
IL28B (major/minor)	15/6	6/6	0.274
Core 70 (wild/mutant)	12/8	6/6	0.718
Core 91 (wild/mutant)	15/5	8/4	0.696
WBC (/mm^3)	5160	4435	0.175
Hb (g/dL)	14.8	14.1	0.022
Platelets (/mm^3)	16.7	14.8	0.345
ALT (IU/L)	51.0	43.5	0.927
γ-GT (IU/L)	34.0	38.0	0.868
Type VI collagen 7S (ng/mL)	4.8	4.8	0.811
Hyaluronic acid (ng/mL)	94.0	105.2	0.671
AFP (ng/mL)	4.5	6.7	0.811
Reduced dose regimen	15	12	0.065

Values are expressed as the median. BMI, body mass index; HCV, hepatitis C virus; Ag, antigen; IL, interleukin; WBC, white blood cells; Hb, hemoglobin; ALT, alanine aminotransferase; γ-GT, γ-glutamyl transferase; AFP, alpha-fetoprotein.

3.5. Contributing Factors for Week 2 Response. Although it was considered that the independent factors contributing to SVR were analyzed by multivariate analysis, there were too many significant variables in view of the small numbers of patients. To validate whether the HCV-RNA reduction at week 2 was an independent factor associated with SVR, the pretreatment factors contributing to week 2 response were analyzed. The results of univariate analysis of pretreatment factors contributing to SVR are shown in Table 6. Response to prior PEG-IFN and ribavirin, cirrhosis, IL28B SNP, core 70 substitution, and hyaluronic acid level, which were significantly related to SVR, were not significant factors contributing to week 2 response. HCV-RNA level and core antigen were the only significant factors contributing to 2-week response. Therefore, week 2 response might be one of the independent factors contributing to SVR.

4. Discussion

Among patients with HCV infection, elderly cirrhotic patients have the highest priority for antiviral treatment because they are at the highest risk of liver-related death such as hepatic failure or hepatocellular carcinoma. Regarding the safety of triple therapy for cirrhotic patients, in the ANRS CO20 CUPIC study [16], although the early discontinuation rate within 16 weeks was 11.7%, a high incidence of serious adverse events (40%), death (1.2%), severe complications (severe infection or hepatic decompensation; 6.4%), and difficult management of anemia (requiring erythropoietin and transfusion) were observed. Furthermore, in an open label expanded access program cohort for evaluating the safety and efficacy of telaprevir-based triple therapy in patients with advanced fibrosis or cirrhosis involving 16 nations worldwide [17], although the early discontinuation rate was 12%, the mortality of the cirrhotic patients was 0.7%. The discontinuation rates in both of these studies might be acceptable for safety and tolerability; however, in common with both studies, age and female gender were independent predictors of severe anemia. In addition, low platelet count (<100,000/mm^3) and low serum albumin level (<35 g/dL) were related to death or severe complications in the CUPIC study. Therefore, it is recommended that patients with factors of both low platelet count and low serum albumin level should not be treated with triple therapy. The telaprevir discontinuation rate in the present study was low (8%) regardless of the inclusion of many elderly and/or cirrhotic patients who are at high risk for severe adverse effects of interferon-based therapy. However, we considered that the reason for the low discontinuation rate was the reduced dose regimen.

Regarding the reduced dose of telaprevir, Sezaki et al. [12] reported a case control study for Japanese patients that compared patients who received telaprevir at a dose of 2250 mg/day and a dose of 1500 mg/day. These investigators reported that the discontinuation rate of patients receiving telaprevir 1500 mg/day was significantly lower than that of the patients receiving telaprevir 2250 mg/day (10% versus 25%), and that the SVR rates of both groups were equivalent (70% versus 83%). Therefore, these investigators suggested that the telaprevir-reduced regimen is safe and effective, especially for elderly and female Japanese patients. However, although in the present study, we reduced not only the telaprevir dose but also the PEG-IFN and ribavirin doses, the discontinuation rate of elderly and cirrhotic patients was high (33%) and significantly higher than that of the other patients. Furthermore, the SVR rate of the elderly and cirrhotic patients was low (44%) and significantly lower than in the other patients. Therefore, we suggest that even the reduced regimen should not be administered to elderly and cirrhotic patients. However, if the telaprevir-based triple therapy was to be applied for elderly cirrhotic patients, both tolerability and the prediction of efficacy must be strictly evaluated.

With respect to the prediction of the efficacy of telaprevir-based triple therapy, other investigators have already reported that amino acid substitution at core 70, IL28B SNP, cirrhosis, alpha-fetoprotein (AFP) level, and prior treatment response are significant pretreatment predictive factors of SVR [6, 18–20]. Regardless of the small number of patients in the present study, we found that prior treatment response, amino acid substitution at core 70, IL28B SNP, cirrhosis, and hyaluronic acid level were also significant predictive factors for SVR. Although the AFP level was not significant in the present study ($P = 0.067$), the AFP level would have been significant if the number of study patients had been much higher. Regarding on-treatment predictive factors, Shimada et al. [21] reported that RVR and very early viral response at week 1 were predictive factors; these investigators noted that the AUCs of the reduction in HCV-RNA levels at week 1 and of the IL28B minor allele were 0.754 and 0.777, respectively, and the predictability of both factors was equivalent. However, they did not evaluate the reduction in HCV-RNA levels at week 2. In the present study, comparison of AUC levels according to on-treatment factors within 4 weeks, including RVR, revealed that the best time point for predicting SVR using viral response was at week 2. Furthermore, the ability of HCV-RNA reduction at week 2 to predict SVR was the best among significant predictive factors, comparable to that of the combination of IL28B SNP and core amino acid substitution at core 70. Although the Japanese guidelines for the management of hepatitis C virus infection [1] do not recommend telaprevir-based triple

therapy in patients having the IL28B minor allele and mutant type of amino acid substitution at core 70, neither of these tests have been approved by the national medical insurance system in Japan. Therefore, the evaluation of HCV-RNA reduction at week 2 may become an alternative to testing IL28B SNPs and core amino acid substitution. However, in order to validate the present results and to determine an optimal cut-off value, a further large-scale study is necessary.

In the present study, the amount of HCV-RNA was measured by the AccuGene method to evaluate virological response within 2 weeks, because the AccuGene method has a wider range and higher sensitivity than the TaqMan method. For the same reason, the amount of HCV core antigen (Ag) was measured by the ARCHITECT method of the third generation HCV core Ag test. In the present study, however, the best cut-off value for predicting SVR using HCV-RNA reduction at week 2 was set at 4.56 logIU/mL. Shimada et al. [21] also set the best cut-off value of predicting SVR using HCV-RNA reduction at week 1 at 4.7 logIU/mL. As the baseline high viral load is defined as more than 5.0 logIU/mL, and HCV-RNA reduction within 2 weeks can be evaluated within the range of either method, it is considered that the difference of sensitivity between the two methods is not significant for evaluating treatment response. Interestingly, although our previous reports indicated that the monitoring of core Ag within 2 weeks is useful for predicting SVR to PEG-IFN and ribavirin combination therapy [22, 23], core Ag was not useful for predictions in telaprevir-based triple therapy. This may indicate that telaprevir is one of the DAAs that strongly inhibit viral RNA replication.

Certain limitations must be considered when interpreting the results of the present study. The present study was small and included both naïve and previously treated patients. In addition, the P value of HCV RNA reduction at week 2 by assessing AUCs was almost similar to that of the various other significant predictors. There may be no significant difference among the AUCs of significant predictors for SVR. In order to validate the present results, further large-scale prospective studies are necessary.

In conclusion, from the analysis of predictors including viral dynamics, it was demonstrated that the best time point for predicting SVR to telaprevir with concomitant PEG-IFN and ribavirin therapy is at week 2, and that HCV-RNA reduction at 2 weeks is the most useful predictor among viral responses within 4 weeks after therapy initiation. As the predictability of HCV-RNA reduction at 2 weeks is equivalent to that of the combination of IL28B SNP and amino acid substitution at core 70, HCV-RNA reduction at week 2 has the potential to be used as an alternative predictor instead of the tests for IL28B SNP and amino acid substitution at core 70.

Conflict of Interests

The authors declare that there is no conflict of interests regarding the publication of this paper.

References

[1] Editors of the Drafting Committee for Hepatitis Management Guidelines: The Japan Society of Hepatology, "Guidelines for the management of hepatitis C virus infection: first edition, May 2012, the Japan Society of Hepatology," *Hepatology Research*, vol. 43, no. 1, pp. 1–34, 2013.

[2] H. Kumada, J. Toyota, T. Okanoue, K. Chayama, H. Tsubouchi, and N. Hayashi, "Telaprevir with peginterferon and ribavirin for treatment-naive patients chronically infected with HCV of genotype 1 in Japan," *Journal of Hepatology*, vol. 56, no. 1, pp. 78–84, 2012.

[3] N. Hayashi, T. Okanoue, H. Tsubouchi, J. Toyota, K. Chayama, and H. Kumada, "Efficacy and safety of telaprevir, a new protease inhibitor, for difficult-to-treat patients with genotype 1 chronic hepatitis C," *Journal of Viral Hepatitis*, vol. 19, no. 2, pp. e134–e142, 2012.

[4] Y. Karino, I. Ozeki, S. Hige et al., "Telaprevir impairs renal function and increases blood ribavirin concentration during telaprevir/pegylated interferon/ribavirin therapy for chronic hepatitis C," *Journal of Viral Hepatitis*, vol. 21, no. 5, pp. 341–347, 2014.

[5] V. Virlogeux, P. Pradat, F. Bailly et al., "Boceprevir and telaprevir-based triple therapy for chronic hepatitis C: virological efficacy and impact on kidney function and model for end-stage liver disease score," *Journal of Viral Hepatitis*, vol. 21, pp. e98–e107, 2014.

[6] N. Akuta, F. Suzuki, M. Hirakawa et al., "Amino acid substitution in hepatitis C virus core region and genetic variation near the interleukin 28B gene predict viral response to telaprevir with peginterferon and ribavirin," *Hepatology*, vol. 52, no. 2, pp. 421–429, 2010.

[7] K. Chayama, C. N. Hayes, H. Abe et al., "IL28B but not ITPA polymorphism is predictive of response to pegylated interferon, ribavirin, and telaprevir triple therapy in patients with genotype 1 hepatitis C," *Journal of Infectious Diseases*, vol. 204, no. 1, pp. 84–93, 2011.

[8] S. Bota, I. Sporea, R. Șirli, A. M. Neghină, A. Popescu, and M. Strāin, "Role of interleukin-28B polymorphism as a predictor of sustained virological response in patients with chronic hepatitis C treated with triple therapy: a systematic review and meta-analysis," *Clinical Drug Investigation*, vol. 33, no. 5, pp. 325–331, 2013.

[9] I. M. Jacobson, J. G. McHutchison, G. Dusheiko et al., "Telaprevir for previously untreated chronic hepatitis C virus infection," *The New England Journal of Medicine*, vol. 364, no. 25, pp. 2405–2416, 2011.

[10] K. E. Sherman, S. L. Flamm, N. H. Afdhal et al., "Response-guided telaprevir combination treatment for hepatitis C virus infection," *The New England Journal of Medicine*, vol. 365, no. 11, pp. 1014–1024, 2011.

[11] T. Hara, N. Akuta, F. Suzuki et al., "A pilot study of triple therapy with telaprevir, peginterferon and ribavirin for elderly patients with genotype 1 chronic hepatitis C," *Journal of Medical Virology*, vol. 85, no. 10, pp. 1746–1753, 2013.

[12] H. Sezaki, F. Suzuki, T. Hosaka et al., "Effectiveness and safety of reduced-dose telaprevir-based triple therapy in chronic hepatitis C patients," *Hepatology Research*, 2014.

[13] P. Simmonds, E. C. Holmes, T.-A. Cha et al., "Classification of hepatitis C virus into six major genotypes and a series of subtypes by phylogenetic analysis of the NS-5 region," *Journal of General Virology*, vol. 74, part 11, pp. 2391–2399, 1993.

[14] N. Akuta, F. Suzuki, H. Sezaki et al., "Association of amino acid substitution pattern in core protein of hepatitis C virus genotype 1b high viral load and non-virological response to interferon-ribavirin combination therapy," *Intervirology*, vol. 48, no. 6, pp. 372–380, 2005.

[15] Y. Tanaka, N. Nishida, M. Sugiyama et al., "Genome-wide association of IL28B with response to pegylated interferon-α and ribavirin therapy for chronic hepatitis C," *Nature Genetics*, vol. 41, no. 10, pp. 1105–1109, 2009.

[16] C. Hézode, H. Fontaine, C. Dorival et al., "Triple therapy in treatment-experienced patients with HCV-cirrhosis in a multicentre cohort of the French Early Access Programme (ANRS CO20-CUPIC)—NCT01514890," *Journal of Hepatology*, vol. 59, no. 3, pp. 434–441, 2013.

[17] M. Colombo, I. Fernández, D. Abdurakhmanov et al., "Safety and on-treatment efficacy of telaprevir: the early access programme for patients with advanced hepatitis C," *Gut*, vol. 63, no. 7, pp. 1150–1158, 2014.

[18] N. Akuta, F. Suzuki, T. Fukushima et al., "Prediction of treatment efficacy and telaprevir-resistant variants after triple therapy in patients infected with hepatitis C virus genotype 1," *Journal of Clinical Microbiology*, vol. 51, no. 9, pp. 2862–2868, 2013.

[19] A. Tsubota, N. Shimada, M. Atsukawa et al., "Impact of IL28B polymorphisms on 24-week telaprevir-based combination therapy for Asian chronic hepatitis C patients with hepatitis C virus genotype 1b," *Journal of Gastroenterology and Hepatology*, vol. 29, no. 1, pp. 144–150, 2014.

[20] N. Shimada, A. Tsubota, M. Atsukawa et al., "α-Fetoprotein is a surrogate marker for predicting treatment failure in telaprevir-based triple combination therapy for genotype 1b chronic hepatitis C Japanese patients with the IL28B minor genotype," *Journal of Medical Virology*, vol. 86, no. 3, pp. 461–472, 2014.

[21] N. Shimada, H. Toyoda, A. Tsubota et al., "Baseline factors and very early viral response (week 1) for predicting sustained virological response in telaprevir-based triple combination therapy for Japanese genotype 1b chronic hepatitis C patients: a multicenter study," *Journal of Gastroenterology*, 2013.

[22] H. Tamai, N. Shingaki, T. Shiraki et al., "Prediction of sustained response to low-dose pegylated interferon alpha-2b plus ribavirin in patients with genotype 1b and high hepatitis C virus level using viral reduction within 2 weeks after therapy initiation," *Hepatology Research*, vol. 41, no. 12, pp. 1137–1144, 2011.

[23] H. Tamai, Y. Mori, N. Shingaki et al., "Low-dose pegylated interferon-α2a plus ribavirin therapy for elderly and/or cirrhotic patients with HCV genotype-1b and high viral load," *Antiviral Therapy*, vol. 19, no. 1, pp. 107–115, 2014.

Portraying Persons Who Inject Drugs Recently Infected with Hepatitis C Accessing Antiviral Treatment: A Cluster Analysis

Jean-Marie Bamvita,[1,2] **Elise Roy,**[3] **Geng Zang,**[1] **Didier Jutras-Aswad,**[1,2]
Andreea Adelina Artenie,[1,4] **Annie Levesque,**[1,4] **and Julie Bruneau**[1,2]

[1] *CRCHUM (Centre de Recherche du Centre Hospitalier de l'Université de Montréal), Tour Saint-Antoine 850, Rue St-Denis, Montréal, QC, Canada H2X 0A9*

[2] *Département de Médecine Familiale, Faculté de Médecine, Université de Montréal, Pavillon Roger-Gaudry, Bureau S-711, 2900 boul. Édouard-Montpetit, Montréal, QC, Canada H3T 1J4*

[3] *Faculté de Médecine et des Sciences de la Santé, Université de Sherbrooke, Campus Longueuil 1111, Rue St-Charles Ouest, Bureau 500, Longueuil, QC, Canada J4K 5G4*

[4] *Family Medicine Department, McGill University, 5858 Chemin de la Côte des Neiges, 3e Étage, Montréal, QC, Canada H3S 1Z1*

Correspondence should be addressed to Julie Bruneau; julie.bruneau@umontreal.ca

Academic Editor: Alessandro Antonelli

Objectives. To empirically determine a categorization of people who inject drug (PWIDs) recently infected with hepatitis C virus (HCV), in order to identify profiles most likely associated with early HCV treatment uptake. *Methods.* The study population was composed of HIV-negative PWIDs with a documented recent HCV infection. Eligibility criteria included being 18 years old or over, and having injected drugs in the previous 6 months preceding the estimated date of HCV exposure. Participant classification was carried out using a TwoStep cluster analysis. *Results.* From September 2007 to December 2011, 76 participants were included in the study. 60 participants were eligible for HCV treatment. Twenty-one participants initiated HCV treatment. The cluster analysis yielded 4 classes: class 1: *Lukewarm health seekers dismissing HCV treatment offer*; class 2: *multisubstance users willing to shake off the hell*; class 3: *PWIDs unlinked to health service use*; class 4: *health seeker PWIDs willing to reverse the fate. Conclusion.* Profiles generated by our analysis suggest that prior health care utilization, a key element for treatment uptake, differs between older and younger PWIDs. Such profiles could inform the development of targeted strategies to improve health outcomes and reduce HCV infection among PWIDs.

1. Introduction

The prevalence of HCV infection is estimated at 130–170 million people worldwide, currently driven by the growing number of infections among people who inject drugs (PWID) [1]. If not treated, the majority (75–85%) evolve to chronic infection; and some (20%) develop intractable and lethal diseases (cirrhosis, liver failure, and hepatoma) [2].

Before the advent of well-tolerated, orally administered HCV treatment regimens, traditional interferon-based antiviral treatment induced significant side effects that were deterring some patients from completing the treatment course.

For patients who achieved sustained viral response equivalent to a cure, HCV treatment was shown to bring additional benefits, such as reduction of risky drug-consumption behaviours [3] and improvement of quality of life [4]. It is likely that, within the next three to five years, well-tolerated, orally administered interferon-free regimens will be available, thus improving the feasibility of treating difficult populations [5]. A recent modeling study by Martin and colleagues suggested that significant decreases in HCV prevalence can be accomplished by increasing simultaneously needle exchange program and opiate substitution therapy coverage on the one hand and HCV treatment coverage on the other hand [6].

In large observational community-based drug users' cohorts, however, the HCV treatment uptake was estimated at <8% or less than 1% annually [7]. Further, despite increasing efforts to attract vulnerable population in treatment, the number of PWIDs treated annually still stagnates [8].

Barriers to HCV treatment were found to be multifactorial and included factors impeding optimal access at the level of the patient, system, and practitioner [7]. Attempts to frame the influence of multidimensional factors and conditions facilitating or impeding health care access and outcomes can be guided by the Behavioral Model of Health Services Utilization, a conceptual framework developed by Andersen [9]. Reasons cited by PWIDs with HCV for not seeking treatment include poor education about their condition and its treatment, an absence of noticeable symptoms, fear of adverse effects of treatment, and other ongoing medical comorbidities and social issues [10]. Beyond individual barriers, factors affecting treatment uptake include financial coverage, housing stability, and assessment by the physician of the risks and benefits of immediate versus delayed treatment for HCV-chronically infected individuals [7]. From a service development perspective, it is important to identify profiles of individuals according to treatment uptake. Such profiles could help inform novel interventions to increase treatment uptake in subgroups with specific characteristics. PWIDs recently infected by HCV who are systematically offered treatment under universal financial coverage represent a unique group to study in order to assess how individual profiles, as opposed to specific risk factors, affect treatment uptake. Cluster analysis has been used in intervention research to unmask unknown heterogeneity between concurrent groups by focusing more on inherent differences between cases than on individual variables [11].

The objective of this study was to empirically identify profiles associated with early HCV treatment uptake among recently HCV infected PWIDs who were systematically offered HCV treatment and were covered by universal health insurance.

2. Methods

2.1. Study Population. The study population was composed of PWIDs recently infected with HCV, enrolled in IMPACT, a study aiming at examining the effect of acute HCV infection and antiviral treatment on the behaviors and quality of life of PWIDs who have access to specific targeted health services. Eligibility criteria included being 18 years old or over, having injected drugs in the previous 6 months or in the 3-month-period preceding the estimated date of HCV infection, and living in the Greater Montreal area. Documented acute HCV infection was defined as either (1) a HCV antibody negative test, followed by either a HCV antibody or RNA positive test within 6 months of the HCV antibody negative test period or (2) an acute symptomatic infection with evidence of hepatitis illness (i.e., jaundice or alanine aminotransferase (ALT) elevation over 400 U/L). Participants were recruited from two main sources: (i) the St. Luc Cohort, a prospective cohort study with semiannual visits designed to examine individual

and contextual factors associated with HCV and HIV infections among current PWIDs (i.e., drug injection in the six months prior to recruitment) [12] and (ii) community and hospital-based collaborating clinics, including the addiction medicine clinic at the Centre Hospitalier de l'Université de Montréal (CHUM).

Eligible individuals were invited to participate in the study and were systematically referred to the CHUM addiction medicine clinic for clinical assessment. PWIDs recently infected with HCV, who did not resolve spontaneously after 20 weeks of estimated infection, were offered HCV treatment regardless of their drug use or social conditions.

The research protocol has been approved by the Institutional Research Ethical Board of the CHUM and includes an authorization to access participants' clinical data, when available. A $30 stipend for travel costs was offered for each completed research visit.

2.2. Variables and Measurement Instruments. The variable of interest was "treatment initiation," defined as receiving a first dose of pegylated interferon. Information was retrieved from the clinical chart and validated with the clinical nurse. Two measurement instruments were used to characterize participants. The SF-36 questionnaire was used to assess health related quality of life (QualityMetric Health Outcomes Scoring Software 4.0). This questionnaire has been extensively used and validated in various patient settings and in the general population [13]. Using factor analysis, items of this questionnaire are conceptually reduced to two main dimensions: physical and mental component of quality of life, which were used for analysis in this study. A short interviewer-administered questionnaire, derived from the St. Luc Cohort questionnaire [14], was used to collect sociodemographic characteristics, information on injection drug use practices, health related factors, and service utilization. Drug use consumption was documented for the prior 6 months.

Given the focus on healthcare utilization, the sample has been described according to the Andersen model, with variables categorized as predisposing, enabling, and need factors [9]. Predisposing factors comprise individual variables associated with service utilization. Enabling factors include contextual, systemic, or structural variables associated with service utilization. Need factors relate to diseases or risky behaviors that could impact on health and well-being. Variables considered in our model were further chosen with respect to the current body of knowledge on HCV treatment access for drug users.

2.3. Analyses. Frequency distribution for categorical variables and mean values along with standard deviations for continuous variables were used for descriptive analyses. Bivariate analyses using Pearson chisquare statistics for categorical variables and independent sample t-test for continuous variables were conducted to compare PWID characteristics according to HCV treatment initiation. Statistically significant differences were assessed at $P < 0.05$; P values were two-sided.

TABLE 1: Characteristics of participants and comparative analyses according to treatment initiation ($n = 60$).

| | Total sample ($N = 60$) | | Frequency distribution | | | | Comparison tests |
| | | | Treatment not initiated $n = 39$ (65%) | | Treatment initiated $n = 21$ (35%) | | P value[*] |
	n	%	n	%	n	%	
Age categories							
<30 years old	28	46.7	21	53.8	7	33.3	
30–39 years old	15	25.0	9	23.1	6	28.6	0.311
>40 years old	17	28.3	9	23.1	8	38.1	0.133
Gender							
Female	15	25.0	11	28.2	4	19.0	0.437
Male	45	75.0	28	71.8	17	81.0	
Education							
Secondary or less	44	73.3	30	76.9	14	66.7	0.397
College or above	16	26.7	9	23.1	7	33.3	
Housing							
Stable housing (home, apartment, room)	25	41.7	18	46.2	7	33.3	
Temporary housing (therapy, prison, shelter)	22	36.7	12	30.8	10	47.6	0.217
Homeless	13	21.7	9	23.1	4	19.0	0.858
Alcohol consumption	36	60.0	23	59.0	13	61.9	0.825
IV drugs consumed							
IV heroine	29	48.3	19	48.7	10	47.6	0.935
IV cocaine	53	88.3	34	87.2	19	90.5	0.705
Vaccines received							
Hepatitis B vaccine	17	28.3	7	17.9	10	47.6	0.015
Quality of life scores							
PCS mean (SD)	46,4	10.2	45.6	9.8	47.9	10.9	0.389
MCS mean (SD)	33,9	13.9	34.0	14.2	33.9	13.8	0.985
Methadone	20	33.3	10	25.6	10	47.6	0.085
Having been followed up in the 6 prior months by a family physician	11	18.3	6	15.4	5	23.8	0.424

[*]Pearson chi-square.

Participant profile was carried out by means of a TwoStep cluster analysis using SPSS Statistics 20.0 package [15, 16]. Variables were introduced in the cluster analysis in an orderly manner, categorical variables first and then continuous variables. The first categorical variable entered was "having initiated HCV treatment." Age categories and housing categories were multicategorical variables. The SF-36 physical and mental component scores were entered as continuous scores in the model. The log-likelihood method was used to determine intersubject distance. The first iteration yielded a two-class cluster model based on Schwarz Bayesian criteria and log-likelihood method, reflecting the overall contribution of participants to the interclass homogeneity. This cluster analysis was discarded because classes were not contrasted enough for interpretation [17]. Finally the number of classes was set at 4 and produced an acceptable model. The quality of the model was estimated as satisfactory by the class cohesion and separation test.

3. Results

From September 2007 to December 2011, 76 participants infected with HCV within the previous six months were recruited in Montreal, Canada. Sixteen (21%) cleared their infection spontaneously and were not included in this investigation. Table 1 presents descriptive characteristics of the 60 participants included in analyses, along with comparison analyses between those who have initiated HCV treatment and those who have not. Overall, 21 participants (35%) had initiated HCV treatment.

The four-class cluster analysis is displayed on Table 2. Classes were labelled according to the most prominent characteristics within classes. The four classes can be described as follows.

Class 1. Lukewarm Health Seekers Dismissing HCV Treatment Offer. This includes younger participants (79% under 30 years

TABLE 2: Participants typology (cluster analysis; $N = 60$).

	Class 1 $n = 14$ (23.3%)	Class 2 $n = 15$ (25.0%)	Class 3 $n = 11$ (18.3%)	Class 4 $n = 20$ (33.3%)	Combined $N = 60$ (100.0%)
Predisposing factors					
Age categories n (%)					
<30 years old	11 (78.6)	13 (86.7)	4 (36.4)	0 (0.0)	28 (46.7)
30–39 years old	3 (21.4)	2 (13.3)	7 (63.6)	3 (15.0)	15 (25.0)
40 years old and over	0 (0.0)	0 (0.0)	0 (0.0)	17 (85.0)	17 (28.3)
Gender n (%)					
Females	12 (85.7)	0 (0.0)	0 (0.0)	3 (15.0)	15 (25.0)
Males	2 (14.3)	15 (100.0)	11 (100.0)	17 (85.0)	45 (75.0)
Education n (%)					
Elementary/secondary	13 (92.9)	12 (80.0)	6 (54.5)	13 (65.0)	44 (73.3)
College or over	1 (7.1)	3 (20.0)	5 (45.5)	7 (35.0)	16 (26.7)
Enabling factor					
Housing n (%)					
Stable housing (home, apartment, room)	9 (64.3)	9 (60.0)	5 (45.5)	2 (10.0)	25 (41.7)
Temporary housing (therapy, prison, shelter)	4 (28.6)	2 (13.3)	0 (0.0)	16 (80.0)	22 (36.7)
Homeless	1 (7.1)	4 (26.7)	6 (54.5)	2 (10.0)	13 (21.7)
Need factors					
IV cocaine consumption n (%)	9 (64.3)	15 (100.0)	11 (100.0)	18 (90.0)	53 (88.3)
IV heroine consumption n (%)	9 (64.3)	15 (100.0)	2 (18.2)	3 (15.0)	29 (48.3)
Alcohol consumption n (%)	8 (57.1)	13 (86.7)	4 (36.4)	11 (55.0)	36 (60.0)
Quality of life (SF-36) (mean (SD)					
PCS mean (SD)	45.7 (6.9)	46.4 (9.4)	46.7 (9.1)	46.8 (13.4)	46.4 (10.2)
MCS mean (SD)	25.3 (12.1)	37.0 (14.8)	37.5 (8.1)	35.7 (15.3)	33.9 (13.9)
Health service utilization					
Methadone program n (%)	5 (35.7)	8 (53.3)	3 (27.3)	4 (20.0)	20 (33.3)
Hepatitis B vaccine n (%)	4 (28.6)	3 (20.0)	0 (0.0)	10 (50.0)	17 (28.3)
Followed up by a family physician n (%)	5 (35.7)	1 (6.7)	0 (0.0)	5 (25.0)	11 (18.3)
Having initiated treatment n (%)	**2 (14.3)**	**8 (53.3)**	**0 (0.0)**	**11 (55.0)**	**21 (35.0)**

old), mostly females (86%), poorly educated (93% without a college degree), living predominantly in stable housing (64%). Compared to other classes, they rank fourth as to cocaine injection (64%) and second as to heroin injection. They have the lowest score on both physical and mental components of quality of life. They represent one of the two highest proportions of participants followed up by a family physician (35%) and the third lowest proportion of HCV treatment uptake (14%).

Class 2. Multisubstance Users Willing to Shake off the Hell. This includes mostly younger participants (87% under 30 years old), exclusively males, poorly educated, living mostly in stable housing. All members (100%) of this class use IV cocaine and IV heroin. They rank first as regard alcohol consumption and have the highest proportion of methadone program involvement. 53% have initiated a HCV treatment, ranking second of the 4 classes.

Class 3. PWIDs Unlinked to Health Service Use. This includes middle-age participants (64% between 30 and 40 years old), exclusively males, with the highest proportion of homelessness of all classes, injecting mostly cocaine. They also report the lowest involvement in health service use. No one in that class has initiated a HCV treatment.

Class 4. Health Seeker PWIDs Willing to Reverse the Fate. This includes the oldest group (all over 30 years old), mostly males, poorly educated, living predominantly (90%) in unstable housing conditions and using IV cocaine use. Participants in this class have the highest score on the physical component of quality of life, the highest proportion of health service use, and the highest proportion of HCV treatment initiation.

4. Discussion

PWIDs face many challenges and experience competing needs when it comes to taking care of their health. Overall, 35% of eligible PWIDs initiated treatment. The proportion of participants treated in our study soon after diagnosis is greater than in most studies among HCV infected active PWIDs [18]. This may indicate that delaying treatment, either for recently or chronically infected individuals, might not be the best option to increase uptake. Findings from a recent clinical trial conducted in Canada support this assumption: a higher overall sustained viral response (65% versus 39%) was found among PWIDs allocated to immediate versus delayed treatment onset [19].

This study was undertaken to draw profiles associated with HCV treatment uptake after recent infection, in a setting where treatment was systematically offered under universal health insurance coverage. Overall, results suggest that educated male and female PWIDs and those who had links with various health care services, as shown by prior hepatitis B vaccination, opiate substitution treatment (OST) participation, and visit to a health care professional, were more likely to initiate HCV treatment after recent infection, regardless of drug-consumption. As in McGowan study [20], participants in classes 2 and 4, who initiated treatment, were also characterized by lower self-rated mental health quality of life. According to Anderson's model, prior healthcare service utilization may enable further health service use [9]. Participants in classes 2 and 4, which together comprise 90% of all participants treated, had higher proportions of methadone program participation, hepatitis B vaccination, and follow-up by family physician. In a study conducted in Australia by Digiusto and Treloar [21], participants who had consulted a general practitioner for medication were more likely to have initiated HCV treatment. Participation to a methadone maintenance treatment has been associated with a higher willingness to be treated [22], to increased treatment uptake [23] and to better outcomes [24]. In a recent study among drug users followed in methadone and community clinics with enhanced HCV treatment access, methadone was not associated with uptake [25].

A salient characteristic of this cluster analysis was the identification of distinct profiles according to treatment uptake, for which standard comparisons were not quite informative. For instance, age was not statistically associated with treatment uptake in bivariate analysis. However, the age distribution in clusters suggests that uptake profiles differ between older and younger drug users. Classes 1 and 2 comprised 24 of the 28 individuals under 30. In contrast, classes 3 and 4 included all but five individuals over 30.

Hence, when contrasting "younger" (classes 1 and 2) and "older" (classes 3 and 4) PWID profiles, results from the cluster analysis suggest that the effect of health care utilization, an important element for treatment uptake, differed between older and younger groups. Younger individuals who initiated treatment reported being in methadone substitution treatment in higher proportions. Vaccination and family physician attendance were reported by a substantial proportion of older individuals initiating treatment, and by none of those who did not. In addition, class profiles showed that housing status, namely, living in a prison, a shelter, or in a therapy setting, was related to treatment uptake among older PWIDs, but not so among younger drug users.

The seemingly positive impact of living in an institutional facility, either prison, therapy, or shelter, on treatment uptake among older participants in our study may indicate enhanced linkages with healthcare services through service providers, relative to other individuals in this cohort [26]. Conversely, class 3 profile includes a majority of homeless individuals, no one having initiated HCV treatment. According to Andersen's

theory, when healthcare access is determined by enabling factors, such as their housing situation among older participants, systemic inequity is an issue [9].

Active use of illicit drugs is a treatment barrier documented in many studies. Active illicit drug use was associated with reluctance to initiate HCV treatment by the patient [27] and by the physician [28]. Alcohol abuse was also found associated with not initiating treatment [29]. In our setting, however, the proportion of participants reporting drug and alcohol use was slightly higher among initiates relative to participants who were not treated, consistent across all classes. Active substance use was not a motive to deny treatment in this study. This finding suggests that active drug use may not be an important factor in the decision to get treated in the absence of systemic and practitioner-level barriers. It is also possible that ongoing drug use was linked to more contact with health services, probably due to multiple health related consequences of drug use overtime.

Results of this study are subject to numerous limitations. First, we acknowledge that our sample may not be representative of drug users in other settings. If there have been some observed shifts in its use, cocaine is still the most prevalent injection drug used in Eastern Canada [30]. Moreover, cocaine use worldwide has remained stable, with indications of increases in Oceania, Asia, Africa, and some countries in South America [31]. Despite close clinical follow-up of participants through laboratory analyses, our results could be biased by the self-reported behavioral data related to alcohol and drug use. In general, self-reported data from PWIDs tend to be accurate [32]. This study could also be subject to interviewer bias, which has been mitigated, if not prevented, by regular retraining of interviewers to uphold the integrity of data collection procedures and avoid imposition of systematic bias. A sample of 60 participants is obviously low. Nonetheless, the quality of the model was estimated to be satisfactory.

5. Conclusion

This study underscores the importance of reaching beyond the individual-level factors in characterizing vulnerable populations in relation to HCV treatment uptake. Looking at profiles instead of individual variables can help tackle health related behaviors of PWIDs recently infected with HCV. This natural experiment represents a novel approach to understanding how specific patient characteristics can be used to develop targeted strategies to improve health outcomes and reduce HCV infection. For example, systemic barriers should be recognized early among those eligible for HCV treatment—such as difficulty in accessing decent accommodation or job—and tackled strategically by linking patients with case manager and social worker services.

Conflict of Interests

The authors declare that there is no conflict of interests regarding the publication of this paper.

Acknowledgments

This study was funded through the following institutions and grant agencies: Fonds de la recherche du Québec-Santé (FRQ-S) and Canadian Institutes for Health Research (CIHR). Dr Jutras-Aswad holds a Junior 1 FRQ-S career award. Jean-Marie Bamvita holds a fellowship award from the National Canadian Research Training Program on HCV. The authors would like to acknowledge the contribution of Élisabeth Deschênes, Rachel Bouchard, and the other staff at HEPCO (Impact) research site. They extend their special thanks to the St. Luc Cohort (Impact) participants, without whom this research would not be possible.

References

[1] C. W. Shepard, L. Finelli, and M. J. Alter, "Global epidemiology of hepatitis C virus infection," *The Lancet Infectious Diseases*, vol. 5, no. 9, pp. 558–567, 2005.

[2] Y. Ueno, J. D. Sollano, and G. C. Farrell, "Prevention of hepatocellular carcinoma complicating chronic hepatitis C," *Journal of Gastroenterology and Hepatology*, vol. 24, no. 4, pp. 531–536, 2009.

[3] W. A. Zule and D. P. Desmond, "Factors predicting entry of injecting drug users into substance abuse treatment," *The American Journal of Drug and Alcohol Abuse*, vol. 26, no. 2, pp. 247–261, 2000.

[4] J. G. McHutchison, J. E. Ware Jr., M. S. Bayliss et al., "The effects of interferon alpha-2b in combination with ribavirin on health related quality of life and work productivity," *Journal of Hepatology*, vol. 34, no. 1, pp. 140–147, 2001.

[5] N. K. Martin, P. Vickerman, A. Miners et al., "Cost-effectiveness of hepatitis C virus antiviral treatment for injection drug user populations," *Hepatology*, vol. 55, no. 1, pp. 49–57, 2012.

[6] N. K. Martin, P. Vickerman, J. Grebely et al., "Hepatitis C virus treatment for prevention among people who inject drugs: modeling treatment scale-up in the age of direct-acting antivirals," *Hepatology*, vol. 58, no. 5, pp. 1598–1609, 2013.

[7] S. H. Mehta, B. L. Genberg, J. Astemborski et al., "Limited uptake of hepatitis C treatment among injection drug users," *Journal of Community Health*, vol. 33, no. 3, pp. 126–133, 2008.

[8] M. Alavi, J. D. Raffa, G. D. Deans et al., "Continued low uptake of treatment for hepatitis C virus infection in a large community-based cohort of inner city residents," *Liver International*, vol. 34, no. 8, pp. 1198–1206, 2014.

[9] R. M. Andersen, "Revisiting the behavioral model and access to medical care: does it matter?" *Journal of Health and Social Behavior*, vol. 36, no. 1, pp. 1–10, 1995.

[10] S. A. Strathdee, M. Latka, J. Campbell et al., "Factors associated with interest in initiating treatment for hepatitis C virus (HCV) infection among young HCV-infected injection drug users," *Clinical Infectious Diseases*, vol. 40, supplement 5, pp. S304–S312, 2005.

[11] D. A. Luke, "Getting the big picture in community science: methods that capture context," *The American Journal of Community Psychology*, vol. 35, no. 3-4, pp. 185–200, 2005.

[12] J. Bruneau, É. Roy, N. Arruda, G. Zang, and D. Jutras-Aswad, "The rising prevalence of prescription opioid injection and its association with hepatitis C incidence among street-drug users," *Addiction*, vol. 107, no. 7, pp. 1318–1327, 2012.

[13] S. J. Coons, S. Rao, D. L. Keininger, and R. D. Hays, "A comparative review of generic quality-of-life instruments," *PharmacoEconomics*, vol. 17, no. 1, pp. 13–35, 2000.

[14] J. Bruneau, F. Lamothe, J. Soto et al., "Sex-specific determinants of HIV infection among injection drug users in Montreal," *CMAJ*, vol. 164, no. 6, pp. 767–773, 2001.

[15] M. J. Norusis, "Cluster Analysis," Chapter 16 in IBM SPSS Statistics 19 Guide to Data Analysis, 2011, http://www.norusis.com/pdf/SPC_v13.pdf.

[16] IBM SPSS Statistics, "Analyse TwoStep Cluster," 2011, http://www-01.ibm.com/support/knowledgecenter/SSLVMB_20.0.0/com.ibm.spss.statistics.help/idh_twostep_main.htm.

[17] M. S. Aldenderfer and R. K. Blasfield, *Chapter 23: Cluster Analysis*, Sage, 2014, http://www.uk.sagepub.com/burns/website%20material/Chapter%2023%20-%20Cluster%20Analysis.pdf.

[18] J. Grebely, J. D. Raffa, C. Lai et al., "Low uptake of treatment for hepatitis C virus infection in a large community-based study of inner city residents," *Journal of Viral Hepatitis*, vol. 16, no. 5, pp. 352–358, 2009.

[19] R. J. Hilsden, G. Macphail, J. Grebely, B. Conway, and S. S. Lee, "Directly observed pegylated interferon plus self-administered ribavirin for the treatment of hepatitis C virus infection in people actively using drugs: a randomized controlled trial," *Clinical Infectious Diseases*, vol. 57, supplement 2, pp. S90–S96, 2013.

[20] C. E. McGowan and M. W. Fried, "Barriers to hepatitis C treatment," *Liver International*, vol. 32, no. 1, pp. 151–156, 2012.

[21] E. Digiusto and C. Treloar, "Equity of access to treatment, and barriers to treatment for illicit drug use in Australia," *Addiction*, vol. 102, no. 6, pp. 958–969, 2007.

[22] C. Treloar, P. Hull, G. J. Dore, and J. Grebely, "Knowledge and barriers associated with assessment and treatment for hepatitis C virus infection among people who inject drugs," *Drug and Alcohol Review*, vol. 31, no. 7, pp. 918–924, 2012.

[23] R. Moirand, M. Bilodeau, S. Brissette, and J. Bruneau, "Determinants of antiviral treatment initiation in a hepatitis C-infected population benefiting from universal health care coverage," *Canadian Journal of Gastroenterology*, vol. 21, no. 6, pp. 355–361, 2007.

[24] S.-M. Alavian, A. Mirahmadizadeh, M. Javanbakht et al., "Effectiveness of methadone maintenance treatment in prevention of hepatitis C virus transmission among injecting drug users," *Hepatitis Monthly*, vol. 13, no. 8, Article ID e12411, 2013.

[25] M. Alavi, J. Grebely, M. Micallef et al., "Assessment and treatment of hepatitis C virus infection among people who inject drugs in the opioid substitution setting: ETHOS study," *Clinical Infectious Diseases*, vol. 57, supplement 2, pp. S62–S69, 2013.

[26] J. D. Farley, V. K. Wong, H. V. Chung et al., "Treatment of chronic hepatitis C in Canadian prison inmates," *Canadian Journal of Gastroenterology*, vol. 19, no. 3, pp. 153–156, 2005.

[27] G. Gazdag, G. Horváth, O. Szabó, and G. S. Ungvari, "Barriers to antiviral treatment in hepatitis C infected intravenous drug users," *Neuropsychopharmacologia Hungarica*, vol. 12, no. 4, pp. 459–462, 2010.

[28] S. Manolakopoulos, M. J. Deutsch, O. Anagnostou et al., "Substitution treatment or active intravenous drug use should not be contraindications for antiviral treatment in drug users with chronic hepatitis C," *Liver International*, vol. 30, no. 10, pp. 1454–1460, 2010.

[29] J. A. Morrill, M. Shrestha, and R. W. Grant, "Barriers to the treatment of hepatitis C: patient, provider, and system factors,"

Journal of General Internal Medicine, vol. 20, no. 8, pp. 754–758, 2005.

[30] E. Roy, P. Leclerc, C. Morissette et al., "Prevalence and temporal trends of crack injection among injection drug users in eastern central Canada," *Drug and Alcohol Dependence*, vol. 133, no. 1, pp. 275–278, 2013.

[31] United Nations Office on Drugs and Crime (UNODC), "Recent statistics and trend analysis of illicit drug markets," 2012, http://www.unodc.org/documents/data-and-analysis/WDR2012/ WDR_2012_Chapter1.pdf.

[32] J. de Irala, C. Bigelow, J. McCusker, R. Hindin, and L. Zheng, "Reliability of self-reported human immunodeficiency virus risk behaviors in a residential drug treatment population," *American Journal of Epidemiology*, vol. 143, no. 7, pp. 725–732, 1996.

Predictors of Health-Related Quality of Life in Outpatients with Cirrhosis: Results from a Prospective Cohort

Maja Thiele,[1,2,3] Gro Askgaard,[4] Hans B. Timm,[5] Ole Hamberg,[4] and Lise L. Gluud[2,6]

[1] *Department of Medicine, Copenhagen University Hospital Koge, 4600 Koege, Denmark*
[2] *Department of Medicine, Copenhagen University Hospital Gentofte, 2900 Hellerup, Denmark*
[3] *Department of Gastroenterology and Hepatology, Odense University Hospital, 5000 Odense, Denmark*
[4] *Department of Hepatology, Copenhagen University Hospital Rigshospitalet, 2100 Copenhagen, Denmark*
[5] *Department of Medicine, Copenhagen University Hospital Glostrup, 2600 Glostrup, Denmark*
[6] *Gastrounit, Copenhagen University Hospital Hvidovre, 2650 Hvidovre, Denmark*

Correspondence should be addressed to Maja Thiele; maja.thiele@rsyd.dk

Academic Editor: Yoichi Hiasa

Background. Cirrhosis may lead to a poor health-related quality of life (HRQOL), which should be taken into consideration when addressing the cirrhotic outpatient. *Methods.* Prospective cohort study evaluating predictors of HRQOL in outpatients with cirrhosis. Patients with overt hepatic encephalopathy at baseline were excluded. HRQOL was evaluated at baseline using the six point Chronic Liver Disease Questionnaire. Predictors of low quality of life scores (<4 points) and mortality were analyzed using multivariable logistic regression. *Results.* In total, 92 patients were included (mean age 61 years, 59% male). Nineteen patients died (mean duration of follow-up 20 months). The mean Child-Pugh score was 6.9. Twenty percent had a poor HRQOL judged by the Chronic Liver Disease Questionnaire score and 45% had covert hepatic encephalopathy. The only predictors of poor HRQOL were the Child-Pugh score ($\beta = 0.45; P = 0.013$), nonalcoholic etiology of cirrhosis ($\beta = -2.34; P = 0.009$), and body mass index ($\beta = -0.20; P = 0.023$). The body mass index predicted poor HRQOL independently of the presence of ascites and albumin level. *Conclusions.* The body mass index was associated with a low HRQOL. This suggests that malnutrition may be an important target in the management of patients with cirrhosis.

1. Introduction

The prognosis of cirrhosis has improved following the development of a number of effective interventions [1–3]. The improvements include the management of gastrointestinal bleeding, hepatorenal syndrome, spontaneous bacterial peritonitis, hepatocellular carcinoma, and hepatic encephalopathy (HE) [4–8]. The health-related quality of life (HRQOL) is therefore becoming increasingly important [9–13]. Most quality of life studies have used generic questionnaires, which allow for comparisons between different groups of patients. These questionnaires will provide an overall picture of the wellbeing of participants. Patients with cirrhosis have specific somatic and cognitive symptoms that may affect their HRQOL [12, 14, 15]. These symptoms may not be captured by generic scales [9, 13, 16, 17]. Questionnaires specifically for patients with chronic liver disease have therefore been developed [14, 18].

Identifying factors associated with HRQOL may help improve patient care and guide future research [12]. This is especially the case for long-term care in an outpatient setting. We therefore performed a prospective cohort study aimed at investigating the prognosis and predictors of HRQOL in patients with cirrhosis followed up at an outpatient setting.

2. Materials and Methods

2.1. Included Subjects. From February 2008 to May 2012 we conducted a prospective cohort study on patients with cirrhosis recruited from two Danish liver outpatient clinics. Patients were eligible for inclusion if they had histological or clinical cirrhosis and were able to read Danish. Patients with overt HE (West Haven Criteria Grades 2 to 4) and concurrent malignancy were excluded. The study protocol conformed to the ethical guidelines of the 1975 Declaration of Helsinki and was approved by the Danish ethics committee.

Patients were identified at their regular visits to the participating clinics or through the Danish case-mix system of diagnostic codes (dkDRG; Diagnosis Related Groups, based on the ICD-10 classification system). Patients identified electronically were invited to participate by telephone. Patients who agreed to participate completed a written informed consent at the inclusion visit.

At inclusion, demographic data, the patient history, and medication were recorded. A full physical examination and a broad screening panel of tests (including liver function tests, haematology, creatinine, and electrolytes) were performed. The Child-Pugh score was calculated. Evidence of covert HE [17] was evaluated clinically and using the continuous reaction time test (CRT), which is a validated computerized psychometric test [19–24]. The test records reaction times to sound stimuli. Test results are expressed as reaction time percentiles (10, 50, and 90). An index value for the reaction time variance (index value = 50 percentile/90 percentile − 10 percentile) is calculated. Lower index values indicate higher reaction time variance with values below 1.900 suggesting HE in patients with cirrhosis.

HRQOL was evaluated using the six-point, 29-item Chronic Liver Disease Questionnaire (CLDQ) [18]. The questionnaire covers six domains: abdominal symptoms, fatigue, worry, activity, and systemic symptoms. The questionnaire was validated in a pilot study cohort of 15 patients (after backward and forward translation into Danish).

2.2. Statistical Analyses. Patient characteristics were summarized as proportions with means and standard deviations/range. The CLDQ score was classed as low (<4) or high (4–6). Predictors of CLDQ scores and mortality were analyzed using binary logistic regression. Multivariable analyses were performed using backward elimination. The predictors were age, gender, body mass index (BMI), etiology of liver cirrhosis, employment, marital status, comorbidities, previous hepatic decompensation, covert hepatic encephalopathy, Child-Pugh score, ascites, ongoing alcohol abuse, albumin, and hyponatremia. Statistical analyses were performed using STATA version 12 (Stata Corp., College Station, Texas, US).

3. Results

3.1. Patient Characteristics. A total of 92 patients were included and followed for a mean duration of 20 months (range 3 to 52 months). Four patients withdrew their consent regarding the CRT test and the HRQOL questionnaire. Five patients did not complete the CRT test or the HRQOL scores because they had to be hospitalized due to worsening of their underlying liver disease. All 92 patients continued in the follow-up cohort and were included in the outcome analysis.

The mean age of included patients was 61 (SD 8.7; range 41 to 83 years) and 54 (59%) were men. The mean

TABLE 1: Patient characteristics at inclusion.

Variable	Mean ± SD (range) N (%)
Followup (months)	19.9 ± 16.0 (3–52)
Male gender	54 (59)
Employed	14 (15)
Married or similar	51 (55)
Age (years)	61.5 ± 8.7 (41–83)
Alcoholic liver cirrhosis	79 (86)
Child-Pugh score	6.8 ± 1.6 (5–12)
Child-Pugh class A/B/C	46/38/8
International normalized ratio	1.28 ± 0.3 (0.9–3.1)
ALT (international units)	32 ± 25 (3–163)
Creatinine (μmol/L)	86 ± 35 (43–221)
Sodium (mmol/L)	137 ± 6 (101–146)
Ammonia (μmol/L)	37 ± 34 (0–91)
Albumin (g/L)	39 ± 6 (27–50)
Ongoing alcohol abuse	39 (42)
Ascites present	26 (28)
Prior decompensation	
Ascites	59 (64)
Hepatic encephalopathy	21 (23)
Varices	41 (45)
Prior variceal bleeding	13 (14)
Comorbidities	
Lung disease	11 (12)
Heart disease*	30 (33)
Kidney disease	12 (13)
Diabetes	18 (20)
Prior malignancy	8 (9)

*includes arterial hypertension and atrial fibrillation. ALT: alanine aminotransferase.

body mass index was 24 (SD 4.0; range 16 to 35). Most patients had cirrhosis due to alcoholic liver disease (Table 1). The remaining patients had autoimmune liver diseases (4), nonalcoholic steatohepatitis (2), chronic hepatitis C infection (3), hemochromatosis (1), or cryptogenic cirrhosis (3).

Fifty-two percent of the patients were classed as Child-Pugh class A. The mean Child-Pugh score was 6.9 (SD 1.7; range 5 to 12). Seventy-seven patients had clinical signs of decompensation prior to inclusion. At baseline, 26 patients (28%) had ascites and 41 patients (45%) were diagnosed as having covert HE. Sixty-one patients were treated with lactulose, 61 with beta-blockers, 57 with loop diuretics, and 35 with spironolactone. Eighty-three received vitamins.

During followup, 19 patients died (21%), including seven classed as Child-Pugh class A at baseline (Table 2). Most patients died from liver related causes. Even though patients with concurrent malignancy were excluded, six fatalities were due to cancer disease. Four of these were hepatocellular carcinoma, stressing the importance of this cancer even in a population consisting largely of patients with alcoholic cirrhosis.

TABLE 2: Causes of death during followup.

Causes	Child-Pugh class
Gastrointestinal bleeding (1), variceal bleeding (2), hepatorenal syndrome (1), metastatic oropharynx cancer (1), and HCC (2).	A
Metastatic lung cancer (2), progressive liver failure (2), HCC (1), sepsis (1), and unknown (1).	B
Gastrointestinal bleeding (1), progressive liver failure (2), HRS (1), and HCC (1).	C

HCC: hepatocellular carcinoma; HRS: hepatorenal syndrome.

TABLE 3: Clinical outcomes during followup.

Event	N (%)
Death	19 (21)
Transplantation	1 (1)
TIPS	2 (2)
Hepatic encephalopathy	25 (27)
Hepatorenal syndrome	6 (7)
Nonvariceal gastrointestinal bleeding	17 (18)
Variceal bleeding	5 (5)
Hepatocellular carcinoma	4 (4)
Spontaneous bacterial peritonitis	6
Bacterial infections	34
Other events, requiring hospitalisation	25

TIPS: transjugular intrahepatic portosystemic shunt.

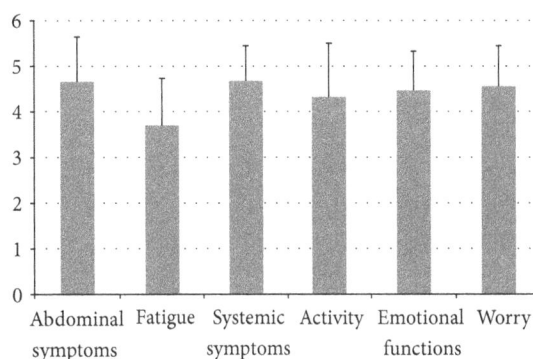

FIGURE 1: Means with standard deviations for the Chronic Liver Disease Questionnaire domains.

One patient underwent successful liver transplantation and two patients received a transjugular intrahepatic portosystemic shunt. Spontaneous bacterial peritonitis was diagnosed in six patients and 34 developed other bacterial infections that required hospitalization. Seventeen patients were admitted with upper gastrointestinal bleeding, 25 developed overt HE, and six developed hepatorenal syndrome. Seven patients were admitted with an ischemic stroke (Table 3).

In univariable logistic regression, the Child-Pugh score and albumin predicted mortality (regression coefficient (β) 0.362; $P = 0.018$ and $\beta = -0.129; P = 0.012$). None of the remaining variables were associated with mortality (Table 4). In multivariable regression analysis, the Child-Pugh score remained the only predictor of mortality after backward elimination.

The mean CLDQ score was 4.4 (SD 0.7; range: 2.8 to 5.9). Eighteen patients (20%) had low CLDQ scores. The most frequent complaint was fatigue (mean score 3.7; SD 1.0; range 1 to 6 points) and most commonly patients had trouble lifting or carrying heavy objects (Figure 1). Univariable analysis found that patients with a low CDLQ score were more likely to have a high Child-Pugh score ($\beta = 0.454; P = 0.013$), other causes of cirrhosis than alcohol ($\beta = -2.343; P = 0.009$), and a low BMI ($\beta = -0.202; P = 0.023$). The association with BMI was independent of the presence of ascites, low albumin or the Child-Pugh score. None of the remaining variables were associated with low CLDQ scores (Table 4). In multivariable analysis, the Child-Pugh score and etiology other than alcohol were independent predictors of CLDQ scores ($\beta = 0.854; P = 0.006$ and $\beta = -2.583; P = 0.039$) but not BMI ($\beta = -0.210; P = 0.060$).

4. Discussion

This prospective cohort study showed that one in five outpatients with cirrhosis had a low health-related quality of life. The finding was surprising considering the high proportion of patients without signs of hepatic decompensation. The severity of the underlying liver disease predicted both poor HRQOL and mortality. The nutritional status estimated by the BMI was a predictor of HRQOL, independent of the presence of ascites or low albumin. Patients with a low BMI were more likely to have a low HRQOL.

The relatively small sample size is the main limitation of the present study and may explain why the Child-Pugh score, non-alcoholic etiology, and BMI were the only predictors of quality of life. However, our results concur with studies showing that the Child-Pugh score is associated with the quality of life. Our results concur with studies showing that the Child-Pugh score is associated with the quality of life [12, 14]. The association between a low BMI and a low quality of life has been identified for patients with other disease categories but not for patients with cirrhosis [25, 26]. The association between a low BMI and a low quality of life score was independent of the severity of the underlying liver disease, presence of ascites, and albumin level. This suggests that interventions aiming at an improved overall nutritional status of cirrhotic patients may improve their quality of life. We recommend following the International Society for Hepatic Encephalopathy and Nitrogen Metabolism consensus statement regarding nutritional management of hepatic encephalopathy in patients with cirrhosis [27]. Frequent small meals rich in vegetables and dairy protein supplemented with a night time snack of complex

TABLE 4: Univariable regression analysis of potential predictors for mortality and health-related quality of life.

Variable	Mortality		CLDQ score <4	
	Regression coefficient β	P value	Regression coefficient β	P value
Age	0.017	0.576	−0.020	0.507
Gender	−0.580	0.264	−0.945	0.091
Body mass index	−0.147	0.083	**−0.202**	**0.023**
Employment	−0.405	0.619	−0.539	0.519
Marital status	0.095	0.855	−0.841	0.133
Nonalcoholic etiology of cirrhosis	−0.891	0.196	**−2.343**	**0.009**
Comorbidities				
Heart disease	0.598	0.267	0.270	0.634
Pulmonary disease	—	—	−0.219	0.798
Renal disease	0.758	0.263	−0.515	0.537
Diabetes	0.557	0.360	−0.644	0.437
Previous malignancy	0.921	0.238	−0.348	0.763
Previous hepatic decompensation				
Ascites	0.459	0.425	−0.270	0.634
Hepatic encephalopathy	0.642	0.267	−0.707	0.315
Esophageal varices	0.118	0.820	−0.879	0.140
Child-Pugh score	**0.362**	**0.018**	**0.454**	**0.013**
Ascites at inclusion	−0.142	0.807	0.752	0.199
Minimal hepatic encephalopathy	−0.013	0.982	0.160	0.778
Hyponatremia	−0.002	0.679	−0.003	0.521
Albumin	**−0.129**	**0.012**	−0.083	0.109
Ongoing alcohol abuse	−0.064	0.903	−0.491	0.379

CLDQ: Chronic Liver Disease Questionnaire.
Results in bold refers to statistically significant predictors of mortality and CLDQ.

carbohydrates may be of benefit to all cirrhotics with a BMI below 25. Accordingly, studies on patients with cirrhosis have found a beneficial effect on the HRQOL of branched chain amino acids and late evening nutritional supplements, which resulted in minor weight gains [28–30].

Our results do not allow for a recommendation of the optimal BMI in chronic liver disease, neither does our study offer a causal explanation of the association between lower BMI and low HRQOL. A low BMI may cause low HRQOL, for example, due to decreased resilience. Alternatively, the body weight of patients with a low HRQOL may decrease, for example, due to inadequate food intake. However, as excess body weight has been associated with increased risk of HCC in chronic liver disease and disease progression in alcoholic liver disease, it can be speculated that BMI in patients with cirrhosis should not exceed 25 [31, 32]. Likewise, avoiding obesity associated with coronary heart disease and diabetes is of great importance, especially as the incidence of NASH cirrhosis is increasing.

The CLDQ is developed and validated in cohorts of patients with all types of liver diseases [18]. We did however find that patients with nonalcoholic etiologies of liver disease had significantly lower HRQOL than patients with alcoholic cirrhosis. The reason for this is unclear and opposes prior findings [14].

In agreement with previous studies, 60% of included patients had covert HE [33, 34]. We found no association between CLDQ scores and HE as judged by the continuous reaction times. Unlike studies on overt HE [9, 13, 16, 35], the evidence on the impact of covert HE on HRQOL is less conclusive [9, 13, 36–39]. However, we cannot exclude that our study would have generated different results if the sample size was larger.

Although most of the included patients had compensated liver disease at baseline, the prognosis was severe. Twenty-one percent of included patients died. Seven of nineteen deaths occurred in patients who were classed as Child-Pugh group A. Most of these patients had previous signs of decompensated liver disease with ascites, variceal bleeding, spontaneous bacterial peritonitis, or overt HE. Our results support the theory that decompensating events as well as Child-Pugh scores predict long-term prognosis in cirrhosis [3]. The increased risk of infections concurs with previous evidence [40, 41]. The relatively high number of strokes may reflect the coagulopathy that is seen in chronic liver disease [42].

In conclusion, this study found that the prognosis of patients with cirrhosis is severe. The finding suggests that these patients should be followed at outpatient clinics as even patients with a low Child-Pugh class may benefit from regular visits. Additional studies are needed to identify the most efficient management strategies in order to improve the prognosis as well as the quality of life. Interventions directed against malnutrition may help achieve this goal.

Abbreviations

BMI: Body mass index
CLDQ: Chronic Liver Disease Questionnaire
CRT: Continuous reaction time test
HE: Hepatic encephalopathy
HRQOL: Health-related quality of life.

Conflict of Interests

There is no conflict of interests.

Authors' Contribution

Maja Thiele is the gurantator of the paper. Conceptualization: Lise Lotte Gluud, Ole Hamberg, Hans B. Timm. Recruitment: All authors. Data collection: Gro Askgaard, Hans B. Timm, Maja Thiele. Statistical analyses: Maja Thiele, Lise Lotte Gluud. Drafted the paper: Maja Thiele, Lise Lotte Gluud, Gro Askgaard. All authors have approved the final version of the paper.

Acknowledgments

The authors would like to thank Mette Munk Lauridsen, M.D., for advice regarding the continuous reaction time test and the specialist nurses Kirsten Passow, Hanne Bennick, Birte Röttig, and Kirsten Larsen for their dedicated work, which facilitated the conduct of the present study. The study was supported by a working grant from the START Fund, Copenhagen University Hospital Gentofte. Results from the study were presented at the 15th ISHEN Symposium (International Society for Hepatic Encephalopathy and Nitrogen Metabolism) and at the 2012 annual meeting of the Danish Society of Gastroenterology and Hepatology.

References

[1] A. Propst, T. Propst, G. Zangerl, D. Ofner, G. Judmaier, and W. Vogel, "Prognosis and life expectancy in chronic liver disease," *Digestive Diseases and Sciences*, vol. 40, no. 8, pp. 1805–1815, 1995.

[2] H. T. Sørensen, A. M. Thulstrup, L. Mellemkjar et al., "Long-term survival and cause-specific mortality in patients with cirrhosis of the liver: a nationwide cohort study in Denmark," *Journal of Clinical Epidemiology*, vol. 56, no. 1, pp. 88–93, 2003.

[3] G. D'Amico, G. Garcia-Tsao, and L. Pagliaro, "Natural history and prognostic indicators of survival in cirrhosis: a systematic review of 118 studies," *Journal of Hepatology*, vol. 44, no. 1, pp. 217–231, 2006.

[4] M. Thiele, A. Krag, U. Rohde, and L. L. Gluud, "Meta-analysis: banding ligation and medical interventions for the prevention of rebleeding from oesophageal varices," *Alimentary Pharmacology and Therapeutics*, vol. 35, no. 10, pp. 1155–1165, 2012.

[5] L. L. Gluud, K. Christensen, E. Christensen, and A. Krag, "Systematic review of randomized trials on vasoconstrictor drugs for hepatorenal syndrome," *Hepatology*, vol. 51, no. 2, pp. 576–584, 2010.

[6] R. Wiest, A. Krag, and A. Gerbes, "Spontaneous bacterial peritonitis: recent guidelines and beyond," *Gut*, vol. 61, no. 2, pp. 297–310, 2012.

[7] EASL-EORTC, "EASL-EORTC Clinical Practice Guidelines: management of hepatocellular carcinoma," *Journal of Hepatology*, vol. 56, pp. 908–943, 2012.

[8] J. S. Bajaj, "Review article: the modern management of hepatic encephalopathy," *Alimentary Pharmacology and Therapeutics*, vol. 31, no. 5, pp. 537–547, 2010.

[9] M. R. Arguedas, T. G. DeLawrence, and B. M. McGuire, "Influence of hepatic encephalopathy on health-related quality of life in patients with cirrhosis," *Digestive Diseases and Sciences*, vol. 48, no. 8, pp. 1622–1626, 2003.

[10] E. Fritz and J. Hammer, "Gastrointestinal symptoms in patients with liver cirrhosis are linked to impaired quality of life and psychological distress," *European Journal of Gastroenterology and Hepatology*, vol. 21, no. 4, pp. 460–465, 2009.

[11] M. Holecek, "Three targets of branched-chain amino acid supplementation in the treatment of liver disease," *Nutrition*, vol. 26, no. 5, pp. 482–490, 2010.

[12] G. Marchesini, G. Bianchi, P. Amodio et al., "Factors associated with poor health-related quality of life of patients with cirrhosis," *Gastroenterology*, vol. 120, no. 1, pp. 170–178, 2001.

[13] I. Les, E. Doval, M. Flavia et al., "Quality of life in cirrhosis is related to potentially treatable factors," *European Journal of Gastroenterology & Hepatology*, vol. 22, pp. 221–227, 2010.

[14] Z. M. Younossi, N. Boparai, L. L. Price, M. L. Kiwi, M. McCormick, and G. Guyatt, "Health-related quality of life in chronic liver disease: the impact of type and severity of disease," *American Journal of Gastroenterology*, vol. 96, no. 7, pp. 2199–2205, 2001.

[15] E. Kalaitzakis, M. Simrén, R. Olsson et al., "Gastrointestinal symptoms in patients with liver cirrhosis: associations with nutritional status and health-related quality of life," *Scandinavian Journal of Gastroenterology*, vol. 41, no. 12, pp. 1464–1472, 2006.

[16] Z.-J. Bao, D.-K. Qiu, X. Ma et al., "Assessment of health-related quality of life in Chinese patients with minimal hepatic encephalopathy," *World Journal of Gastroenterology*, vol. 13, no. 21, pp. 3003–3008, 2007.

[17] J. S. Bajaj, J. Cordoba, K. D. Mullen et al., "Review article: the design of clinical trials in hepatic encephalopathy—an International Society for Hepatic Encephalopathy and Nitrogen Metabolism (ISHEN) consensus statement," *Alimentary Pharmacology and Therapeutics*, vol. 33, no. 7, pp. 739–747, 2011.

[18] Z. M. Younossi, G. Guyatt, M. Kiwi, N. Boparai, and D. King, "Development of a disease specific questionnaire to measure health related quality of life in patients with chronic liver disease," *Gut*, vol. 45, no. 2, pp. 295–300, 1999.

[19] S.-E. Christensen, P. Elsass, and H. Vilstrup, "Number connection test and continuous reaction times in non-encephalopathic patients: a comparative study," *Journal of Applied Toxicology*, vol. 1, no. 5, pp. 262–263, 1981.

[20] P. Elsass, "Continuous reaction times in cerebral dysfunction," *Acta Neurologica Scandinavica*, vol. 73, no. 3, pp. 225–246, 1986.

[21] P. Elsass, S. E. Christensen, E. L. Mortensen, and H. Vilstrup, "Discrimination between organic and hepatic encephalopathy by means of continuous reaction times," *Liver*, vol. 5, no. 1, pp. 29–34, 1985.

[22] P. Elsass, S. E. Christensen, and L. Ranek, "Continuous reaction time in patients with hepatic encephalopathy. A quantitative

measure of changes in consciousness," *Scandinavian Journal of Gastroenterology*, vol. 16, no. 3, pp. 441–447, 1981.

[23] M. M. Lauridsen, H. Gronbaek, E. B. Naeser et al., "Gender and age effects on the continuous reaction times method in volunteers and patients with cirrhosis," *Metabolic Brain Disease*, vol. 27, no. 4, pp. 559–565, 2012.

[24] M. M. Lauridsen, P. Jepsen, and H. Vilstrup, "Critical flicker frequency and continuous reaction times for the diagnosis of minimal hepatic encephalopathy. A comparative study of 154 patients with liver disease," *Metabolic Brain Disease*, vol. 26, no. 2, pp. 135–139, 2011.

[25] J. C. Hoekstra, J. H. M. Goosen, G. S. de Wolf, and C. C. P. M. Verheyen, "Effectiveness of multidisciplinary nutritional care on nutritional intake, nutritional status and quality of life in patients with hip fractures: a controlled prospective cohort study," *Clinical Nutrition*, vol. 30, no. 4, pp. 455–461, 2011.

[26] A. Nourissat, M. P. Vasson, Y. Merrouche et al., "Relationship between nutritional status and quality of life in patients with cancer," *European Journal of Cancer*, vol. 44, no. 9, pp. 1238–1242, 2008.

[27] P. Amodio, C. Bemeur, R. Butterworth et al., "The nutritional management of hepatic encephalopathy in patients with cirrhosis: international society for hepatic encephalopathy and nitrogen metabolism consensus," *Hepatology*, vol. 58, pp. 325–336, 2013.

[28] Y. Nakaya, K. Okita, K. Suzuki et al., "BCAA-enriched snack improves nutritional state of cirrhosis," *Nutrition*, vol. 23, no. 2, pp. 113–120, 2007.

[29] G. Marchesini, G. Bianchi, M. Merli et al., "Nutritional supplementation with branched-chain amino acids in advanced cirrhosis: a double-blind, randomized trial," *Gastroenterology*, vol. 124, no. 7, pp. 1792–1801, 2003.

[30] L. D. Plank, E. J. Gane, S. Peng et al., "Nocturnal nutritional supplementation improves total body protein status of patients with liver cirrhosis: a randomized 12-month trial," *Hepatology*, vol. 48, no. 2, pp. 557–566, 2008.

[31] Y. Chen, X. Wang, J. Wang, Z. Yan, and J. Luo, "Excess body weight and the risk of primary liver cancer: an updated meta-analysis of prospective studies," *European Journal of Cancer*, vol. 48, no. 14, pp. 2137–2145, 2012.

[32] S. Naveau, V. Giraud, E. Borotto, A. Aubert, F. Capron, and J.-C. Chaput, "Excess weight risk factor for alcoholic liver disease," *Hepatology*, vol. 25, no. 1, pp. 108–111, 1997.

[33] R. K. Dhiman, R. Kurmi, K. K. Thumburu et al., "Diagnosis and prognostic significance of minimal hepatic encephalopathy in patients with cirrhosis of liver," *Digestive Diseases and Sciences*, vol. 55, no. 8, pp. 2381–2390, 2010.

[34] S. Prasad, R. K. Dhiman, A. Duseja, Y. K. Chawla, A. Sharma, and R. Agarwal, "Lactulose improves cognitive functions and health-related quality of life in patients with cirrhosis who have minimal hepatic encephalopathy," *Hepatology*, vol. 45, no. 3, pp. 549–559, 2007.

[35] J. S. Bajaj, J. B. Wade, D. P. Gibson et al., "The multi-dimensional burden of cirrhosis and hepatic encephalopathy on patients and caregivers," *American Journal of Gastroenterology*, vol. 106, no. 9, pp. 1646–1653, 2011.

[36] F. Moscucci, S. Nardelli, I. Pentassuglio et al., "Previous overt hepatic encephalopathy rather than minimal hepatic encephalopathy impairs health-related quality of life in cirrhotic patients," *Liver International*, vol. 31, no. 10, pp. 1505–1510, 2011.

[37] E. Wunsch, B. Szymanik, M. Post, W. Marlicz, M. Mydłowska, and P. Milkiewicz, "Minimal hepatic encephalopathy does not impair health-related quality of life in patients with cirrhosis: a prospective study," *Liver International*, vol. 31, no. 7, pp. 980–984, 2011.

[38] H.-H. Tan, G. H. Lee, K. T. J. Thia, H. S. Ng, W. C. Chow, and H. F. Lui, "Minimal hepatic encephalopathy runs a fluctuating course: results from a three-year prospective cohort follow-up study," *Singapore Medical Journal*, vol. 50, no. 3, pp. 255–260, 2009.

[39] H. Schomerus and W. Hamster, "Quality of life in cirrhotics with minimal hepatic encephalopathy," *Metabolic Brain Disease*, vol. 16, no. 1-2, pp. 37–41, 2001.

[40] V. Arvaniti, G. D'Amico, G. Fede et al., "Infections in patients with cirrhosis increase mortality four-fold and should be used in determining prognosis," *Gastroenterology*, vol. 139, no. 4, pp. 1246.e5–1256.e5, 2010.

[41] J. S. Bajaj, J. G. O'Leary, F. Wong et al., "Bacterial infections in end-stage liver disease: current challenges and future directions," *Gut*, vol. 61, pp. 1219–1225, 2012.

[42] A. Tripodi and P. M. Mannucci, "The coagulopathy of chronic liver disease," *The New England Journal of Medicine*, vol. 365, no. 2, pp. 147–156, 2011.

Seroepidemiology of Hepatitis B and C Viruses in the General Population of Burkina Faso

Issoufou Tao,[1,2] Tegwindé R. Compaoré,[1,2] Birama Diarra,[1,2] Florencia Djigma,[1,2] Theodora M. Zohoncon,[1,2] Maléki Assih,[1,2] Djeneba Ouermi,[1,2] Virginio Pietra,[1,3] Simplice D. Karou,[1,2,4] and Jacques Simpore[1,2,3]

[1] Centre de Recherche Biomoléculaire Pietro Annigoni (CERBA), BP 364, Ouagadougou 01, Burkina Faso
[2] Laboratoire de Biologie Moléculaire et de Génétique (LABIOGENE), Université de Ouagadougou, BP 7021, Burkina Faso
[3] Centre Médical Saint Camille (SCMC), BP 364, Ouagadougou 01, Burkina Faso
[4] École Supérieure des Techniques Biologiques et Alimentaires (ESTBA-UL), Université de Lomé, BP 1515, Togo

Correspondence should be addressed to Simplice D. Karou; simplicekarou@hotmail.com

Academic Editor: Annarosa Floreani

Objectives. In Burkina Faso, few studies reported the prevalence of HBV and HCV in the general population. This study aimed to evaluate the prevalence of hepatitis B and C viruses in the general population and to determine the most affected groups in relation to the risk factors associated with the infection. *Method.* A voluntary testing opened to anyone interested was held at Saint Camille Medical Centre in Ouagadougou. Rapid tests were carried out on 995 persons who voluntarily answered a range of questions before the venous blood sampling. *Results.* The results revealed that the antigen HBs carriers in the general population represented 14.47% (144/995) and the prevalence of HCV was 1.00% (10/995). The difference between HBV's prevalence in men (18.58%) and that in women (11.60%) was statistically significant ($P = 0.002$). The most affected groups were undergraduated students (19.57%) and persons working in the informal sector (15.98%). The least affected group was high level students (8.82%). *Conclusion.* Burkina Faso is a country with a high prevalence of HBV, while the incidence of HCV is still low in the general population. Therefore, more campaigns on the transmission routes of HBV and HCV are needed to reduce the spread of these viruses in sub-Saharan Africa.

1. Introduction

According to the World Health Organization, more than 240 million people are infected with the hepatitis B virus (HBV) worldwide, and the majority is living in the developing countries [1]. Yearly, there are more than 600000 deaths due to the complications related to the infection. HBV's association with liver diseases, such as the primary liver carcinoma and cirrhosis, is clearly established [2, 3]. The HBV prevalence is around 15% in Southeast Asia [4]. In Africa, the virus is highly endemic [5]. Because of its high HBV prevalence, Burkina Faso has been classified by WHO in 2002 as an area of high endemicity [6].

Hepatitis C virus (HCV) in Burkina Faso causes about 900 deaths per year. This virus is also a major risk factor for the liver cancer [7]. HBV and HCV are easily transmissible through sexual, parenteral, and vertical routes [8]. Several behavioral, environmental, and cultural factors may also be responsible for their infections [9]. In Africa, after the vertical and the sexual transmissions, HBV and HCV infections are due to cultural practices (levirate, sorority, sexual rituals, scarification, piercing, and tattoos) or medical surgeries [10, 11]. HBV and HCV are easily transmitted than the Human herpes virus 8 (HHV-8) [12]. They are even cited as risk factors associated with the infection by HHV-8 and HIV [13, 14].

In Burkina Faso, many studies have reported different prevalence for HBV and HCV among target groups. In fact, authors reported that 12.1% patients in the health district of Nanoro [15], 18% among blood donors of Nouna, 11%

TABLE 1: Sociodemographic data in relation to the HBV infection throughout the population.

Characteristics	Profession						Marital status			
	Civil servant	Informal sector	High school students	Undergraduate students	Housewives	Trader	Single	Married	Widow	Divorced
Total	211	169	155	152	112	52	535	439	14	7
HBV (+) number	35	32	15	37	17	8	80	59	4	1
%	14.22	15.98	8.82	19.57	13.17	13.33	14.95	15.52	28.57	14.28
OR (95% IC)	—	—	—	—	—	—	—	—	—	—
P values				0.10					0.43	

4. Data Analysis

Statistical analysis was performed with Epi Info version 6 and SPSS version 20 software. P values ≤ 0.05 were considered significant.

5. Results

The surface antigen HBs and the anti-HCV antibodies screening concerned 995 individuals of which 586 (58.89%) were women and 409 (41.10%) were male. The ages ranged from 8 to 75 years (with a mean of 41.5 ± 12.6 years). According to the marital status, 53.80% (535/995) were single, 439 (44.10%) were married, and the rest were divorced or widowed. For the professional status, the majority was civil servants, followed by the informal sector workers, the undergraduate students, and the high level students (Table 1). With regard to the professional status, the most affected groups by HBV infection were undergraduate students and individuals working in the informal sector. Table 2 displays the sociocultural practices in relation to HBV infection. According to the table, 68.73% of the population was circumcised, or doing piercing, tattooing, or scarification, or had a genital mutilation; 35.60% had unprotected sex. In relation to the clinical background, 14.40% of the studied population had undergone medical surgery and 13.60% had at least once been hospitalized (Table 3). The present results also showed that the mature age, marital status, gender, and job insecurity (informal sector) are some risk factors for HBV infection. Indeed, 15.52% of married people were HBV carriers against 14.95% for singles. Analysis done on gender showed a significant difference ($P = 0.002$) between the rates of infection among men (28.58%) and women (11.60%). The most affected age class was 31–40 years with an infection rate of 16.33%. The least affected age group was 41–50 years with an infection rate of 11.27% (Table 4). There were no significant differences between HBV prevalence in people who benefited from a blood transfusion and those who have not ($P = 0.81$) nor between those having undergone surgery and those who have not ($P = 0.25$). However, there was a significant difference between the prevalence of HBV among genital mutilated or circumcised people (16.18%) and uncircumcised or genital nonmutilated individuals (11.22%): $P = 0.04$. In general, cultural practices appeared to be risk factors associated with HBV infection. Only 1.00% of the population was concerned

among blood donors of Ouagadougou [16], and 9.3% among pregnant women of Ouagadougou [14] were infected by HBV. For the HCV infection, studies report 4.4% among blood donors of Regional Center of Blood Transfusion of Ouagadougou [17] and 0.6% among health professionals in the district of Nanoro [15]. However, there are very few studies on the prevalence of HBV and HCV across the general population of Burkina Faso. HBV constitutes a public health problem; Burkina Faso's Ministry of Health adopted strategies such as strengthening the prevention of infections in the health care facilities and blood safety measures, as well as the integration of HBV vaccine through the expanded program on immunization (EPI) [15]. This study aimed to (1) evaluate the seroprevalence of HBV and HCV in the general population of Burkina Faso, (2) determine the most affected groups by the infections with hepatitis B and hepatitis C, and (3) study the risk factors associated with the HBV and HCV infection.

2. Methodology

The study was conducted during an awareness campaign against hepatitis organized by "SOS Hépatites Burkina." "SOS Hépatites Burkina" is an association of professionals that educates people about hepatitis. The campaign and the study took place in the Saint Camille Medical Centre in Ouagadougou. It involved 995 people composed of 586 women and 409 men. Testing was free and voluntary, and sampling was preceded by individual counseling. The subjects responded to a range of questions concerning their age, marital status, criminal record, profession, serostatus for HIV, intravenous drugs use, and health history. Biological parents or relatives have given their consent for infants. The results were made available during single post test counseling. The presence of the HBs antigen and anti-VHC antibodies were both determined by the rapid tests ABON.

3. Ethical Issues

The study was approved by the institutional ethics committee of the Centre for Biomolecular Research Pietro Annigoni and that of Saint Camille Medical Centre. All the persons who participated in this study gave their informed consent.

TABLE 2: The sociocultural practices in relation to the HBV infection in the population.

| | Transcutaneous examination or acupuncture | | Cultural practices | | Unprotected sex | | Prison | |
| | + | − | Excision, circumcision, and tattooing | | + | − | + | − |
			Circumcised and female mutilated genital	Piercing, scarification, and tattooing				
Total	37	958	649	34	354	641	04	991
HBV (+) N	03	141	105	04	54	90	0.00	144
(%)	8.10	14.71	32.28	11.76	15.25	14.04		14.53
OR (95% IC)	1	1.5 0.1–1.6	—		1.1 0.7–1.5	1	—	
P values	0.34		—		0.63		—	

TABLE 3: Clinical background in relation to the HBV infection in the population.

| | Blood transfusion | | Surgery | | Hospitalized | | HBV mothers | | HIV | | HCV | |
	+	−	+	−	+	−	+	−	+	−	+	−
Total	37	958	143	852	135	860	28	967	9	986	10	985
HBV (+) N	6	138	16	128	21	123	6	138	2	142	0	144
(%)	16.21	14.40	11.18	15.02	15.55	14.30	21.42	14.27	22.22	14.4	0.00	14.21
OR (95% IC)	1.15 0.4–2.8	1	1	0.7 0.4–1.2	1.1 0.6–1.8	1	1.6 0.1–1.6	1	1.6 0.3–8.2	1	—	
P values	0.81		0.25		0.69		0.27		0.62		—	

with the infection of HCV. Civil servants were the most affected (2.03%), while individuals from the informal sector represented the least affected group (0, 49%).

6. Discussion

This study aimed to assess the prevalence of HBV in the general population of Ouagadougou. Data analysis confirmed the high prevalence (14.5%) of hepatitis B and the low one of hepatitis C (1.00%) in the general population of Burkina Faso. The very low prevalence of HCV did not allow us to draw correlations and discuss it. HBV prevalence is in the range of 10–17% reported in adults in Nigeria [18, 19]. These results also show a higher HBV prevalence than in the target groups as reported by other studies. Indeed, Pietra et al. [15] reported a prevalence of HbsAg of 12.1% in the health professionals of Nanoro district; Collenberg et al. in 2006 [16] reported an HBV's prevalence of 14.3% (Nouna) and 17.3% (Ouagadougou) in blood donors and pregnant women. However, a prevalence of 12.9% was recorded in 2013 in blood donors of the National Blood Transfusion Center of Burkina Faso [20]. Several studies agreed that HBV prevalence is lower in rural than in urban areas [2, 16, 21]. The significant difference ($P = 0.002$) between HBV infections in men and women reported in this study is consistent with the results obtained by Deng et al. [22] in 2013 in China (6.54% versus 3.87%) and Makuwa et al. [21] in Gabon in 2009 (16.2% versus 9.9%). This study reports an HBV/AIDS coinfection of 22.22%. This is a common coinfection, given the fact that the two viruses share the same transmission routes [11, 23,

24]. This study also reports an HBV infection in 21.42% of children under 12 years of age who are born from HIV and HBV positive mothers. At this stage, the study cannot demonstrate the evidence of a vertical transmission or a horizontal infection. In fact, some traditional practices could explain the high prevalence of HBV in children, particularly the mothers using saliva to heal baby wound. It is in this sense that Kiire confirmed that horizontal transmission is the main route of transmission of HBV in babies [25]. However, vertical transmission probably plays an important role, as in Burkina no action (HBV screening during pregnancy, vaccination at birth) is taken to fight against it. The lack of significant difference in the prevalence of HBV among people when taking into account their health background (blood transfusion, surgery, and hospitalization) can be explained by the improvement of blood safety and the health management system in Burkina Faso. In fact, HIV, hepatitis B and hepatitis C, and the bacterium *Treponema pallidum subspecies pallidum* are routinely detected in blood donations [20]. However, the prevalence of 16.21% of HBV among transfused persons against 14.40% in nontransfused shows that the contamination by residual risk of blood transfusion remains. The age group of 30–40 years of age is the most affected (16.33%), followed by 20 to 30 years (15.9%). These results show that young people are most affected by HBV infection. These results are similar to those of Makuwa et al., [21] who reported a prevalence of 22.22% among young men in the same age group in urban areas of Gabon. The low prevalence of individuals in the age group above 50 years of age could indicate that several people in this group might have died from cirrhosis or liver cancer due to lack of medical

TABLE 4: HBV infection by gender and age classes.

| | Gender | | Age classes | | | | |
	Male	Female	<20	21–30	31–40	41–50	≥50
Total	409	586	155	358	251	133	98
HBV (+)	76	68	19	57	41	15	12
(%)	18.58	11.60	12.25	15.92	16.33	11.27	12.24
OR (95% IC)	1.7 (1.2–2.4)	1	—	—	—	—	—
P values	0.002				—		

care. We note a higher prevalence of HBV (15.52%) among married individuals compared to single individuals (14.95%). This study also reports a high prevalence of HBV among widowed (28.57%). The lowest prevalence occurs among the high school student's group (8.82%). Undergraduate students are the most affected group with a prevalence of 19.57%. This could be explained by the fact that they are at the prime of life and are likely to have risky sexual behaviors. Finally, this study reported a high prevalence (16.00%) of HBV in persons who were circumcised, or had a genital mutilation, or had a piercing, a tattoo, or a scarification. This confirms that these cultural practices are risk factors associated with HBV infection [26].

7. Conclusion

This study reports a high prevalence of HBV infection in Burkina Faso. Many people do not have information on the importance of vaccination against HBV as primary prevention. They also ignore the support possibilities of medical chronic hepatitis. Better organization and increased awareness campaigns on HBV and HCV will reduce their prevalence. Moreover, the reduction of the HBV vaccine cost will lower the spread of the hepatitis B virus. In the short term, we suggest working with control structures against HIV to organize forums to raise awareness on HIV, HBV, and HCV.

Conflict of Interests

The authors declare that there is no conflict of interests regarding the publication of this paper.

Acknowledgments

The authors wish to thank the staff of Saint Camille Medical Center and CERBA. They would like to thank "SOS Hépatites Burkina" and Miss Justine YARA. They would also like to thank the IEC (Italian Episcopal Conference) and WAEMU through their PACER2 program for their financial support.

References

[1] WHO, Hépatite B. Aide mémoire 2013, no. 204, 2013.

[2] S. Kakumu, K. Sato, and T. Morishita, "Prevalence of hepatitis B, hepatitis C, and GB virus C/hepatitis G virus infections in liver disease patients and Inhabitants in Ho Chi Minh," Vietnam Journal of Medical Virology, vol. 54, pp. 243–248, 1998.

[3] A. M. Hammad and M. H. E. D. Zaghloul, "Hepatitis G virus infection in Egyptian children with chronic renal failure (single centre study)," Annals of Clinical Microbiology and Antimicrobials, vol. 8, article 36, 2009.

[4] A. P. Catterall and I. M. Murray-Lyon, "Strategies for hepatitis B immunisation," Gut, vol. 33, no. 5, pp. 576–579, 1992.

[5] J. Hou, Z. Liu, and F. Gu, "Epidemiology and prevention of hepatitis B virus infection," International Journal of Medical Sciences, vol. 2, no. 1, pp. 50–57, 2005.

[6] WHO, "Relevé Epidémiologique hebdomadaire," vol. 77, no. 6, pp. 41–48, 2002.

[7] WHO, "Department of Measurement and Health Information. Estimated total deaths by cause and WHO Member State, 2002".

[8] B. Pozzetto and O. Garraud, "Emergent viral threats in blood transfusion," Transfusion Clinique et Biologique, vol. 18, no. 2, pp. 174–183, 2011.

[9] A. Kramvis and M. C. Kew, "Epidemiology of hepatitis B virus in Africa, its genotypes and clinical associations of genotypes," Hepatology Research, vol. 37, no. 1, pp. S9–S19, 2007.

[10] W. F. Carman, "Infections associated with medical intervention: hepatitis viruses and HGV," British Medical Bulletin, vol. 54, no. 3, pp. 731–748, 1998.

[11] J. Simpore, V. Pietra, S. Pignatelli et al., "Effective program against mother-to-child transmission of HIV at Saint Camille Medical Centre in Burkina Faso," Journal of Medical Virology, vol. 79, no. 7, pp. 873–879, 2007.

[12] J. G. Feldman, H. Minkoff, S. Landesman, and J. Dehovitz, "Heterosexual transmission of hepatitis C, hepatitis B, and HIV-1 in a sample of inner-city women," Sexually Transmitted Diseases, vol. 27, no. 6, pp. 338–342, 2000.

[13] S. Plancoulaine, L. Abel, M. Van Beveren et al., "Human herpesvirus 8 transmission from mother to child and between siblings in an endemic population," The Lancet, vol. 356, no. 9235, pp. 1062–1065, 2000.

[14] J. Simpore, M. Granato, R. Santarelli et al., "Prevalence of infection by HHV-8, HIV, HCV and HBV among pregnant women in Burkina Faso," Journal of Clinical Virology, vol. 31, no. 1, pp. 78–80, 2004.

[15] V. Pietra, D. Kiema, D. Sorgho et al., "Prevalence of Hepatitis B virus markers and hepatitis C virus antibodies in health staff in the District of Nanoro, Burkina Faso," Science and Technology, Science Santé, vol. 31, no. 1-2, 2008.

[16] E. Collenberg, T. Ouedraogo, J. Ganamé et al., "Seroprevalence of six different viruses among pregnant women and blood donors in rural and urban Burkina Faso: a comparative analysis," Journal of Medical Virology, vol. 78, no. 5, pp. 683–692, 2006.

[17] M. T. Zeba, M. Sanou, C. Bisseye et al., "Characterization of hepatitis C virus genotype among blood donors at the regional blood transfusion centre of Ouagadougou, Burkina Faso," Blood Transfusion, vol. 12, supplement 1, pp. s54–s57, 2014.

[18] J. A. Mustapha and D. Glancy, "Rapidly progressive dyspnea," *Proceedings of the Baylor University Medical Center*, vol. 15, pp. 95–96, 2002.

[19] E. I. Ugwuja and N. C. Ugwu, "Seroprevalence of hepatitis B surface antigen and liver function tests among adolescents in Abakaliki, South Eastern Nigeria," *Internet Journal of Tropical Medicine*, vol. 6, no. 2, 2010.

[20] I. Tao, C. Bisseye, B. M. Nagalo et al., "Screening of hepatitis G and Epstein-Barr viruses among voluntary non remunerated blood donors (VNRBD) in Burkina Faso, West Africa," *Mediterranean Journal of Hematology and Infectious Diseases*, vol. 5, no. 1, Article ID e2013053, 2013.

[21] M. Makuwa, A. Mintsa-Ndong, S. Souquière, D. Nkoghé, E. M. Leroy, and M. Kazanji, "Prevalence and molecular diversity of hepatitis B virus and hepatitis delta virus in urban and rural populations in northern Gabon in Central Africa," *Journal of Clinical Microbiology*, vol. 47, no. 7, pp. 2265–2268, 2009.

[22] Q. J. Deng, Y. Q. Pan, C. Y. Wang et al., "Prevalence and Risk Factors for hepatitis B in Hua County, Henan Province," *Beijing Da Xue Xue Bao*, vol. 45, pp. 965–970, 2013.

[23] O. Iroezindu, C. A. Daniyam, O. O. Agbaji et al., "Prevalence of hepatitis B e antigen Among human immunodeficiency virus and hepatitis B virus co-infected patients in Jos, Nigeria," *Journal of Infections in Developing Countries*, vol. 7, pp. 951–959, 2013.

[24] M. Mohammadi, G. Talei, A. Sheikhian et al., "Survey of hepatitis B virus Both (HBsAg) and hepatitis C virus (HCV- Ab) coinfection Among HIV positive patients," *Virology Journal*, vol. 6, article 202, 2009.

[25] C. F. Kiire, "The epidemiology and prophylaxis of hepatitis B in sub-Saharan Africa: a view from tropical and subtropical Africa," *Gut*, vol. 38, no. 2, pp. S5–S12, 1996.

[26] A. C. Eke, U. A. Eke, C. I. Okafor, I. U. Ezebialu, and C. Ogbuagu, "Prevalence, correlates and pattern of hepatitis B surface antigen in a low resource setting," *Virology Journal*, vol. 8, article 12, 2011.

Circulating Cytokines and Histological Liver Damage in Chronic Hepatitis B Infection

Kittiyod Poovorawan,[1] Pisit Tangkijvanich,[2] Chintana Chirathaworn,[3] Naruemon Wisedopas,[4] Sombat Treeprasertsuk,[1] Piyawat Komolmit,[1] and Yong Poovorawan[5]

[1] *Division of Gastroenterology, Department of Medicine, Faculty of Medicine, Chulalongkorn University, Bangkok 10330, Thailand*
[2] *Department of Biochemistry, Faculty of Medicine, Chulalongkorn University, Bangkok 10330, Thailand*
[3] *Department of Microbiology, Faculty of Medicine, Chulalongkorn University, Bangkok 10330, Thailand*
[4] *Department of Pathology, Faculty of Medicine, Chulalongkorn University, Bangkok 10330, Thailand*
[5] *Department of Pediatrics, Center of Excellence in Clinical Virology, Faculty of Medicine, Chulalongkorn University, Bangkok 10330, Thailand*

Correspondence should be addressed to Yong Poovorawan; yong.p@chula.ac.th

Academic Editor: Piero Luigi Almasio

Each phase of hepatitis B infection stimulates distinct viral kinetics and host immune responses resulting in liver damage and hepatic fibrosis. Our objective has been to correlate host inflammatory immune response including circulating Th1 and Th2 cytokines in patients with chronic hepatitis B infection with liver histopathology. Sixty-four patients with chronic hepatitis B without previous treatment were recruited. The liver histology and histological activity index were assessed for various degrees of necroinflammation and hepatic fibrosis. We determined circulating levels of the Th1 and Th2 cytokines. Forty-six males and 18 females at a median age of 34.5 years were studied. HBeAg was present in 28/64 (43.75%) of the patients. In patients negative for HBeAg, IL-10 and IFN-gamma were significantly correlated with degrees of necroinflammation ($r = 0.34$, $r = 0.38$, resp.; $P < 0.05$). Moreover, TNF-alpha was significantly correlated with degrees of fibrosis ($r = 0.35$; $P < 0.05$), and IL-10 and TNF-alpha were significantly correlated with significant fibrosis ($r = 0.39$, $r = 0.35$, resp.; $P < 0.05$). These correlations were found in the HBeAg negative group as opposed to the HBeAg positive group. In HBeAg negative patients, circulating cytokines IL-10 and IFN-gamma were correlated with degrees of necroinflammation, whereas IL-10 and TNF-alpha were correlated with significant fibrosis.

1. Introduction

Chronic hepatitis B infection is a major cause of chronic liver disease worldwide. Each phase of hepatitis B infection stimulates distinct viral kinetics and host immune responses resulting in liver damage and hepatic fibrosis [1]. Vaccine induced immune response in humans has provided excellent long term protection and result decline prevalence of hepatitis B virus (HBV) infection in long term [2, 3]. In contrast to host immune response in chronic hepatitis B infection, due to immune tolerance, only a small proportion of chronic hepatitis B (CHB) patients could clear the infection [4]. Histological damage and risk of HCC in CHB patients depend on various parameters such as duration of infection, coinfection with other hepatitis viruses, and alcohol consumption [5]. Cytokines are known to play a significant role in host immune responses. In chronic hepatitis B patients, the concentration of circulating Th17 cells (producing IL-17) increased with disease progression from CHB (mean, 4.34%) to acute-on-chronic liver failure (mean, 5.62%) patients as compared to healthy controls (mean, 2.42%) [6]. Furthermore, higher serum levels of IL-10 and IL-12 in HBeAg positive patients are correlated with early, spontaneous HBeAg seroconversion [7]. T cells play a major role in the immunopathogenesis associated with chronic hepatitis B. T cells destroy infected hepatocytes and suppress HBV replication [8]. Our objective has been to correlate host inflammatory immune response including circulating Th1 and Th2 cytokines in patients with chronic hepatitis B infection with the liver histopathology observed.

2. Materials and Methods

A cross-sectional prospective study was conducted on chronic HBV patients who were evaluated for treatment at Chulalongkorn King Memorial Hospital from 2010 to 2012. The research protocol was approved by the Institutional Review Board (IRB number 515/53) of the Faculty of Medicine, Chulalongkorn University. The objective of the study was explained to the patients, and subsequently, written consent was obtained.

2.1. Patients. Sixty-four patients with chronic hepatitis B without previous treatment were recruited. Clinical, demographic, and laboratory data were collected. Patients with evidence of HCV or HIV coinfection, alcoholic liver disease, and chronic liver disease due to other causes and acute viral hepatitis B were excluded from the study.

2.2. Specimen Collection. From January 2010 to January 2012, 64 samples were collected from patients with chronic HBV infection. Samples were collected as clotted blood and sera were separated within 6 hours. All specimens were kept at $-70°C$ until tested.

2.3. Clinical Assessment. Based on their HBeAg status, patients were classified into an HBeAg positive and an HBeAg negative group. Liver biopsy was performed by percutaneous needle biopsy (16-gauge, Menghini). Specimen length of at least 1.5 cm and at least 10 portal tracks is required for an adequate evaluation [9].

Histology and histological activity index (HAI) were graded according to degrees of necroinflammation applying the following score: 0 = no inflammation, 1–4 = minimal inflammation, 5–8 = mild inflammation, 9–12 = moderate inflammation, and 13–18 = marked inflammation as described by Knodell et al. [10]. Hepatic fibrosis was staged on a 5-point scale (F0: no fibrosis; F1: minimal fibrosis; F2: fibrosis with a few septa; F3: numerous bridging fibroses without cirrhosis; F4: cirrhosis or advanced severe fibrosis) as described in the Metavir score. F0-F1 was defined as nonsignificant fibrosis and F2–F4 as significant fibrosis.

2.4. Liver Stiffness Measurement. Transient elastography was performed by a well-trained nurse using FibroScan 502 (Echosens, Paris, France). The median value of 10 validated scores was considered the elastic modulus of the liver, and it was expressed in kilopascals (kPa).

2.5. Laboratory Method. Circulating levels of Th1 cytokines comprising IL-2, IL-12p70, and interferon-gamma (IFN-gamma) and Th2 cytokines including IL-4, IL-5, IL-10, IL-13, and also TNF-alpha and GMCSF were measured by

ELISA (Bio-Plex Cytokine Assays). We quantitatively determined the HBsAg titer by ELISA method (Elecsys, Roche Diagnostics, Indianapolis, IN, USA), and the HBV DNA concentration was measured by quantitative real time PCR (The Abbott m2000sp Real Time System).

We determined serum anti-HCV and anti-HIV by enzyme immunoassay (Architect, Abbott Diagnostics, Germany).

2.6. Statistical Analysis. Continuous variables were compared between groups using unpaired t-test and one-way ANOVA. Categorical variables were compared between groups using chi-square/Fisher's exact test. Pearson's correlation coefficient was used to describe the correlation between two continuous, normally distributed variables. Spearman's correlation was used where variables were not normally distributed. All statistical analyses were performed using SPSS version 16.

3. Results

Forty-six males and 18 females at a median age of 34.5 years were studied. HBeAg was present in 28 of 64 (43.75%) patients. In the study population, HBeAg negative patients were older than those positive for HBeAg. HBV DNA, HBsAg titer, and ALT concentrations were significantly higher in the HBeAg positive group. Degrees of hepatic necroinflammation, liver fibrosis, and liver stiffness measured by FibroScan were not significantly different between both groups (Table 1).

Among all patients, cytokine levels were not correlated with ALT, DNA levels, and liver stiffness measurement by FibroScan. The correlation between IL-5 and HBsAg titer was negative ($r = -0.239$; $P < 0.05$).

In HBeAg negative patients, inflammatory cytokine IL-5 and IL-12p70 levels were significantly higher than in HBeAg positive patients (0.726 versus 0.508 and 2.17 versus 0.217, resp.; $P < 0.05$). Other mean serum cytokine levels were not statistically different (Table 2).

In the HBeAg negative group, IL-10 and IFN-gamma were significantly correlated with degrees of necroinflammation ($r = 0.336$, $r = 0.380$, resp.; $P < 0.05$). while other cytokines were not correlated (Figure 1). In the HBeAg positive group, none of the cytokines was correlated with degrees of necroinflammation (Figure 2). After multivariate analysis with baseline characteristic, laboratory data, and other cytokines, IL-10 was the only one parameter which significantly correlated with degrees of necroinflammation (Table 3).

TNF-alpha was significantly correlated with degrees of fibrosis ($r = 0.35$; $P < 0.05$), and IL-10 and TNF-alpha were significantly correlated with significant fibrosis in HBeAg negative patients ($r = 0.39$, $r = 0.35$, resp.; $P < 0.05$). After multivariate analysis with baseline characteristic, associated laboratory data and other cytokines, there was no significant correlation between IL-10, TNF-alpha, and significant fibrosis. In the HBeAg positive group, none of the cytokines was correlated with fibrosis.

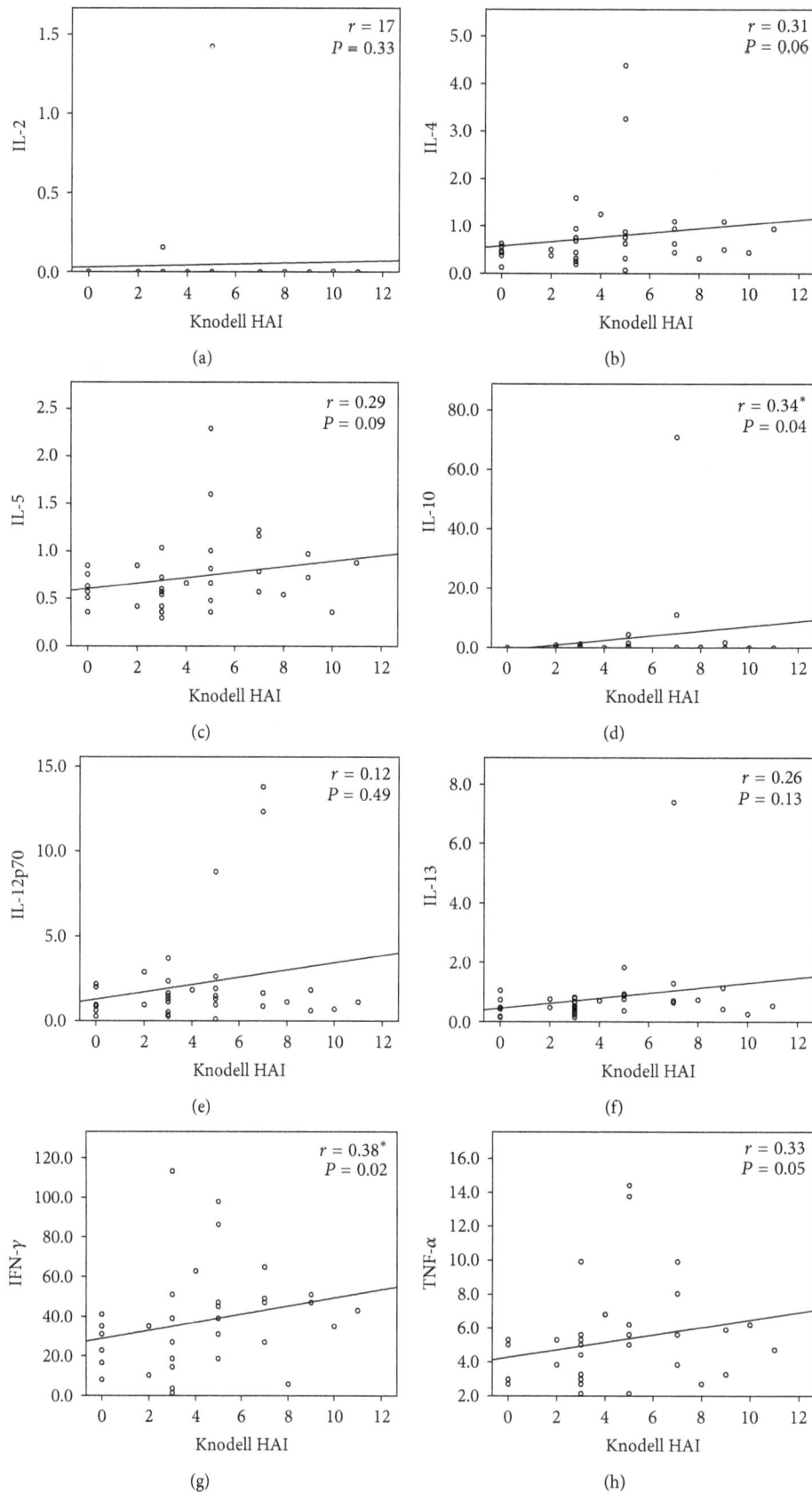

FIGURE 1: Correlation between circulating cytokine levels (pg/mL) and degrees of necroinflammation (Knodell histological activity index) in the HBeAg negative group (N = 36). [†]Spearman's rank correlation coefficient, [*]statistically significant.

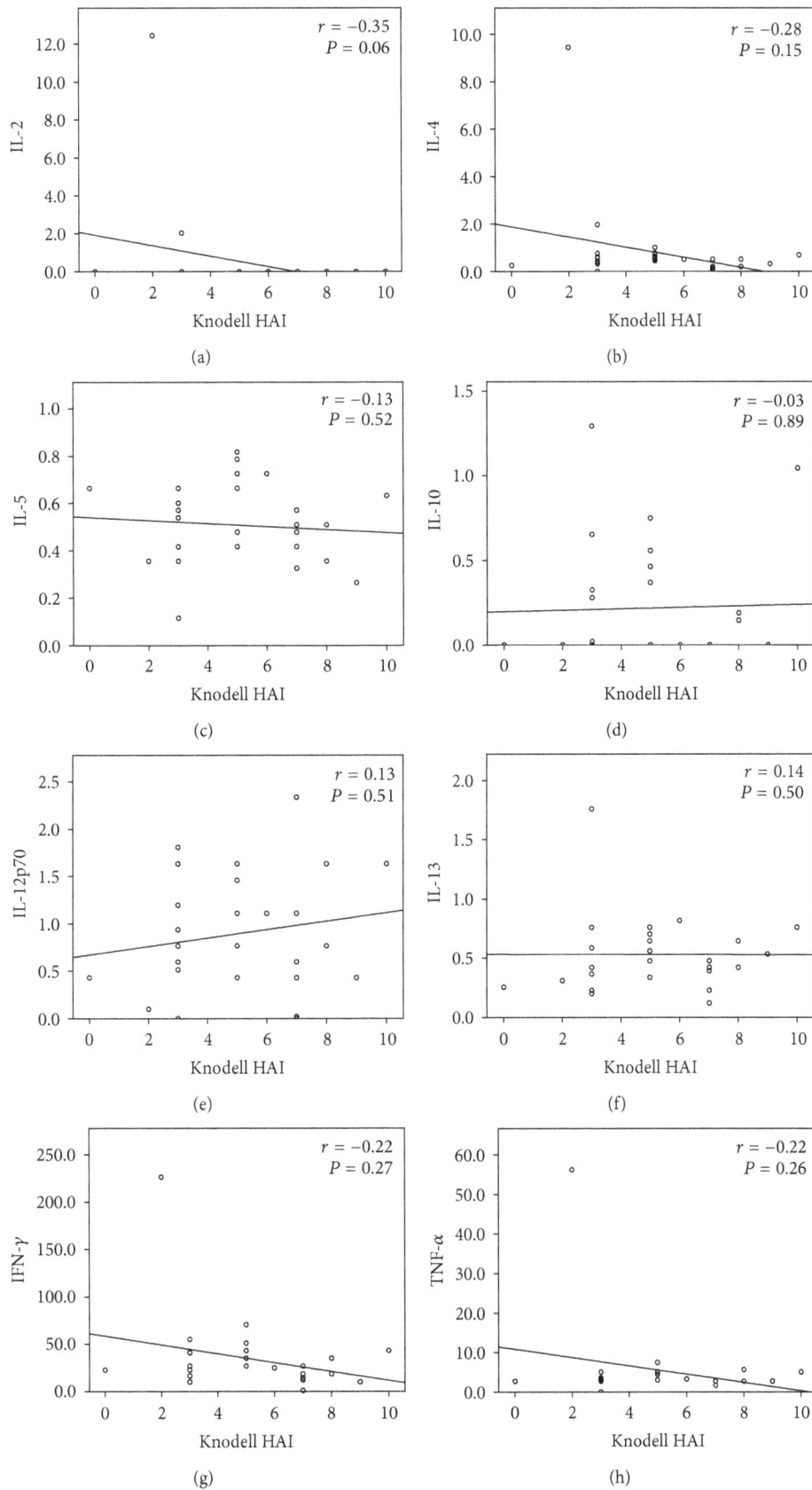

FIGURE 2: Correlation between circulating cytokine levels (pg/mL) and degrees of necroinflammation (Knodell histological activity index) in the HBeAg positive group ($N = 28$). [†]Spearman's rank correlation coefficient.

TABLE 1: Comparison of demographic, clinical, and ALT level, histopathology, and liver stiffness characteristics between HBeAg positive and HBeAg negative patients[*].

	HBeAg positive ($n = 28$)	HBeAg negative ($n = 36$)	P value
Age > 40yrs	3/28 (10.7%)	21/36 (58.3%)	<0.01
Age (yrs)	30.9 ± 7.9	42 ± 10.2	0.02
Male gender	17/28 (60.7%)	28/36 (77.8%)	0.14
Mean BMI	25.1 ± 4.8	23.7 ± 3.8	0.43
Underlying of DM	0	2/36 (5.6%)	0.27
ALT > 60 U/L	20/28 (71.4%)	16/36 (44.4%)	0.03
HBV DNA (logIU/mL)	7.08 ± 1.39	5.34 ± 1.35	<0.01
HBsAg titer (IU/mL)	20380.8 ± 21308	5477 ± 7557.3	<0.01
Knodell HAI ≥ 4	17/28 (60.7%)	17/36 (47.2%)	0.28
Significant fibrosis	11/28 (39.3%)	21/36 (58.3%)	0.13
Liver stiffness (Kpa)	7.13 ± 2.49	7.76 ± 3.72	0.09

[*] Plus-minus values are means ± SD for all comparisons.

TABLE 2: Comparison of cytokine levels between HBeAg positive and HBeAg negative patients[*].

(pg/mL)	HBeAg positive ($n = 28$)	HBeAg negative ($n = 36$)	P value
IL-2	0.517 ± 2.37	0.726 ± 0.38	0.24
IL-4	0.79 ± 1.74	0.77 ± 0.83	0.95
IL-5	0.508 ± 0.16	0.726 ± 0.38	<0.01[**]
IL-10	0.217 ± 0.35	2.607 ± 11.9	0.29
IL-12p70	0.898 ± 0.60	2.17 ± 3.06	0.03[**]
IL-13	0.529 ± 0.31	0.803 ± 1.18	0.24
GMCSF	1.131 ± 0.1.75	1.56 ± 1.84	0.35
IFN-gamma	34.8 ± 40.72	37.36 ± 25.43	0.76
TNF-alpha	5.446 ± 10.09	5.196 ± 2.93	0.89

[*] Plus-minus values are means ± SD for all comparisons.
[**] Statistically significant.

4. Discussion

Chronic hepatitis B infection results in a complex interplay between virus and host immune response. T-cell immune response is correlated with fibrosis and hepatic inflammation in HBV chronic hepatitis and cirrhotic patients [11]. The phase of disease is determined by clinical characteristics of liver inflammation and virus replication in the host. Chronic hepatitis B (CHB) infection progresses through various phases in relation to the host, that is, immune tolerant, immune active, and inactive carrier. The immune response in each phase of disease depends on complex mechanisms. Recent data have demonstrated that even the immune tolerant phase of CHB is not associated with an immune profile of T-cell tolerance [12].

Cytokines contribute to the immune response and have a specific response to each disease [13]. T-helper cytokines in CHB patients and healthy controls were different. For example, serum IL-33 was significantly higher in healthy controls at the baseline but decreased after antiviral treatment [14]. Some data have demonstrated that the circulating cytokine profile in chronic hepatitis B is related to the HBeAg status, virus replication, and stage of liver disease [15, 16]. Inflammatory cytokine IL-5 and IL-12p70 levels were significantly higher in the HBeAg negative group. A previous

study has demonstrated that IL-5 as well as IL-4 levels were increased in acute self-limited hepatitis B [17]. IL-12 was found to significantly augment the HBcAg-specific secretion of IFN-gamma in CHB children and, thus, to increase the probability of HBeAg seroconversion in CHB patients [7, 18]. Treatment of CHB patients with a combined regimen of IL-12 and lamivudine enhanced T-cell reactivity to HBV and IFN-gamma production. However, IL-12 did not suppress HBV replication in HBeAg positive patients and did not uphold inhibition of HBV replication after lamivudine withdrawal [19].

Interleukin-10 (IL-10) generally suppresses cellular immune responses by modulating the function of T cells and antigen-presenting cells [20]. In contrast to CHB patients, IL-10 was related to the HBeAg status, virus replication, and liver disease progression [16]. This study confirmed the correlation between IL-10 and histological liver damage in HBeAg negative CHB patients. Furthermore, a recent study has demonstrated that the IL-10 level can also serve as a predictor of HBeAg seroconversion in CHB patients [7].

IFN-gamma and TNF-alpha were thought to be important immune mediators in the host defense against hepatitis B virus (HBV) infection. These cytokines can induce apoptosis in liver cells expressing HBV [21]. TNF-alpha mediates an innate antiviral response that targets the integrity of HBV

TABLE 3: Multivariate analyses of the association between degrees of necroinflammation and other parameters.

Parameters	Standardized coefficients	P value
Age	−0.13	0.51
BMI	0.02	0.93
ALT	0.38	0.13
HBV DNA	0.07	0.82
HBsAg titer	−0.16	0.6
IL-2	−0.38	0.19
IL-4	0.35	0.51
IL-5	0.16	0.66
IL-10	0.96	0.04*
IL-12p70	−1.69	0.06
IL-13	0.67	0.16
GMCSF	−0.70	0.18
IFN-gamma	0.27	0.48
TNF-alpha	0.76	0.09

*Statistically significant.

nucleocapsids [22]. IFN-gamma suppresses hepatitis B virus replication and significantly reduces expression of the large HBV surface protein (LHBs) and hepatocytes' microscopical appearance of ground glass [23].

This study has established that circulating cytokines IL-10 and IFN-gamma are correlated with degrees of necroinflammation in HBeAg negative patients, whereas IL-10 and TNF-alpha are correlated with significant fibrosis. These correlations were found in the HBeAg negative group as opposed to the HBeAg positive group. However, further research should be performed to determine the exact roles of each cytokine in liver necroinflammation and fibrogenesis.

Conflict of Interests

The authors declare that there is no conflict of interests regarding the publication of this paper.

Acknowledgments

This work was supported by the Chulalongkorn University liver Research Unit, The Higher Education Research Promotion and National Research University Project of Thailand (HR1155A-55), Thailand Research Fund (DPG5480002), Office of the Commission on Higher Education, Center of Excellence in Clinical Virology, Chulalongkorn University, CU Centenary Academic Development Project, and Chulalongkorn Hospital. The authors also would like to thank the entire staff of the Center of Excellence in Clinical Virology, Medicine, Biochemistry, Faculty of Medicine, Chulalongkorn University and Hospital, for their assistance in this research. Finally, the authors would like to thank Ms. Petra Hirsch for reviewing the paper.

References

[1] D. Ganem and A. M. Prince, "Hepatitis B virus infection—natural history and clinical consequences," *The New England Journal of Medicine*, vol. 350, no. 11, pp. 1118–1129, 2004.

[2] Y. Poovorawan, V. Chongsrisawat, A. Theamboonlers, H. L. Bock, M. Leyssen, and J.-M. Jacquet, "Persistence of antibodies and immune memory to hepatitis B vaccine 20 years after infant vaccination in Thailand," *Vaccine*, vol. 28, no. 3, pp. 730–736, 2010.

[3] N. Chimparlee, S. Oota, S. Phikulsod, P. Tangkijvanich, and Y. Poovorawan, "Hepatitis B and hepatitis C Virus in Thai blood donors," *Southeast Asian Journal of Tropical Medicine and Public Health*, vol. 42, no. 3, pp. 609–615, 2011.

[4] R. S. Tedder, S. Ijaz, N. Gilbert et al., "Evidence for a dynamic host-parasite relationship in e-negative hepatitis B carriers," *Journal of Medical Virology*, vol. 68, no. 4, pp. 505–512, 2002.

[5] A. S. F. Lok and B. J. McMahon, "Chronic hepatitis B: update 2009," *Hepatology*, vol. 50, no. 3, pp. 661–662, 2009.

[6] J.-Y. Zhang, Z. Zhang, F. Lin et al., "Interleukin-17-producing CD4+ T cells increase with severity of liver damage in patients with chronic hepatitis B," *Hepatology*, vol. 51, no. 1, pp. 81–91, 2010.

[7] J.-F. Wu, T.-C. Wu, C.-H. Chen et al., "Serum levels of interleukin-10 and interleukin-12 predict early, spontaneous hepatitis B virus e antigen seroconversion," *Gastroenterology*, vol. 138, no. 1, pp. 165–172, 2010.

[8] Y. Shimizu, "T cell immunopathogenesis and immunotherapeutic strategies for chronic hepatitis B virus infection," *The World Journal of Gastroenterology*, vol. 18, no. 20, pp. 2443–2451, 2012.

[9] D. C. Rockey, S. H. Caldwell, Z. D. Goodman, R. C. Nelson, and A. D. Smith, "Liver biopsy," *Hepatology*, vol. 49, no. 3, pp. 1017–1044, 2009.

[10] R. G. Knodell, K. G. Ishak, W. C. Black et al., "Formulation and application of a numerical scoring system for assessing histological activity in asymptomatic chronic active hepatitis," *Hepatology*, vol. 1, no. 5, pp. 431–435, 1981.

[11] J.-T. Tang, J.-Y. Fang, W.-Q. Gu, and E.-L. Li, "T cell immune response is correlated with fibrosis and inflammatory activity in hepatitis B cirrhotics," *The World Journal of Gastroenterology*, vol. 12, no. 19, pp. 3015–3019, 2006.

[12] P. Kennedy, E. Sandalova, J. Jo et al., "Preserved T-cell function in children and young adults with immune-tolerant chronic hepatitis B," *Gastroenterology*, vol. 143, no. 3, pp. 637–645, 2012.

[13] A. Bertoletti, M. M. D'Elios, C. Boni et al., "Different cytokine profiles of intrahepatic T cells in chronic hepatitis B and hepatitis C virus infections," *Gastroenterology*, vol. 112, no. 1, pp. 193–199, 1997.

[14] J. Wang, Y. Cai, H. Ji et al., "Serum IL-33 levels are associated with liver damage in patients with chronic hepatitis B," *Journal of Interferon & Cytokine Research*, vol. 32, no. 6, pp. 248–253, 2012.

[15] S. Khan, A. Bhargava, N. Pathak, K. K. Maudar, S. Varshney, and P. K. Mishra, "Circulating biomarkers and their possible role in pathogenesis of chronic hepatitis B and C viral infections," *Indian Journal of Clinical Biochemistry*, vol. 26, no. 2, pp. 161–168, 2011.

[16] H. Bozkaya, M. Bozdayi, R. Turkyilmaz et al., "Circulating IL-2, IL-10 and TNF-α in chronic hepatitis B: their relations to HBeAg status and the activity of liver disease," *Hepato-Gastroenterology*, vol. 47, no. 36, pp. 1675–1679, 2000.

[17] A. Penna, G. del Prete, A. Cavalli et al., "Predominant T-helper 1 cytokine profile of hepatitis B virus nucleocapsid-specific T cells in acute self-limited hepatitis B," *Hepatology*, vol. 25, no. 4, pp. 1022–1027, 1997.

[18] A. Szkaradkiewicz, A. Jopek, and J. Wysocki, "Effects of IL-12 and IL-18 on HBcAg-specific cytokine production by CD4 T lymphocytes of children with chronic hepatitis B infection," *Antiviral Research*, vol. 66, no. 1, pp. 23–27, 2005.

[19] E. I. Rigopoulou, D. Suri, S. Chokshi et al., "Lamivudine plus interleukin-12 combination therapy in chronic hepatitis B: antiviral and immunological activity," *Hepatology*, vol. 42, no. 5, pp. 1028–1036, 2005.

[20] M. Ejrnaes, C. M. Filippi, M. M. Martinic et al., "Resolution of a chronic viral infection after interleukin-10 receptor blockade," *Journal of Experimental Medicine*, vol. 203, no. 11, pp. 2461–2472, 2006.

[21] H. Shi and S.-H. Guan, "Increased apoptosis in HepG2.2.15 cells with hepatitis B virus expression by synergistic induction of interferon-γ and tumour necrosis factor-α," *Liver International*, vol. 29, no. 3, pp. 349–355, 2009.

[22] R. Puro and R. J. Schneider, "Tumor necrosis factor activates a conserved innate antiviral response to hepatitis B virus that destabilizes nucleocapsids and reduces nuclear viral DNA," *Journal of Virology*, vol. 81, no. 14, pp. 7351–7362, 2007.

[23] K. Reifenberg, E. Hildt, B. Lecher et al., "IFNγ expression inhibits LHBs storage disease and ground glass hepatocyte appearance, but exacerbates inflammation and apoptosis in HBV surface protein-accumulating transgenic livers," *Liver International*, vol. 26, no. 8, pp. 986–993, 2006.

Knowledge of Hepatitis B Virus Infection, Immunization with Hepatitis B Vaccine, Risk Perception, and Challenges to Control Hepatitis among Hospital Workers in a Nigerian Tertiary Hospital

Olusegun Adekanle,[1] Dennis A. Ndububa,[1] Samuel Anu Olowookere,[2] Oluwasegun Ijarotimi,[1] and Kayode Thaddeus Ijadunola[2]

[1]*Department of Medicine, Obafemi Awolowo University/Obafemi Awolowo University Teaching Hospitals Complex, Ile-Ife 220005, Osun State, Nigeria*
[2]*Department of Community Health, Obafemi Awolowo University/Obafemi Awolowo University Teaching Hospitals Complex, Ile-Ife 220005, Osun State, Nigeria*

Correspondence should be addressed to Olusegun Adekanle; olusegunadekanle@yahoo.co.uk

Academic Editor: Annarosa Floreani

Background. Studies had reported high rate of hepatitis B infection among hospital workers with low participation in vaccination programmes, especially those whose work exposes them to the risk of HBV infection. The study assessed knowledge of hepatitis B virus infection, risk perception, vaccination history, and challenges to control hepatitis among health workers. *Methods.* A descriptive cross-sectional study. Consenting health care workers completed a self-administered questionnaire that assessed respondents' general knowledge of HBV, vaccination history and HBsAg status, risk perception, and challenges to control hepatitis. Data was analysed using descriptive and inferential statistics. *Results.* Three hundred and eighty-two health care workers participated in the study. There were 182 males and 200 females. The respondents comprised 94 (25%) medical doctors, 168 (44%) nurses, 68 (18%) medical laboratory technologists, and 52 (14%) pharmacists. Over 33% had poor knowledge with 35% not immunized against HBV. Predictors of good knowledge include age less than 35 years, male sex, being a medical doctor, previous HBsAg test, and complete HBV immunisation. Identified challenges to control hepatitis include lack of hospital policy (91.6%), poor orientation of newly employed health workers (75.9%), and low risk perception (74.6%). *Conclusion.* Hospital policy issues and low risk perception of HBV transmission have grave implications for the control of HBV infection.

1. Background

Hepatitis B virus (HBV) is a hepadnavirus. Chronic hepatitis B infection is endemic in Asia and Africa with more than 75% of the world's chronic HBsAg carriers being of Asian and African origins [1]. The burden of the virus is however a global one, even as black children from HBV endemic areas adopted by whites have been implicated in infection of white families [2]. In addition, HBV is transmitted by the sexual route [3] and marriage across races could expose people from low incidence areas to HBV. There is high prevalence of HBV infection among blacks [4], as well as high rate of infection among hospital workers [5]. Moreover, hospital workers have low participation in vaccination programmes, especially those whose work exposes them to the risk of HBV infection [6, 7].

A good knowledge of HBV virus means and modes of infection as well as adequate vaccination may reduce infection rate. The knowledge of HBV is generally low among the populace in a study carried out among Turkish community in Netherland [8]. On the other hand, studies carried out among health care workers in Sudan and Morocco revealed that most of them had a good knowledge of blood as a medium of infection but lacked adequate vaccine coverage [9, 10]. HBV could be transmitted through many other routes, and inadequate knowledge of HBV among health workers may reflect their behavioural pattern to vaccination and safety measures.

Presently, Obafemi Awolowo University Teaching Hospitals Complex has no written policy on hepatitis control; hence, there is no compulsion for health workers to take standard precaution against this deadly virus. Apart from the annual world hepatitis day marked in the hospital, little awareness is created to guard against this virus. Previous studies in Nigeria have focused on medical students and theatre and laboratory workers and few of such studies with limited number of participants on health workers in other areas of the hospital service. Few or no studies have been conducted among all health professionals in any hospital to assess their knowledge base of HBV. It therefore becomes necessary to conduct a baseline assessment of health workers knowledge of HBV and their risk perception and relate the findings to their behavioural pattern toward HBV prevention and hence the need for this study.

2. Methods

This was a descriptive cross-sectional study conducted at the Obafemi Awolowo University Teaching Hospitals Complex, Ile-Ife, Nigeria. The hospital is a 576-bed tertiary health centre, 200 kilometres northeast of Lagos. The study was conducted in two of the principal hospitals (Ife State Hospital and Wesley Guild Hospital) which serve as referral centres for the neighbouring states of Oyo, Kwara, Ondo, Ekiti, and Kogi.

The study population included the clinical members of staff, namely, doctors, nurses, pharmacists, and medical laboratory technologists. The study was conducted between January and April 2013.

The required sample size of 382 was calculated using an appropriate statistical formula for estimating the minimum sample size in descriptive health studies [$n = Z^2 pq/d^2$] [11], where 53.8% of health care workers completed HBV vaccination [7]. The total number of categories of clinical staff (i.e., medical doctors, nurses, laboratory technologists, and pharmacists) at the selected hospitals was collected at the establishment department. The number allocated to each group of clinical staff was determined proportionately using the formula: $n/N \times 382$, where n is the number of occupational groups and N is the total number of clinical staffs.

Eligible persons after an informed consent completed a self-administered pretested questionnaire. The questionnaire assessed the respondents' general knowledge of hepatitis B virus, mode of transmission, risk perception, and challenges to control HBV among respondents. For those with positive HBsAg serostatus, the questionnaire inquired about action taken. The questionnaire also assessed compliance with treatment among those who were on treatment as well as vaccination history of those who were negative to HBsAg. The questionnaires were distributed consecutively to members of each occupational group during the break period after

completion of a written consent form. The respondents were allowed to fill the questionnaire in their spare time at their convenience. Questionnaire information was anonymised.

The Ethics and Research Committee of the Obafemi Awolowo University Teaching Hospitals Complex approved the study with protocol numbers IRB/IEC/0004553 and NHREC/27/02/2009a.

The data collected was entered and kept in a password-protected computer.

The data obtained was analysed using SPSS version 16. Simple descriptive and inferential statistics were done. Test of significance was conducted using appropriate statistical methods. Multivariate analysis was performed using logistic regression to evaluate sociodemographic variables and other variables that are independently associated with HBV knowledge as well as HBV vaccine uptake. Adjusted odd ratio (AOR) and 95% CI were presented and used as measures of the strength of association. Significant level was put at $P < 0.05$.

3. Results

Out of 500 health workers approached none declined participation but 90 did not return their questionnaire. 28 questionnaires were excluded from analysis because of non-completeness. A total of 382 questionnaires with completed data were analysed (response rate of 76%). The mean age of the study participants was 33.8 ± 8.9 years (age range 20–59 years). There were 182 males and 200 females, with M : F ratio of about 1 : 1. The respondents are comprised of 94 (25%) medical doctors, 168 (44%) nurses, 68 (18%) medical laboratory technologists, and 52 (14%) pharmacists. The medical doctors included 45 (12%) house physicians, 44 (12%) resident doctors, and 5 (1%) consultant physicians/surgeons. Two hundred and sixteen (57%) were married, and the rest 166 (43%) were single. Most, 379 (99%), had tertiary level of education (Table 1). Reported prevalence of HBsAg among the respondents was 6.7%.

Majority, 367 (96%), of the participants were aware of HBV, and this was not statistically significant among the professional groups (doctors 93/94 (99%) versus nurses 159/168 (95%) versus lab technologists 64/68 (94%) versus pharmacists 51/52 (98%); $P > 0.05$). The knowledge of the transmission of HBV was good for blood as a medium for all categories of professionals. However, knowledge of other body fluids as source of infection varies among respondents. For instance, doctors had a reasonable good knowledge of saliva as a medium of infection 55/94 (59%) while this knowledge was poor among other professionals. On the other hand, only doctors had a poor knowledge that vaginal/seminal fluid could be a source of infection 25/94 (27%). Also the knowledge of exchange of used needles among patients as well as infected mothers with HBV transmitting the virus to their unborn babies was good for all professionals.

On the knowledge of the population at risk, nurses and laboratory technologists were the least aware that men having sex with men (MSM) could transmit HBV, 111/168 (66%) and 44/68 (65%), respectively, compared with the highest response among doctors 91/94 (98%), $P < 0.05$.

TABLE 1: Sociodemographic characteristics of respondents.

| Characteristics | Sex | | Total (%) |
	Male (%)	Female (%)	
Age group (years)			
18–34	110 (49)	114 (51)	224 (59)
35 and above	72 (46)	86 (54)	158 (41)
Marital status			
Single	97 (58)	69 (42)	166 (43)
Married	85 (39)	131 (61)	216 (57)
Highest level of education			
Secondary	3 (100)	0 (0)	3 (0.8)
Tertiary	179 (47)	200 (53)	379 (99)
Occupation			
Medical doctor	73 (78)	21 (22)	94 (25)
Nurse	40 (24)	128 (76)	168 (44)
Laboratory technologist	43 (63)	25 (37)	68 (18)
Pharmacist	26 (50)	26 (50)	52 (14)
Religion			
Christianity	143 (45)	175 (55)	318 (83)
Islam	39 (61)	25 (39)	64 (17)
Ethnicity			
Yoruba	156 (46)	184 (54)	340 (89)
Igbo	15 (63)	9 (38)	24 (6)
Hausa/Urhobo	11 (61)	7 (39)	18 (5)
HBsAg result			
Positive	9 (4.9)	9 (4.5)	18 (4.7)
Negative	119 (65.4)	130 (65)	249 (65.2)
Not done	54 (29.7)	61 (30.5)	115 (30.1)

Also laboratory technologists reported the least awareness of commercial sex workers 49/68 (72%), multiple sex partners 47/68 (69%), patients with sickle cell anaemia who have had multiple blood transfusions 19/68 (28%), and health care workers 59/68 (87%) as population at risk of HBV infection. This compared with 93/94 (99%), 91/94 (97%), 70/94 (75%), and 94/94 (100%) respectively, among doctors, $P < 0.05$. Also, pharmacists were the least who were aware that long distance drivers were at risk of HBV infection 13/52 (25%) compared with the other professionals, $P < 0.05$ (Table 2). All the respondents had reasonably good knowledge of the chronic complications of HBV. However, medical doctors had better knowledge of these chronic complications than the other professionals, $P < 0.05$ (Table 2).

In reported HBsAg test, nurses were the least group that knew their present HBsAg status 82/118 (70%). All the respondents were aware of hepatitis B vaccine with compliance with vaccination regime being the lowest among nurses than the other groups (87/168, 52%). Only 248 (65%) of our respondents were fully immunised with HBV vaccine. However, all participants were willing to receive HBV vaccine if given the opportunity (Table 3).

In the multivariate logistic regression model the predictors of good knowledge of HBV were age <35 years, male sex,

being a medical doctor, previous HBsAg test, and complete immunisation with HBV vaccine (Table 4).

Also, factors determining HBV vaccine uptake among participants included male sex and having had a previous HBsAg test (Table 5).

Identified challenges to control hepatitis included inappropriate hospital policy (91.6%), poor orientation of newly employed health workers (75.9%), and low risk perception (74.6%) (Table 6).

4. Discussion

The study assessed knowledge of hepatitis B virus, risk perception, vaccination, and challenges to control hepatitis among health workers in a Nigerian tertiary hospital.

The reported prevalence of HBsAg was low in this study when most seroprevalence studies have between 10 and 15% of the Nigerian population being positive to HBsAg [12]. The reason for the low figure may have been because this is a questionnaire administered study rather than a seroprevalence study. Many people who think they are negative may be infected without a serotest. Besides, hepatitis infection is usually higher among health workers than the general population [5].

The awareness level of 96% for HBV among the respondents was similar to that reported by Okwara et al. [13]. This may probably have been as a result of the educational programmes on hepatitis received from the place of work and the news media as well as patients and staff members with complications of chronic hepatitis B virus infection that present regularly to the hospital. Some respondents did not know about the chronic complications of HBV like liver cirrhosis and liver cancer. This shows the lack of in-depth knowledge about HBV among these health workers beyond ordinary awareness. This finding agrees with the reports by other authors in Nigeria [13, 14].

There was a good knowledge of blood as a medium of infection in this study which is similar to reports by both Bakry and Djeriri et al., among Sudanese and Moroccans health workers [9, 10]. The knowledge of the respondents on saliva and tear was poor compared with blood as a medium. Kabir et al. have similarly noted a poor knowledge of the routes of HBV infection among Iranian medical specialists [15]. There was a poor knowledge of the vaginal route of HBV infection among doctors in this study contrary to reports in the literature. Studies have shown that HBV can be transmitted through the sexual route [3, 15, 16], as well as among family members in the household [16]. It thus seems that the major areas health workers lacked adequate knowledge is in the obscured routes of transmitting HBV.

The prevalence of HBsAg is increased in individuals with multiple sexual partners, sickle cell anaemic patients, long distance truck drivers, and injection drug users as well as men who have sex with men (MSM) [17–21]. The knowledge of these among health workers will call for caution and strict adherence to universal precaution among health workers having direct contact with them. However, in this survey, the result showed a poor knowledge of this among some categories of health workers. Only the doctors had a good

TABLE 2: Knowledge, routes, and means of infection and at risk population of HBV.

Variables	Medical doctors (%)	Nurses (%)	Lab technologists (%)	Pharmacists (%)	P value
Aware of HBV (yes)	93/94 (99)	159/168 (95)	64/68 (94)	51/52 (98)	0.829
HBV causes liver cancer? (Yes)	92/94 (98)	107/168 (64)	44/68 (65)	30/52 (58)	0.001
HBV causes liver cirrhosis (yes)	91/94 (97)	132/168 (79)	56/68 (82)	40/52 (77)	0.001
Infection routes					
Blood (yes)	92/94 (98)	163/168 (97)	64/68 (94)	51/52 (98)	0.587
Tear (yes)	37/94 (39)	41/168 (24)	16/68 (24)	13/52 (25)	0.046
Saliva (yes)	55/94 (59)	75/168 (45)	28/68 (41)	23/52 (44)	0.127
Vaginal/seminal fluid (yes)	25/94 (27)	126/168 (75)	49/68 (72)	43/52 (83)	0.001
Means of HBV infection					
Exchange of needle (yes)	94/94 (100)	143/168 (85)	56/68 (82)	50/52 (96)	0.001
Vertical transmission (yes)	86/94 (92)	129/168 (77)	51/68 (75)	34/52 (65)	0.001
At risk population					
*MSM (yes)	91/94 (97)	111/168 (66)	44/68 (65)	38/52 (73)	0.001
Sex workers (yes)	93/94 (99)	133/168 (79)	49/68 (72)	46/52 (89)	0.001
Health workers (yes)	94/94 (100)	154/168 (92)	59/68 (87)	49/52 (94)	0.001
Long distance drivers (yes)	89/94 (95)	63/168 (38)	18/68 (27)	13/52 (25)	0.001
Injection drug users (yes)	94/94 (100)	140/168 (83)	43/68 (63)	41/52 (79)	0.001
Sickle cell anaemic patients (yes)	70/94 (75)	71/168 (42)	19/68 (28)	15/52 (29)	0.001
Multiple sexual partners (yes)	91/94 (97)	130/168 (77)	47/68 (69)	44/52 (85)	0.001

*MSM: men having sex with men.

TABLE 3: HBV serostatus, awareness, and vaccination history of respondents.

Variable	Medical doctors (%)	Nurses (%)	Lab technologists (%)	Pharmacists (%)	P value
Ever screened for HBV (yes)	76/94 (81)	118/168 (70)	55/68 (81)	18/52 (35)	0.001
Knows present status	66/76 (87)	82/118 (70)	46/55 (84)	14/18 (78)	0.024
Took action on positive HBV test (yes)	1/2 (50)	7/12 (58)	3/5 (60)	1/1 (100)	1.000
Completed HBV vaccination after negative HBV test	59/64 (92)	61/70 (87)	27/41 (66)	13/13 (100)	0.002
Proportion on treatment	1/2 (50)	7/12 (58)	2/3 (67)	1/1 (100)	1.000
Proportion that completed treatment	1/1 (100)	4/7 (57)	2/3 (67)	1/1 (100)	1.000
Proportion that cleared HBV	1/1 (100)	1/4 (25)	2/3 (67)	1/1 (100)	0.571
Aware of HBV vaccine (yes)	93/94 (99)	164/168 (98)	65/68 (96)	50/52 (96)	0.474
Received 3 doses of HBV vaccine	80/94 (85)	87/168 (52)	46/68 (68)	35/52 (67)	0.001
Screened for HBsAg before vaccination	43/86 (50)	54/127 (43)	38/56 (68)	8/45 (18)	0.001
Willingness to receive HBV vaccination	82/84 (98)	144/155 (93)	61/63 (97)	48/49 (98)	0.349

knowledge of this. This finding contrasted with that by Kabir et al. among medical specialists [15].

The proportion of the respondents that ever screened for HBV infection was particularly low among the nurses and pharmacists. The implication of this is that health workers who are infected with HBV may present with any of the chronic complications of HBV such as hepatocellular carcinoma or liver cirrhosis as is usually observed in the general population. Furthermore, the implication of a negative HBsAg test was not known to some respondents as very few sought vaccination.

There seems to be a high level of vaccine awareness and low vaccination coverage among health workers in Nigeria. Only 54% of health workers completed HBV vaccination in this hospital in a previous HBV vaccination exercise [7], while 65% of respondents reported complete HBV vaccine in this study. This is despite the fact that the hospital carries out occasional vaccination programmes. This pattern is similar to reports from other centres: Kesieme in south-south geopolitical zone of Nigeria reported 87% awareness level but only 27% vaccination coverage [22], while, in north central Nigeria, Okeke et al. reported that only 48% completed their HBV vaccination with an awareness level of 92% [23]. The reason between the level of awareness and vaccination in the study by Okeke et al. was due to lack of opportunity and forgetting to be vaccinated, while Okwara reported high response among those that had tertiary education. About 99% of our respondents had tertiary education with a vaccination rate of 65%. This supports the findings of Okwara et al. [13], even though we did not inquire into reasons why they did not take vaccine. In addition, we also found that being a male and having had a previous HBsAg test were strongly associated with HBV vaccination.

TABLE 4: Multivariate analysis of factors associated with good knowledge of HBV among the respondents.

Variable	AOR	95% CI	P value
Age group (years)			
18–34	1.746	1.130–2.700	0.012
≥35	1		
Sex			
Male	1.984	1.172–3.359	0.011
Female	1		
Marital status			
Married	0.747	0.485–1.151	0.187
Single	1		
Occupation			
Medical doctor	24.057	6.731–85.978	0.001
Nurse	1.110	0.593–2.079	0.744
Lab technologist	0.841	0.407–1.737	0.640
Pharmacist	1		
Ever screened for HBsAg			
Yes	2.021	1.205–3.389	0.008
No	1		
Doses of vaccine taken			
Appropriate	2.000	1.290–3.103	0.002
Inappropriate	1		

TABLE 5: Multivariate analysis of factors associated with HBV vaccine uptake among health workers.

Variable	AOR	95% CI	P value
Age group (years)			
18–34	1.681	0.947–2.986	0.076
≥35	1		
Sex			
Male	1.756	1.067–2.890	0.027
Female	1		
Marital status			
Married	1.718	0.917–3.218	0.091
Single	1		
Occupation			
Medical doctor	1.037	0.172–6.242	0.968
Nurse	0.501	0.212–1.184	0.115
Lab technologist	0.420	0.158–1.114	0.081
Pharmacist	1		
Ever screened for HBsAg			
Yes	3.689	2.078–6.547	0.001
No	1		

TABLE 6: Challenges to control of hepatitis B infection among health workers.

*Challenges	Frequency (N = 382)	%
Inappropriate hospital policy	350	91.6
Poor orientation of new health workers	290	75.9
Low risk perception	285	74.6
Poor knowledge	124	32.5
Poor implementation of hospital policy	112	29.3
Fear of side effects of vaccine/injection	85	22.3

*Multiple response.

anti-HBs tests can give a false vaccine protection to infected people thereby making them prone to the chronic complications of the virus. Therefore, a mandatory Nigerian government and hospital policy of HBsAg screening and vaccination may need to be put in place for workers and patients protection.

The number that had treatment or those that visited a doctor after a positive HBsAg test was small. This again may reflect their poor knowledge of HBV infection and its long term complications as has been shown in this study.

In this study, factors that favoured a good HBV knowledge were slightly different from that reported by Karaivazoglou et al. among health care workers in Greece [25], while they reported occupation, higher education, and HBsAg vaccination; this study in addition identified younger age, male sex, and having had a previous HBsAg test as indices of good knowledge of HBV.

Several studies have highlighted the importance of the control of viral hepatitis through health education, hepatitis B vaccination of at risk population, and treatment of infected persons [7, 9, 26–28]. Thus, the lack of adequate hospital policy to enforce mandatory hepatitis B test as well as its poor implementation may hinder the effective control of HBV. Many workers that started HBV vaccine did not complete probably due to fear or side effects of the vaccine.

The reported positive association between knowledge of HBV and vaccine uptake as well as poor orientation of new members of staff among the respondents may result from low risk perception which increases possibility of HBV infection through obscure routes. It therefore implied that all health care workers should be educated on HBV and the necessity of following the HBV vaccine regimen.

Limitation to this study is that it is a cross-sectional study; therefore, cause-effect relationship may be difficult to establish. Some respondents could also have given socially acceptable responses to some questions even though they were reassured about the purpose of the study.

5. Conclusion

The hospital workers of this institution have low perceived risk of HBV infection and low vaccination coverage despite a high awareness of HBV vaccine. Therefore, a policy of mandatory HBsAg screening and vaccination may need to be put in place to protect both staff and patients of the institution. Free HBsAg screening for newly employed staff

The situation is however different outside Nigeria with higher vaccine coverage among health workers [24, 25]. This may therefore translate to routine HBsAg and anti-HBs tests and vaccination for Nigerian health workers who wish to practice in other countries of the world.

Only 37% were screened for HBsAg before vaccination. The government of Nigeria as well as the institution's policy is to vaccinate everyone without a prior HBsAg test. However, the liver unit of the hospital advise that screening is done before vaccination so that only those who will benefit take the vaccine. The practice of vaccination without HBsAg and before vaccination may need to be incorporated into the policy to make it effective.

Conflict of Interests

The authors do not have any conflict of interests.

Acknowledgments

The authors are grateful to the management of Obafemi Awolowo University Teaching Hospitals and health workers that participated in the study.

References

[1] C.-L. Lai, R.-N. Chien, N. W. Y. Leung et al., "A one-year trial of lamivudine for chronic hepatitis B," *The New England Journal of Medicine*, vol. 339, no. 2, pp. 61–68, 1998.

[2] F. G. J. Cobelens, H. J. van Schothorst, P. M. E. Wertheim-van Dillen, R. J. Ligthelm, I. S. Paul-Steenstra, and P. P. A. M. van Thiel, "Epidemiology of hepatitis B infection among expatriates in Nigeria," *Clinical Infectious Diseases*, vol. 38, no. 3, pp. 370–376, 2004.

[3] P. Luksamijarulkul, A. Mooktaragosa, and S. Luksamijarulkul, "Risk factors for hepatitis B surface antigen positivity among pregnant women," *Journal of the Medical Association of Thailand*, vol. 85, no. 3, pp. 283–288, 2002.

[4] O. Adekanle, D. A. Ndububa, O. O. Ayodeji, B. Paul-Odo, and T. A. Folorunso, "Sexual transmission of the hepatitis B virus among blood donors in a tertiary hospital in Nigeria," *Singapore Medical Journal*, vol. 51, no. 12, pp. 944–947, 2010.

[5] A. C. Belo, "Prevalence of hepatitis B virus markers in surgeons in Lagos, Nigeria," *East African Medical Journal*, vol. 77, no. 5, pp. 283–285, 2000.

[6] R. C. Ibekwe and N. Ibeziako, "Hepatitis B vaccination status among health workers in Enugu, Nigeria," *Nigerian Journal of Clinical Practice*, vol. 9, no. 1, pp. 7–10, 2006.

[7] A. O. Fatusi, O. A. Fatusi, A. O. Esimai, A. A. Onayade, and O. S. Ojo, "Acceptance of hepatitis B vaccine by workers in a Nigerian teaching hospital," *East African Medical Journal*, vol. 77, no. 11, pp. 608–612, 2000.

[8] Y. J. J. Van Der Veen, H. A. C. M. Voeten, O. De Zwart, and J. H. Richardus, "Awareness, knowledge and self-reported test rates regarding Hepatitis B in Turkish-Dutch: a survey," *BMC Public Health*, vol. 10, article 512, 2010.

[9] S. H. Bakry, A. F. Mustafa, A. S. Eldalo, and M. A. Yousif, "Knowledge, attitude and practice of health care workers toward Hepatitis B virus infection, Sudan," *International Journal of Risk and Safety in Medicine*, vol. 24, no. 2, pp. 95–102, 2012.

[10] K. Djeriri, H. Laurichesse, J. L. Merle et al., "Hepatitis B in Moroccan health care workers," *Occupational Medicine*, vol. 58, no. 6, pp. 419–424, 2008.

[11] L. Kish, *Survey Sampling*, John Wiley & Sons, New York, NY, USA, 1965.

[12] D. A. Ndububa, O. S. Ojo, O. O. Adeodu et al., "Primary hepatocellular carcinoma in Ile-Ife, Nigeria: a prospective study of 154 cases," *Nigerian Journal of Medicine*, vol. 10, no. 2, pp. 59–63, 2001.

[13] E. C. Okwara, O. O. Enwere, C. K. Diwe, J. E. Azike, and A. E. Chukwulebe, "Theatre and laboratory workers' awareness of and safety practices against hepatitis B and C infection in

a suburban university teaching hospital in Nigeria," *The Pan African Medical Journal*, vol. 13, p. 2, 2012.

[14] S. C. Nwokediuko, "Chronic hepatitis B: management challenges in resource-poor countries," *Hepatitis Monthly*, vol. 11, no. 10, pp. 786–793, 2011.

[15] A. Kabir, S. V. Tabatabaei, S. Khaleghi et al., "Knowledge, attitudes and practice of iranian medical specialists regarding hepatitis B and C," *Hepatitis Monthly*, vol. 10, no. 3, pp. 176–182, 2010.

[16] A. P. Jimenez, N. S. El-Din, M. El-Hoseiny et al., "Community transmission of hepatitis B virus in Egypt: results from a case-control study in Greater Cairo," *International Journal of Epidemiology*, vol. 38, no. 3, pp. 757–765, 2009.

[17] M. R. H. Roushan, M. Mohraz, and A. A. Velayati, "Possible transmission of hepatitis B virus between spouses and their children in Babol, Northern Iran," *Tropical Doctor*, vol. 37, no. 4, pp. 245–247, 2007.

[18] M. Nouraie, S. Nekhai, and V. R. Gordeuk, "Sickle cell disease is associated with decreased HIV but higher HBV and HCV comorbidities in US hospital discharge records: a cross-sectional study," *Sexually Transmitted Infections*, vol. 88, no. 7, pp. 528–533, 2012.

[19] M. A. Matos, R. M. Bringel Martins, D. D. Da Silva França et al., "Epidemiology of hepatitis B virus infection in truck drivers in Brazil, South America," *Sexually Transmitted Infections*, vol. 84, no. 5, pp. 386–389, 2008.

[20] R. V. Houdt, S. M. Bruisten, A. G. C. L. Speksnijder, and M. Prins, "Unexpectedly high proportion of drug users and men having sex with men who develop chronic hepatitis B infection," *Journal of Hepatology*, vol. 57, no. 3, pp. 529–533, 2012.

[21] A.-S. Mansson, T. Moestrup, E. Nordenfelt, and A. Widell, "Continued transmission of hepatitis B and C viruses, but no transmission of human immunodeficiency virus among intravenous drug users participating in a syringe/needle exchange program," *Scandinavian Journal of Infectious Diseases*, vol. 32, no. 3, pp. 253–258, 2000.

[22] E. B. Kesieme, K. Uwakwe, E. Irekpita, A. Dongo, K. J. Bwala, and B. J. Alegbeleye, "Knowledge of hepatitis B vaccine among operating room personnel in Nigeria and their vaccination status," *Hepatitis Research and Treatment*, vol. 2011, Article ID 157089, 5 pages, 2011.

[23] E. N. Okeke, N. G. Ladep, E. I. Agaba, and A. O. Malu, "Hepatitis B vaccination status and needle stick injuries among medical students in a Nigerian university," *Nigerian Journal of Medicine*, vol. 17, no. 3, pp. 330–332, 2008.

[24] T. Paul, A. Maktabi, K. Almas, and S. Saeed, "Hepatitis B awareness and attitudes amongst dental health care workers in Riyadh, Saudi Arabia," *Odonto-Stomatologie Tropicale*, vol. 22, no. 86, pp. 9–12, 1999.

[25] K. Karaivazoglou, C. Triantos, M. Lagadinou et al., "Acceptance of hepatitis B vaccination among health care workers in Western Greece," *Archives of Environmental and Occupational Health*, vol. 69, no. 2, pp. 107–111, 2014.

[26] R. Mihigo, D. Nshimirimana, A. Hall, M. Kew, S. Wiersma, and C. J. Clements, "Control of viral hepatitis infection in Africa: are we dreaming?" *Vaccine*, vol. 31, no. 2, pp. 341–346, 2013.

[27] H. Ohara, I. Ebisawa, and H. Naruto, "Prophylaxis of acute viral hepatitis by immune serum globulin, hepatitis b vaccine, and health education: a sixteen year study of Japan overseas cooperation volunteers," *The American Journal of Tropical Medicine and Hygiene*, vol. 56, no. 1, pp. 76–79, 1997.

[28] B. J. Bojuwoye, "The burden of viral hepatitis in Africa," *West African Journal of Medicine*, vol. 16, no. 4, pp. 198–203, 1997.

A Novel Structurally Stable Multiepitope Protein for Detection of HCV

Alexsandro S. Galdino,[1] **José C. Santos,**[2] **Marilen Q. Souza,**[2] **Yanna K. M. Nóbrega,**[3] **Mary-Ann E. Xavier,**[4] **Maria S. S. Felipe,**[2] **Sonia M. Freitas,**[4] **and Fernando A. G. Torres**[2]

[1]*Laboratório de Biotecnologia de Microrganismos, Universidade Federal de São João Del-Rei, 35501-296 Divinópolis, MG, Brazil*
[2]*Departamento de Biologia Celular, Universidade de Brasília, 70910-900 Brasília, DF, Brazil*
[3]*Laboratório de Doenças Imunogenéticas e Crônico-degenerativas, Universidade de Brasília, 70910-900 Brasília, DF, Brazil*
[4]*Laboratório de Biofísica, Universidade de Brasília, 70910-900 Brasília, DF, Brazil*

Correspondence should be addressed to Fernando A. G. Torres; ftorres@unb.br

Academic Editor: Piero Luigi Almasio

Hepatitis C virus (HCV) has emerged as the major pathogen of liver diseases in recent years leading to worldwide blood-transmitted chronic hepatitis, liver cirrhosis, and hepatocellular carcinoma. Accurate diagnosis for differentiation of hepatitis C from other viruses is thus of pivotal importance for proper treatment. In this work we developed a recombinant multiepitope protein (rMEHCV) for hepatitis C diagnostic purposes based on conserved and immunodominant epitopes from *core*, NS3, NS4A, NS4B, and NS5 regions of the virus polyprotein of genotypes 1a, 1b, and 3a, the most prevalent genotypes in South America (especially in Brazil). A synthetic gene was designed to encode eight epitopes *in tandem* separated by a flexible linker and bearing a his-tag at the C-terminal end. The recombinant protein was produced in *Escherichia coli* and purified in a single affinity chromatographic step with >95% purity. Purified rMEHCV was used to perform an ELISA which showed that the recombinant protein was recognized by IgG and IgM from human serum samples. The structural data obtained by circular dichroism (CD) spectroscopy showed that rMEHCV is a highly thermal stable protein at neutral and alkaline conditions. Together, these results show that rMEHCV should be considered an alternative antigen for hepatitis C diagnosis.

1. Introduction

Hepatitis C virus (HCV) is an important human pathogen affecting 3% of the human population [1]. Chronic infection is a major cause of liver cirrhosis and hepatocellular carcinoma [2]. Seroprevalence studies suggest that at least 170 million individuals have been infected worldwide [1]. The incidence of new HCV infections has decreased in affluent countries owing to screening of blood products, but an increase of global patients is still expected [2, 3]. The HCV genome is represented by a single-stranded positive RNA molecule which encodes a polyprotein of 3010–3033 amino acid residues [4]. The HCV polyprotein is co- and posttranslationally processed to produce several structural and nonstructural polypeptides [5]. Six genotypes and several HCV subtypes are well characterized, with an overall nucleotide diversity of 31%–33% between genotypes and 20%–25% between subtypes [6]. Genotypes 1, 2, and 3 are widely distributed throughout the world and are responsible for almost all cases in America, Europe, and Japan [7]. In Brazil, approximately 2 million acute cases of hepatitis C have been reported [8] with genotype 1 responsible for 60 to 75% of HCV infections [9–11]. Genotype 3 is the second-most prevalent and genotype 2 represents less than 5% of cases.

Several Enzyme Immune Assay (EIA) based diagnostic kits are available in the market for detection of HCV antibodies in the plasma; these are based on peptide antigens (third generation) or recombinant antigens (fourth generation) from both structural and nonstructural regions of the viral protein. The requirement of multiple peptides and/or multiple recombinant proteins for reliable diagnosis of HCV infection may add to the final cost of these EIA kits. Alternatively, the development of multiepitope proteins is an attractive approach to reduce the complexity and the final costs of such diagnostic kits [12]. In this work we have designed a single recombinant multiepitope protein (rMEHCV) consisting of several immunodominant and conserved specific epitopes from structural and nonstructural proteins derived from genotypes 1, 2, and 3, the most prevalent in South America. The recombinant protein was successfully produced and tested for HCV detection in infected patients in Brazil.

2. Material and Methods

2.1. Strains and Reagents. *Escherichia coli* BL21 (λDE3) pLysS (F$^-$ ompT hsdS$_B$ (r$_B^-$ m$_B^-$) gal dcm (DE3) pLysS [Cam^r]) and expression vector pET21a were purchased from Novagen. NiSepharose™ 6 Fast Flow resin (GE Healthcare) was used to purify rMEHCV. Restriction enzymes were purchased from New England Biolabs. Illustra™ Plasmid Prep Mini Spin Kit was purchased from GE Healthcare. Secondary antibody-enzyme conjugates, monoclonal anti-poly histidine-alkaline phosphatase (AP) antibody and monoclonal anti-human IgG-HRPO, and HRPO substrate Sigma Fast™ OPD (o-phenylenediamine dihydrochloride) Peroxidase Substrate Tablet Set were purchased from Sigma-Aldrich. Infected human sera samples were kindly provided by WAMA Diagnóstica (São Carlos, Brazil) and are listed in Table 1. Other reagents of analytical grade were obtained from standard commercial sources.

2.2. Design of the Synthetic Gene, Cloning, and Expression. The overall structure of the synthetic gene encoding rMEHCV was based on the construct previously described elsewhere [12] with the inclusion of immunodominant sequences of genotypes prevalent in South America (1a, 1b, and 3a). The sequences used were obtained from GenBank: *core*(1a), *core*(3a), NS3(1a), NS4A(1a), NS4B(1a), and NS5(1a) (accession # AF009606, M62321, and M67463), NS4(1b) and NS5(1b) (accession # D90208, M58335) and from the website https://euhcvdb.ibcp.fr/euHCVdb/. The length of individual epitopes varied from 16–48 amino acid residues and each one was separated by a flexible linker (Gly-Ser-Gly-Ser-Gly). The synthetic gene was custom synthesized by Epoch Biosciences with codon adaptation for *E. coli* and was cloned as a *Nde*I/*Xho*I fragment into pET21a in-frame with a C-terminal histidine tag in order to allow protein purification by affinity chromatography. The resulting plasmid was used to transform *E. coli* BL21 (DE3) competent cells and selection was performed on LB agar plates containing 100 μg/mL ampicillin. An individual colony was inoculated in 5 mL 4YT (32 g/L Bactotryptone, 20 g/L yeast extract, 5 g/L NaCl, pH 7.2) containing 100 μg/mL ampicillin and allowed to grow overnight at 37°C under agitation (200 rpm). One milliliter of the preculture was transferred to 20 mL 4YT in a 250 mL E-flask. The culture was grown in the same conditions described above until an OD$_{600}$ of 0.6 when 1 mM IPTG was added. The induced culture was harvested by centrifugation at 6000 ×g for 15 min at 4°C and the pellet was stored at −80°C.

TABLE 1: Infected human sera used in this work.

Sera	Pathologies
1, 2, and 3	HCV (+)
4, 5, and 6	HCV (−)
7 and 8	HAV (hepatitis A)
9, 10, and 11	HAV and HBV (hepatitis B)
12	HBV
13 and 14	RUB (rubella) and CMV (cytomegalovirus)
15	HBV
16	RUB, CMV, and TOX (toxoplasmosis)
17	RUB and TOX
18	CMV and TOX
19	HBV

2.3. Purification of rMEHCV. The frozen pellet was resuspended in 1 mL Lysis Buffer (8 M urea, 50 mM NaH$_2$PO$_4$, 300 mM NaCl, 10 mM imidazole, pH 8.0) following incubation at 4°C for 16 h. After that, cell suspension was sonicated (5 pulses of 10 seconds with 1-minute intervals) using Vibra Cell sonicator (Sonics & Materials, Inc.) and incubated on ice for 2 h following centrifugation at 6000 ×g for 15 min at 4°C. The supernatant was added to 0.5 mL Ni-Sepharose 6 Fast Flow resin (Sigma-Aldrich) (resuspended in Lysis Buffer) which was then incubated at 4°C for 90 min on a vertical disc rotator. After incubation the resin was sedimented and washed four times with 1 mL Washing Buffer (4 M urea, 50 mM NaH$_2$PO$_4$, 300 mM NaCl, 20 mM imidazole, pH 8.0). Protein was eluted in three fractions using 0.5 mL Elution Buffer (50 mM NaH$_2$PO$_4$, 300 mM NaCl, 500 mM imidazole, pH 8.0).

2.4. Gel Electrophoresis and Western Blotting. Protein integrity and molecular mass calculation were evaluated by running samples on 12% SDS-PAGE [13]. Proteins were stained with Coomassie Brilliant Blue R-250 (Sigma-Aldrich). For Western Blotting, a monoclonal anti-poly-histidine clone His-1 alkaline phosphatase conjugate (Sigma-Aldrich) was diluted 1:1000 in PBS, and nitroblue tetrazolium salt and 5-bromo-4-chloro-3-indolyl phosphate (NBT/BCIP kit, Invitrogen) were used for signal development.

2.5. In-House Enzyme-Linked Immunosorbent Assay (ELISA). The wells of polystyrene plates (Greiner Bio-One) were sensitized with 20 ng purified rMEHCV dissolved in 100 μL 0.1 M sodium carbonate-bicarbonate buffer (pH 9.6). After incubation at 4°C for 16 h the coated wells were washed with PBST (PBS supplemented with 0.2% Tween 20, pH 7.2) and blocked for 2 h at 37°C with PBS containing 5% (w/v) dried skim milk powder and washed again with PBST. Subsequently, 100 μL of a dilution (100 μL PBST, 5% (w/v) dried skim milk powder, and 5 μL serum) was placed into the wells resulting in a final dilution of approximately 1/20. After incubation for 1 h at 37°C, the wells were washed with PBST and 100 μL of peroxidase-labeled goat anti-human immunoglobulin G conjugate (Sigma-Aldrich) diluted at 1:25,000 in PBS containing

Core(1a)   Core(3a)
MSTNPKPQRKTKRNTNRRPQDVKFPGGGQIVGGVYLLPRRGPRL GSGSG MSTLPKPQRKTKR

                                                        NS4A(1b)
NTIRRPQDVKFPGGGQIVGGVYVLPRRGPRL GSGSG IIPDREVLYREFDEMEECASHLPYIE

                                                        NS3(1a)
QGMQLAEQFKQKALGL GSGSG YMSKAHGVDPNIRTGVRTITTGSPITYSTYGKFLADGGCSG

                                                        NS4A(1a)
GAYDIII GSGSG IIPDREVLYQEFDEMEECSQHLPYIEQGMMLAEQFKQKALGL GSGSG PPL

NS5(1b)   NS4B(1a)   NS5(1a)
LESWKDPDYVPPVVH GSGSG IAFASRGNHVSPTHYV GSGSG PPLVETWKKPDYEPPVVH LE-

H$_{6x}$

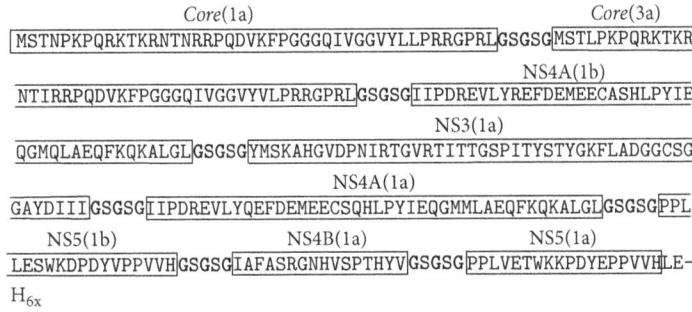

FIGURE 1: Primary structure of rMEHCV. Epitopes derived from structural (core) and nonstructural proteins (NS3, NS4A, NS4B, and NS5) from HCV genotypes 1, 2, and 3 are boxed. Each epitope is separated by a flexible linker (bold). A histidine tag (H$_{6x}$) is present at the C-terminal end.

5% (w/v) dried skim milk powder was added following incubation for 1 h at 37°C. The wells were again washed with 200 μL OPD by incubating for 30 min at room temperature. The optical densities (OD) were read at 450 nm. The results from the in-house kit were compared to those obtained from the Hepanóstika HCV Ultra® (Beijing, China) commercial kit.

2.6. Circular Dichroism Spectroscopy. Circular dichroism (CD) assays were carried out using Jasco J-815 spectropolarimeter (Jasco, Tokyo, Japan) equipped with a Peltier-type temperature controller and thermostatized cuvette holder linked to a thermostatic bath. Far-UV spectra were recorded using 0.2 cm path length quartz cuvettes at a protein concentration of 0.084 mg/mL in 5 mM Tris-HCl (pH 7.0 and 8.0). Five consecutive measurements were accumulated and the averaged spectra were recorded. The observed ellipticities were converted into molar ellipticity $[\theta]$ based on molecular mass per residue of 115 Da [14]. The data was corrected for the baseline contribution of Tris-HCl buffer considered to estimate the secondary structure content using the CD Spectra Deconvolution (CDNN) [15]. Thermal denaturation experiments were performed by temperature increase from 25 to 95°C followed by changes in dichroic signal at 208 nm ($[\theta]_{208}$). The thermal denaturing curves were normalized and expressed considering the unfolded protein fraction (f_U) according to (1). The equilibrium constants for unfolding process and thermodynamic parameters enthalpy (ΔH_m), entropy (ΔS_m), and the Gibbs free energy (ΔG^{25}) were calculated from (2), (3), and (4), respectively [16]:

$$f_U = \frac{(y_N - y)}{(y_N - y_U)}, \tag{1}$$

$$K_{eq} = \frac{f_U}{(1 - f_U)}, \tag{2}$$

$$R \ln K_{eq} = -\Delta H \left(\frac{1}{T}\right) + \Delta S, \tag{3}$$

$$\Delta G = \Delta H - T\Delta S, \tag{4}$$

where y_N and y_U represent the amount of y protein present in native and unfolded state, respectively. R is the universal gas constant (1,987 cal K^{-1} mol^{-1}) and T the temperature in Kelvin (K). The melting temperature (T_m), where the unfolding occurs, was calculated from the nonlinear fitting of unfolding curves using Origin software 8.0 (Microcal Software Inc., Northampton, MA program).

3. Results

3.1. Design of rMEHCV. In order to design a multiepitope protein that could be of diagnostic use, linear and conserved immunodominant epitopes which are known to elicit anti-HCV antibodies were selected based on data from the literature [9–12]. These epitopes are located on five distinct regions of the HCV polyprotein. Due to the sequence variation among genotypes 1a, 1b, and 3a, eight epitopes—core(1a), core(3a), NS4A(1b), NS3(1a), NS4A(1a), NS5(1b), NS4B(1a), and NS5(1a)—were chosen representing genotypes circulating worldwide, especially in South America. Multiple sequence alignments of the HCV genotypes of different isolates allowed the identification of conserved immunodominant epitopes which were assembled *in tandem* and connected by flexible glycine-serine linkers. This would allow the epitopes to be freely available for interaction with their cognate antibodies thus contributing to the overall sensitivity and specificity of the diagnostic test. The primary amino acid sequence of rMEHCV was predicted to encode a ~34.4 kDa protein which is shown in Figure 1.

3.2. Expression and Purification of the rMEHCV. The gene coding for rMEHCV was cloned into the bacterial expression vector pET21a for inducible expression under the control of the T7 bacteriophage promoter. After transformation of *E. coli* BL21 (DE3) a selected clone was analyzed for rMEHCV expression by SDS-PAGE after induction with IPTG. As shown in Figure 2(a), an inducible protein band with a molecular mass of ~35 kDa was observed. The cell lysate was incubated with Ni-NTA resin in the presence of 8 M urea and samples were collected during different steps of the purification and analyzed by SDS-PAGE. Elution of the bound proteins was achieved with 500 mM imidazole and

(a)

(b)

(c)

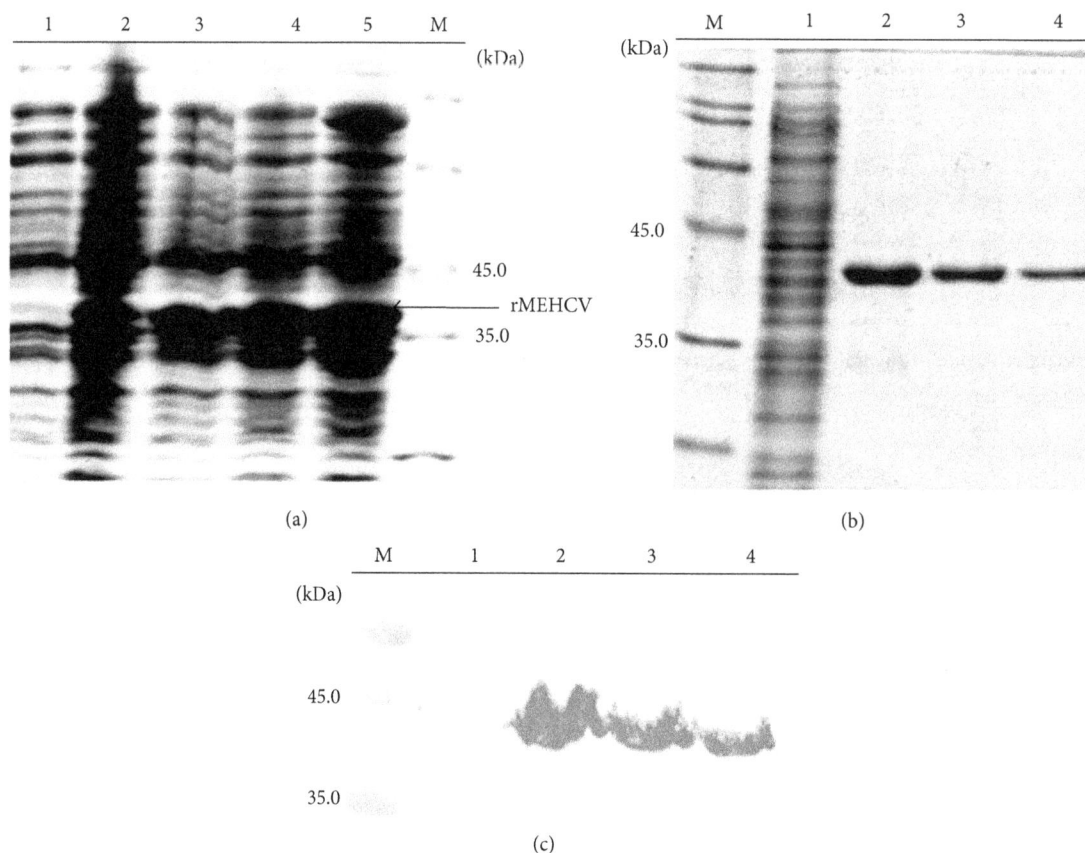

FIGURE 2: Expression and purification of rMEHCV. (a) Cell lysates from a selected clone induced by IPTG visualized on a Coomassie Blue stained 12% SDS-PAGE. Lane 1, cell lysates from uninduced culture. Lanes 2–5, cell lysates from induced culture after 2, 4, 6, and 8 h, respectively; Lane M, unstained protein molecular weight marker (Fermentas Life Sciences). The arrow indicates the position of the band corresponding to rMEHCV. (b) Fractions collected after Ni-NTA chromatography visualized on 12% SDS-PAGE. Lane M, molecular weight markers (Weight Standard, Broad Range, BioRad). Lane 1, flow-through, Lanes 2–4, purified rMEHCV after elution with 500 mM imidazole. (c) Western blot analysis of the purified rMEHCV. The monoclonal antibody, anti-polyhistidine alkaline phosphatase conjugate, was used after dilution 1:1000 in PBS (pH 7.2). Lane M, PAGE™ Ruler (Fermentas Life Science). Lanes 1–4 correspond to the same fractions shown in (b).

resulted in highly purified rMEHCV (Figure 2(b)). The 6x histidine tag at the C-terminal end of rMEHCV was used to identify the recombinant protein by Western Blotting. The affinity-purified protein was blotted and probed with commercially available monoclonal anti-polyhistidine antibody which recognized the purified protein as being rMEHCV (Figure 2(c)).

3.3. Human Anti-Hepatitis C Virus Antibodies Recognize rME-HCV. After protein purification, an in-house ELISA was developed for the assessment of rMEHCV as a potential antigen for HCV detection. In order to standardize the amount of protein required to obtain a suitable signal, different amounts of purified rMEHCV were coated onto ELISA plates. After blocking, 10 μL sera samples (anti-HCV positive and negative) were added. The results showed that 0.02 μg/mL of the recombinant protein provided the optimal signal, that is, OD > 0.8 (data not shown). Therefore, 20 ng/well (in 100 μL) rMEHCV was utilized for setting up the in-house anti-HCV test kit. To establish the specificity of rMEHCV, 17 human

positive and 10 negative sera samples for anti-HCV were evaluated in triplicate. The results showed that the test kit was able to distinguish positive and negative sera, showing no false-negative or false-positive results (Figure 3(a)) as compared to a commercial kit (Hepanóstika HCV Ultra) (Figure 3(b)) which essentially yielded the same results. In addition, to establish if rMEHCV does not exhibit any false-positives in the presence of sera samples from humans infected with non-HCV pathogens, 13 sera samples from patients carrying common infections, hepatitis A, hepatitis B, rubella, cytomegalovirus, and toxoplasmosis, were evaluated using the in-house anti-HCV test kit and all samples scored negative (Figure 4).

3.4. Structural Analysis by Circular Dichroism (CD). In order to gain more insight into the structure of rMEHCV we performed CD analysis. The Far-UV CD spectra of rMEHCV at 25°C, pH 7.0 and 8.0 presented a negative dichroic band at 208 nm, a broad and of low intensity negative band at 220–228 nm, and positive prominent CD signal at 195 nm

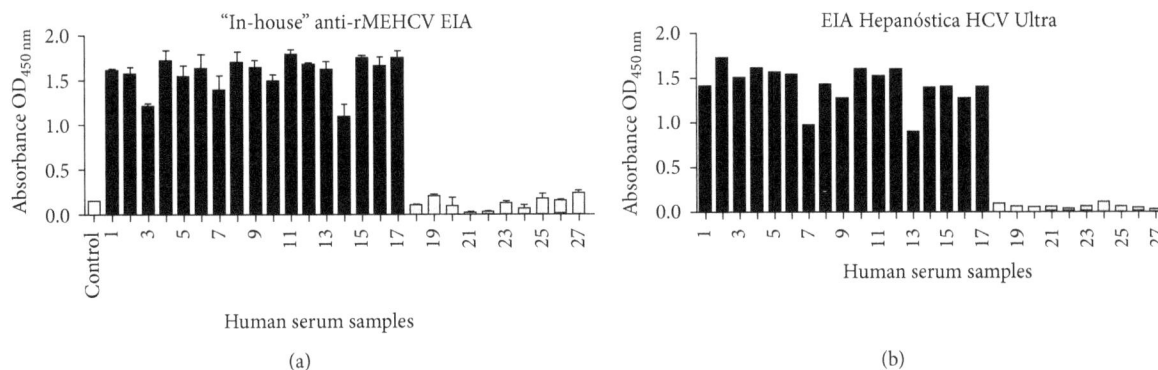

FIGURE 3: Specificity test for rMEHCV. (a) Detection of HCV using an in-house EIA. Each well of the EIA plates was coated with 20 ng purified rMEHCV and assayed with 17 positive and 10 negative human sera samples. The white bar represents the control "blank" test (0 ng protein coated + serum # 1 + conjugated secondary antibody), and the black bars and gray bars represent the sera positive and negative for anti-HCV, respectively. The bars represent the average of triplicates of each serum with its respective standard deviation. (b) Analysis of samples tested in (a) with a commercial kit (Hepanóstika HCV Ultra kit). The sera were diluted 1/10.

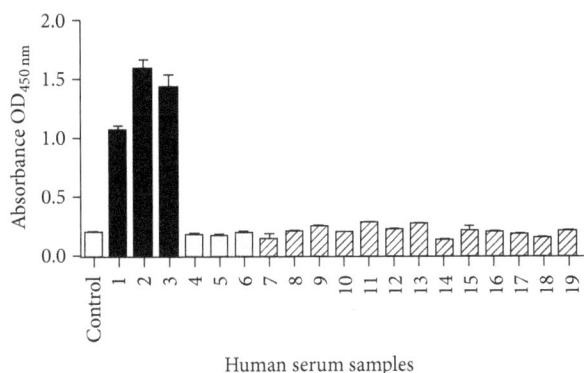

FIGURE 4: Cross-reactivity test of rMEHCV using in-house EIA. Human sera samples were diluted 1/20 and secondary antibody was diluted 1/25,000. The bars represent the standard deviation of triplicates. The white bar represents the control "blank" test (0 ng protein coated + serum # 1 + conjugated secondary antibody), and the black, gray, and crosshatched bars represent positive sera, negative for anti-HCV and positive for other diseases, respectively. Sample numbering follows the list shown in Table 1.

(Figure 5(a)), suggesting predominantly the presence of β-sheet and a low content of α-helix structures. It was confirmed by the estimated secondary structure contents of rMEHCV at pH 7.0 of 12.5% α-helix, 56.0% β-sheet (parallel, antiparallel, and turns), and 32.6% random-coil structures. At pH 8.0 almost the same pattern of secondary structure was observed, as depicted in Figure 5(a). Although the alkaline conditions did not promote considerable secondary structure alterations at 25°C, compared with those at pH 7.0, the thermal denaturation assays indicated the pH dependent structural changes of protein, as judged by differences in unfolding processes (Figures 5(b) and 5(c)). The Far-UV spectra at pH 7.0 show a gradual decrease of the dichroic signal (upward until ~zero), as a function of temperature, suggesting the whole protein unfolding process (Figure 5(b)). In contrast, despite

dichroic signal decreasing from about −6,000 to −3,500 degree·cm^2·dmol^{-1}, at pH 8.0 indicating the secondary structure changes (Figure 5(c)), the whole pattern of protein denaturation could not be verified. It was in agreement with equilibrium thermal folding/unfolding process of rMEHCV from 25 to 95°C, monitored by Far-UV CD at 208 nm. At pH 7.0 the rMEHCV unfolded process occurs as two-state model from native to unfold protein (Figure 6), whereas at pH 8.0 two distinctive transitions involving the native and molten globule intermediates, but not the whole denatured protein, were observed (data not shown). The nonlinear fitted unfolding curve at pH 7.0 (Figure 6) shows the inflection points corresponding to the melting temperatures of 66.3°C. The thermodynamic parameters, calculated according to the van't Hoff approximation (Figure 7) at pH 7.0, were ΔH_m 115.8 kcal·mol^{-1}, ΔS_m 341.47 cal·mol^{-1}K^{-1} and the Gibbs free energy (ΔG^{25}) 14.02 kcal·mol^{-1} which indicates high stability of protein in this condition. Additionally, the protein seems to be more stable at pH 8.0, as indicated by the not observed unfolding pattern until 95°C under this condition.

4. Discussion

Hepatitis C is a worldwide public health problem. In Brazil, it has been shown that from those individuals who test positive for HCV infection approximately 80% have the chronic form of the disease. Based on these data, it is estimated that there are 400,000 to 3,800,000 cases of chronic hepatitis C in Brazil alone [8]. Because of the increase in the number of cases detected worldwide in recent years, the demand for diagnostic tests for HCV has increased accordingly. The method of choice for HCV detection is generally based on EIA because of its ease of use, low variability, easy automation, and low costs. Over the years, several generations of EIA tests have been developed with the aim of increasing sensitivity and specificity. The first generation anti-HCV tests were developed in the late 80s [17]. These tests contained a single recombinant antigen derived from the NS4 region and lacked

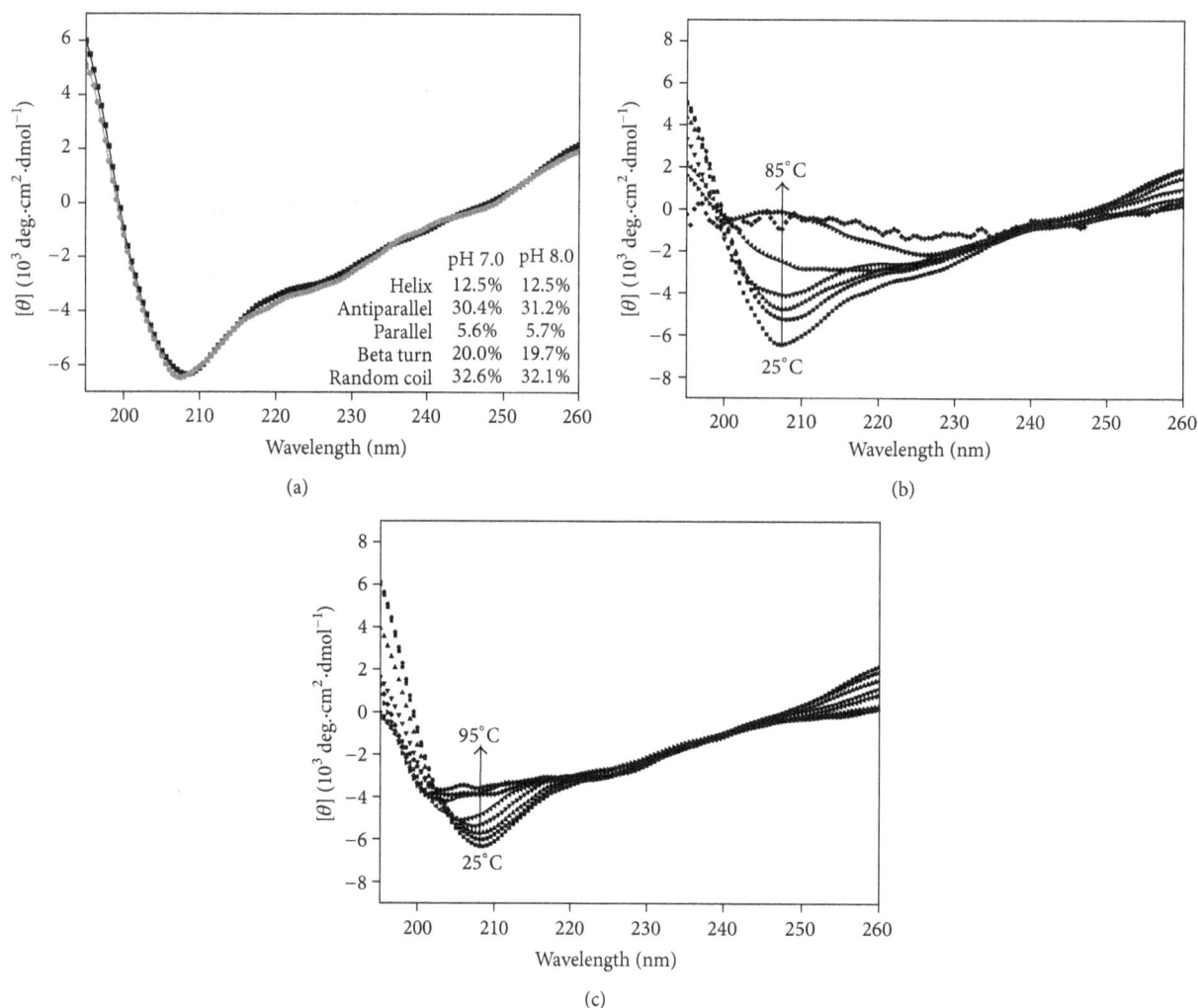

	pH 7.0	pH 8.0
Helix	12.5%	12.5%
Antiparallel	30.4%	31.2%
Parallel	5.6%	5.7%
Beta turn	20.0%	19.7%
Random coil	32.6%	32.1%

FIGURE 5: Structural analysis of rMEHCV by circular dichroism. (a) Far-UV CD spectra of rMEHCV (2.5 μM) at 25°C in 5 mM Tris-HCl pH 7.0 (gray line) and pH 8.0 (black line). The table inset shows the secondary structure content of protein in both pHs; (b) Far-UV CD spectra of rMEHCV (2.5 μM) in 5 mM Tris-HCl (pH 7.0) as a function of temperature. The arrow indicates the increase of temperature from 25 to 85°C, in which the complete loss of CD signal was observed; (c) Far-UV CD spectra of rMEHCV (2.5 μM) in 5 mM Tris-HCl (pH 8.0). The arrow indicates the increase of temperature from 25 to 95°C, in which the CD signal reducing until ~3,500 deg·cm^2·dmol^{-1} was observed.

optimal sensitivity and specificity. In order to circumvent these limitations, second generation tests contained antigens derived from the HCV *core*, NS3 and NS4 regions [18]. This resulted in higher levels of sensitivity but a small increase in specificity which nonetheless shortened seroconversion [19]. Third generation anti-HCV tests included an antigen from the NS5 region which resulted in a progressive increase in sensitivity [20] but not all patients with active infection could be identified with these tests [21].

With the advent of recombinant DNA technology, EIA tests were significantly improved because higher antigen concentration could be used. Also, due to the fact that certain antigens are not readily recognized by antiserum belonging to different serovars it is desirable that diagnostic kits should be able to detect as many genotypes as possible. Genetic information is an important parameter to direct the patients for a specific treatment. For example, treatment with

interferon-α and ribavirin has an efficiency of 40–45% in patients infected with HCV genotype 1, whereas in those infected with genotypes 2 and 3 the efficiency increases up to 70–80% [10].

The urgent need for a diagnostic test which offers increased degrees of sensibility and specificity prompted us to develop a recombinant multiepitope protein bearing HCV-specific immunodominant epitopes. Several studies have reported the successful use of multiepitope protein for diagnosis of infectious diseases such as leishmaniasis [22], hepatitis B [23], hepatitis C [12], toxoplasmosis [24], tuberculosis [25], leprosy [26], leptospirosis [27], dengue [28], and Chagas disease [29]. A multiepitope protein (r-HCV-F-MEP) for hepatitis C diagnosis has been previously developed bearing 5 immunodominant regions comprising genotypes circulating worldwide and one Indian isolate [12]. From a clinical perspective, the multiepitope protein developed in

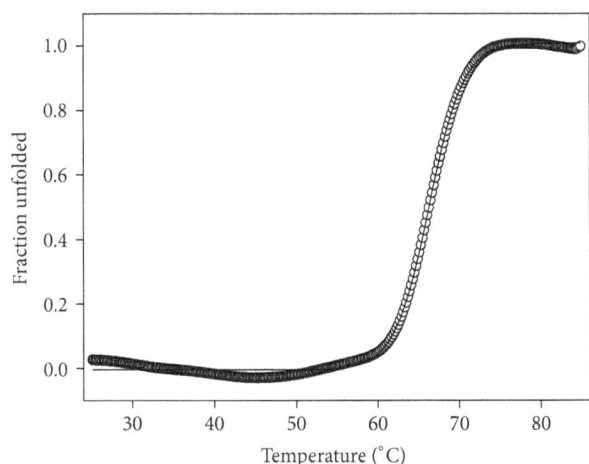

FIGURE 6: Heat-induced unfolding curve of rMEHCV ($2.5\,\mu M$) monitored by CD spectroscopy at 208 nm in 5 mM Tris-HCl pH 7.0. The black line corresponds to the sigmoid fitting of experimental data. The fraction unfolded data are calculated considering the changes in molar ellipticities at 208 nm and equations described in Material and Methods. The melting temperature, T_m, corresponding to the inflection point of the sigmoid is $66.32°C$.

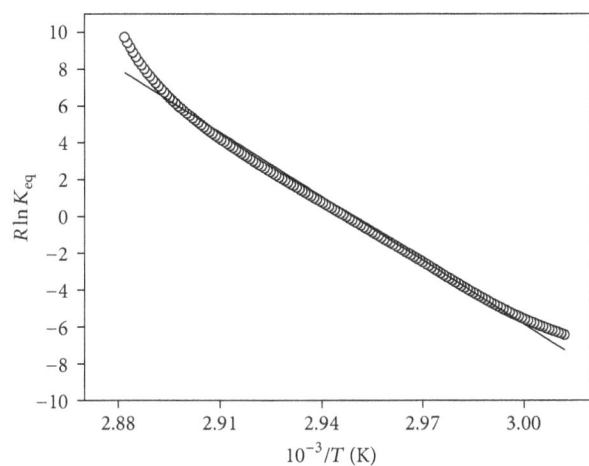

FIGURE 7: Van't Hoff plot of rMEHCV ($2.5\,\mu M$) in 5 mM Tris-HCl (pH 7.0). The black line corresponds to the linear fitting of the experimental data obtained from the unfolding curve.

our work (rMEHCV) aimed at the detection of the most representative HCV serotypes particularly found in Brazil. This was achieved by the inclusion of sequences from the *core*, NS3, NS4A, NS4B, and NS5 regions from genotypes 1a, 1b, and 3a. Genotypes 1, 2, and 3 are found in all continents and constitute the majority of HCV isolates [9]. Genotype 4 is more common in the North and Center-West Africa, while genotypes 5 and 6 are most common in South Africa and Asia, respectively [10]. In Brazil, genotypes 1 and 3 are the most prevalent [11].

We based our construct on the immunodominant regions previously proposed [12] but focused on genotypes 1a, 1b, and 3a. Furthermore, we include extra copies of the immunodominant regions from proteins NS4a and NS5 in order to cover both genotypes 1a and 1b which have some sequence differences in these particular regions.

Since the major goal of this study was to develop a recombinant protein for use in diagnostic kit, the ability of rMEHCV to detect anti-HCV antibodies was tested in an in-house EIA. In this assay the recombinant protein was used as the capture antigen and human sera samples infected or not with HCV were tested. Our results showed that rMEHCV was recognized by all HCV-infected samples with a 100% agreement with a commercial kit. In addition, when exposed to sera samples from patients having other (non-HCV) infections no cross-reaction was observed, thus demonstrating the specificity of rMEHCV, a desirable feature for HCV diagnosis.

The secondary structure content and structural stability of rMEHCV under different pH and temperatures were also studied. These parameters are important given that epitopes should be stable under diagnostic assay conditions. The structural stability of rMEHCV was investigated by circular dichroism spectroscopy in neutral and alkaline conditions. It is known that the CD spectrum of the typical α-helix exhibits two prominent negative bands. One of them occurs at 208 nm, generally of reduced intensity in short helices, and the other at 222 nm, related to strong hydrogen-bonding environment and independent of the length of the helix. The typical β-sheet proteins exhibit a negative band near 218 nm and a positive band near 195 nm, in which the position and magnitude are generally variable. In contrast, unordered polypeptides exhibit a negative band near 200 nm [14, 30]. In this work, the Far-UV CD spectroscopy results indicate that rMEHCV is a structured protein at neutral and alkaline conditions. It seems to contain a small amount of helical structure with low intensity CD signal at 222 nm and high amount of β-sheet structures, indicated just by the positive band at 195 nm, once it does not present the typical maximum at around 218 nm (Figure 5(a)).

While rMEHCV exhibits similar amount of secondary structure at pH 7.0 and 8.0 (Figure 5(a)), the thermal-induced conformational transitions were much less for the latter indicating more stability at pH 8.0 (Figure 5(c)) than at pH 7.0 (Figure 5(b)). The CD_{208nm} measurement of rMEHCV at pH 7.0 (Figure 6) revealed a typical thermal reversible two-state transition from native to unfolded state [16, 30, 31]. It was also indicated by CD rescanning under protein sample cooling (95 to 25°C), after its complete thermal unfolding until 95°C (data not shown). The high values of thermodynamic parameters obtained from the unfolded curve at this pH 7.0, mainly ΔG^{25} of 14.02 kcal·mol^{-1}, indicate a remarkable stability of rMEHCV. It depends on the enthalpy changes that correspond to the binding energy of noncovalent interactions, and the entropy changes associated with the increase of conformational freedom in the polypeptide chain and hydration of exposed groups on unfolded state. Furthermore, the transition temperature (T_m) from native to unfolded state occurs at temperatures above 66°C, compatible with the high stable thermophilic proteins [32, 33]. As seen in this neutral condition the protein was completely unfolded at 95°C. In contrast, at pH 8.0 the conformational changes of the protein could be verified throughout the temperature range of 25 to 95°C (Figure 5(c)), which preserve part of its secondary structure despite temperature increase. This unfolding process involves the presence of intermediates that is larger than the native protein and has an intact secondary structure, known as a molten globule state [31, 34], indicated through the maintenance of dichroic signal of $-3,500$ degree·cm^2·dmol^{-1} at 95°C. It is known that the presence of molten globule intermediate in unfolded process depends not only on the amino acid composition and protein structural arrangement but also on the environmental conditions [30, 31, 34]. Overall, the most abundant amino acids residues composing rMEHCV are glycine (14.6%) and proline (9.2%) which could in part explain the high stability of the protein at both pHs due to favoring of high content of polypeptide fold in globular protein. Furthermore, protein stability can be also explained by two main points: (i) the structural arrangement of rMEHCV due to differences in charged residues as a function of pH; (ii) the high stability at pH 8.0, which is the closest pH to the theoretical isoelectric point of the protein (pI of ~9.0—http://web.expasy.org/protparam/), where globular proteins tend to present maximum stability [16, 35, 36]. The results presented here indicated that the net charges and ionic pairs, due to the high content of charged amino acid residues, induced on the pH 8.0, could also favor a more compact state. This condition results in the stabilization of the protein as a molten globule state, even at the high temperature of 95°C.

It is noteworthy that the N-terminus of rMEHCV contains 28/37 of the total number of lysine and arginine residues in the protein, while the C terminus has 11/14 histidine residues and 18/30 of the acidic residues. At neutral pH, most of these residues are charged, whereas at pH 8.0 all histidines are uncharged. The highest conformational stability of rMEHCV near the pI is likely the result of protein self-association tendency driven by favorable electrostatic interactions on the molecule surface. Additionally, the difference of stability at pH 7.0, compared to pH 8.0, may be also due to the charge balance resulting from histidine residues ionization in the unfolded state relative to the native state, and the possible high number of ionic pairs.

Therefore, we have shown that the secondary structure of rMEHCV in both pHs at 25°C was similar; however the protein was more stable at pH 8.0 as compared to neutral pH. The molecule unfolded at 95°C and at neutral pH, but it can assume an intermediate molten globule structure and a compact denatured state with significant secondary or tertiary structure at pH 8.0. Together, the results presented here showed that rMEHCV is a highly thermal stable protein at neutral and alkaline conditions and could be used under those conditions for HCV diagnosis.

5. Conclusions

The high epitope density derived from different HCV genotypes coupled with a simple purification procedure prompts rMEHCV as a promising alternative for hepatitis C diagnosis, with potential for development of an inexpensive diagnostic test with high degree of specificity.

Conflict of Interests

None of the authors has any other conflict of interests related to this paper.

Authors' Contribution

Alexsandro S. Galdino and José C. Santos contributed equally to this work.

Acknowledgments

This work was supported by Fundação de Amparo à Pesquisa do Distrito Federal Grants 193.000.582/2009 and 193.000.490/2011; Conselho Nacional de Desenvolvimento Científico e Tecnológico Grants 563855/2010-0, 309244/2013-7, and 564000/2010-8. J. C. Santos had a fellowship from CNPq (Brazil).

References

[1] E. Szabó, G. Lotz, C. Páska, A. Kiss, and Z. Schaff, "Viral hepatitis: new data on hepatitis C infection," *Pathology and Oncology Research*, vol. 9, no. 4, pp. 215–221, 2003.

[2] J. F. Perz and M. J. Alter, "The coming wave of HCV-related liver disease: dilemmas and challenges," *Journal of Hepatology*, vol. 44, no. 3, pp. 441–443, 2006.

[3] T. Poynard, M.-F. Yuen, V. Ratziu, and C. L. Lai, "Viral hepatitis C," *The Lancet*, vol. 362, no. 9401, pp. 2095–2100, 2003.

[4] D. Moradpour, F. Penin, and C. M. Rice, "Replication of hepatitis C virus," *Nature Reviews Microbiology*, vol. 5, no. 6, pp. 453–463, 2007.

[5] B. Hoffman and Q. Liu, "Hepatitis C viral protein translation: mechanisms and implications in developing antivirals," *Liver International*, vol. 31, no. 10, pp. 1449–1467, 2011.

[6] P. Simmonds, J. Bukh, C. Combet et al., "Consensus proposals for a unified system of nomenclature of hepatitis C virus genotypes," *Hepatology*, vol. 42, no. 4, pp. 962–973, 2005.

[7] F. Davidson, P. Simmonds, J. C. Ferguson et al., "Survey of major genotypes and subtypes of hepatitis C virus using RFLP of sequences amplified from the $5'$ non-coding region," *The Journal of General Virology*, vol. 76, no. 5, pp. 1197–1204, 1995.

[8] Ministério da Saúde. Secretaria de Vigilância em Saúde. Departamento de Vigilância Epidemiológica, *Hepatites virais: O Brasil está atento/Ministério da Saúde*, Departamento de Vigilância Epidemiológica, Ministério da Saúde, Brasília, Brazil, 3rd edition, 2008.

[9] S. Campiotto, J. R. R. Pinho, F. J. Carrilho et al., "Geographic distribution of hepatitis C virus genotypes in Brazil," *Brazilian Journal of Medical and Biological Research*, vol. 38, no. 1, pp. 41–49, 2005.

[10] R. M. B. Martins, S. A. Teles, N. R. Freitas et al., "Distribution of hepatitis C virus genotypes among blood donors from midwest region of Brazil," *Revista do Instituto de Medicina Tropical de São Paulo*, vol. 48, no. 1, pp. 53–55, 2006.

[11] R. Paraná, L. Vitvitski, F. Berby et al., "HCV infection in northeastern Brazil: unexpected high prevalence of genotype 3a and absence of African genotypes," *Arquivos de Gastroenterologia*, vol. 37, no. 4, pp. 213–216, 2001.

[12] C. A. Dipti, S. K. Jain, and K. Navin, "A novel recombinant multiepitope protein as a hepatitis C diagnostic intermediate of high sensitivity and specificity," *Protein Expression and Purification*, vol. 47, no. 1, pp. 319–328, 2006.

[13] U. K. Laemmli, "Cleavage of structural proteins during the assembly of the head of bacteriophage T4," *Nature*, vol. 227, no. 5259, pp. 680–685, 1970.

[14] A. J. Adler, N. J. Greenfield, and G. D. Fasman, "Circular dichroism and optical rotatory dispersion of proteins and polypeptides," *Methods in Enzymology*, vol. 27, no. 1, pp. 675–735, 1973.

[15] G. Böhm, R. Muhr, and R. Jaenicke, "Quantitative analysis of protein far UV circular dichroism spectra by neural networks," *Protein Engineering*, vol. 5, no. 3, pp. 191–195, 1992.

[16] C. N. Pace and J. M. Scholtz, "Measuring the conformational stability of a protein," in *Protein Structure: A Practical Approach*, pp. 299–321, Oxford University Press, Oxford, UK, 2nd edition, 1997.

[17] G. Kuo, Q.-L. Choo, H. J. Alter et al., "An assay for circulating antibodies to a major etiologic virus of human non-A, non-B hepatitis," *Science*, vol. 244, no. 4902, pp. 362–364, 1989.

[18] Z. Younossi and J. McHutchison, "Serological tests for HCV infection," *Viral Hepatology Reviews*, vol. 2, no. 1, pp. 161–173, 1996.

[19] B. Hosein, C. T. Fang, M. A. Popovsky, J. Ye, M. Zhang, and C. Y. Wang, "Improved serodiagnosis of hepatitis C virus infection with synthetic peptide antigen from capsid protein," *Proceedings of the National Academy of Sciences of the United States of America*, vol. 88, no. 9, pp. 3647–3651, 1991.

[20] J.-H. Kao, M.-Y. Lai, Y.-T. Hwang et al., "Chronic hepatitis C without anti-hepatitis C antibodies by second-generation assay: a clinicopathologic study and demonstration of the usefulness of a third-generation assay," *Digestive Diseases and Sciences*, vol. 41, no. 1, pp. 161–165, 1996.

[21] H. I. Atrah and M. M. Ahmed, "Hepatitis C virus seroconversion by a third generation ELISA screening test in blood donors," *Journal of Clinical Pathology*, vol. 49, no. 3, pp. 254–255, 1996.

[22] A. R. Faria, L. D. C. Veloso, W. Coura-Vital et al., "Novel recombinant multiepitope proteins for the diagnosis of asymptomatic *Leishmania infantum*-infected dogs," *PLoS Neglected Tropical Diseases*, vol. 9, no. 1, Article ID e3429, 2015.

[23] M. Q. de Souza, A. S. Galdino, J. C. dos Santos et al., "A recombinant multiepitope protein for hepatitis B diagnosis," *BioMed Research International*, vol. 2013, Article ID 148317, 7 pages, 2013.

[24] J. Dai, M. Jiang, Y. Wang, L. Qu, R. Gong, and J. Si, "Evaluation of a recombinant multiepitope peptide for serodiagnosis of *Toxoplasma gondii* infection," *Clinical and Vaccine Immunology*, vol. 19, no. 3, pp. 338–342, 2012.

[25] Z. Cheng, J.-W. Zhao, Z.-Q. Sun et al., "Evaluation of a novel fusion protein antigen for rapid serodiagnosis of tuberculosis," *Journal of Clinical Laboratory Analysis*, vol. 25, no. 5, pp. 344–349, 2011.

[26] M. S. Duthie, W. Goto, G. C. Ireton et al., "Use of protein antigens for early serological diagnosis of leprosy," *Clinical and Vaccine Immunology*, vol. 14, no. 11, pp. 1400–1408, 2007.

[27] X. Lin, Y. Chen, and J. Yan, "Recombinant multiepitope protein for diagnosis of leptospirosis," *Clinical and Vaccine Immunology*, vol. 15, no. 11, pp. 1711–1714, 2008.

[28] N. K. Tripathi, A. Shrivastva, P. Pattnaik et al., "Production, purification and characterization of recombinant dengue multiepitope protein," *Biotechnology and Applied Biochemistry*, vol. 46, no. 2, pp. 105–113, 2007.

[29] R. L. Houghton, D. R. Benson, L. Reynolds et al., "Multiepitope synthetic peptide and recombinant protein for the detection of antibodies to *Trypanosoma cruzi* in patients with treated or untreated Chagas' disease," *The Journal of Infectious Diseases*, vol. 181, no. 1, pp. 325–330, 2000.

[30] D. H. A. Corrêa and C. H. I. Ramos, "The use of circular dichroism spectroscopy to study protein folding, form and function," *African Journal of Biochemistry Research*, vol. 3, no. 5, pp. 164–173, 2009.

[31] S. M. Kelly, T. J. Jess, and N. C. Price, "How to study proteins by circular dichroism," *Biochimica et Biophysica Acta—Proteins and Proteomics*, vol. 1751, no. 2, pp. 119–139, 2005.

[32] S. Kumar, C.-J. Tsai, and R. Nussinov, "Factors enhancing protein thermostability," *Protein Engineering*, vol. 13, no. 3, pp. 179–191, 2000.

[33] S. Kumar and R. Nussinov, "How do thermophilic proteins deal with heat?" *Cellular and Molecular Life Sciences*, vol. 58, no. 9, pp. 1216–1233, 2001.

[34] K. Kuwajima, "The molten globule state as a clue for understanding the folding and cooperativity of globular-protein structure," *Proteins: Structure, Function and Genetics*, vol. 6, no. 2, pp. 87–103, 1989.

[35] K. A. Dill, "Dominant forces in protein folding," *Biochemistry*, vol. 29, no. 31, pp. 7133–7155, 1990.

[36] R. A. Staniforth, M. G. Bigotti, F. Cutruzzolà, C. T. Allocatelli, and M. Brunori, "Unfolding of apomyoglobin from *Aplysia limacina*: the effect of salt and pH on the cooperativity of folding," *Journal of Molecular Biology*, vol. 275, no. 1, pp. 133–148, 1998.

29

Atherosclerosis as Extrahepatic Manifestation of Chronic Infection with Hepatitis C Virus

Theodoros Voulgaris and Vassilios A. Sevastianos

4th Department of Internal Medicine, "Evangelismos" General Hospital, 45-47 Ipsilantou Street, 106 76 Athens, Greece

Correspondence should be addressed to Vassilios A. Sevastianos; vsevastianos@gmail.com

Academic Editor: Man-Fung Yuen

Chronic hepatitis C virus infection is associated with significant morbidity and mortality, as a result of progression towards advanced natural course stages including cirrhosis and hepatocellular carcinoma. On the other hand, the SVR following successful therapy is generally associated with resolution of liver disease in patients without cirrhosis. Patients with cirrhosis remain at risk of life-threatening complications despite the fact that hepatic fibrosis may regress and the risk of complications such as hepatic failure and portal hypertension is reduced. Furthermore, recent data suggest that the risk of HCC and all-cause mortality is significantly reduced, but not eliminated, in cirrhotic patients who clear HCV compared to untreated patients and nonsustained virological responders. Data derived from studies have demonstrated a strong link between HCV infection and the atherogenic process. Subsequently HCV seems to represent a strong, independent risk factor for coronary heart disease, carotid atherosclerosis, stroke, and, ultimately, CVD related mortality. The advent of new direct acting antiviral therapy has dramatically increased the sustained virological response rates of hepatitis C infection. In this scenario, the cardiovascular risk has emerged and represents a major concern after the eradication of the virus which may influence the life expectancy and the quality of patients' life.

1. Introduction

Over 160 million people worldwide are chronically infected with the HCV virus [1]. Besides the liver related complications of HCV infection such as liver cirrhosis and hepatocellular carcinoma, chronic infection is associated in several studies with extrahepatic disorders, including metabolic derangements. Though not many studies exist, robust data connect HCV infection with atherosclerosis and consequently its complications as stroke and coronary heart disease. In our days when the HCV infection can be treated in more than 90% of HCV infected patients, it is most important for clinicians to deal with the extrahepatic derangements which can diminish patients' life expectancy and alter their quality of life [2].

2. Pathophysiology Aspects

The pathophysiological basis of the evidenced correlation between HCV infection and atherosclerosis is incompletely understood. Chronic HCV infection is an inflammatory state not only affecting the liver. HCV infection represents a chronic inflammatory state where an imbalance between TH1 and TH2 is observed [3]. Studies have demonstrated that patients with chronic HCV infection exhibit higher IL-6 and TNF-alpha, INFγ, and IL-2 levels and a higher ratio of proinflammatory/anti-inflammatory cytokines [4]. Atherosclerosis is widely known to be a result of persistent inflammatory changes. HCV promoted inflammatory cytokines may contribute to the development of atherosclerosis through the enhancement of intracellular adhesion molecules, expression of anti-endothelium antibodies, and generation of oxidative stress (OXS) and insulin resistance (IR) [5]. What is more severe is that fibrosis and the associated cascade of proinflammatory and profibrogenic pathways generated in the liver might promote carotid atherosclerosis [6]. Furthermore, HCV RNA sequences have been isolated within carotid plaques and this in turn may suggest the possibility of an active infection of the carotid plaque itself [7].

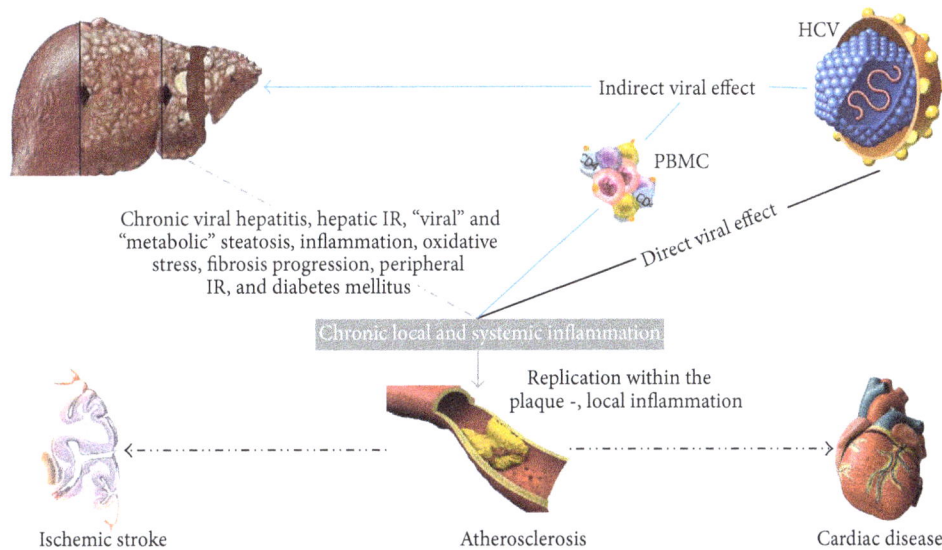

FIGURE 1: Possible mechanisms connecting HCV infection and cardiovascular disease. HCV is considered a "metabolic" virus and is associated with metabolic disorders, in particular insulin resistance and type 2 diabetes mellitus, which are proatherogenic conditions. By inducing hepatic injury and activating peripheral blood mononuclear cells (PBMC), HCV increases circulating levels of proinflammatory cytokines, leading to peripheral IR and hyperinsulinemia. Furthermore, a key feature of HCV infection is associated with hyperhomocysteinaemia, hypoadiponectinaemia, oxidative stress, lipid peroxidation, and all components of the metabolic syndrome. Therefore, "viral" induced and "metabolic" steatosis, together with the direct stimulus of increased insulin levels on hepatic stellate cells (HSCs) likely stimulate the progression of fibrosis within the liver parenchyma. Furthermore, systemic inflammation, the procoagulative state, and direct viral effects on the vascular wall may contribute to the development and progression of the atherogenic process.

Moreover, another important mechanism by which chronic HCV infection can promote the development of atherosclerotic plaques is its well described correlation with proatherogenic conditions such as insulin resistance [8, 9] and diabetes type 2 [10]. IR induces a broad range of toxic systemic effects, including dyslipidemia, hypertension, hyperglycemia, increased production of advanced glycosylation end products, increased inflammatory tone, and a prothrombotic and prooxidative state. Patients with IR are highly vulnerable to the development of accelerated atherosclerosis as well its clinical sequelae, including coronary artery disease and myocardial infarction, carotid artery disease, and ischemic stroke. Multiple explanations have been proposed in order to elucidate the mechanism of the development of IR in HCV infection. It seems more possible that both host and viral factors correlate to IR occurrence. Primarily it was assumed that chronic inflammation and the observed in HCV infection upregulation of inflammatory markers such as TNF-alpha and IL-6 and the deregulation of adipocytokines (leptin, adiponectin) were a leading step, but recent studies failed to prove this assumption. It is now believed that the HCV virus itself and moreover the HCV core protein are the main driving factor by their interactions with SOCS3 or SOCS7 expression and PPAR-γ and PPAR-a [11, 12]. As far as type 2 diabetes and hyperglycemia is concerned its relationship with atherosclerosis is well established and its pathophysiological basis has been extensively studied. Oxidative stress, abnormal NO-mediated vasodilation, and increased macrophage lipid uptake, leading to foam cell formation, are only some features of the complex pathway by which hyperglycemia promotes atheromatosis [13].

Finally, liver steatosis, observed in HCV infection, and its association with hyperhomocysteinaemia are also factors predisposing to atherosclerosis [17]. Steatosis is a common finding in HCV infected patients especially among patients infected with Genotype 3 (GT 3) which seems to have a direct steatogenic effect as steatosis in infection with GT 3 is well correlated with the levels of intrahepatic viral replication [35]. Even if HCV related steatosis has not been proven to directly cause atheromatosis at least four studies have, independently of the metabolic syndrome, directly linked steatosis to atheromatosis [36]. It is not therefore irrational to hypothesize that this effect can be attributed to HCV related steatosis also. It should be mentioned that HCV patients tend to have a more favorable lipid profile possibly due to the straightforward interaction of the HCV virion, which uses the LDL receptor to infect hepatocytes, with the host lipid metabolism [35] (Figure 1).

3. HCV and Atheromatosis

In 2002 for the first time a study by Ishizaka et al. proposed a link between HCV infection and carotid atherosclerosis [14]. Since then several studies by various researchers, executed in different countries, provided evidence that HCV infection is independently associated with carotid plaques with a prevalence from 38% to 64% [37, 38] as also an independent predictor of increased carotid intimal medial thickness (IMT) (Table 1).

TABLE 1: Characteristics of studies associating HCV infection and atheromatosis.

Author, year, country	Study design	Association	Enrolled patients	Comments	Method of carotid atheromatosis assessment
Ishizaka et al., 2002 [14], Japan	Cross-sectional population based	Positive	4784/104 HCV infected	First study in this field, measuring IMT	Ultrasonography IMT measurement
Tomiyama et al., 2003 [15], Japan	Cohort study	Positive	7514/87 HCV infected	Increase arterial stiffness measured by pulse wave velocity	Pulse wave velocity
Mostafa et al., 2010 [16], Egypt	Cross-sectional	Positive	329 anti-HCV positive/724 anti-HCV negative	Patients with active disease had higher risk compared to past infection	Ultrasonography IMT measurement
Petta et al., 2012 [6], Italy	Case control	Positive	174 genotype 1 infected/174 controls	Association between fibrosis and the presence of plaques	Ultrasonography IMT > 1.3 mm
Adinolfi et al., 2012 [17], Italy	Case control	Positive	803/326 HCV infected	Association between HCV steatosis and atheromatosis	Ultrasonography IMT: >1 mm or plaques ≥ 1.5 mm
Huang et al., 2013 [18], China	Meta-analysis	Positive		Strongly correlates HCV infection to carotid atheromatosis	
Masia et al., 2011 [19], Spain	Cohort study	Negative	138 HIV/63 HCV/HIV coinfected	No matching between exposed and control patients for any variable	Ultrasonography IMT > 1.0 mm
Caliskan et al., 2009 [20], Turkey	Prospective 59 months follow-up	Negative	36 HCV infected/36 controls	No matching between exposed and control patients for any variable	Ultrasonography IMT > 1.0 mm
Tien et al., 2009 [21], USA	Cross-sectional	Negative	1675/53 HCV monoinfected	HIV/HCV coinfection may be associated with a greater risk of carotid plaques	Ultrasonography Focal CIMT > 1.5 mm in any of the imaged segment
Völzke et al., 2004 [22], Germany	Cross-sectional	Negative	4310/15 HCV infected	Very small number of HCV infected patients	Ultrasonography IMT measurement

A study published in 2003 by Tomiyama et al., where 87 anti-HCV positives and 7427 anti-HCV negative subjects were enrolled, showed that HCV infected subjects had increased arterial stiffness compared to HCV negative controls [15].

Moreover a large Egyptian study by Mostafa et al. which included 329 anti-HCV positives and 725 anti-HCV negative patients showed that patients with active disease, when adjustment for known cardiovascular risk factor was executed, had a higher risk for atherosclerosis compared to subjects with past infection [16].

A recent study by Petta et al. not only confirmed the higher incidence of carotids plaques in HCV infected patients but also correlated the presence of carotid plaques with the severity of liver fibrosis as it was estimated by liver biopsy [6]. The study enrolled 174 GT 1 biopsy proven HCV patients and 174 control matched subjects. Multivariate logistic regression analysis showed that older age (odds ratio [OR] 1.047, 95% confidence interval [CI] 1.014–1.082, $P = 0.005$) and severe hepatic fibrosis (OR 2.177, 95% CI 1.043–4.542, $P = 0.03$) were independently linked to the presence of carotid plaques. In patients <55 years, 15/67 cases with F0–F2 fibrosis (22.3%) had carotid plaques, compared with 11/21 (52.3%) with F3-F4 fibrosis ($P = 0.008$). By contrast, in patients >55 years the prevalence of carotid plaques was similar in those with

or without severe fibrosis (25/43, 58.1% versus 22/43, 51.1%; $P = 0.51$).

Finally, a study executed by Adinolfi et al. in Italy suggested that HCV-related steatosis is both a good marker for identifying atherosclerosis-prone individuals and an early mediator of atherosclerosis [39]. The writers came to the conclusion that HCV-related steatosis modulates atherogenic factors such as inflammation and the dysmetabolic milieu, therefore favoring the development of atherosclerosis. Once more, in this study, it was observed by the researchers that chronic HCV infection predisposes individuals to the premature development of atherosclerosis and advanced carotid changes.

On the contrary a small number of studies [19–21] failed to prove such an association, though it must be underlined that a meta-analysis executed by Huang et al., which included 11 studies among them the studies of Tien, Calsikan, and Masia, studies which failed to prove such an association, revealed that HCV infection is significantly associated with carotid atherosclerotic burden [40].

Taking into account the abovementioned data HCV infection must be considered as a risk factor for carotid atheromatosis. In the era of new and more efficacious treatments for chronic HCV infection the burden of the nonliver related complications of the HCV infection may become of great significance for the prior HCV infected patients' life expectancy. As a result of this, as it was also stated by Petta et al. [6], it may be indicated that HCV patients aged 55 or more, those with severe fibrosis, and those with HCV related liver steatosis should undergo ultrasonography screening for carotid atherosclerotic disease.

4. HCV and Stroke

Recent data have pointed out a correlation between HCV infection and increase risk for cerebrovascular disease. In a large study executed in the United States where 10,259 anti-HCV seropositive patients and 10,259 matched anti-HCV seronegatives were included, the Hazard Ratio (HR) of death from stroke was 2.20 [41]. In another study executed in Taiwan which enrolled 23,785 subjects (1,307 anti-HCV positive subjects) the HR for cerebrovascular death was 2.18 for seropositives to anti-HCV, compared to the seronegative patients of the study [42].

This positive correlation was also underlined in a recent study where 820 subjects were enrolled, where the multivariate analysis showed an OR of 2.04 for stroke among HCV patients compared to anti-HCV negative patients [26]. Finally, a large meta-analysis of the latest studies conducted in this field suggested that HCV infection [18] significantly increased the risk of stroke (OR = 1.97; 95% CI: 1.64–2.30).

Moreover it was proposed from a single study that HCV load is linearly correlated with the risk of stroke among HCV patients [43]. Of special note is a recent study conducted in Taiwan by Hsu et al. that came to the conclusion that not only did HCV infected patients have a 23% increased risk of stroke compared to age and sex-matched subjects without HCV infections but interferon-based therapy may reduce the long term risk of stroke in patients with HCV infection [44].

This data are furthermore supported by a recent study by Enger et al. [28] where it was demonstrated that HCV patients are in an increased risk of events such as unstable angina and transient ischemic attacks as it was pointed out in their study published in 2014 where 22733 HCV seropositives were enrolled.

To our knowledge only two studies, one including only 21 anti-HCV positive subjects, an obviously very small number of patients capable of extracting confident results [22], and another which was criticized because of the heterogeneity of the study population as far as age, sex, and hypertension status of the study subjects was concerned [45], failed to demonstrate such a positive correlation.

When all data are taken into account it can be safely argued that HCV infection increases the risk of cerebrovascular events and moreover data point to the direction that HCV eradication treatment can prevent these events, a fact highly important in our days when new and more effective treatment strategies against the HCV infection exist.

5. HCV and Cardiovascular Risk

Despite the existence of conflicting evidence, a link between HCV infection and increase cardiovascular risk can be discerned [5, 46]. The pioneer study in this field was published in 2004 by Vassalle et al. where the authors suggested that seropositivity represented an independent predictor for CAD with an odds ratio of 4.2 (95% CI: 1.4 to 13.0, $P = 0.05$) [23]. A large scale epidemiological study conducted in the United States by Butt et al. among (82083 HCV infected and 89582 HCV uninfected subjects) veterans over a 5-year period showed a significantly higher prevalence of cardiac disease among HCV infected patients [24].

In another study by Alyan et al. where 139 HCV seropositive and 225 HCV seronegative patients with angiographically documented CAD were enrolled, HCV infection was documented to be an independent predictor for increased coronary atherosclerosis, as demonstrated by higher Reardon severity score [25].

Recently a retrospective study including 78 HCV positive patients compared to 742 HCV negative subjects was executed, which observed higher ischemic heart events in the HCV positive patients than in the HCV negative patients (22% versus 13%, resp., $P = 0.031$) [26]. Additionally in a recent study where HCV monoinfected, genotype 1, naive, and nonobese (BMI < 30) patients and nondiabetics were included and compared to controls, an intermediate cardiovascular risk, as measured by the Framingham score, was observed [27].

As it was already stated Enger et al. [28] in a recent study came to the conclusion that HCV infected patients are in an increased risk of unstable angina. Moreover the results of the latest study published in 2013 by Satapathy et al. indicated that CAD is significantly more prevalent as also severe (stenosis > 75%) in HCV seropositive patients compared to age-, race-, and sex-matched controls undergoing evaluation by coronary angiogram for suspected CAD. The HCV infected patients were also presented, in a greater scale, with significant multi-vessel coronary artery disease (≥2 vessels). The authors notice that it is not clear whether the observed association between CAD and CHC infection is related to the known metabolic complications related to insulin resistance in patients with chronic HCV infection, or due to under treatment with antiplatelet and lipid-lowering agents because of concerns for gastrointestinal bleeding or hepatotoxicity [29].

Finally, a large recent study conducted in the US added more confirmatory data towards the direction of a positive association. Pothineni et al. in their study among a total of 8,251 HCV antibody positive, 1,434 HCV RNA positive, and 14,799 HCV negative patients came to the conclusion that there is an increased incidence of CHD events in patients with HCV seropositivity and the incidence is much higher in patients with detectable HCV RNA compared with patients with remote infection who are only antibody positive [30].

On the other hand, few studies [33, 34] and a recent review by Wong et al. [31] failed to demonstrate a clear-cut association between HCV infection and CAD. A large study executed in the UK by Forde et al. did not show any correlation between HCV and MI [32], though it must be underlined that there was a short period of follow-up of the subjects and moreover chronic HCV infection was poorly proved (the authors stated that they may have included patients who spontaneously cleared the HCV virus) and additionally it was a retrospective observational study

TABLE 2: Characteristics of studies associating HCV infection and CAD.

Author, year, country		Association	Subjects	Comment
Vassalle et al., 2004 [23], Italy	Case control	Positive	491 with CAD (6.3% HCV seropositive)/195 controls (2% HCV seropositive)	First study that suggested HCV seropositivity as one of the risk factors affecting the onset and development of CAD
Butt et al., 2009 [24], USA	Prospective observational cohort study, 5 yr follow-up	Positive	82,083 HCV infected/89,582 HCV uninfected subjects	HCV infection is associated with a higher risk of CAD after adjustment for traditional risk factors
Alyan et al., 2008 [25], Turkey	Case control	Positive	139 HCV seropositive/225 HCV seronegative patients	HCV infection is an independent predictor for increased coronary atherosclerosis (higher Reardon severity score)
Adinolfi et al., 2013 [26], Italy	Retrospective cohort study	Positive	820/78 HCV infected	A secondary analysis showed that HCV patients had higher prevalence of past ischemic heart disease
Oliveira et al., 2013 [27], Brazil	Cross-sectional comparative study	Positive	62 HCV infected/11 controls	HCV infection was related to higher FRS as well as to higher pro-anti-inflammatory cytokine profile
Enger et al., 2014 [28], USA	Retrospective matched cohort study	Positive	22,733 HCV infected/68,198 comparators	Arterial events, especially unstable angina and transient ischemic attack, were more frequently seen in HCV patients
Satapathy et al., 2013 [29], USA	Retrospective, case control study	Positive	63 HCV infected patients/63 controls	The prevalence and severity of CAD were higher in HCV patients who were evaluated for CAD by angiogram compared with matched non-HCV patients
Pothineni et al., 2014 [30], USA	Retrospective cohort study	Positive	8,251 HCV antibody positive/1,434 HCV RNA positive/14,799 HCV negative patients	Increased incidence of CHD events in patients with HCV seropositivity; the incidence is much higher in patients with detectable HCV RNA compared with patients with remote infection who are only antibody positive
Wong et al., 2014 [31], USA	Systematic review	Unclear association		Systematic review
Forde et al., 2012 [32], UK	Retrospective, population cohort, 3.9 yr follow-up	Negative	4809 HCV seropositive/71 668 seronegative	No correlation between HCV and MI but short period of follow-up of the subjects and moreover chronic HCV infection was poorly proved
Arcari et al., 2006 [33], USA	Case control	Negative	292 case subjects/290 controls, overall 52 HCV positive	No association was found between HCV positivity and acute myocardial infarction
Momiyama et al., 2005 [34], Japan	Case control	Negative	524 with CAD (3.4% HCV infected)/106 controls	

where residual confounding by unmeasured confounders is possible. As far as the study of Arcari et al. which also failed to prove a correlation is concerned, not only was the sample size of the HCV infected patients too small but moreover there was no additional confirmatory PCR-RNA executed, a fact that may have further decreased the sample [33].

Even if some studies failed to prove this correlation it is not illogical to conclude that chronic HCV infection appears to be linked with excess cardiovascular risk (Table 2). Based on the abovementioned data HCV infection must be considered as a pre-atherogenetic state of an increased cardiovascular risk.

6. Conclusion

From a clinical point of view HCV infected patients not suitable for treatment or who have failed treatment options must be monitored for carotid atheromatosis, in order to prevent cardiovascular events. There are no formed guidelines but patients with severe liver fibrosis, HCV related steatosis, or of aged >55, who according to research data are of high risk for carotid atheromatosis, are the most eligible candidates for assessment of the existence of carotid atheromatosis.

Based on the bibliography, ultrasonography of the carotid arteries with IMT measurement should be offered to those HCV infected patients, in order to assess carotid atheromatosis as it is the test most commonly used in the studies conducted in this field.

In order to ameliorate HCV infected patients quality of life and to prevent extrahepatic complications, patients with well proven carotid atheromatosis should be offered primary prevention. It must be highlighted that not all patients are amenable of receiving primary prevention with antiplatelet therapy and lipid lowering agents. The risk of bleeding as also the liver related toxicity of lipid lowering agents must be balanced against the risk of a cardiovascular event.

Due to the lack of studies executed in this field, more data are needed in order to further specify which patients should be screened for carotid atheromatosis. The impact of HCV genotype as also that of the virus load should be further assessed.

In the era of new and more efficacious treatments for chronic HCV infection the burden of the nonliver related complications of the HCV infection may become of great significance for the prior HCV infected patient's life expectancy. As a consequence, it is a necessity to investigate if treatment does reverse the nonliver derangements such as carotid atheromatosis observed in HCV infected patients. Recent data have proven the reversion of liver fibrosis after the successful treatment of HCV infection [47, 48] and the diminished risk not only of HCC development but also of liver-related complications [49–51]. Moreover, the eradication of the virus inhibits the inflammatory cascade [52, 53]. It was already stated that patients with higher fibrosis scores showed a greater prevalence of carotid atheromatosis. It is not irrational then to hypothesize that carotid atheromatosis may also reverse the liver fibrosis and the superimposed inflammation tends to return to normal state but for the present time remains a scientific question whose answer must be provided by well-designed large randomized controlled studies.

Conflict of Interests

The authors declare that there is no conflict of interests regarding the publication of this paper.

References

[1] D. Lavanchy, "Evolving epidemiology of hepatitis C virus," *Clinical Microbiology and Infection*, vol. 17, no. 2, pp. 107–115, 2011.

[2] F. Negro, D. Forton, A. Craxì, M. S. Sulkowski, J. J. Feld, and M. P. Manns, "Extrahepatic morbidity and mortality of chronic hepatitis C," *Gastroenterology*, vol. 149, no. 6, pp. 1345–1360, 2015.

[3] P. M. Jacobson Brown and M. G. Neuman, "Immunopathogenesis of hepatitis C viral infection: Th1/Th2 responses and the role of cytokines," *Clinical Biochemistry*, vol. 34, no. 3, pp. 167–171, 2001.

[4] Z. Abbas and T. Moatter, "Interleukin (IL) 1beta and IL-10 gene polymorphism in chronic hepatitis C patients with normal or elevated alanine aminotransferase levels," *The Journal of the Pakistan Medical Association*, vol. 53, no. 2, pp. 59–62, 2003.

[5] L. E. Adinolfi, R. Zampino, L. Restivo et al., "Chronic hepatitis C virus infection and atherosclerosis: clinical impact and mechanisms," *World Journal of Gastroenterology*, vol. 20, no. 13, pp. 3410–3417, 2014.

[6] S. Petta, D. Torres, G. Fazio et al., "Carotid atherosclerosis and chronic hepatitis C: a prospective study of risk associations," *Hepatology*, vol. 55, no. 5, pp. 1317–1323, 2012.

[7] M. Boddi, R. Abbate, B. Chellini et al., "Hepatitis C virus RNA localization in human carotid plaques," *Journal of Clinical Virology*, vol. 47, no. 1, pp. 72–75, 2010.

[8] R. Moucari, T. Asselah, D. Cazals-Hatem et al., "Insulin resistance in chronic hepatitis C: association with genotypes 1 and 4, serum HCV RNA level, and liver fibrosis," *Gastroenterology*, vol. 134, no. 2, pp. 416–423, 2008.

[9] J. M. Hui, A. Sud, G. C. Farrell et al., "Insulin resistance is associated with chronic hepatitis C and virus infection fibrosis progression," *Gastroenterology*, vol. 125, no. 6, pp. 1695–1704, 2003.

[10] C.-S. Wang, S.-T. Wang, W.-J. Yao, T.-T. Chang, and P. Chou, "Hepatitis C virus infection and the development of type 2 diabetes in a community-based longitudinal study," *American Journal of Epidemiology*, vol. 166, no. 2, pp. 196–203, 2007.

[11] M. W. Douglas and J. George, "Molecular mechanisms of insulin resistance in chronic hepatitis C," *World Journal of Gastroenterology*, vol. 15, no. 35, pp. 4356–4364, 2009.

[12] E. Bugianesi, F. Salamone, and F. Negro, "The interaction of metabolic factors with HCV infection: does it matter?" *Journal of Hepatology*, vol. 56, supplement 1, pp. S56–S65, 2012.

[13] G. Pasterkamp, "Methods of accelerated atherosclerosis in diabetic patients," *Heart*, vol. 99, no. 10, pp. 743–749, 2013.

[14] N. Ishizaka, Y. Ishizaka, E. Takahashi et al., "Association between hepatitis C virus seropositivity, carotid-artery plaque, and intima-media thickening," *The Lancet*, vol. 359, no. 9301, pp. 133–135, 2002.

[15] H. Tomiyama, T. Arai, K.-I. Hirose, S. Hori, Y. Yamamoto, and A. Yamashina, "Hepatitis C virus seropositivity, but not hepatitis B virus carrier or seropositivity, associated with increased pulse wave velocity," *Atherosclerosis*, vol. 166, no. 2, pp. 401–403, 2003.

[16] A. Mostafa, M. K. Mohamed, M. Saeed et al., "Hepatitis C infection and clearance: impact on atherosclerosis and cardiometabolic risk factors," *Gut*, vol. 59, no. 8, pp. 1135–1140, 2010.

[17] L. E. Adinolfi, L. Restivo, R. Zampino et al., "Chronic HCV infection is a risk of atherosclerosis. Role of HCV and HCV-related steatosis," *Atherosclerosis*, vol. 221, no. 2, pp. 496–502, 2012.

[18] H. Huang, R. Kang, and Z. Zhao, "Hepatitis C virus infection and risk of stroke: a systematic review and meta-analysis," *PLoS ONE*, vol. 8, no. 11, Article ID e81305, 2013.

[19] M. Masia, S. Padilla, C. Robledano, J. M. Ramos, and F. Gutierrez, "Evaluation of endothelial function and subclinical atherosclerosis in association with hepatitis C virus in HIV-infected patients: a cross-sectional study," *BMC Infectious Diseases*, vol. 11, article 265, 2011.

[20] Y. Caliskan, H. Oflaz, H. Püsüroglu et al., "Hepatitis C virus infection in hemodialysis patients is not associated with insulin resistance, inflammation and atherosclerosis," *Clinical Nephrology*, vol. 71, no. 2, pp. 147–157, 2009.

[21] P. C. Tien, M. F. Schneider, S. R. Cole et al., "Association of hepatitis C virus and HIV infection with subclinical atherosclerosis in the women's interagency HIV study," *AIDS*, vol. 23, no. 13, pp. 1781–1784, 2009.

[22] H. Völzke, C. Schwahn, B. Wolff et al., "Hepatitis B and C virus infection and the risk of atherosclerosis in a general population," *Atherosclerosis*, vol. 174, no. 1, pp. 99–103, 2004.

[23] C. Vassalle, S. Masini, F. Bianchi, and G. C. Zucchelli, "Evidence for association between hepatitis C virus seropositivity and coronary artery disease," *Heart*, vol. 90, no. 5, pp. 565–566, 2004.

[24] A. A. Butt, W. Xiaoqiang, M. Budoff, D. Leaf, L. H. Kuller, and A. C. Justice, "Hepatitis C virus infection and the risk of coronary disease," *Clinical Infectious Diseases*, vol. 49, no. 2, pp. 225–232, 2009.

[25] O. Alyan, F. Kacmaz, O. Ozdemir et al., "Hepatitis C infection is associated with increased coronary artery atherosclerosis defined by modified reardon severity score system," *Circulation Journal*, vol. 72, no. 12, pp. 1960–1965, 2008.

[26] L. E. Adinolfi, L. Restivo, B. Guerrera et al., "Chronic HCV infection is a risk factor of ischemic stroke," *Atherosclerosis*, vol. 231, no. 1, pp. 22–26, 2013.

[27] C. P. M. S. Oliveira, C. R. Kappel, E. R. Siqueira et al., "Effects of hepatitis C virus on cardiovascular risk in infected patients: a comparative study," *International Journal of Cardiology*, vol. 164, no. 2, pp. 221–226, 2013.

[28] C. Enger, U. M. Forssen, D. Bennett, D. Theodore, S. Shantakumar, and A. McAfee, "Thromboembolic events among patients with hepatitis C virus infection and cirrhosis: a matched-cohort study," *Advances in Therapy*, vol. 31, no. 8, pp. 891–903, 2014.

[29] S. K. Satapathy, Y. J. Kim, A. Kataria et al., "Higher prevalence and more severe coronary artery disease in hepatitis C virus-infected patients: a case control study," *Journal of Clinical and Experimental Hepatology*, vol. 3, no. 3, pp. 186–191, 2013.

[30] N. V. K. C. Pothineni, R. Delongchamp, S. Vallurupalli et al., "Impact of hepatitis C seropositivity on the risk of coronary heart disease events," *American Journal of Cardiology*, vol. 114, no. 12, pp. 1841–1845, 2014.

[31] R. J. Wong, F. Kanwal, Z. M. Younossi, and A. Ahmed, "Hepatitis C virus infection and coronary artery disease risk: a systematic review of the literature," *Digestive Diseases and Sciences*, vol. 59, no. 7, pp. 1586–1593, 2014.

[32] K. A. Forde, K. Haynes, A. B. Troxel et al., "Risk of myocardial infarction associated with chronic hepatitis C virus infection: a population-based cohort study," *Journal of Viral Hepatitis*, vol. 19, no. 4, pp. 271–277, 2012.

[33] C. M. Arcari, K. E. Nelson, D. M. Netski, F. J. Nieto, and C. A. Gaydos, "No association between hepatitis C virus seropositivity and acute myocardial infarction," *Clinical Infectious Diseases*, vol. 43, no. 6, pp. e53–e56, 2006.

[34] Y. Momiyama, R. Ohmori, R. Kato, H. Taniguchi, H. Nakamura, and F. Ohsuzu, "Lack of any association between persistent hepatitis B or C virus infection and coronary artery disease," *Atherosclerosis*, vol. 181, no. 1, pp. 211–213, 2005.

[35] A. Lonardo, L. E. Adinolfi, P. Loria, N. Carulli, G. Ruggiero, and C. P. Day, "Steatosis and hepatitis C virus: mechanisms and significance for hepatic and extrahepatic disease," *Gastroenterology*, vol. 126, no. 2, pp. 586–597, 2004.

[36] S. Fargion, M. Porzio, and A. L. Fracanzani, "Nonalcoholic fatty liver disease and vascular disease: state-of-the-art," *World Journal of Gastroenterology*, vol. 20, no. 37, pp. 13306–13324, 2014.

[37] G. Targher, L. Bertolini, R. Padovani, S. Rodella, G. Arcaro, and C. Day, "Differences and similarities in early atherosclerosis between patients with non-alcoholic steatohepatitis and chronic hepatitis B and C," *Journal of Hepatology*, vol. 46, no. 6, pp. 1126–1132, 2007.

[38] Y. Ishizaka, N. Ishizaka, E. Takahashi et al., "Association between hepatitis C virus core protein and carotid atherosclerosis," *Circulation Journal*, vol. 67, no. 1, pp. 26–30, 2003.

[39] L. E. Adinolfi, L. Restivo, and A. Marrone, "The predictive value of steatosis in hepatitis C virus infection," *Expert Review of Gastroenterology and Hepatology*, vol. 7, no. 3, pp. 205–213, 2013.

[40] H. Huang, R. Kang, and Z. Zhao, "Is hepatitis C associated with atherosclerotic burden? A systematic review and meta-analysis," *PLoS ONE*, vol. 9, no. 9, Article ID e106376, 2014.

[41] U. Forssen, A. McAfee, C. Enger, D. Bennett, and S. Shantakumar, "Risk of thromboembolic events (TEs) among patients infected with hepatitis C," *Hepatology*, vol. 50, article 672A, 2009.

[42] C.-C. Liao, T.-C. Su, F.-C. Sung, W.-H. Chou, and T.-L. Chen, "Does hepatitis C virus infection increase risk for stroke? A population-based cohort study," *PLoS ONE*, vol. 7, no. 2, Article ID e31527, 2012.

[43] M.-H. Lee, H.-I. Yang, S.-N. Lu et al., "Chronic hepatitis C virus infection increases mortality from hepatic and extrahepatic diseases: a community-based long-term prospective study," *Journal of Infectious Diseases*, vol. 206, no. 4, pp. 469–477, 2012.

[44] C.-S. Hsu, J.-H. Kao, Y.-C. Chao et al., "Interferon-based therapy reduces risk of stroke in chronic hepatitis C patients: a population-based cohort study in Taiwan," *Alimentary Pharmacology & Therapeutics*, vol. 38, no. 4, pp. 415–423, 2013.

[45] Z. M. Younossi, M. Stepanova, F. Nader, Z. Younossi, and E. Elsheikh, "Associations of chronic hepatitis C with metabolic and cardiac outcomes," *Alimentary Pharmacology and Therapeutics*, vol. 37, no. 6, pp. 647–652, 2013.

[46] U. Vespasiani-Gentilucci, P. Gallo, A. De Vincentis, G. Galati, and A. Picardi, "Hepatitis C virus and metabolic disorder interactions towards liver damage and atherosclerosis," *World Journal of Gastroenterology*, vol. 20, no. 11, pp. 2825–2838, 2014.

[47] E. L. Ellis and D. A. Mann, "Clinical evidence for the regression of liver fibrosis," *Journal of Hepatology*, vol. 56, no. 5, pp. 1171–1180, 2012.

[48] S. L. George, B. R. Bacon, E. M. Brunt, K. L. Mihindukulasuriya, J. Hoffman, and A. M. Di Bisceglie, "Clinical, virologic, histologic, and biochemical outcomes after successful HCV therapy: a 5-year follow-up of 150 patients," *Hepatology*, vol. 49, no. 3, pp. 729–738, 2009.

[49] V. Mallet, H. Gilgenkrantz, J. Serpaggi et al., "Brief communication: the relationship of regression of cirrhosis to outcome in chronic hepatitis C," *Annals of Internal Medicine*, vol. 149, no. 6, pp. 399–403, 2008.

[50] H. Yoshida, R. Tateishi, Y. Arakawa et al., "Benefit of interferon therapy in hepatocellular carcinoma prevention for individual patients with chronic hepatitis C," *Gut*, vol. 53, no. 3, pp. 425–430, 2004.

[51] S. Bruno, T. Stroffolini, M. Colombo et al., "Sustained virological response to interferon-α is associated with improved outcome in HCV-related cirrhosis: a retrospective study," *Hepatology*, vol. 45, no. 3, pp. 579–587, 2007.

[52] K. W. Chew, L. Hua, D. Bhattacharya et al., "The effect of hepatitis C virologic clearance on cardiovascular disease biomarkers in human immunodeficiency virus/hepatitis C virus coinfection," *Open Forum Infectious Diseases*, vol. 1, no. 3, Article ID ofu104, 2014.

[53] M. A. Khattab, M. Eslam, M. Shatat et al., "Changes in adipocytokines and insulin sensitivity during and after antiviral therapy for hepatitis C genotype 4," *Journal of Gastrointestinal and Liver Diseases*, vol. 21, no. 1, pp. 59–65, 2012.

30

Seroprevalence and Predictors of Hepatitis B Virus Infection among Pregnant Women Attending Routine Antenatal Care in Arba Minch Hospital, South Ethiopia

Tsegaye Yohanes,[1] Zerihun Zerdo,[1] and Nega Chufamo[2]

[1]Department of Medical Laboratory Science, Arba Minch University, P.O. Box 21, Arba Minch, Ethiopia
[2]School of Medicine, Department of Obstetrics and Gynecology, Arba Minch University, P.O. Box 21, Arba Minch, Ethiopia

Correspondence should be addressed to Tsegaye Yohanes; tsegaye.yohanes@yahoo.com

Academic Editor: Man-Fung Yuen

Hepatitis B virus (HBV) is a serious cause of liver disease affecting millions of people throughout the world. When HBV is acquired during pregnancy, prenatal transmission can occur to the fetus. Therefore, this study is aimed at estimating seroprevalence and associated factors of HBV infection among pregnant women attending Antenatal Clinic (ANC) of Arba Minch Hospital, Southern Ethiopia. A facility based cross-sectional study was conducted on 232 pregnant women visiting ANC from February to April, 2015. Data regarding sociodemographic and associated factors were gathered using questionnaire. Serum samples were tested for hepatitis B surface antigen (HBsAg) by Enzyme Linked Immunosorbent Assay. Data was analyzed using SPSS version 20. The overall seroprevalence of HBV infection was 4.3% (95% CI: 2.2–6.9%). Multivariate analysis showed that history of abortion (AOR = 7.775; 95% CI: 1.538–39.301) and having multiple sexual partners (AOR = 7.189; 95% CI: 1.039–49.755) were independent predictors of HBsAg seropositivity. In conclusion, the prevalence of HBV infection is intermediate. Therefore, screening HBV infection should be routine part of ANC; health information on having single sexual partner for women of childbearing age and on following aseptic techniques during abortion should be provided to health facilities working on abortion.

1. Introduction

Hepatitis B virus is a potentially life-threatening cause of liver disease in the world. It both causes chronic infection and puts people at high risk of death from cirrhosis and liver cancer [1]. Globally, it is estimated that more than 2 billion people are still living with HBV infection. Over 350 million are believed to be chronically infected with the virus and are thought to be at a high risk of developing chronic hepatitis, cirrhosis, and primary hepatocellular carcinoma. About 1.2 million die annually from chronic hepatitis, cirrhosis, and hepatocellular carcinoma [2, 3].

Viral hepatitis during pregnancy is associated with high risk of maternal complications and high rate of vertical transmission. Fetal and neonatal hepatitis acquired from mother during pregnancy lead to impaired cognitive and physical development in latter life of the children [4]. The risk of vertical transmission depends on the time at which pregnant woman acquired HBV infection and on her statuses of HBsAg and hepatitis B early antigen (HBeAg) [5]. In the absence of immunoprophylaxis 10–20% of women seropositive for HBsAg transmit the virus to their neonates. Vertical transmission rate reaches approximately 90% when women are seropositive for both HBsAg and HBeAg [6].

The prevalence of chronic HBV infection is categorized as high (≥8%), intermediate (2–7%), and low (<2%) [7]. In developed countries, the incidence of hepatitis is around 0.1% whereas in developing countries it ranges from 3 to 20% and even higher in some areas [8]. In Africa and Asia, the prevalence of HBV is > 8% and 2 billion people have markers of current or past infection with HBV [9]. About half of new infections result from vertical transmission during pregnancy, a statistic that is linked to the fact that HBV screening is not part of routine antenatal care in the area [10].

Immunization is estimated to avert between 2 and 3 million deaths globally each year. In Ethiopia, routine immunization was launched in 1980. Ethiopia has successfully introduced hepatitis B vaccine in the form of pentavalent combination vaccine into the routine schedule in 2007. Children under the age of one year are the target group for the vaccination [11]. There is no widely available treatment for chronic hepatitis B and the other sequelae of HBV infection in the country, and if they are available, this treatment cost falls on the individual patient [12, 13].

In Ethiopia, the prevalence of liver disease is high and accounts for 12% of the hospital admissions and 31% of mortality rate [14]. The prevalence of HBV infection among pregnant mothers in Addis Ababa was 7% and 50% had evidence of infection at the age of 20 years [15]. In similar studies conducted among pregnant women in Jimma, the prevalence of HBV infection was 3.7% [16] while it was 4.9% and 8.1% among pregnant women in Dessie and Mekelle, respectively [17, 18].

Several studies around the world recommended that pregnant women should be screened for hepatitis B before delivery, as this offers an opportunity to prevent another generation from being chronically infected by the virus. However, in Ethiopia laboratory diagnosis of HBV infection is not part of routine care in ANC of all health facilities. Moreover, there is little information concerning seroprevalence of HBV infection among pregnant women and the existing data indicate that it differ from region to region as indicated above. Therefore, the present study is aimed to estimate seroprevalence of HBV infection and to identify associated risk factors among pregnant women attending ANC in Arba Minch Hospital, South Ethiopia.

2. Methods

2.1. Study Setting and Periods. The study was conducted from February to April 2015 in Antenatal Clinic of Arba Minch Hospital, which is found in Arba Minch Town. Arba Minch is located 505 kilometers in the southern part of Addis Ababa. The town is located in an altitude of 1200–1300 meters above sea level, with average annual temperature of 29°C. Arba Minch Hospital serves more than 2 million people in South Nations Nationalities and Peoples Regional State in Ethiopia.

2.2. Study Design and Sample Size. A facility based cross-sectional study design was used to enroll 232 pregnant women attending ANC in Arba Minch General Hospital. The sample size was determined using single population proportion formula to estimate the prevalence of HBV infection and *Toxoplasma gondii* infection among pregnant mothers attending ANC in Arba Minch General Hospital (larger project). The sample size is calculated based on the following assumptions: prevalence of HBV [18] and *T. gondii* [19] infections as 8.1% and 83.6%, respectively; 95% level of confidence; 5% margin of error. Finally, 10% of nonresponse rate was added to the calculated sample size. Accordingly the minimum calculated sample size for HBV and *T. gondii* infections was 126 and 232. Finally we took the larger sample size calculated ($n = 232$).

2.3. Study Population and Sampling Technique. The present study was conducted among pregnant women attending ANC in Arba Minch Hospital and mentally fit to respond the questions. Systematic sampling technique was used to recruit pregnant mothers in the study. A total of 696 pregnant women attended the ANC clinic during the past three months before study was initiated. This number was divided for the sample size to get the sample interval (k value) which is 3. Therefore, every 3rd mother attending the clinic was enrolled in the study until the calculated sample size was achieved within three months of data collection.

2.4. Data Collection. A pretested and structured questionnaire was used to collect information on sociodemographic, risky sexual behavior, history of hospital admission, history of abortion, and contact with HBV infected individuals. The data was collected through face-to-face interview by using nurses working in the ANC clinic of the hospital. Following the interview, approximately 2 mL of venous blood was collected from each consenting study participant by experienced phlebotomist. The blood was processed according to the standard operating procedures. Briefly, serum was separated from red blood cells and stored at −20°C prior to assay. Finally, the serum was tested for HBsAg using ELISA test kit (DIALAB) at Arba Minch National blood bank center laboratory, strictly following the manufacturer's instruction.

2.5. Data Analysis. After checking for completeness and consistency of the collected information, the data was entered into computer, cleaned, and analyzed using SPSS version 20.0 software package. Descriptive statistic was performed to describe demographic profile of the study participants. Bivariate and multivariate logistic regressions were used to assess the association between potential risk factors considered and HBV infection. Variables with p value < 0.25 by the bivariate analysis were entered into multivariate model. At multivariate logistic regression, p value < 0.05 was set as statistically significant for all variables.

2.6. Ethical Considerations. Ethical clearance was approved and obtained from Arba Minch University College of Medicine and Health Science Research Ethical Review Committee. Official permission was sought from Arba Minch Zonal Health Bureau and Arba Minch Hospital Administration. Moreover, written informed consent was obtained from all study participants prior to interview and blood collection. Confidentiality of the collected information and laboratory test results was maintained. Individual test results were communicated with the attending physician for further management of the cases.

3. Results

3.1. Sociodemographic Characteristics. A total of 232 pregnant women who had been attending Arba Minch Hospital ANC clinic from February 2015 to April 2015 were included in the study. The mean age of the participants was 25.98 years dominantly within the age range of 25–29 years and standard deviation (SD) was 4.49. Higher proportions of the subjects were married and urban dwellers. Majority of the participants wcrc housewives and had studied up to primary level education (Table 1).

3.2. Seroprevalence and Associated Factors of HBV Infection. Of 232 pregnant women tested for HBsAg, 10 (4.3%) were found to be seropositive, giving the overall prevalence of 4.3% (95% CI: 2.2–6.9%). Pregnant women of age group of 25–29 years comprised 101 (43.5%) of the total study participants, of which 4 (4%) were seropositive. HBsAg seropositivity was observed to be higher in first trimester (5.1%) and the least in the second trimester (4.0%) but this difference was not statistically significant ($p > 0.05$). Moreover, none of the sociodemographic factors was significantly associated with HBsAg seropositivity (Table 2).

Sixteen (6.9%) of pregnant women attending ANC clinic had were reported to have history of blood transfusion and 2 (12.5%) of them were seropositive. However, blood transfusion was not significantly associated ($p = 0.605$) with prevalence of HBV infection among pregnant women attending ANC clinic in Arba Minch General Hospital. About 219 (94.4%) and 54 (23.3%) pregnant women had the practice of ear piercing and abortion, respectively. The respective prevalence of HBV infection among pregnant women who pierced their ear and aborted previously was 3.7% ($n = 8$) and 13% ($n = 7$). The significant association was observed between HBV infection and women who aborted previously ($p = 0.013$). Fifty-seven (24.6%) of the study participants had also a history of hospital admission and only 2 (3.5%) of them were seropositive. Concerning respondents of previous history of contracting Sexually Transmitted Disease (STD), of 10 pregnant women who had the disease, 2 (22.2%) were seropositive. The prevalence of HBsAg among women who suffered from STD was significantly higher than those who did not suffer from STD in univariate logistic regression ($p = 0.020$) but this association was not maintained after controlling the effect of confounding variables in multivariate logistic regression ($p = 0.450$). In this study, 12 (5.2%) pregnant women had previous history of multiple sexual partners and 2 (16.7%) of them were seropositive. Sexual practice with more than one individual significantly ($p = 0.046$) increases the transmission of HBV among pregnant women attending ANC clinic (Table 2).

4. Discussion

The seroprevalence of HBsAg among pregnant women attending ANC clinic in Arba Minch General Hospital was 4.3%. According to WHO classification, the prevalence of HBsAg was intermediate among pregnant mothers [20]. Unless preventive measures through vaccination are taken to tackle the risk of transmission, the unborn babies are at a higher risk of contracting HBV infection. The infection was significantly higher among pregnant mothers who had aborted previously and had history of sex with multiple sexual partners. Health facilities or organizations working on abortion of pregnancies play great role in the transmission of the virus which might be associated with using unsterile equipment during the abortion process. Moreover, unsafe

TABLE 1: Sociodemographic characteristics of pregnant women ($n = 232$) attending Antenatal Clinic at Arba Minch Hospital, 2015.

Sociodemographic characteristics	Count N	Percentage %
Age		
15–19	16	6.9%
20–24	69	29.7%
25–29	101	43.5%
30–34	35	15.1%
35–39	11	4.7%
Residence		
Urban	214	92.2%
Rural	18	7.8%
Marital status		
Married	224	96.6%
Single	6	2.6%
Divorced	0	0.0%
Widowed	2	0.9%
Educational status		
Unable to read and write	47	20.3%
Primary	79	34.1%
Secondary	71	30.6%
Tertiary	35	15.1%
Occupation		
Government	67	28.9%
Housewife	140	60.3%
Others◊	25	10.8%
Trimesters		
First (<14 weeks)	39	16.8%
Second (14–28 weeks)	124	53.4%
Third (>28 weeks)	69	29.7%
Gravidity		
Primigravidae	85	36.6%
Multigravidae	147	63.4%

◊ includes students, merchants, and farmers.

sexual practice with multiple sexual partners is the major way of transmission of HBV among women of the childbearing age.

The prevalence of HBsAg among pregnant women attending ANC clinic in Arba Minch General Hospital was comparable with studies conducted in Bahir Dar (3.8%) [21], Jimma (3.7%) [16] and Dessie (4.9%) [17], Dares Salaam in Tanzania (3.9%) [22], and Lagos Nigeria (4.2%) [23]. In contrast to our study, the highest prevalence was reported from Benin (12.5%) [24], Cameron (10.2%) [25], and Mali (8%) [26]. On the other hand, the lowest prevalence was reported from two studies from India [27, 28]. The difference between the present studies and the above studies might be due to difference in socioeconomy and behavioral and cultural practices of age between 15 and 45 years.

In agreement with other studies [29, 30] HBsAg seropositivity was not significantly different by age. There was no difference in seropositivity of HBsAg between urban and rural pregnant mothers in the present study and it is in

TABLE 2: Bivariate and multivariate analyses of factors associated with HBV infection in the study participants, Arba Minch Hospital, 2015.

Variables	Seroprevalence		COR (95% CI)	p value	AOR (95% CI)	p value
	Positive n (%)	Negative n (%)				
Age						
15–19	1 (6.2%)	15 (93.8%)	1.617 (0.169–15.458)	0.677		
20–24	3 (4.3%)	66 (95.7%)	1.102 (0.239–5.087)	0.901		
25–29	4 (4.0%)	97 (96.0%)	1			
30–34	1 (2.9%)	34 (97.1%)	0.713 (0.077–6.606)	0.766		
35–39	1 (9.1%)	10 (90.9%)	2.425 (0.247–23.850)	0.448		
Residence						
Urban	9 (4.2%)	205 (95.8%)	1			
Rural	1 (5.6%)	17 (94.4%)	1.340 (0.160–11.212)	0.787		
Educational status						
Unable to read and write	2 (4.3%)	45 (95.7%)	0.833 (0.147–4.734)	0.837		
Primary	4 (5.1%)	75 (94.9%)	1			
Secondary	2 (2.8%)	69 (97.2%)	0.543 (0.096–3.061)	0.489		
Tertiary	2 (5.7%)	33 (94.3%)	1.136 (0.198–6.514)	0.886		
Occupation						
Government	2 (3.0%)	65 (97.0%)	0.585 (0.118–2.893)	0.511		
Housewife	7 (5.0%)	133 (95.0%)	1			
Others	1 (4.0%)	24 (96.0%)	0.792 (0.093–6.728)	0.831		
Trimesters						
First (<14 weeks)	2 (5.1%)	37 (94.9%)	1.286 (0.240–6.908)	0.769		
Second (14–28 weeks)	5 (4.0%)	119 (96.0%)	1			
Third (>28 weeks)	3 (4.3%)	66 (95.7%)	1.082 (0.251–4.670)	0.916		
Gravidity						
Primigravidae	4 (4.7%)	81 (95.3%)	1.160 (0.318–4.234)	0.822		
Multigravidae	6 (4.1%)	141 (95.9%)	1			
Blood transfusion						
No	8 (3.7%)	208 (96.3%)	1		1	
Yes	2 (12.5%)	14 (87.5%)	3.714 (0.720–19.172)	0.117$^\oplus$	1.689 (0.232–12.296)	0.605
Ear piercing						
No	2 (15.4%)	11 (84.6%)	1		1	
Yes	8 (3.7%)	211 (96.3%)	0.209 (0.039–1.101)	0.065$^\oplus$	0.220 (0.022–2.161)	0.194
Nose piercing						
No	9 (4.1%)	213 (95.9%)	1			
Yes	1 (10.0%)	9 (90.0%)	2.630 (0.300–23.054)	0.383		
Body tattooing						
No	8 (3.7%)	209 (96.3%)	1		1	
Yes	2 (13.3%)	13 (86.7%)	4.019 (0.774–20.879)	0.098$^\oplus$	5.372 (0.617–46.751)	0.128
Tooth extraction						
No	8 (4.5%)	171 (95.5%)	1			
Yes	2 (3.8%)	51 (96.2%)	0.838 (0.173–4.073)	0.827		
Hospital admission						
No	8 (4.6%)	167 (95.4%)	1			
Yes	2 (3.5%)	55 (96.5%)	0.759 (0.156–3.682)	0.732		
History of surgery						
No	9 (4.2%)	204 (95.8%)	1			
Yes	1 (5.3%)	18 (94.7%)	1.259 (0.151–10.506)	0.831		
Contact with liver disease patient						
No	9 (4.1%)	211 (95.9%)	1			
Yes	1 (8.3%)	11 (91.7%)	2.131 (0.248–18.353)	0.491		

TABLE 2: Continued.

Variables	Seroprevalence		COR (95% CI)	p value	AOR (95% CI)	p value
	Positive n (%)	Negative n (%)				
History of abortion						
No	3 (1.7%)	175 (98.3%)	1		1	
Yes	7 (13.0%)	47 (87.0%)	8.688 (2.163–34.891)	0.002⊕	7.775 (1.538–39.301)	0.013*
History of alcohol drinking						
No	7 (3.6%)	187 (96.4%)	1		1	
Yes	3 (7.9%)	35 (92.1%)	3.562 (0.956–13.276)	0.058⊕	1.674 (0.339–8.257)	0.527
Delivery by TBA						
No	9 (4.2%)	204 (95.8%)	1			
Yes	1 (5.3%)	18 (94.7%)	1.259 (0.151–10.506)	0.831		
History of STD						
No	8 (3.6%)	215 (96.4%)	1		1	
Yes	2 (22.2%)	7 (77.8%)	7.679 (1.371–42.995)	0.020⊕	2.430 (0.243–24.295)	0.450
Multiple sexual partners						
No	8 (3.6%)	212 (96.4%)	1		1	
Yes	2 (16.7%)	10 (83.3%)	5.300 (0.993–28.275)	0.051⊕	7.189 (1.039–49.755)	0.046*

⊕Candidate variable for multivariate analysis at $p < 0.25$; *variable significant by the multivariate analysis at $p < 0.05$. COR: crude odds ratio, AOR: adjusted odds ratio, CI: confidence interval, TBA: traditional birth attendant, and STD: Sexually Transmitted Disease.

agreement with a study reported from Sana'a, Yemen [30]. In contrast to our study, study from Eastern Sudan has shown significantly higher prevalence of HBsAg among pregnant mothers from urban area than the rural counterparts [31]. This difference might be due to the varied numbers of urban and rural study participants as compared to our study.

According to this study, the prevalence of HBsAg was significantly higher among pregnant women who had history of abortion. Unplanned pregnancy is related to unprotected sexual intercourse which results in abortion and also increases the risk of HBV infection if such partners are infected. Also, instrumentation during abortion and related activities may serve as sources of exposure; all these circumstances may increase the likelihood of acquiring the infection. This is in agreement with a study reported from Lagos Nigeria [23] but in contrast with similar study carried out in North West of Iran [32].

In the current study, the rate of HBV infection was significantly higher and about seven times more likely to occur in those who had history of multiple sexual partners as compared to those who did not have multiple sexual partners. The significant association of having multiple sexual partners with HBV infection was also documented by other investigators [18, 33]. In contrast, some studies have shown that there was no significant association between abortion and seropositivity of HBsAg among pregnant mothers [22, 34]. Hepatitis B virus infection is sexually transmitted and the transmission increases with the duration of sexual activity and number of sexual partners [35, 36].

Blood transfusion is one of the means of transmission of bloodborne pathogen like HBV but it was not significantly associated with HBsAg seropositivity in the present study. This finding corroborates the report from Nigeria [37]. However, blood transfusion was significantly associated with transmission of HBV in a number of studies [21, 23, 28]. Improving the quality of laboratory screening of blood for

HBV is one of the components in reducing the risk for transfusion-transmitted HBV. The possible explanation for absence of significant association between HBV infection and blood transfusion might be improved screening of HBV infection from blood donors before transfusion in Ethiopia.

The rate of vertical transmission of HBV infection is influenced by the time of pregnancy at which acute HBV infection occurs in the mothers [5]. In our study, the highest seroprevalence of HBV infection was found in those pregnant women at the first trimester as compared to second and third trimesters. However, there was no statistically significant difference in the prevalence of HBsAg seropositivity in different gestational age of pregnant mothers and it was in agreement with other studies [29, 38].

5. Conclusions

In conclusion, the prevalence of HBsAg among pregnant mothers attending ANC clinic in Arba Minch general hospital was intermediate. Abortion and unsafe sexual practice with more than one sexual partner play significant role in the transmission of the virus from infected person to healthy women of childbearing age. Therefore, screening pregnant women for HBV infection should be part of the routine care in ANC clinic in Arba Minch general hospital and in other similar settings. Health information on safe sex to women of childbearing age should be given to interrupt the transmission. In addition, health facilities working on abortion should strictly follow the aseptic techniques in order to save the life of both aborting mother and subsequent children of that mother.

Conflict of Interests

The authors declare that they do not have any conflict of interests.

Authors' Contribution

Tsegaye Yohanes conceived the study, participated in the study design and data analysis, and drafted the paper. Zerihun Zerdo and Nega Chufamo participated in the study design, data acquisition, and data analysis. All authors contributed to the writing of the paper and approved the final paper.

Acknowledgments

The authors would like to thank staff members of Arba Minch Hospital ANC clinic for their cooperation during data collection. They are grateful to Arba Minch Blood Bank center staff for their cooperation. They are also grateful to the study participants. This research was financially supported by Arba Minch University.

References

[1] World Health Organization, "Hepatitis B," Fact Sheet 204, World Health Organization, Geneva, Switzerland, 2015, http://www.who.int/mediacentre/factsheets/fs204/en/.

[2] M. J. U. Dahoma, A. A. Salim, R. Abdool et al., "HIV and substance abuse: the dual epidemics challenging Zanzibar," African Journal of Drug & Alcohol Studies, vol. 5, no. 2, pp. 131–139, 2006.

[3] R. M. Merrill and B. D. Hunter, "Sero-prevalence of markers for hepatitis B viral infection," International Journal of Infectious Diseases, vol. 15, no. 2, pp. e78–e121, 2011.

[4] A. O. Olaitan and L. G. Zamani, "Prevalence of hepatitis B virus and hepatitis C virus in ante-natal patients in Gwagwalada—Abuja, Nigeria," Report and Opinion, vol. 2, no. 7, pp. 48–50, 2010.

[5] N.-C. Vu Lam, P. B. Gotsch, and R. C. Langan, "Caring for pregnant women and newborns with hepatitis B or C," American Family Physician, vol. 82, no. 10, pp. 1225–1229, 2010.

[6] American College of Obstetricians and Gynecologists, "Viral hepatitis in pregnancy," Obstetrics & Gynecology, vol. 110, no. 4, pp. 941–956, 2007, ACOG Practice Bulletin No. 86.

[7] Centers for Disease Control and Prevention, "Recommendations for identification and public health management of persons with chronic hepatitis B virus infection," Morbidity and Mortality Weekly Report, vol. 57, pp. 1–20, 2008.

[8] S. Shukla, G. Mehta, M. Jais et al., "A prospective study on acute viral hepatitis in pregnancy; seroprevalence, and fetomaternal outcome of 100 cases," Journal of Bioscience and Technology, vol. 2, no. 3, pp. 279–286, 2011.

[9] N. Leung, "Chronic hepatitis B in Asian women of childbearing age," Hepatology International, vol. 3, supplement 1, pp. 24–31, 2009.

[10] MCHP-Maternal and Child Health Integrated Program, "Intersecting Epidemics: An Overview of the Causes of Maternal Death and Infectious Diseases," 2014, http://www.mchip.net/sites/default/files/Maternal%20Health_Infectious%20Diseases%20Overview%20Briefer.pdf.

[11] FMOH, National Expanded Programme on Immunization Comprehensive Multi-Year Plan 2011–2015, Federal Ministry of Health, Addis Ababa, Ethiopia, 2010.

[12] A. Bane, A. Patil, and M. Khatib, "Healthcare cost and access to care for viral hepatitis in Ethiopia," International Journal of Innovation and Applied Studies, vol. 9, no. 4, pp. 1718–1723, 2014.

[13] W. J. Edmunds, A. Dejene, Y. Mekonnen, M. Haile, W. Alemnu, and D. J. Nokes, "The cost of integrating hepatitis B virus vaccine into national immunization programmes: a case study from Addis Ababa," Health Policy and Planning, vol. 15, no. 4, pp. 408–416, 2000.

[14] E. Tsega, "Epidemiology, prevention and treatment of viral hepatitis with emphasis on new developments," Ethiopian Medical Journal, vol. 38, no. 2, pp. 131–141, 2000.

[15] A. Abebe, D. J. Nokes, A. Dejene, F. Enquselassie, T. Messele, and F. T. Cutts, "Seroepidemiology of hepatitis B virus in Addis Ababa, Ethiopia: transmission patterns and vaccine control," Epidemiology and Infection, vol. 131, no. 1, pp. 757–770, 2003.

[16] M. Awole and S. Gebre-Selassie, "Seroprevalence of HBsAg and its risk factors among pregnant women in Jimma, Southwest Ethiopia," Ethiopian Journal of Health Development, vol. 19, no. 1, pp. 45–50, 2005.

[17] M. Seid, B. Gelaw, and A. Assefa, "Sero-prevalence of HBV and HCV infections among pregnant women attending antenatal care clinic at Dessie Referral Hospital, Ethiopia," Advances in Life Sciences and Health, vol. 1, no. 2, pp. 109–120, 2014.

[18] A. Semaw, H. Awet, and M. Yohannes, "Sero-prevalence of hepatitis B surface antigen and associated factors among pregnant mothers attending antenatal care service, Mekelle, Ethiopia: evidence from institutional based quantitative cross-sectional study," World Academy of Science, Engineering and Technology: Medical and Health Sciences, vol. 2, no. 9, 2015.

[19] E. Zemene, D. Yewhalaw, S. Abera, T. Belay, A. Samuel, and A. Zeynudin, "Seroprevalence of Toxoplasma gondii and associated risk factors among pregnant women in Jimma town, Southwestern Ethiopia," BMC Infectious Diseases, vol. 12, article 337, 2012.

[20] WHO/EPI, "Protocol for assessing prevalence of hepatitis B infection in antenatal patients," Tech. Rep. WHO/EPI/GEN/90.6, World Health Organization, Geneva, Switzerland, 1990, http://www.who.int/iris/handle/10665/61617.

[21] Y. Zenebe, W. Mulu, M. Yimer, and B. Abera, "Sero-prevalence and risk factors of hepatitis B virus and human immunodeficiency virus infection among pregnant women in Bahir Dar city, Northwest Ethiopia: a cross sectional study," BMC Infectious Diseases, vol. 14, no. 1, article 118, 2014.

[22] S. Rashid, C. Kilewo, and S. Aboud, "Seroprevalence of hepatitis B virus infection among antenatal clinic attendees at a tertiary hospital in Dar es Salaam, Tanzania," Tanzania Journal of Health Research, vol. 1, no. 16, pp. 1–8, 2014.

[23] O. C. Ezechi, O. O. Kalejaiye, C. V. Gab-Okafor et al., "Seroprevalence and factors associated with Hepatitis B and C co-infection in pregnant Nigerian women living with HIV Infection," The Pan African Medical Journal, vol. 17, article 197, 2014.

[24] O. Ugbebor, M. Aigbirior, F. Osazuwa, E. Enabudoso, and O. Zabayo, "The prevalence of hepatitis B and C viral infections among pregnant women," North American Journal of Medical Sciences, vol. 3, no. 5, pp. 238–241, 2011.

[25] J. J. Noubiap, J. R. Nansseu, S. T. Ndoula, J. J. Bigna, A. M. Jingi, and J. Fokom-Domgue, "Prevalence, infectivity and correlates of hepatitis B virus infection among pregnant women in a rural district of the Far North Region of Cameroon," BMC Public Health, vol. 15, article 454, 2015.

[26] B. MacLean, R. F. Hess, E. Bonvillain et al., "Seroprevalence of hepatitis B surface antigen among pregnant women attending the hospital for women & children in Koutiala, Mali," South African Medical Journal, vol. 102, no. 1, pp. 47–49, 2012.

[27] K. S. Saraswathi and F. Aljabri, "The study of prevalence of Hepatitis B surface antigen during pregnancy in a tertiary care hospital, South India," *Der Pharmacia Lettre*, vol. 4, no. 3, pp. 983–985, 2012.

[28] C. Pande, S. K. Sarin, S. Patra et al., "Prevalence, risk factors and virological profile of chronic hepatitis b virus infection in pregnant women in India," *Journal of Medical Virology*, vol. 83, no. 6, pp. 962–967, 2011.

[29] O. M. Kolawole, A. A. Wahab, D. A. Adekanle, T. Sibanda, and A. I. Okoh, "Seroprevalence of hepatitis B surface antigenemia and its effects on hematological parameters in pregnant women in Osogbo, Nigeria," *Virology Journal*, vol. 9, article 317, 2012.

[30] E. A. Murad, S. M. Babiker, G. I. Gasim, D. A. Rayis, and I. Adam, "Epidemiology of hepatitis B and hepatitis C virus infections in pregnant women in Sana'a, Yemen," *BMC Pregnancy and Childbirth*, vol. 13, article 127, 2013.

[31] T. M. Abdallah, M. H. Mohamed, and A. A. Ali, "Seroprevalence and epidemiological factors of hepatitis B virus (HBV) infection in Eastern Sudan," *International Journal of Medicine and Medical Sciences*, vol. 3, no. 7, pp. 239–241, 2011.

[32] M. Motazakker, M. S. Nagadeh, F. Khalili et al., "Hepatitis B virus infection among pregnant women attending health care centers of Urmia," *Journal of Guilan University of Medical Sciences*, vol. 23, no. 89, pp. 45–50, 2014.

[33] C. E. Onwuakor, V. C. Eze, I. U. Nwankwo, and J. O. Iwu, "Seroprevalence of hepatitis B surface antigen (HBsAg) amongst pregnant women attending antenatal clinic at the Federal Medical Centre Umuahia, Abia State, Nigeria," *American Journal of Public Health Research*, vol. 2, no. 6, pp. 255–259, 2014.

[34] A. C. Eke, U. A. Eke, C. I. Okafor, I. U. Ezebialu, and C. Ogbuagu, "Prevalence, correlates and pattern of hepatitis B surface antigen in a low resource setting," *Virology Journal*, vol. 8, article 12, 2011.

[35] V. U. Usanga, L. Abia-Bassey, P. C. Inyang-Etoh, S. M. Udoh, F. Ani, and E. Archibong, "Prevalence of sexually transmitted diseases in pregnant and non-pregnant women in Calabar, cross river state, Nigeria," *The Internet Journal of Gynecology and Obstetrics*, vol. 14, no. 2, pp. 1–7, 2009.

[36] G. Fisseha, "Young women sexual behaviour and self-reported sexually transmitted diseases in northern ethiopia: a cross sectional study," *European Journal of Preventive Medicine*, vol. 3, no. 3, pp. 55–62, 2015.

[37] J. O. Alegbeleye, T. K. Nyengidik, and J. I. Ikimal, "Maternal and neonatal seroprevalence of hepatitis B surface antigen in a hospital based population in South-South, Nigeria," *International Journal of Medicine and Medical Sciences*, vol. 5, no. 5, pp. 241–246, 2013.

[38] G. R. Pennap, E. T. Osanga, and A. Ubam, "Seroprevalence of hepatitis B surface antigen among pregnant women attending antenatal clinic in federal medical center Keffi, Nigeria," *Research Journal of Medical Sciences*, vol. 5, no. 2, pp. 80–82, 2011.

31

Prevalence of Hepatitis C Virus Genotypes in District Bannu, Khyber Pakhtunkhwa, Pakistan

Shamim Saleha,[1] Anwar Kamal,[1] Farman Ullah,[2] Nasar Khan,[1] Asif Mahmood,[1] and Sanaullah Khan[3]

[1] Department of Microbiology, Kohat University of Science and Technology (KUST), Khyber Pakhtunkhwa, Kohat 26000, Pakistan
[2] Department of Biotechnology and Genetic Engineering, Kohat University of Science and Technology (KUST), Khyber Pakhtunkhwa, Kohat 26000, Pakistan
[3] Department of Zoology, Kohat University of Science and Technology (KUST), Khyber Pakhtunkhwa, Kohat 26000, Pakistan

Correspondence should be addressed to Shamim Saleha; shamimsaleha@yahoo.com

Academic Editor: Annagiulia Gramenzi

Determination of an individual's hepatitis C virus (HCV) genotypes prior to antiviral therapy has become increasingly important for the clinical management and prognosis of HCV infection. Therefore, this study was conducted to investigate the prevalence of HCV genotypes in HCV infected patients of district Bannu in Khyber Pakhtunkhwa region of Pakistan. Serum samples of 117 seropositive patients were screened for HCV-RNA by using reverse transcriptase-nested polymerase chain reaction (RT-nested PCR) and then PCR positive samples were subjected to HCV genotyping. Out of 117 seropositive samples, 110 samples were found positive by PCR analysis. Genotype 3a was the most prevalent one detected in 38% of patients, followed by genotype 3b in 21% of patients, and then genotype 2a in 12% of patients. However 21% of HCV-PCR positive samples could not be genotyped by method used in this study. Genotype 3a was the most prevalent genotype in patients of all age groups and its prevalence was found high among patients with increasing age (>34 years). Moreover, genotypes 3a and 3b were found to be the most prevalent genotypes in patients with history of shaving by barbers, receiving multiple injections, and dental procedures. In conclusion there is need of further investigation of genotypes of HCV by using more sensitive assays and considering large sample size in district Bannu.

1. Introduction

HCV infection is among life threatening public health problems worldwide, with over 170–200 million infected people [1] including about 17 million from Pakistan [2]. HCV is considered the leading cause of liver cirrhosis and hepatocellular carcinoma. It has been estimated to cause approximately 27% of cirrhosis and 25% of hepatocellular carcinoma cases worldwide [3]. Each year about 350,000 people die due to HCV [4].

HCV is a small enveloped, positive sense single stranded RNA virus and has been classified as a separate genus *hepacivirus* in the Flaviviridae family [5]. The HCV genome is approximately 9.6 kb, encoding a polyprotein of about 3010 amino acids and is flanked by short untranslated regions (UTRs) regions at the $5'$ and $3'$ terminus [6]. This polyprotein is posttranslationally processed by viral and cellular proteins to generate the structural proteins (C, E1, E2, and p7) and nonstructural proteins (NS2, NS3, NS4A, NS4B, NS5A, and NS5B), [7].

HCV shows high degree of genetic heterogeneity; consequently six major genotypes and multiple subtypes of HCV have been identified so far in world [8]. Distribution of HCV genotypes and subtypes in different regions of the world is variable. The common subtypes found in North and South America, Europe, Russia, China, Japan, Australia, and New Zealand are 1a, 1b, 2a, 2c, and 3a [3]. Genotype 4 is predominant in Egypt, North Africa, Central Africa, and Middle East [9]. Genotype 5 in South Africa [10] and genotype 6 in Southeast Asia [11] have been identified. Genotype 3 is the most prevalent genotype in India, Bangladesh, Pakistan, and Nepal [12–15]. Subtypes of genotypes 1, 2, 3,

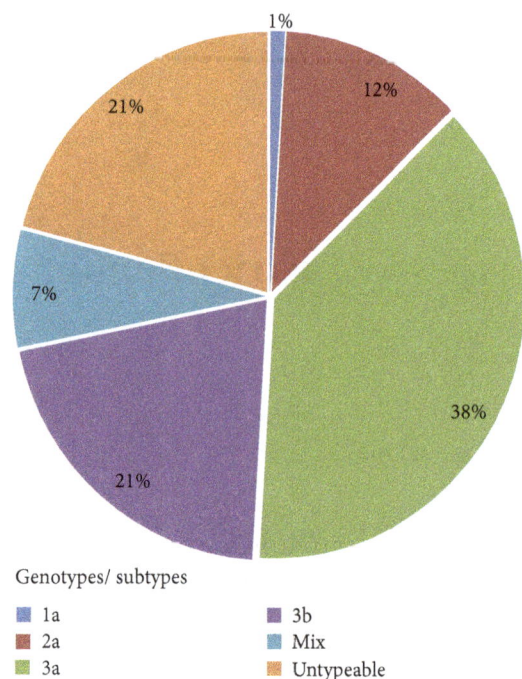

Figure 1: Prevalence of HCV genotypes in district Bannu.

and 6 have been found prevalent in Thailand [16], Vietnam, Indonesia, and Burma [1] respectively. Genotype 1b is the most prevalent genotype in China; however genotype 2 has also been reported from some regions of China [1].

In Pakistan, the prevalence of HCV infection has been estimated to be 8% and is increasing gradually due to deficiency in basic health care recourses and lack of the general public awareness about safety measures [8]. Some studies have been conducted on prevalence of HCV genotypes in Khyber Pukhtunkhwa region of Pakistan [17–20]. However, little has been reported on prevalence of HCV genotypes in district Bannu in Khyber Pukhtunkhwa region of Pakistan. Therefore, this study was conducted to find out baseline information on the prevalence of HCV genotypes in district Bannu. Accurate HCV genotyping can be used in better understanding of HCV infection, for creating awareness in the general public and subsequently for implementation of preventive and therapeutic strategies.

2. Materials and Methods

2.1. Ethical Consideration. All the procedures used in this study were approved by the Ethics Committees of Department of Microbiology, Kohat University of Science and Technology. The informed consent was signed by the patients for participating in the study.

2.2. Inclusion Criteria. An inclusion criterion for patients was to be seropositive for anti-HCV by third generation enzyme linked immunosorbent assay (ELISA). The information regarding age, gender, and possible routes of transmission was obtained from each participating patient. Total 117

blood samples were collected from patients attending district hospital Bannu and Khalifa hospital Bannu.

2.3. DNA Extraction. Serum was separated from each blood sample at 3000 ×g for 5 min and then labeled and stored deep-frozen at −20°C. RNA was extracted using RNA extraction Kit (Ultrascript, Anagen Technologies Inc., USA) as per manufacturer's instructions.

2.4. Genotyping. Extracted RNA was reverse transcribed into complementary DNA (cDNA). For this $10\,\mu$L of HCV extracted RNA was incubated at 37°C for 50 min along with primer specific for core region and 200 U of Moloney Murine Leukemia Virus reverse transcriptase (M-MLV RTase) (Fermentas USA), 5X first strand buffer (MMulv buffer) dNTPs and ddH_2O. In the first round of Nested PCR, cDNA was amplified by using sense and antisense primers for qualitative analysis. The PCR program was as follows: initial denaturation was at 94°C for 5 min, followed by 45 cycles, each of 45 sec denaturation at 92°C, 45 sec annealing at 55°C, and 1 min extension at 72°C, with final extension at 72°C for 10 min. In second round of Nested PCR, genotype-specific PCR was performed by using allele specific primers for core region reported by Ohno et al. [21] at same PCR program that was adopted for first round Nested PCR. The final PCR products obtained after each round of Nested PCR were subjected to electrophoresis and separated on 2% agarose gel. After staining with ethidium bromide, the gel was visualized under UV-transilluminator. To determine genotype specific bands, the banding pattern was photographed in Gel Documentation System (ENDURO GDS).

3. Results

Out of 117 anti-HCV positive sera by ELISA, 110 samples were found positive by PCR analysis, with greater representation of males 81 (73.6%) as compared to females 29 (26.4%) as shown in Table 1. Genotyping of 110 HCV-PCR positive samples determined four different genotypes including 1a, 2a, 3a, and 3b (Figure 1). However, HCV genotypes 1b, 2b, 4, 5, and 6 were not detected among patients studied. Genotype 3a was the most prevalent one detected in 42 (38%) patients, followed by genotype 3b in 23 (21%) patients and then genotype 2a in 13 (12%) patients. Genotype 1a was the least prevalent and was detected in only in 1 (1%) patient while in 8 (7%) patients mixed genotypes of HCV were detected. Moreover, 23 (21%) HCV-PCR positive samples could not be genotyped by using the method as described previously [21].

The studied patients were categorized in three different age groups and then prevalence of age associated HCV genotypes was determined (Table 1). Genotype 3a was most prevalent genotype in all age groups patients and its prevalence was found high among patients with increasing age (>34 years). High prevalence of genotype 3b was observed in age groups 35–54 and 55–74 years. Similarly, high prevalence of genotype 2a was also observed in age group 55–74 years. Moreover, genotype 1a was found in only one patient, who had age of 23 years and subsequently belonged to age group 15–34 years.

TABLE 1: Prevalence of HCV genotypes among the patients of different age groups.

Age groups	Genotypes						Total	% age
	1a	2a	3a	3b	Mix	Untypeable		
15–34	1	1	7	5	4	3	21	19.1
35–54	0	3	17	9	3	12	44	40
55–74	0	9	18	9	1	8	45	40.9
Total	1	13	42	23	8	23	110	100

TABLE 2: Possible routes of transmission of HCV genotypes among the patients.

Possible routes of transmission	Genotypes						Total	% age
	1a	2a	3a	3b	Mix	Untypeable		
Multiple therapeutic injections received	0	3	19	10	1	6	39	35.4
Dental procedures	1	5	6	5	2	3	22	20
Blood transfusion	0	1	2	0	1	3	7	6.4
Shaving by barber	0	4	15	7	4	10	40	36.4
Tattooing	0	0	0	1	0	1	2	1.8
Total	1	13	42	23	8	23	110	100

In our study, those patients who had history of visit to barber shop, intravenous drug addiction, and dental procedures were recorded major risk factors responsible for HCV transmission in district Bannu as shown in Table 2. Patients with history of visit to barber shop and receiving multiple therapeutic injections accounted for 40 (36.4%) and 39 (35.4%), respectively, followed by patients with history of dental procedures 22 (20%). History of blood transfusion and tattooing was recorded in 7 (6.4%) and 2 (1.8%) patients, respectively.

Genotype 3a and genotype 3b were found to be the most prevalent genotypes in patients with history of shaving by barbers, receiving multiple injections, and dental procedures. However, genotype 2a and genotype 1a were more commonly found in patients with history of dental procedures (Table 2).

4. Discussion

The molecular epidemiological studies have reported that significant regional differences appear to be present in the frequency distribution of HCV genotypes. Moreover, determination of HCV genotypes in geographically diverse regions facilitates therapeutic decisions and preventive strategies [22]. It has been reported that there are variations in disease outcome and response to antiviral therapy of HCV genotypes [23]. However, in Pakistan treatment of HCV infected patients is based on qualitative or quantitative viral detection and genotypes are not determined prior to treatment. Therefore variable response rates of HCV infected patients to antiviral therapy cannot be detected. The present study was conducted to determine baseline data on the prevalence of HCV genotypes in a district in Khyber Pakhtunkhwa region of Pakistan. The baseline information will help in better understanding of HCV infection, awareness in the general public and subsequent control strategies.

The distribution of HCV genotypes was found variable among studied patients. The genotype 3a was found to be the most prevalent genotype followed by 3b and 2a and genotype 1a was found to be less prevalent (Figure 1). Results of the present study are in conformity with results of previous studies reported from different regions of the Khyber Pakhtunkhwa in Pakistan [20–25]. Previous studies conducted in India, Bangladesh, and Nepal also reported that the genotype 3 is the most prevalent genotype [12–14]. In this study the assay used could not determine HCV genotypes among a considerable number of HCV patients (23%). Untypeable genotypes have previously been reported in another study conducted in Pakistan [25]. However, there is a need to use more reliable and sensitive assay for genotyping of HCV in untypeable samples.

The distribution of HCV genotypes may be variable among the patients of different age groups. Studies have reported that genotypes 1b and 2 were more prevalent in older patients, whereas genotype 1a was observed more frequently in the younger population [26, 27]. Another study reported that in France genotype 5 was frequently detected in patients aged more than 50 years [28]. In Iran genotype 3a was the most frequently detected in patients less than 40 years [29]. In this study, we observed the distribution of HCV genotypes among different age groups. The prevalence of genotypes 2a and 3a was found increasing with increasing age of patients. Genotype 3b was found more prevalent in age groups more than 35 years. Moreover, genotype 1a was least prevalent genotype detected in a patient of a younger age group less than 34 years. The findings of this study are important for therapeutic management of HCV infected patients.

Various studies have suggested that HCV genotypes are associated with different routes of transmission. Analysis of possible routes in transmission of HCV genotypes in district Bannu is shown in Table 2. The HCV genotypes reported in present study were isolated from participating patients with known route of transmission. In our study genotypes 3a and 3b were more frequently observed in patients with previous history of shaving by barbers followed by multiple injections received and dental procedures. Whereas genotypes 1a and 2a were more commonly observed in patients who had history of dental procedures. HCV genotype 2a was also common in patients with previous history of visit to barbers and receiving multiple injections.

The possible routes of transmission of HCV genotypes have also been reported in other studies. The high prevalence of HCV genotype 3 is attributed to intravenous drug addicts in the United States and Europe [30]. Moreover present study and other studies from Pakistan have also reported increased prevalence of genotype 3 in those patients who had received multiple therapeutic unsafe and unnecessary injections by untrained health practitioners particularly in rural areas. These untrained health practitioners usually use nondisposable syringe or used syringe and needles for more than one patient at the public health-care centers [24–32]. However, high prevalence of genotypes 3a, 3b, and 2a among patients of district Bannu with history of shaving by barbers and dental procedures has not been reported in the United States and Europe. In present study we observed in district Bannu that uneducated barbers common practice is to reuse of unsterilized razors and scissors for multiple customers. Similarly untrained health practitioners at dental clinics are usually in practice of using used and unsterilized dental equipment for multiple individuals. Consequently, these barbers and health practitioners are promoting the risk of transmission of HCV infection from one person to another in this district. In a patient with genotype 1a the possible route of transmission observed in the present study was dental procedure. This is consistent with result of a previous study from Pakistan where most of patients with genotype 1a had a history of dental procedures [24].

5. Conclusion

Our study provides baseline information on the prevalence of HCV genotypes in district Bannu in Khyber Pukhtunkhwa region of Pakistan. The most prevalent HCV genotype was 3a isolated from patients in district Bannu, followed by genotypes 3b and 2a. The frequency distribution of these genotypes was found variable according to the age groups of the patients studied. The possible routes of transmission for these genotypes observed were shaving by barbers, receiving multiple injections, and dental procedures. Further studies are needed to investigate HCV genotypes in district Bannu by using more sensitive assays and considering large population size.

Conflict of Interests

There is no conflict of interests regarding the publication of this paper.

Acknowledgments

This study was financially supported by Department of Microbiology, Kohat University of Science and Technology, Khyber Pukhtunkhwa, Pakistan. The authors acknowledge all patients who participated in the study.

References

[1] S. Butt, M. Idrees, H. Akbar et al., "The changing epidemiology pattern and frequency distribution of hepatitis C virus in Pakistan," *Infection, Genetics and Evolution*, vol. 10, no. 5, pp. 595–600, 2010.

[2] M. Idrees, S. Rafique, I. Rehman et al., "Hepatitis C virus genotype 3a infection and hepatocellular carcinoma: Pakistan experience," *World Journal of Gastroenterology*, vol. 15, no. 40, pp. 5080–5085, 2009.

[3] M. J. Alter, "Epidemiology of hepatitis C virus infection," *World Journal of Gastroenterology*, vol. 13, no. 17, pp. 2436–2441, 2007.

[4] A. Hatzakis, S. Wait, J. Bruix et al., "The state of hepatitis B and C in Europe: report from the hepatitis B and C summit conference," *Journal of Viral Hepatitis*, vol. 18, no. 1, pp. 1–16, 2011.

[5] C. H. Hagedorn, E. H. van Beers, and C. de Staercke, "Hepatitis C virus RNA-dependent RNA polymerase (NS5B polymerase)," *Current Topics in Microbiology and Immunology*, vol. 242, p. 327, 2000.

[6] N. Kato, "Molecular virology of hepatitis C virus," *Acta Medica Okayama*, vol. 55, no. 3, pp. 133–159, 2001.

[7] M. Liew, M. Erali, S. Page, D. Hillyard, and C. Wittwer, "Hepatitis C genotyping by denaturing high-performance liquid chromatography," *Journal of Clinical Microbiology*, vol. 42, no. 1, pp. 158–163, 2004.

[8] M. Idrees, A. Lal, M. Naseem, and M. Khalid, "High prevalence of hepatitis C virus infection in the largest province of Pakistan," *Journal of Digestive Diseases*, vol. 9, no. 2, pp. 95–103, 2008.

[9] A. R. N. Zekri, A. A. Bahnassy, H. M. A. El-Din, and H. M. Salama, "Consensus siRNA for inhibition of HCV genotype-4 replication," *Virology Journal*, vol. 6, article 13, 2009.

[10] R. W. Chamberlain, N. Adams, A. A. Saeed, P. Simmonds, and R. M. Elliott, "Complete nucleotide sequence of a type 4 hepatitis C virus variant, the predominant genotype in the Middle East," *Journal of General Virology*, vol. 78, no. 6, pp. 1341–1347, 1997.

[11] A. S. Abdulkarim, N. N. Zein, J. J. Germer et al., "Hepatitis C virus genotypes and hepatitis G virus in hemodialysis patients from Syria: identification of two novel hepatitis C virus subtypes," *The American Journal of Tropical Medicine and Hygiene*, vol. 59, no. 4, pp. 571–576, 1998.

[12] N. N. Zein, "Clinical significance of hepatitis C virus genotypes," *Clinical Microbiology Reviews*, vol. 13, no. 2, pp. 223–235, 2000.

[13] D. Amarapurkar, M. Dhorda, A. Kirpalani, A. Amarapurkar, and S. Kankonkar, "Prevalence of hepatitis C genotypes in Indian patients and their clinical significance," *Journal of Association of Physicians of India*, vol. 49, pp. 983–985, 2001.

[14] S. Singh, V. Malhotra, and S. K. Sarin, "Distribution of hepatitis C virus genotypes in patients with chronic hepatitis C infection in India," *Indian Journal of Medical Research*, vol. 119, no. 4, pp. 145–148, 2004.

[15] I. Rehman, M. Idrees, M. Ali et al., "Hepatitis C virus genotype 3a with phylogenetically distinct origin is circulating in Pakistan," *Genetic Vaccines and Therapy*, vol. 9, article 2, 2011.

[16] H. Okamoto, Y. Sugiyama, S. Okada et al., "Typing hepatitis C virus by polymerase chain reaction with type-specific primers: Application to clinical surveys and tracing infectious sources," *Journal of General Virology*, vol. 73, no. 3, pp. 673–679, 1992.

[17] A. Ali, H. Ahmed, and M. Idrees, "Molecular epidemiology of Hepatitis C virus genotypes in Khyber Pakhtoonkhaw of Pakistan," *Virology Journal*, vol. 7, pp. 203–210, 2010.

[18] I. M. Idrees, H. Ahmed, M. Ali, L. Ali, and A. Ahmed, "Hepatitis C virus genotypes circulating in district Swat of Khyber Pakhtoonkhaw, Pakistan," *Virology Journal*, vol. 8, article 16, 2011.

[19] A. Z. Safi, Y. Waheed, J. Sadat, S. Salahuddin, U. Saeed, and M. Ashraf, "Molecular study of HCV detection, genotypes and their routes of transmission in North West Frontier Province, Pakistan," *Asian Pacific Journal of Tropical Biomedicine*, vol. 2, no. 7, pp. 532–536, 2012.

[20] S. Q. Afridi, M. N. Zahid, M. Z. Shabbir et al., "Prevalence of HCV genotypes in district Mardan," *Virology Journal*, vol. 10, article 90, 2013.

[21] T. Ohno, M. Mizokami, M. G. Saleh et al., "Usefulness and limitation of phylogenetic analysis for hepatitis C virus core region: Application to isolates from Egyptian and Yemeni patients," *Archives of Virology*, vol. 141, no. 6, pp. 1101–1113, 1996.

[22] G. L. Davis, R. Esteban-Mur, V. Rustgi et al., "Interferon alfa-2b alone or in combination with ribavirin for the treatment of relapse of chronic hepatitis C," *The New England Journal of Medicine*, vol. 339, no. 21, pp. 1493–1499, 1998.

[23] G. Dusheiko, J. Main, H. Thomas et al., "Ribavirin treatment for patients with chronic hepatitis C: results of a placebo-controlled study," *Journal of Hepatology*, vol. 25, no. 5, pp. 591–598, 1996.

[24] M. Idrees and S. Riazuddin, "Frequency distribution of hepatitis C virus genotypes in different geographical regions of Pakistan and their possible routes of transmission," *BMC Infectious Diseases*, vol. 8, article 69, 2008.

[25] S. Ali, I. Ali, S. Azam, and B. Ahmad, "Frequency distribution of HCV genotypes among chronic hepatitis C patients ofkhyber pakhtunkhwa," *Virology Journal*, vol. 8, article 193, 2011.

[26] M. Cenci, M. Massi, M. Alderisio, G. De Soccio, and O. Recchia, "Prevalence of hepatitis C virus (HCV) genotypes and increase of type 4 in Central Italy: an update and report of a new method of HCV genotyping," *Anticancer Research*, vol. 27, no. 2, pp. 1219–1222, 2007.

[27] A. Petruzziello, N. Coppola, A. M. Diodato et al., "Age and gender distribution of hepatitis C virus genotypes in the metropolitan area of Naples," *Intervirology*, vol. 56, no. 3, pp. 206–212, 2013.

[28] C. Henquell, C. Cartau, A. Abergel et al., "High prevalence of hepatitis C virus type 5 in central France evidenced by a prospective study from 1996 to 2002," *Journal of Clinical Microbiology*, vol. 42, no. 7, pp. 3030–3035, 2004.

[29] F. J. Sefidi, H. Keyvani, S. H. Monavari, S. M. Alavian, S. Fakhim, and F. Bokharaei-Salim, "Distribution of hepatitis C virus genotypes in Iranian chronic infected patients," *Hepatitis Monthly*, vol. 13, no. 1, pp. e7991–e7998, 2013.

[30] M. Martinot-Peignoux, F. Roudot-Thoraval, I. Mendel et al., "Hepatitis C virus genotypes in France: relationship with epidemiology, pathogenicity and response to interferon therapy," *Journal of Viral Hepatitis*, vol. 6, no. 6, pp. 435–443, 1999.

[31] Y. Waheed, T. Shafi, S. Z. Safi, and I. Qadri, "Hepatitis C virus in Pakistan: a systematic review of prevalence, genotypes and risk factors," *World Journal of Gastroenterology*, vol. 15, no. 45, pp. 5647–5653, 2009.

[32] W. Jafri, N. Jafri, J. Yakoob et al., "Hepatitis B and C: Prevalence and risk factors associated with seropositivity among children in Karachi, Pakistan," *BMC Infectious Diseases*, vol. 6, article 101, 2006.

Prevalence and Seroincidence of Hepatitis B and Hepatitis C Infection in High Risk People Who Inject Drugs in China and Thailand

J. Brooks Jackson,[1] Liu Wei,[2] Fu Liping,[3] Apinun Aramrattana,[4] David D. Celentano,[5] Louise Walshe,[5] Yi Xing,[1] Paul Richardson,[1] Ma Jun,[3] Geetha Beauchamp,[6] Deborah Donnell,[6] Yuhua Ruan,[7] Liying Ma,[7] David Metzger,[8] and Yiming Shao[7]

[1] *Department of Pathology, Johns Hopkins University, Baltimore, MD 21287, USA*
[2] *Guangxi Center for Disease Control and Prevention, Nanning 530028, China*
[3] *Xinjiang Center for Disease Control and Prevention, Urumqi 83001, China*
[4] *Research Institute for Health Sciences, Chiang Mai University, Chiang Mai 50200, Thailand*
[5] *Department of Epidemiology, Johns Hopkins Bloomberg School of Public Health, Baltimore, MD 21205, USA*
[6] *Fred Hutchinson Cancer Research Center, Seattle, WA 98109, USA*
[7] *State Key Laboratory for Infectious Disease Prevention and Control, National Center for AIDS/STD Control and Prevention, Chinese Center for Disease Control and Prevention, Collaborative Innovation Center for Diagnosis and Treatment of Infectious Diseases, Beijing 102206, China*
[8] *University of Pennsylvania, Philadelphia, PA 19104, USA*

Correspondence should be addressed to J. Brooks Jackson; bjackso@jhmi.edu

Academic Editor: Annarosa Floreani

We determined the prevalence and incidence of HBV and HCV infection in people who inject drugs (PWIDs) at high risk for HIV in China and Thailand and determined the association of HBV and HCV incidence with urine opiate test results and with short-term versus long-term buprenorphine-naloxone (B-N) treatment use in a randomized clinical trial (HPTN 058). 13.8% of 1049 PWIDs in China and 13.9% of 201 PWIDs in Thailand were HBsAg positive at baseline. Among HBsAg negative participants, the HBsAg incidence rate was 2.7/100 person years in China and 0/100 person years in Thailand. 81.9% of 1049 PWIDs in China and 59.7% of 201 in Thailand were HCV antibody positive at baseline. The HCV confirmed seroincidence rate among HCV antibody negative PWIDs was 22/100 person years in China and 4.6/100 person years in Thailand. Incident HBsAg was not significantly different in the short-term versus long-term B-N arm in China or Thailand. Participants with positive opiate results in at least 75% of their urines during the time period were at increased risk of incident HBsAg (HR = 5.22; 95% CI, 1.08 to 25.22; $P = 0.04$) in China, but not incident HCV conversion in China or Thailand.

1. Background and Objectives

Transmission of hepatitis C virus (HCV), hepatitis B virus (HBV), and human immunodeficiency virus (HIV-1) has been causally associated with the injection of drugs of abuse by people who inject drugs (PWIDs) due to sharing of needles and injection equipment contaminated by infected blood. HCV and HBV seroprevalence rates among PWIDs have varied considerably depending on the geographic region and time period of the PWID populations tested.

HCV seroprevalence rates among most PWIDs populations worldwide have been reported to be often higher than 50% with widely varying rates of 3–95% for HIV/HCV coinfection [1]. In China, HCV prevalence rates among the general population have been estimated to be approximately 3.2% [2] with HCV prevalence rates of between 34% and

99% among PWID populations [2]. In Thailand, an HCV prevalence rate of 70% among PWIDs has been reported [3]. HCV coinfection complicates HIV treatment options and has been reported to increase the probability of progression to a new AIDS-defining clinical event or to death and is associated with a smaller CD4-cell recovery increase in response to HIV therapy [4].

Hepatitis B surface antigen (HBsAg) prevalence rates in China have been relatively high with an estimated 7.18% rate in the general population in 2006 [5]. In Thailand, the HBsAg prevalence rate among HIV infected Thai patients has been reported to be 8.7% [6]. Like HCV coinfection, HBV coinfection is associated with increased risk of HIV progression and death [7] and also complicates HIV treatment options as several antiretroviral drugs have activity against both HIV and HBV.

Between 2007 and 2011 we conducted an open-label randomized clinical trial of buprenorphine-naloxone (B-N) treatment of opiate dependence as a strategy for prevention of HIV in opiate dependent injectors in Chiang Mai, Thailand; Heng County and Nanning city, Guangxi, China; and Urumqi, Xinjiang, China. All PWIDs enrolled were HIV negative adults and had injected opiates at least 12 times in the last 28 days and had a positive urine test for opiates. Approximately 44%, 14%, 7%, and 53% of PWIDs in the study reported sharing needles or works during the 6 months prior to enrollment in Heng County, Nanning, Urumqi, and Chiang Mai, respectively.

Participants were randomized in a 1:1 ratio to a short-term arm consisting of detoxification using B-N combined with 12 months of behavioral and drug and risk counseling (BDRC) or to a long-term arm consisting of taking B-N three times per week and BDRC for 12 months. Rates of HIV-infection (determined at screening, and at 26 and 52 weeks of follow-up) and death were compared one year after completing the interventions. During the first year, 39% of monthly visits in the long-term arm versus 69% in the short-term arm had positive urine drug screens (OR = 0.3, $P < 0.001$) [8]. The objective of this substudy was to determine the seroprevalence and incidence of HCV antibody and HBsAg among these initially HIV negative PWIDs and to determine the association of HBV and HCV incidence with urine opiate test results and with short-term versus long-term B-N treatment use at follow-up.

At the time of enrolment, participants in China gave consent for storage of specimens for future testing, whereas participants in Thailand were not asked and only protocol testing was performed. Approvals for HCV and HBV testing of these specimens among these initially HIV negative PWIDs were obtained from the local Institutional Review Boards in China, Thailand, and Johns Hopkins University in the United States. In Thailand, participants found to be negative for HBsAg and HBsAb at baseline were offered HBV vaccination, whereas in China, all participants found to be HBsAg negative were offered HBV vaccine, so some may have been HBsAb positive.

2. Methods

Serum samples from 1049 HIV antibody negative PWIDs in Heng County, Nanning, and Urumqi, China (963 men and 86 women) were tested at baseline and between 26 and 52 weeks later for HBsAg using a commercial enzyme immunoassay (EIA) (Abbott Murex HBsAg version 3.0) and for HCV antibody using two different HCV EIA assays (Ortho HCV antibody version 3.0 and Wantai HCV antibody assay) at baseline and between 26 and 156 weeks later. If the HBsAg test was initially nonreactive, then the participant was considered to be negative for HBsAg. If the HBsAg test was initially reactive, then it was repeated in duplicate. If at least two of 3 tests were reactive, then the participant was considered to be positive for HBsAg. For HCV testing, if both HCV EIA antibody assays were nonreactive, then the participant was considered not to be HCV infected. If either assay was reactive, then the Ortho HCV assay was repeated in duplicate. If two of 3 Ortho HCV assays were reactive, then the participant was considered to be HCV infected. Samples that were repeatedly reactive for HCV antibody at a follow-up visit were tested for HCV RNA by the Roche COBAS AmpliPrep/COBAS TaqMan HCV assay. Not all participants had follow-up testing performed in China due to early closure of the study by the Data Safety Monitoring Board on account of futility due to a low HIV incidence (the primary study endpoint).

In Thailand, serum samples from approximately 201 HIV antibody negative PWIDs (188 men and 13 women) were tested at baseline for HBsAb and HBsAg using the AxSYM assay (Abbott Laboratories). Seventy-three of 201 participants who were found to be HBsAg and HBsAb negative were offered HBV vaccine of whom 68 received all 3 HBV vaccinations. They were tested at 26 and 52 weeks after enrollment for HBsAg using a commercial assay (AxSYM version 2, Abbott Laboratories) and all 201 participants were tested for HCV antibody (AxSYM HCV test Version 3, Abbott Laboratories). If the HBsAg test was initially nonreactive, then the participant was considered to be negative for HBsAg. If the HBsAg test was initially reactive, then it was repeated in duplicate. If at least two of 3 tests were reactive, then the participant was considered to be positive for HBsAg. For HCV testing, if the HCV EIA antibody AxSYM assay was initially nonreactive, then the participant was considered not to be HCV infected. If the assay was reactive, then the sample was retested using another assay (Murex anti HCV version 4.0, Abbott Laboratories). If both tests were reactive, the individual was considered HCV antibody positive. If the Murex HCV antibody test was negative, then the result was considered indeterminate.

Urine tests for opiate use were performed every 4 weeks during the first 52 weeks and then semi-annually (weeks 78, 104, 130, and 156). In all 4 sites, the same commercial test for detection of urine opiates with a sensitivity (cut off) of 300 ng/mL was used according to the manufacturer's directions (Integrated E-Z Split Key Cup, Acon Laboratories, San Diego, CA).

TABLE 1: HBV and HCV prevalence and incidence rates for HBV and HCV at 3 sites in China and one site in Thailand; (95% confidence intervals).

	3 sites in China	Chiang Mai, Thailand
HBsAg prevalence at baseline	13.8% (11.7, 15.9)	13.9% (9.1, 18.7)
HCV Ab prevalence at baseline	81.9% (80.7, 83.1)	59.7% (56.2, 63.2)
HBsAg incidence	2.7/100 py (1.2, 5.1)	0/100 py (0.00, 10.1)
HCV Ab incidence	22/100 py (14.7, 31.6)	4.6/100 py (1.9, 9.0)

TABLE 2: Demographics data for HBsAg negative participants at 3 sites in China and one site in Thailand.

	3 sites in China N = 607	Chiang Mai, Thailand N = 55
Age (mean, range)	33 (18–54)	37 (18–65)
Males	92% (556)	96% (53)
Married/living with partner	48% (291)	78% (43)

TABLE 3: Demographics data for HCV uninfected participants negative at 3 sites in China and one site in Thailand.

	3 sites in China N = 132	Chiang Mai, Thailand N = 78
Age (mean, range)	30 (18–54)	38 (19–65)
Males	96% (127)	91% (71)
Married/living with partner	52% (68)	76% (59)

2.1. Statistical Analysis. Seroincidence rates and confidence intervals were calculated based on a Poisson distribution, with time of infection set to time of first antibody positive test. Cox proportional hazards models were used to compute hazard ratios using time to first positive test among those negative at baseline, censoring participants at their final test visit for HBV and HCV, respectively. Associations with positive urine opiate tests were assessed using the proportion of positive opiate urine tests calculated over each 26 week testing interval for each participant. All analyses were conducted using SAS 9.2 (SAS, Inc).

3. Results

As shown in Table 1, 145 (13.8%) of 1049 PWIDs in China were HBsAg positive at baseline [80 (19.5%) of 411 PWIDs in Heng County, Guangxi, 16 (9.9%) of 161 in Nanning Guangxi, and 49 (10.3%) of 477 in Urumqi, Xinjiang]. Of the 904 HBsAg negative participants at baseline, 607 (67%) were tested at follow-up; 9 had detectable HBsAg, demonstrating an HBsAg incidence rate of 2.7/100 person years. The demographic data (age, gender, marital status) for HBsAg negative participants by country at baseline are shown in Table 2.

In PWIDs in China, the incidence of becoming HBsAg positive in the short- versus long-term B-N treatment was 4.34/100 person years versus 1.15/100 person years (HR = 3.55;

95% CI 0.74 to 17.08, $P = 0.11$) with the Kaplan Meier curve shown by treatment arm in Figure 1(a). In the first 26 weeks of the study, across both arms of the study 40% of the initially HBsAg negative participants in China had at least 75% of their urine samples test positive for opiates and 44% between 26 and 52 weeks. Those with positive urine opiate results in at least 75% of their urines during the time period were at increased risk of incident HBsAg (HR = 5.22; 95% CI, 1.08 to 25.22; $P = 0.04$).

In terms of HCV antibody, 859 (81.9%) of 1049 PWIDs in China were HCV antibody positive at baseline [322 (78.4%) of 411 PWIDs in Heng County, Guangxi; 150 (93.2%) of 161 in Nanning, Guangxi; and 387 (81.1%) of 477 in Urumqi, Xinjiang]. The percentage of women and men who were HCV antibody positive at baseline was 94% and 81%, respectively. The percentage of those who were HCV antibody positive at baseline of less than or equal to 34 years of age compared with more than 34 years of age was 77% and 88%, respectively. Of the 190 HCV antibody negative participants, 132 had follow up samples at 26–156 weeks of which 41 had detectable HCV antibody by repeating EIA testing). The demographic data (age, gender, and marital status) for HCV antibody negative participants by country at baseline are shown in Table 3. HCV RNA PCR testing confirmed HCV infection in 29 of 41 antibody repeatedly reactive samples yielding an overall confirmed seroincidence rate of 22/100 person years with the Kaplan Meier curve shown in Figure 1(b). Heng County, Guangxi, had an incidence rate of 20.9 per 100 years [95% CI, 10.8 to 36.4]; Nanning, Guangxi, 27.7 per 100 years [95% CI, 0.7 to 154]; and Urumqi, Xinjiang, 22.6 per 100 person years [95% CI, 12.9 to 36.7].

Overall, in China, short-term versus long-term B-N treatment was not associated with HCV infection (HR = 0.95; 95% CI, 0.45 to 1.97; $P = 0.9$) with the Kaplan Meier curve shown in Figure 1 by treatment arm. In the first 26 weeks of the study, 42% of the initially HCV uninfected participants in China had at least 75% of their urine test positive for opiates; between 26 and 52 weeks this decreased to 34%, and post intervention increased to 62% at week 78 and 58% at week 104. Those with positive opiate results in at least 75% of their urines during the time period did not appear at increased risk of incident HCV infection (HR = 1.044; 95% CI, 0.48 to 2.23; $P = 0.91$).

In Thailand, 28 (13.9%) of 201 PWIDs were HBsAg positive at baseline. Of the 173 HBsAg and HBsAb negative participants, 55 (31.8%) had follow-up samples six months later of which none had detectable HBsAg or 0/100 person years. In terms of HCV, 120 (59.7%) of 201 PWIDs were HCV antibody positive at baseline in Thailand. The percentage of women and men who were HCV antibody positive at baseline was 46% and 61%, respectively. The percentage of those who were HCV antibody positive at baseline of less than or equal to 34 years of age compared with more than 34 years of age was 65% and 56%, respectively. Of the 81 HCV antibody negative participants, 78 had follow-up samples of which 8 had detectable HCV antibody for an incidence rate of 4.59 per 100 person years [95% CI, 2.0 to 9.0]. Short-term versus long-term B-N treatment was not associated with HCV infection in Thailand (HR = 1.39; 95% CI, 0.33 to 5.83, $P = 0.65$) with the

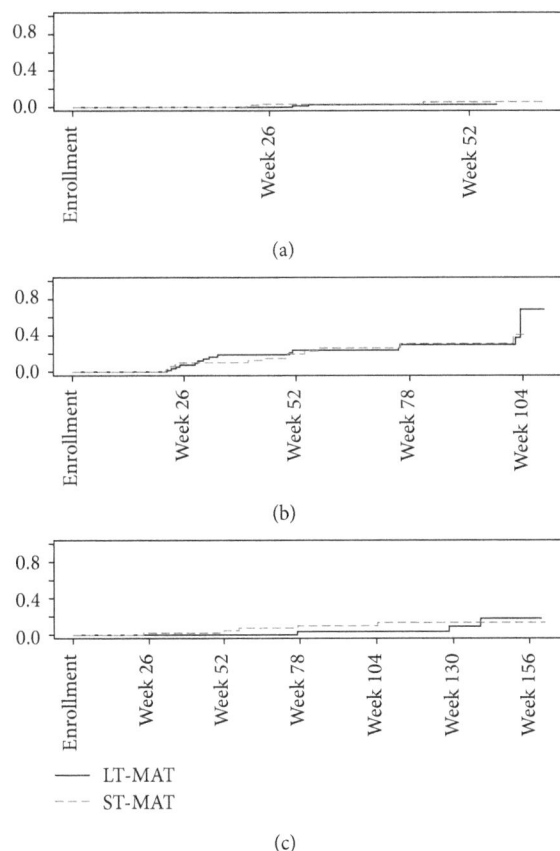

FIGURE 1: (a) Cumulative probability of Hepatitis B in China. (b) Cumulative probability of Hepatitis C in China. (c) Cumulative Probability of Hepatitis C in Thailand.

Kaplan Meier curve shown by treatment arm in Figure 1(c). Those with positive opiate results in at least 75% of their urines during the time period did not appear at increased risk of incident HCV infection (HR = 2.85; 95% CI, 0.55 to 14.58; $P = 0.21$).

Among the HIV antibody negative participants who were either HCV uninfected or HBsAg negative at baseline, there were no HIV incident cases in Thailand (0/55) and 6 incident HIV cases in China among the 607 HBsAg negative participants in follow-up for an HIV incidence rate of 0.81/100 person years (interquartile range 0.30, 1.76). These 6 cases were among 586 participants who remained HBsAg negative in follow-up.

There was one HIV incident case among 132 participants in follow-up in China who was HCV uninfected at baseline for an incidence rate of 0.66/100 person years (interquartile range (0.02, 3.70). This one HIV incident case was among 29 subjects who became HCV infected during follow-up.

4. Discussion

The prevalence and incidence of HBsAg and HCV infection among HIV negative PWIDs in 3 sites in China and one site in Thailand were very high. The baseline HBsAg prevalence in China and Thailand was nearly identical at 13.8% and

13.9%, respectively, nearly twice as high as that reported in the general population [5]. HBV vaccine and HBV immunoglobulin to prevent perinatal transmission have been available for a couple of decades. However, the mean age and range of Thai participants who were HbSAg positive at baseline were 37 and 23 to 48 years, respectively, and for Chinese participants who were HbSAg positive at baseline were 32 and 18 to 49 years, respectively. Given this older cohort, it is likely they did not receive HBV vaccination perinatally as newborns. This difference probably reflects the additional risk of injection use above that caused by perinatal transmission in these populations. However, the relatively low HBsAg incidence rates of 2.7/100 person years in China and 0/100 persons years in Thailand are not surprising given the high background rates of HBV infection and clearance in high hepatitis endemic areas [9] and the fact that a number of HBsAg negative participants at baseline agreed to the receipt of HBV vaccine. For example, in Thailand, all HBsAg negative and HBsAb negative participants received HBV vaccine, which probably explains the zero incidence of HBV infection, whereas in China at least 29% (260 of 940) HBsAg negative PWIDs at baseline did not receive HBV vaccine. Given that HBsAb was not measured in the Chinese participants at any time in the study, some HBsAg negative participants at baseline may have been immune at baseline and/or after vaccination. However, there appear to be a number of susceptibles who became HBsAg positive either because they did not receive the vaccine or were given the vaccine, but they became infected shortly after enrollment as all of the incident cases occurred by week 26.

In terms of hepatitis C, approximately 82% and 60% of PWIDs in this study in China and Thailand, respectively, were HCV antibody positive at baseline which is consistent with reported prevalence rates in these countries [1, 2]. The HCV incidence rates were 22/100 person years in China compared with 4.6/100 person years in Thailand which may reflect the higher prevalence rate at baseline or higher risk injection practices associated with increased sharing and/or higher frequency of injection in China.

Those participants with positive opiate urine tests in at least 75% of the urines over the study period were at increased risk of incident HBsAg conversion, but they were not at increased risk for HCV antibody conversion. HBsAg and HCV antibody incidence rates were not significantly associated with short-term versus long-term B-N treatment arms, although in China, the HBsAg incidence rate was more than 3-fold higher in the short-term B-N arm and nearly 5-fold higher in those participants with positive opiate results in at least 75% of their urines at follow-up.

Why there was not a significantly higher HCV incidence associated with positive urine opiate tests is not clear. Perhaps the number of susceptible participants in this high HCV prevalence population was too small to discern a difference, or the efficiency of HCV transmission is so high through needle sharing that differences in incident infection will not be significant given that 39% of monthly visits in the long term B-N arm had positive urine drug screens. Another possible explanation is that many of the Thai participants were mostly from ethnic minorities whose networks appeared small and closed. Perhaps HCV had not reached some of these closed networks. Many of the PWIDs also smoked opium or may have injected opium less frequently which would give positive urine results, yet be associated with a lower risk of HCV transmission.

These findings support the concept that decreased injection drug use, as evidenced by negative urine opiate tests associated with the long term B-N arm, will likely lead to decreased HBsAg incidence rates.

Conflict of Interests

The authors declare that they have no potential conflict of interests.

Acknowledgments

Study drug was provided by Reckitt Benckiser Pharmaceuticals, Inc. Work on this document was supported by Grant nos. UM1 068619, UM1-AI-069482, UM1-AI-069406, UM1-AI068613, and UMI-AI-069411 from the National Institute of Allergy and Infectious Diseases (NIAID), with additional support from the National Institute on Drug Abuse (NIDA). The content is solely the responsibility of the authors and does not necessarily represent the official views of the NIAID, NIDA, or the National Institutes of Health. J. Brooks Jackson, Liu Wei, Fu Liping, and Apinun Aramrattana are the first coauthors.

References

[1] C. Aceijas and T. Rhodes, "Global estimates of prevalence of HCV infection among injecting drug users," *International Journal of Drug Policy*, vol. 18, no. 5, pp. 352–358, 2007.

[2] L. J. Liu and L. Wei, "Epidemiology of hepatitis C virus," *Infectious Disease Information*, vol. 20, pp. 261–264, 2007 (Chinese).

[3] V. Verachai, T. Phutiprawan, A. Theamboonlers et al., "Prevalence and genotypes of hepatitis C virus infection among drug addicts and blood donors in Thailand," *Southeast Asian Journal of Tropical Medicine and Public Health*, vol. 33, no. 4, pp. 849–851, 2002.

[4] G. Greub, B. Ledergerber, M. Battegay et al., "Clinical progression, survival, and immune recovery during antiretroviral therapy in patients with HIV-1 and hepatitis C virus coinfection: The swiss HIV cohort study," *The Lancet*, vol. 356, no. 9244, pp. 1800–1805, 2000.

[5] F. M. Lu, T. Li, S. Liu, and H. Zhuang, "Epidemiology and prevention of hepatitis B virus infection in China," *Journal of Viral Hepatitis*, vol. 17, supplement 1, pp. 4–9, 2010.

[6] S. Sungkanuparph, A. Vibhagool, W. Manosuthi et al., "Prevalence of hepatitis B virus and hepatitis C virus co-infection with human immunodeficiency virus in Thai patients: a tertiary-care-based study," *Journal of the Medical Association of Thailand*, vol. 87, no. 11, pp. 1349–1354, 2004.

[7] H. M. Chun, M. P. Roediger, K. H. Hullsiek et al., "Hepatitis B virus coinfection negatively impacts HIV outcomes in HIV seroconverters," *Journal of Infectious Diseases*, vol. 205, no. 2, pp. 185–193, 2012.

[8] D. Metzger, D. Donnell, B. Jackson et al., "One year of counseling supported buprenorphine-naloxone treatment for HIV prevention in opiate dependent injecting drug users showed efficacy in reducing opiate use and injection frequency: HPTN 058 in Thailand and China. Abstract THPE191," in *Proceedings of the 19th International AIDS Conference*, Washington, DC, USA, July 2012.

[9] C. L. Fan, L. Wei, D. Jiang et al., "Spontaneous viral clearance after 6–21 years of hepatitis B and C viruses coinfection in high HBV endemic area," *World Journal of Gastroenterology*, vol. 9, no. 9, pp. 2012–2016, 2003.

Histological and Clinical Characteristics of Patients with Chronic Hepatitis C and Persistently Normal Alanine Aminotransferase Levels

Bakht Roshan[1] and Grace Guzman[2]

[1] Department of Medicine, Section of Hepatology, University of Illinois at Chicago, 840 South Wood Street, Suite 130, Chicago, IL 60612, USA

[2] Department of Pathology (MC847), University of Illinois at Chicago, 840 South Wood Street, Suite 130, Chicago, IL 60612, USA

Correspondence should be addressed to Bakht Roshan; bakhtroshan@gmail.com

Academic Editor: Annarosa Floreani

Patients with chronic hepatitis C virus (HCV) infection and persistently normal alanine aminotransferase (PNALT) are generally described to have mild liver disease. The aim of this study was to compare clinical and histological features in HCV-infected patients with PNALT and elevated ALT. Patients presenting to the University of Illinois Medical Center, Chicago, who had biopsy proven HCV, an ALT measurement at the time of liver biopsy, at least one additional ALT measurement over the next 12 months, and liver biopsy slides available for review were identified. PNALT was defined as ALT ≤ 30 on at least 2 different occasions over 12 months. Of 1200 patients with HCV, 243 met the study criteria. 13% (32/243) of patients had PNALT while 87% (211/243) had elevated ALT. Significantly more patients with PNALT had advanced fibrosis (F3 and F4) compared to those with elevated ALT ($P = 0.007$). There was no significant difference in the histology activity index score as well as mean inflammatory score between the two groups. In conclusion, in a well-characterized cohort of patients at a tertiary medical center, PNALT did not distinguish patients with mild liver disease.

1. Introduction

Hepatitis C virus (HCV) infection is reported to have a prevalence of approximately 3% worldwide [1]. Almost 80% of those infected go on to develop chronic infection. Majority of patients with chronic HCV have a mild, asymptomatic elevation in serum transaminase levels with no significant clinical symptoms. Around 25% of patients with chronic HCV have persistently normal alanine aminotransferase (PNALT) [2].

Definition of normal alanine aminotransferase (ALT) has changed over time and reference range for normal ALT differs based on different laboratory cutoffs. Prati et al. [3] in 2002 suggested new cutoffs with 30 U/L (international unit) for men and 19 U/L for women compared to 40 U/L and 30 U/L for men and women, respectively. This resulted in improved sensitivity but decreased specificity. Similarly, definition of PNALT differs widely. A 2009 American Association for the Study of Liver Disease (AASLD) practice guideline suggested an ALT value of 40 U/L on 2-3 different occasions separated by at least a month over a period of 6 months [4]. Others have used 3 different ALT levels equal to or below upper limit of normal (ULN) separated by at least 1 month and sometimes over a period of 18 months [5]. Thus, there is no consensus on a universal definition of PNALT.

It was generally thought that people with PNALT have a mild liver disease and the degree of liver fibrosis is minimal [6–14]. Based on this, people with PNALT were initially monitored conservatively without treatment. Later on, it was realized that a considerable number of such patients developed significant inflammation and fibrosis over time [15]. More recently, treatment has been recommended along the same lines for patients with PNALT as patients with elevated ALT [4].

TABLE 1: ALT range expressed in international unit (U/L).

Interval	Biopsy	3 months	6 months	12 months
PNALT (median)	9–30 (24)	9–28 (20)	10–30 (22)	11–30 (21)
Elevated ALT (median)	16–987 (56)	14–57 (27)	12–1248 (45)	10–231 (43)

Although more data is becoming available about the relationship of liver enzymes and course of chronic HCV infection, data regarding HCV infection and PNALT is relatively scarce. Because of variation in the definition of PNALT, fewer studies have looked at the relationship of PNALT with chronic HCV infection using updated normal ALT definitions [16].

Department of Hepatology at the University of Illinois (U of I) medical center, Chicago, had a database of over 1200 patients with chronic HCV infection. Medical records of these patients were reviewed in an effort to characterize patients with chronic HCV infection and PNALT. Histological and clinical parameters for patients with PNALT as well as elevated ALT were analyzed.

2. Materials and Methods

Database of patients with HCV infection presenting to U of I medical center, Chicago, was reviewed. These patients had a liver biopsy done between 1996 and 2007. Patients with biopsy proven HCV infection and a detectable HCV ribonucleic acid (RNA) in blood were chosen. Of these, patients with an ALT at liver biopsy, at least one additional over the next 12 months, and liver biopsy slides available for review were identified.

Most of the liver biopsy procedures were done at U of I medical center and in cases where biopsies were done at outside facility they were read again at U of I medical center. Two expert hepatologists, who were masked to clinical data, assigned Knodell et al. [17] score to liver biopsies. Intervals for ALT measurement were chosen around the time of liver biopsy as well as 3, 6, and 12 months after biopsy. Patients with end-stage renal disease like those on dialysis and stage IV chronic kidney disease with creatinine clearance of 15–29, those who received organ transplant, those with co-infection with HIV, those who were positive for Hepatitis B surface antigen (HBsAg), and those receiving antiviral therapy for chronic HCV were excluded.

PNALT was defined as ALT ≤ 30 U/L on at least 2 different occasions over 12 months. Strict PNALT was defined as ALT $\leq$ 30 U/L for males and $\leq$19 U/L for females.

Demographic data including age at biopsy, gender, and race were recorded. Clinical data included body mass index (BMI), alcohol use, tobacco use, and presence of diabetes mellitus (DM). HCV virus was further characterized by recording HCV RNA levels, genotype, and duration of infection. Histological data included individual markers of inflammation like portal tract inflammation, piece meal necrosis, and lobular inflammation as well as fibrosis according to Knodell et al. scoring system. Inflammatory score (sum of portal tract inflammation, piece meal necrosis, and lobular inflammation) and histologic activity index (HAI) score (sum of inflammatory score and fibrosis) were calculated. Histologic data from PNALT was then compared with patients from elevated ALT group. Finally, clinical characteristics of PNALT with advanced fibrosis were compared with PNALT but with no advanced fibrosis.

Statistical analysis was performed using SPSS (SPSS Inc., Chicago, IL). Independent sample t-test and chi-squared test were used to calculate P values where appropriate.

3. Results

A total of 243 patients out of a database of 1200 patients with HCV satisfied the study criteria. Main reasons to exclude a large number of patients were a lack of detectable RNA despite biopsy report, outside biopsy report but slides not available for review, single or no ALT value, and patients undergoing treatments. Those analyzed were further divided into PNALT, strict PNALT, and elevated ALT group. 32 (13%) of these patients were identified as PNALT group and 211 (87%) were identified as elevated ALT group. Only 13 (5%) patients satisfied criterion for strict PNALT and this group was not analyzed further. The range of ALT values at different time intervals was specified (Table 1). 24 (75%) of PNALT patients were females while 85 (40%) with elevated ALT were females. 13 (41%) with PNALT were African American (AA) compared to 87 (41%) with elevated ALT, 14 (44%) were Caucasian (W) compared to 79 (38%) with elevated ALT, and 5 (15%) were Hispanic (H) compared to 44 (21%) with elevated ALT. There was no statistically significant difference in the racial distribution between PNALT and elevated ALT group.

There was a higher frequency of women in the PNALT group compared to the elevated ALT group ($P = 0.001$). Diabetes and alcohol use were more common among patients with elevated ALT compared to PNALT ($P = 0.04$ and 0.049, resp.). Most notably, patients with PNALT had a higher rate of cirrhosis ($P = 0.007$). There were no differences in age at biopsy, tobacco use, BMI, RNA level, and duration of infection between PNALT and elevated ALT groups (Table 2).

Further evaluation of liver histology showed no statistically significant difference in mean fibrosis score, mean portal tract inflammation score, mean piecemeal necrosis score (PMN), mean lobular inflammation score, mean histologic activity index (HAI) score, and mean inflammatory score between PNALT group and elevated ALT group (Table 3). Comparison of clinical characteristics of PNALT group with advanced fibrosis with PNALT group without advanced fibrosis showed that only platelet count was significantly different between the two groups (Table 4). Tables 5 and 6 characterize the distribution of HCV genotypes based on PNALT and HAI score, respectively.

TABLE 2: Clinical data/distribution of patients.

	PNALT ($n = 32$)	Elevated ALT ($n = 211$)	Total ($n = 243$)	P value
Gender M/F	8/24	126/85	134/109	0.001
Race (W/AA/H)	14/13/5	79/87/44	93/100/49*	0.717
Alcohol (Y/N)	6/26	77/134	83/160	0.049
Tobacco (Y/N)	6/26	30/181	36/207	0.501
DM (Y/N)	2/30	46/165	48/195	0.04
Mean age at biopsy in years (n)	50 (31)	47 (211)	242*	0.153
Mean BMI (n)	26 (27)	25 (177)	204*	0.5
Mean RNA level in IU/mL (n)	1883693 (30)	4439614 (159)	189*	0.09
Duration of infection in years (n)	26 (21)	25 (152)	173*	0.768
Fibrosis (F0-1/F2-4)	10/22	84/127	94/149	0.354
Fibrosis (F0-2/F3-4)	24/8	192/19	216/27	0.007

*Data not available for all patients.

TABLE 3: Histological data.

	PNALT (mean ± SD)	Elevated ALT (mean ± SD)	P value
Fibrosis	2 ± 1	1.7 ± 1	0.067
Portal tract inflammation	1.66 ± 1	1.77 ± 1	0.46
PMN	1.47 ± 1	1.48 ± 1	0.96
Lobular inflammation	0.72 ± 1	0.9 ± 1	0.175
HAI score	6 ± 3	6 ± 3	0.94
Inflammatory score	4 ± 2	4 ± 2	0.7

TABLE 4: PNALT with advanced fibrosis versus PNALT without advanced fibrosis.

	PNALT with advanced fibrosis	PNALT without advanced fibrosis	Total number of patients $n = 32$	P value
Mean age at biopsy in years (n)	48 (8)	50 (23)	31*	0.7
ALT at biopsy in U/L (n)	23 (7)	21 (24)	31*	0.5
ALT at 12 months in U/L (n)	21 (4)	21 (19)	23*	0.88
Mean RNA level in IU (n)	134288 (6)	2321044 (24)	30*	0.127
Mean BMI (n)	27 (6)	26 (21)	27*	0.634
AST (n)	41 (7)	28 (24)	31*	0.061
Platelet count (n)	81000 (5)	257000 (21)	26*	0.001

*Data not available for all patients.

TABLE 5: HCV genotype characteristics.

Genotype	PNALT (n)	Elevated ALT (n)	Total (%)	P value
1	3	16	19 (11)	
1a	10	60	70 (39)	
1b	8	49	57 (31)	
2a	1	5	6 (3)	0.8
2b	0	13	13 (7)	
3a	1	13	14 (8)	
4	0	2	2 (1)	
Total	23	158	181 (100)	

TABLE 6: HCV genotype and HAI score.

Genotype	HAI score			Total (%)	P value
	≤6	7–12	>13		
1	16	3	0	19 (11)	
1a	45	25	0	70 (39)	
1b	38	16	3	57 (31)	
2a	4	2	0	6 (3)	0.34
2b	6	7	0	13 (7)	
3a	9	5	0	14 (8)	
4	2	0	0	2 (1)	
Total (%)	**120 (66)**	**58 (32)**	**3 (2)**	**181 (100)**	

TABLE 7: ALT value and HAI score within PNALT.

	HAI score			Total	P value
	≤6	7–12	>13		
ALT value					
<19	7	1	0	8	
20–30	15	8	1	24	0.4
Total	**22**	**9**	**1**	**32**	

4. Discussion

The natural history of chronic HCV infection with PNALT is poorly understood [18–20]. We attempt to describe the characteristics of patients with PNALT, which constitutes almost 25–30% of patients with chronic HCV infection. There are few significant findings from this work. Firstly, a high proportion of patients with PNALT had advanced fibrosis, and degree of inflammation was not significantly different than chronic HCV infection with abnormal ALT. Secondly, it was difficult to identify a substantially large set of patients with HCV infection and PNALT given that there is a significant fluctuation in the ALT level over time [9, 15]. Thirdly, patients with multiple comorbidities were excluded leaving a small cohort size.

We chose duration of 12 months to observe the levels of ALT instead of 6 months period. It is becoming clear that 6 months is probably too short given that in some cases ALT level may fluctuate after initial period of stability [7, 21–24]. Most patients with PNALT were females, which is consistent with earlier findings [7–9]. Abstinence from alcohol and lack of DM were associated with PNALT. There was no association with race. Similarly, age at biopsy, BMI, RNA level, and duration of infection were not significantly different between the two groups. HCV genotype distribution showed that a majority (81%) of patients belonged to genotype 1 and it is a well-characterized fact [25]. There was no significant difference in terms of distribution of genotypes between the 2 groups (Table 5). Also there was no significant difference in HAI according to genotype distribution (Table 6). HCV genotyping was performed in 181/243 (75%) patients and was missing in 62 (25%) patients. The likely reason was transition from paper to electronic records in 1990s and loss of some data.

Within PNALT, those with advanced fibrosis differed from those without advanced fibrosis by platelet count only. Other variables as shown in Table 4 did not achieve a significance level. Similarly, PNALT patients were divided based on low-normal ALT (<19) and high-normal ALT (20–30) for comparing HAI scores among them but no significance was seen (Table 7).

The most interesting finding was the comparison of histological data. Studies to date have been mentioning a milder disease for PNALT in terms of fibrosis and necroinflammation [7–9, 26–28]. Our study indicated that fibrosis and necroinflammation were comparable in both groups. Some studies have pointed to this fact as well [14, 29, 30]. This is an interesting finding given that despite significant inflammation (comparable to abnormal ALT) the ALT levels in some of these patients have been consistently low. The exact etiology of PNALT despite significant inflammation is not clear. Similarly, advanced fibrosis was more common in PNALT group as compared to the elevated ALT group ($P = 0.007$). It is thought that ALT levels normalize in patients with advanced fibrosis [31] and that is why some authors will advocate doing liver biopsy in patients with HCV infection and normal ALT levels [32]. It is interesting to note that the 6 patients with PNALT who had cirrhosis also had evidence of thrombocytopenia. Thrombocytopenia is a well-established marker of cirrhosis [33]. Our results indicate that platelet count can be used as a marker to predict fibrosis in patients with PNALT.

There were several limitations to this study. First, it was a retrospective study. Cases were excluded because only a single measurement was available. For instance, almost all patients in the study group had an ALT measured around biopsy but only slightly more than half had ALT measured around 12 months. This is why ALT was recorded around 3 months and

6 months as well. Second, sample size was relatively small and might not be a true representative of patients with PNALT. This might in particular be valid for PNALT with advanced fibrosis as 8 (25%) out of 32 patients with PNALT had F3-F4 while only 19 (9%) out of 211 patients with elevated ALT had F3-F4 ($P = 0.007$). It is not clear if the outcome would have been the same if denominator for PNALT was high.

Small sample size was caused mainly as described before as well as comorbid conditions like advanced kidney disease, HIV, HBsAg positive, and being on antiviral treatment. For example, 11 patients with PNALT were excluded as they had ESRD; ALT levels are known to be lower in ESRD [34, 35] secondary to an impaired immune response in patients with ESRD [36]. Third, ALT levels were measured at irregular intervals. This raises concern that those with PNALT and severe liver fibrosis may have been in biochemical remission. For example, of the 8 patients with severe liver fibrosis (stages 3 and 4) and PNALT, only 2 patients had 4 ALT measurements over 12 months (over the period of 0, 3, 6, and 12 months), while 3 patients had 3 ALT measurements over 12 months, and the remaining 3 patients had only 2 ALT measurements over the 12 months period. Thus, it is not possible to say with certainty that all patients with PNALT and severe liver damage had uniformly low ALT all along.

5. Conclusion

In conclusion, histological changes observed in HCV patients with PNALT will argue that ALT is not a reliable indicator of hepatic inflammation or fibrosis. In fact, PNALT was associated with advanced fibrosis in the current study. Female gender, absence of DM, and abstinence from alcohol were associated with PNALT. Platelet count could be used to predict fibrosis in patients with PNALT. These findings indicate the need for more studies with higher number of PNALT patients to look at the relationship of PNALT with changes occurring at histological and molecular levels.

Conflict of Interests

The authors declare that there is no conflict of interests regarding the publication of this paper.

References

[1] S. Pol, A. Vallet-Pichard, M. Corouge, and V. O. Mallet, "Hepatitis C: epidemiology, diagnosis, natural history and therapy," *Contributions to Nephrology*, vol. 176, pp. 1–9, 2012.

[2] N. Boyer and P. Marcellin, "Natural history of hepatitis C and the impact of anti-viral therapy," *Forum: Trends in Experimental and Clinical Medicine*, vol. 10, no. 1, pp. 4–18, 2000.

[3] D. Prati, E. Taioli, A. Zanella et al., "Updated definitions of healthy ranges for serum alanine aminotransferase levels," *Annals of Internal Medicine*, vol. 137, no. 1, pp. 1–10, 2002.

[4] M. G. Ghany, D. B. Strader, D. L. Thomas, and L. B. Seeff, "Diagnosis, management, and treatment of hepatitis C: an update," *Hepatology*, vol. 49, no. 4, pp. 1335–1374, 2009.

[5] S. Zeuzem, M. Diago, E. Gane et al., "Peginterferon alfa-2a (40 kilodaltons) and ribavirin in patients with chronic hepatitis C and normal aminotransferase levels," *Gastroenterology*, vol. 127, no. 6, pp. 1724–1732, 2004.

[6] C. Puoti, L. Bellis, A. Galossi et al., "Antiviral treatment of HCV carriers with persistently normal ALT levels," *Mini-Reviews in Medicinal Chemistry*, vol. 8, no. 2, pp. 150–152, 2008.

[7] M. Persico, E. Persico, R. Suozzo et al., "Natural history of hepatitis C virus carriers with persistently normal aminotransferase levels," *Gastroenterology*, vol. 118, no. 4, pp. 760–764, 2000.

[8] M. Martinot-Peignoux, N. Boyer, D. Cazals-Hatem et al., "Prospective study on anti-hepatitis C virus-positive patients with persistently normal serum alanine transaminase with or without detectable serum hepatitis C virus RNA," *Hepatology*, vol. 34, no. 5, pp. 1000–1005, 2001.

[9] M. L. Shiffman, M. Diago, A. Tran et al., "Chronic hepatitis C in patients with persistently normal alanine transaminase levels," *Clinical Gastroenterology and Hepatology*, vol. 4, no. 5, pp. 645–652, 2006.

[10] D. B. Strader, T. Wright, D. L. Thomas, and L. B. Seeff, "Diagnosis, management, and treatment of hepatitis C," *Hepatology*, vol. 39, no. 4, pp. 1147–1171, 2004.

[11] P. Mathurin, "Slow progression rate of fibrosis in hepatitis C virus patients with persistently normal alanine transaminase activity," *Hepatology*, vol. 27, no. 3, pp. 868–872, 1998.

[12] P. Marcellin, S. Levy, and S. Erlinger, "Therapy of hepatitis C: patients with normal aminotransferase levels," *Hepatology*, vol. 26, supplement 1, no. 3, pp. 133S–136S, 1997.

[13] N. C. Tassopoulos, "Treatment of patients with chronic hepatitis C and normal ALT levels," *Journal of Hepatology*, vol. 31, supplement 1, pp. 193–196, 1999.

[14] C. Puoti, L. Bellis, R. Guarisco, O. D. Unto, L. Spilabotti, and O. M. Costanza, "HCV carriers with normal alanine aminotransferase levels: healthy persons or severely ill patients? Dealing with an everyday clinical problem," *European Journal of Internal Medicine*, vol. 21, no. 2, pp. 57–61, 2010.

[15] T. Okanoue, M. Minami, A. Makiyama, Y. Sumida, K. Yasui, and Y. Itoh, "Natural course of asymptomatic hepatitis C virus-infected patients and hepatocellular carcinoma after interferon therapy," *Clinical Gastroenterology and Hepatology*, vol. 3, supplement 2, pp. S89–S91, 2005.

[16] F. M. Sanai, A. Helmy, C. Dale et al., "Updated thresholds for alanine aminotransferase do not exclude significant histological disease in chronic hepatitis C," *Liver International*, vol. 31, no. 7, pp. 1039–1046, 2011.

[17] R. G. Knodell, K. G. Ishak, and W. C. Black, "Formulation and application of a numerical scoring system for assessing histological activity in asymptomatic chronic active hepatitis," *Hepatology*, vol. 1, no. 5, pp. 431–435, 1981.

[18] L. B. Seeff, "The natural history of chronic hepatitis C virus infection," *Clinics in Liver Disease*, vol. 1, no. 3, pp. 587–602, 1997.

[19] L. B. Seeff, "Natural history of chronic hepatitis C," *Hepatology*, vol. 36, supplement 1, no. 5, pp. S35–S46, 2002.

[20] R. Zapata, "Clinical aproach to the patient with chronic hepatitis C infection and normal aminotransferases," *Annals of Hepatology*, vol. 9, no. 1, supplement, pp. 72–79, 2010.

[21] S. C. Gordon, J. W. Fang, A. L. Silverman, J. G. McHutchison, and J. K. Albrecht, "The significance of baseline serum alanine aminotransferase on pretreatment disease characteristics and response to antiviral therapy in chronic hepatitis C," *Hepatology*, vol. 32, no. 2, pp. 400–404, 2000.

[22] J. Jamal, "Clinical features of hepatitis C-infected patients with persistently normal alanine transaminase levels in

the Southwestern United States," *Hepatology*, vol. 30, no. 5, pp. 1307–1311, 2000.

[23] C. Puoti, R. Castellacci, F. Montagnese et al., "Histological and virological features and follow-up of hepatitis C virus carriers with normal aminotransferase levels: the Italian prospective study of the asymptomatic C carriers (ISACC)," *Journal of Hepatology*, vol. 37, no. 1, pp. 117–123, 2002.

[24] C. Puoti, R. Guarisco, L. Bellis, and L. Spilabotti, "Diagnosis, management, and treatment of hepatitis C," *Hepatology*, vol. 50, no. 1, pp. 322–325, 2009.

[25] N. N. Zein, J. Rakela, E. L. Krawitt, K. R. Reddy, T. Tominaga, and D. H. Persing, "Hepatitis C virus genotypes in the United States: epidemiology, pathogenicity, and response to interferon therapy," *Annals of Internal Medicine*, vol. 125, no. 8, pp. 634–639, 1996.

[26] C. Puoti, R. Castellacci, and F. Montagnese, "Hepatitis C virus carriers with persistently normal aminotransferase levels: healthy people or true patients?" *Digestive and Liver Disease*, vol. 32, no. 7, pp. 634–643, 2000.

[27] C. Puoti, A. Magrini, T. Stati et al., "Clinical, histological, and virological features of hepatitis C virus carriers with persistently normal or abnormal alanine transaminase levels," *Hepatology*, vol. 26, no. 6, pp. 1393–1398, 1997.

[28] S. Zeuzem, A. Alberti, W. Rosenberg et al., "Review article: management of patients with chronic hepatitis C virus infection and "normal" alanine aminotransferase activity," *Alimentary Pharmacology and Therapeutics*, vol. 24, no. 8, pp. 1133–1149, 2006.

[29] J. L. Dienstag and J. G. McHutchison, "American gastroenterological association medical position statement on the management of hepatitis C," *Gastroenterology*, vol. 130, no. 1, pp. 225–230, 2006.

[30] C. Puoti, "HCV carriers with persistently normal aminotransferase levels: normal does not always mean healthy," *Journal of Hepatology*, vol. 38, no. 4, pp. 529–532, 2003.

[31] D. C. Rockey, S. H. Caldwell, Z. D. Goodman, R. C. Nelson, and A. D. Smith, "Liver biopsy," *Hepatology*, vol. 49, no. 3, pp. 1017–1044, 2009.

[32] C. Puoti, R. Guarisco, L. Spilabotti et al., "Should we treat HCV carriers with normal ALT levels? the "5Ws" dilemma," *Journal of Viral Hepatitis*, vol. 19, no. 4, pp. 229–235, 2012.

[33] S.-N. Lu, J.-H. Wang, S.-L. Liu et al., "Thrombocytopenia as a surrogate for cirrhosis and a marker for the identification of patients at high-risk for hepatocellular carcinoma," *Cancer*, vol. 107, no. 9, pp. 2212–2222, 2006.

[34] H. A. Azevedo, C. A. Villela-Nogueira, R. M. Perez et al., "Similar HCV viral load levels and genotype distribution among end-stage renal disease patients on hemodialysis and HCV-infected patients with normal renal function," *Journal of Nephrology*, vol. 20, no. 5, pp. 609–616, 2007.

[35] A. M. Contreras, I. Ruiz, G. Polanco-Cruz et al., "End-stage renal disease and hepatitis C infection: comparison of alanine aminotransferase levels and liver histology in patients with and without renal damage," *Annals of Hepatology*, vol. 6, no. 1, pp. 48–54, 2007.

[36] M. R. Hassan, N. R. N. Mustapha, F. M. Zawawi, B. S. P. Earnest, K. Voralu, and S. P. Pani, "A comparison of genotype and markers of disease severity of chronic hepatitis C in patients with and without end-stage renal disease," *Singapore Medical Journal*, vol. 52, no. 2, pp. 86–89, 2011.

Permissions

All chapters in this book were first published in HEPRT, by Hindawi Publishing Corporation; hereby published with permission under the Creative Commons Attribution License or equivalent. Every chapter published in this book has been scrutinized by our experts. Their significance has been extensively debated. The topics covered herein carry significant findings which will fuel the growth of the discipline. They may even be implemented as practical applications or may be referred to as a beginning point for another development.

The contributors of this book come from diverse backgrounds, making this book a truly international effort. This book will bring forth new frontiers with its revolutionizing research information and detailed analysis of the nascent developments around the world.

We would like to thank all the contributing authors for lending their expertise to make the book truly unique. They have played a crucial role in the development of this book. Without their invaluable contributions this book wouldn't have been possible. They have made vital efforts to compile up to date information on the varied aspects of this subject to make this book a valuable addition to the collection of many professionals and students.

This book was conceptualized with the vision of imparting up-to-date information and advanced data in this field. To ensure the same, a matchless editorial board was set up. Every individual on the board went through rigorous rounds of assessment to prove their worth. After which they invested a large part of their time researching and compiling the most relevant data for our readers.

The editorial board has been involved in producing this book since its inception. They have spent rigorous hours researching and exploring the diverse topics which have resulted in the successful publishing of this book. They have passed on their knowledge of decades through this book. To expedite this challenging task, the publisher supported the team at every step. A small team of assistant editors was also appointed to further simplify the editing procedure and attain best results for the readers.

Apart from the editorial board, the designing team has also invested a significant amount of their time in understanding the subject and creating the most relevant covers. They scrutinized every image to scout for the most suitable representation of the subject and create an appropriate cover for the book.

The publishing team has been an ardent support to the editorial, designing and production team. Their endless efforts to recruit the best for this project, has resulted in the accomplishment of this book. They are a veteran in the field of academics and their pool of knowledge is as vast as their experience in printing. Their expertise and guidance has proved useful at every step. Their uncompromising quality standards have made this book an exceptional effort. Their encouragement from time to time has been an inspiration for everyone.

The publisher and the editorial board hope that this book will prove to be a valuable piece of knowledge for researchers, students, practitioners and scholars across the globe.

List of Contributors

Sandeep R. Varma, R. Sundaram, S. Gopumadhavan, Satyakumar Vidyashankar and Pralhad S. Patki
Research and Development, The Himalaya Drug Company, Bangalore 562 123, India

Li Ma, Malgorzata G. Norton, Zhong Zhao, Lilin Zhong, Pei Zhang and Evi B. Struble
Laboratory of Plasma Derivatives, Division of Hematology, Office of Blood Research and Review, Center for Biologics Evaluation and Research, FDA 1401 Rockville Pike, Rockville, MD 20852, USA

Iftekhar Mahmood
Division of Hematology, Office of Blood Research and Review, Center for Biologics Evaluation and Research, FDA 1401 Rockville Pike, Rockville, MD 20852, USA

Adnan Said
Division of Gastroenterology and Hepatology, University of Wisconsin School of Medicine and
Public Health and William S. Middleton VAMC, Madison, WI 53705, USA

Janice H. Jou
Division of Gastroenterology and Hepatology, Oregon Health Sciences University and Portland VAMC, Portland, OR 97239, USA

G. F. Oxenkrug and P. Summergrad
Psychiatry and Inflammation Program, Department of Psychiatry, Tufts Medical Center, Tufts University, Boston, MA 02111, USA

W. A. Turski
Department of Experimental and Clinical Pharmacology, Medical University, 20-090 Lublin, Poland

W. Zgrajka
Department of Toxicology, Institute of Rural Health, 20-090 Lublin, Poland

J. V. Weinstock
Division of Gastroenterology/Hepatology, Tufts Medical Center, Tufts University, Boston, MA 02111, USA

Joseph Kluck
Department of Pharmacy, Philadelphia Veterans Affairs Medical Center, 3900Woodland Avenue, Philadelphia, PA 19104, USA
Department of Pharmacy, Hospital of the University of Pennsylvania, 3400 Spruce Street, Philadelphia, PA 19104, USA

Rose M. O'Flynn
Department of Pharmacy, Philadelphia Veterans Affairs Medical Center, 3900Woodland Avenue, Philadelphia, PA 19104, USA

David E. Kaplan and Kyong-Mi Chang
Gastroenterology Section, Philadelphia Veterans Affairs Medical Center, 3900Woodland Avenue, Philadelphia, PA 19104, USA
Division of Gastroenterology, University of Pennsylvania Perelman School of Medicine, 421 Curie Boulevard, 9th Floor, Philadelphia, PA 19104, USA

Chhagan Bihari and Archana Rastogi
Department of Pathology, Institute of Liver and Biliary Sciences (ILBS), D-1 Vasant Kunj, New Delhi 110070, India

Shiv Kumar Sarin
Department of Hepatology, Institute of Liver and Biliary Sciences (ILBS), New Delhi 110070, India

Sara Romani
Gastroenterology and Liver Diseases Research Center, Shahid Beheshti University of Medical Sciences, Tehran, Iran
2Department of Microbiology, Faculty of Biological Sciences, Shahid Beheshti University, Tehran, Iran

Mahsa Khanyaghma, Shaghayegh Derakhshani, Seyed Reza Mohebbi, Afsaneh Sharifian and Mohammad Reza Zali
Gastroenterology and Liver Diseases Research Center, Shahid Beheshti University of Medical Sciences, Tehran, Iran

Seyed Masoud Hosseini
Department of Microbiology, Faculty of Biological Sciences, Shahid Beheshti University, Tehran, Iran

Shabnam Kazemian
Basic and Molecular Epidemiology of Gastroenterology Disorders Research Center, Shahid Beheshti University of Medical Sciences,

Pedram Azimzadeh
Gastroenterology and Liver Diseases Research Center, Shahid Beheshti University of Medical Sciences, Tehran, Iran
Basic and Molecular Epidemiology of Gastroenterology Disorders Research Center, Shahid Beheshti University of Medical Sciences, Tehran, Iran

Shinji Shimoda, Kosuke Sumida, Sho Iwasaka, Satomi Hisamoto and Koichi Akashi
Department of Medicine and Biosystemic Science, Graduate School of Medical Science, Kyushu University, Fukuoka 812-8252, Japan

Hironori Tanimoto and Hideyuki Nomura
The Center for Liver Disease, Shin-Kokura Hospital, Kitakyushu 803-8505, Japan

Kazufumi Dohmen
Department of Internal Medicine, Chihaya Hospital, Fukuoka 813-8501, Japan

Kazuhiro Takahashi
Department of Medicine, Hamanomachi Hospital, Fukuoka 810-8539, Japan

Akira Kawano
Department of Medicine, Kitakyushu Municipal Medical Center, Kitakyushu 802-0077, Japan

Eiichi Ogawa, Norihiro Furusyo and Jun Hayashi
Department of General Internal Medicine, Kyushu University Hospital, Fukuoka 812-8582, Japan

Hiroshi Abe, Nobuyoshi Seki, Tomonori Sugita, Yuta Aida, Haruya Ishiguro, Tamihiro Miyazaki, Munenori Itagaki, Satoshi Sutoh and Yoshio Aizawa
Division of Gastroenterology and Hepatology, Department of Internal Medicine, Jikei University School of Medicine Katsushika Medical Center, Katsushika-ku, Tokyo 125-8506, Japan

Hamid UllahWani, Saad Al Kaabi, Manik Sharma, Rajvir Singh, Anil John, Moutaz Derbala, and Muneera J. Al-Mohannadi
Department of Medicine, Division of Gastroenterology, Hamad Medical Corporation (HMC), 2 South 2, P.O. Box 3050, Doha, Qatar

Mostafa M. Sira and Behairy E. Behairy
Department of Pediatric Hepatology, National Liver Institute, Menofiya University, Shebin El-koom, Menofiya 32511, Egypt

Azza M. Abd-Elaziz
Department ofMicrobiology and Immunology, National Liver Institute, Menofiya University, Shebin El-koom, Menofiya 32511, Egypt

Sameh A. Abd Elnaby and Ehab E. Eltahan
Department of Pediatrics, Faculty of Medicine, Menofiya University, Shebin El-koom, Menofiya 32511, Egypt

David Isaacs and Nader Abdelaziz
Brighton and Sussex Medical School, Brighton BN1 9PX, UK

Majella Keller and Jeremy Tibble
Medicine, Royal Sussex County Hospital, Brighton BN2 5BE, UK

Inam Haq
Brighton and Sussex Medical School, Brighton BN1 9PX, UK
Medicine, Royal Sussex County Hospital, Brighton BN2 5BE, UK

Shrruti Grover, Archana Rastogi, Jyotsna Singh, Apurba Rajbongshi and Chhagan Bihari
Department of Pathology, Institute of Liver and Biliary Sciences D-1, Vasant Kunj, New Delhi 110070, India

Kranthi Kosaraju, Sameer Singh Faujdar and Aashima Singh
Department of Microbiology, Kasturba Medical College and Hospital, Manipal University, Madhav Nagar, Manipal 576104, Karnataka, India

Ravindra Prabhu
Department of Nephrology, Kasturba Medical College and Hospital, Manipal University, Madhav Nagar, Manipal 576104, Karnataka, India

Joseph D. Comber and Aykan Karabudak, Xiaofang Huang and Ramila Philip
Immunotope, Inc., Doylestown, PA 18902, USA

Vivekananda Shetty
Baylor College of Medicine, Houston, TX 77030, USA

James S. Testa
Celldex Therapeutics, Hampton, NJ 08827, USA

Nazir Ibrahim and Amr Idris
Internal Medicine and Gastroenterology Departments, Syrian Private University, P.O. Box 36822, Damascus, Syria
Internal Medicine Department, Syrian Private University, Mazzeh Street, P.O. Box 36822, Damascus, Syria

Mehdi Zobeiri
Internal Medicine Department, Imam Reza Hospital, Kermanshah University of Medical Sciences, Kermanshah, Iran

Nobukazu Yuki
Department of Gastroenterology, Osaka National Hospital, Hoenzaka 2-1-14, Chuo-ku, Osaka 540-0006, Japan

Shinji Matsumoto and Toshikazu Yamaguchi
BML, Inc., Kawagoe 350-1101, Japan

Michio Kato
Department of Gastroenterology, Minamiwakayama National Hospital, Tanabe 646-8558, Japan

Chhagan Bihari Archana Rastogi and Nalini Gupta
Department of Pathology, Institute of Liver and Biliary Sciences, D-1, Vasant Kunj, New Delhi 110070, India

Priyanka Saxena
Department of Hematology, Institute of Liver and Biliary Sciences, D-1, Vasant Kunj, New Delhi 110070, India

Devraj Rangegowda, Ashok Chowdhury and Shiv Kumar Sarin
Department of Hepatology, Institute of Liver and Biliary Sciences, D-1, Vasant Kunj, New Delhi 110070, India

Roba M. Talaat and Mahmoud F. Dondeti
Molecular Biology Department, Genetic Engineering and Biotechnology Research Institute (GEBRI), University of Sadat City, Sadat City 22857, Egypt

Soha Z. El-Shenawy
Biochemistry Department, National Liver Institute (NLI), Menoufiya University, Shebeen El-Kom, Menoufiya 32511, Egypt

Omaima A. Khamiss
Animal Biotechnology Department, Genetic Engineering and Biotechnology Research Institute (GEBRI), University of Sadat City, Sadat City 22857, Egypt

Fatemeh Farshadpour
Department of Microbiology and Parasitology, School of Medicine, Bushehr University of Medical Sciences, Bushehr 7514633341, Iran
Persian Gulf Tropical Medicine Research Center, Bushehr University of Medical Sciences, Bushehr 7514633341, Iran

Reza Taherkhani
Department ofMicrobiology and Parasitology, School ofMedicine, Bushehr University ofMedical Sciences, Bushehr 7514633341, Iran
3Persian Gulf Biomedical Research Center, Bushehr University of Medical Sciences, Bushehr 7514633341, Iran

Manoochehr Makvandi
Health Research Institute, Infectious and Tropical Disease Research Center, Ahvaz Jundishapur University of Medical Sciences, Ahvaz 6135715794, Iran

Hideyuki Tamai, Ryo Shimizu, Naoki Shingaki, Yoshiyuki Mori, Shuya Maeshima, Junya Nuta, Yoshimasa Maeda, KosakuMoribata, Yosuke Muraki, Hisanobu Deguchi, Izumi Inoue, Takao Maekita, Mikitaka Iguchi, Jun Kato, and Masao Ichinose
Second Department of Internal Medicine, Wakayama Medical University, 811-1 Kimiidera, Wakayama, Wakayama Prefecture 641-0012, Japan

Jean-Marie Bamvita, Didier Jutras-Aswad and Julie Bruneau
CRCHUM (Centre de Recherche du Centre Hospitalier de l'Université de Montréal), Tour Saint-Antoine 850, Rue St-Denis, Montréal, QC, Canada H2X 0A9
D´epartement de Médecine Familiale, Facultéde Médecine, Université de Montréal, Pavillon Roger-Gaudry, Bureau S-711, 2900 boul. ´Edouard-Montpetit, Montréal, QC, Canada H3T 1J4

Elise Roy
Faculté de Médecine et des Sciences de la Santé, Universitéde Sherbrooke, Campus Longueuil 1111, Rue St-Charles Ouest, Bureau 500, Longueuil, QC, Canada J4K 5G4

Geng Zang
CRCHUM (Centre de Recherche du Centre Hospitalier de l'Université de Montréal), Tour Saint-Antoine 850, Rue St-Denis, Montréal, QC, Canada H2X 0A9

Andreea Adelina Artenie and Annie Levesque
CRCHUM (Centre de Recherche du Centre Hospitalier de l'Université de Montréal), Tour Saint-Antoine 850, Rue St-Denis, Montréal, QC, Canada H2X 0A9
Family Medicine Department, McGill University, 5858 Chemin de la Côte des Neiges, 3e Ètage, Montréal, QC, Canada H3S 1Z1

Maja Thiele
Department of Medicine, Copenhagen University Hospital Koge, 4600 Koege, Denmark
Department of Medicine, Copenhagen University Hospital Gentofte, 2900 Hellerup, Denmark
Department of Gastroenterology and Hepatology, Odense University Hospital, 5000 Odense, Denmark

Gro Askgaard and Ole Hamberg,
Department of Hepatology, Copenhagen University Hospital Rigshospitalet, 2100 Copenhagen, Denmark

Hans B. Timm
Department of Medicine, Copenhagen University Hospital Glostrup, 2600 Glostrup, Denmark

Lise L. Gluud
Department of Medicine, Copenhagen University Hospital Gentofte, 2900 Hellerup, Denmark
Gastrounit, Copenhagen University Hospital Hvidovre, 2650 Hvidovre, Denmark

Issoufou Tao, Tegwindé R. Compaoré, Birama Diarra, Florencia Djigma, Theodora M. Zohoncon, Maléki Assih and Djeneba Ouermi
Centre de Recherche Biomoléculaire Pietro Annigoni (CERBA), BP 364, Ouagadougou 01, Burkina Faso
Laboratoire de Biologie Moléculaire et de Génétique (LABIOGENE), Université de Ouagadougou, BP 7021, Burkina Faso

Virginio Pietra
Centre de Recherche Biomoléculaire Pietro Annigoni (CERBA), BP 364, Ouagadougou 01, Burkina Faso
Centre Médical Saint Camille (SCMC), BP 364, Ouagadougou 01, Burkina Faso

Simplice D. Karou
Centre de Recherche Biomoléculaire Pietro Annigoni (CERBA), BP 364, Ouagadougou 01, Burkina Faso
Laboratoire de Biologie Moléculaire et de Génétique (LABIOGENE), Université de Ouagadougou, BP 7021, Burkina Faso
Ècole Supérieure des Techniques Biologiques et Alimentaires (ESTBA-UL), Universitéde Lomé, BP 1515, Togo

Jacques Simpore
Centre de Recherche Biomoléculaire Pietro Annigoni (CERBA), BP 364, Ouagadougou 01, Burkina Faso
Laboratoire de Biologie Moléculaire et de Génétique (LABIOGENE), Université de Ouagadougou, BP 7021, Burkina Faso

Centre Médical Saint Camille (SCMC), BP 364, Ouagadougou 01, Burkina Faso

Kittiyod Poovorawan, Sombat Treeprasertsuk and Piyawat Komolmit
Division of Gastroenterology, Department of Medicine, Faculty of Medicine, Chulalongkorn University, Bangkok 10330,Thailand

Pisit Tangkijvanich
Department of Biochemistry, Faculty of Medicine, Chulalongkorn University, Bangkok 10330, Thailand

Chintana Chirathaworn
Department of Microbiology, Faculty of Medicine, Chulalongkorn University, Bangkok 10330, Thailand

Olusegun Adekanle, Dennis A. Ndububa and Oluwasegun Ijarotimi
Department of Medicine, Obafemi Awolowo University/ Obafemi Awolowo University Teaching Hospitals Complex, Ile-Ife 220005, Osun State, Nigeria

Samuel Anu Olowookere and Kayode Thaddeus Ijadunola
Department of Community Health, Obafemi Awolowo University/Obafemi Awolowo University Teaching Hospitals Complex, Ile-Ife 220005, Osun State, Nigeria

Naruemon Wisedopas
Department of Pathology, Faculty of Medicine, Chulalongkorn University, Bangkok 10330, Thailand

Yong Poovorawan
Department of Pediatrics, Center of Excellence in Clinical Virology, Faculty of Medicine, Chulalongkorn University, Bangkok 10330,Thailand

Alexsandro S. Galdino
Laboratório de Biotecnologia de Microrganismos, Universidade Federal de São João Del-Rei, 35501-296 Divinópolis, MG, Brazil

José C. Santos, Marilen Q. Souza, Maria S. S. Felipe and Fernando A. G. Torres
Departamento de Biologia Celular, Universidade de Brasília, 70910-900 Brasília, DF, Brazil

Yanna K. M. Nóbrega
Laboratório de Doenças Imunogenéticas e Crônico-degenerativas, Universidade de Brasília, 70910-900 Brasília, DF, Brazil

Mary-Ann E. Xavier and SoniaM. Freitas
Laboratório de Biofísica, Universidade de Brasília, 70910-900 Brasília, DF, Brazil

Theodoros Voulgaris and Vassilios A. Sevastianos
4th Department of Internal Medicine, "Evangelismos" General Hospital, 45-47 Ipsilantou Street, 106 76 Athens, Greece

Tsegaye Yohanes and Zerihun Zerdo
Department ofMedical Laboratory Science, Arba MinchUniversity, P.O. Box 21, Arba Minch, Ethiopia

Nega Chufamo
School of Medicine, Department of Obstetrics and Gynecology, Arba Minch University, P.O. Box 21, Arba Minch, Ethiopia

Shamim Saleha, Anwar Kamal, Nasar Khan and Asif Mahmood
Department of Microbiology, Kohat University of Science and Technology (KUST), Khyber Pakhtunkhwa, Kohat 26000, Pakistan

Farman Ullah
Department of Biotechnology and Genetic Engineering, Kohat University of Science and Technology (KUST), Khyber Pakhtunkhwa, Kohat 26000, Pakistan

Sanaullah Khan
Department of Zoology, Kohat University of Science and Technology (KUST), Khyber Pakhtunkhwa, Kohat 26000, Pakistan

J. Brooks Jackson, Yi Xing and Paul Richardson
Department of Pathology, Johns Hopkins University, Baltimore, MD 21287, USA

Liu Wei
Guangxi Center for Disease Control and Prevention, Nanning 530028, China

Fu Liping and Ma Jun
Xinjiang Center for Disease Control and Prevention, Urumqi 83001, China

Apinun Aramrattana
Research Institute for Health Sciences, Chiang Mai University, Chiang Mai 50200,Thailand

David D. Celentano and LouiseWalshe
Department of Epidemiology, Johns Hopkins Bloomberg School of Public Health, Baltimore, MD 21205, USA

Geetha Beauchamp and Deborah Donnell
Fred Hutchinson Cancer Research Center, Seattle, WA 98109, USA

Yuhua Ruan, Liying Ma and Yiming Shao
State Key Laboratory for Infectious Disease Prevention and Control, National Center for AIDS/STD Control and Prevention, Chinese Center for Disease Control and Prevention, Collaborative Innovation Center for Diagnosis and Treatment of Infectious Diseases, Beijing 102206, China

David Metzger
University of Pennsylvania, Philadelphia, PA 19104, USA

Bakht Roshan
Department of Medicine, Section of Hepatology, University of Illinois at Chicago, 840 South Wood Street, Suite 130, Chicago, IL 60612, USA

Grace Guzman
Department of Pathology (MC847), University of Illinois at Chicago, 840 South Wood Street, Suite 130, Chicago, IL 60612, USA

www.ingramcontent.com/pod-product-compliance
Lightning Source LLC
Chambersburg PA
CBHW080534200326
41458CB00012B/4429